T3-BHM-495

Veterinary Virology

Second Edition

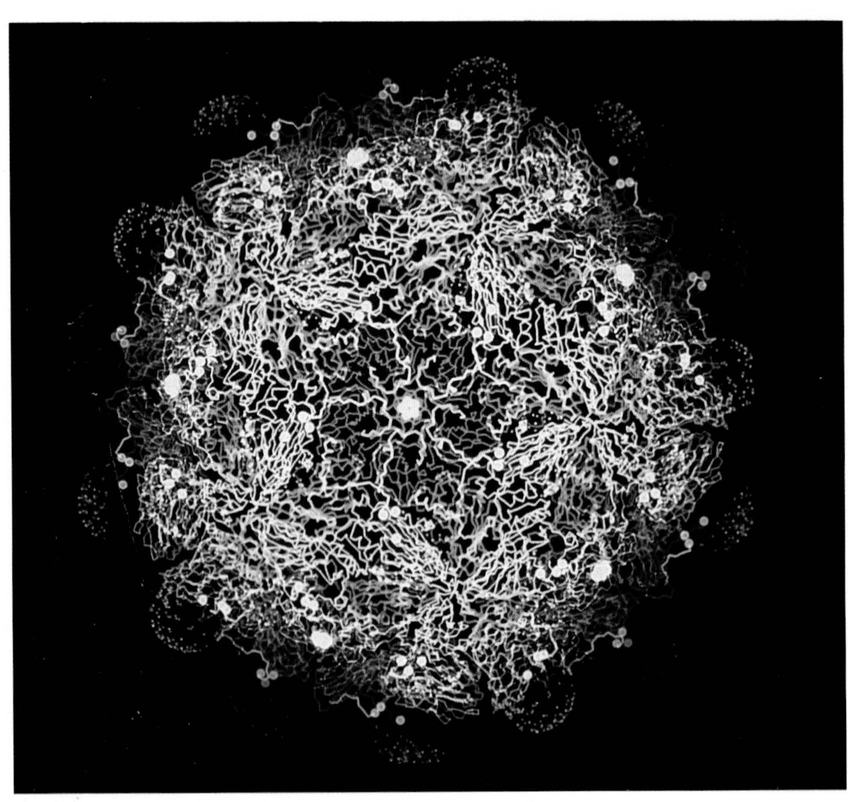

Virion of foot-and-mouth disease virus at 2.9 Å resolution, showing the α-carbon backbones of the capsid proteins with the view down the fivefold axis of symmetry. VP1, blue; VP2, green; VP3, red; VP4, yellow. The central "rosette" comprises five pale yellow balls, which represent the disulfide bonds between the VP3 chains that line the 11 Å hole at the fivefold axis. The course of the C terminus of VP1 is shown in white, crossing VP3 at a constant radius from the fivefold axis to lie on the VP1 of the adjacent protomer. Clouds of blue dots at the periphery represent the approximate locations of the residues of VP1 that contain the major antigenic determinant. (Courtesy Dr. F. Brown.)

Veterinary Virology

Second Edition

FRANK J. FENNER
The John Curtin School of Medical Research
The Australian National University
Canberra, ACT, Australia

E. PAUL J. GIBBS
College of Veterinary Medicine
University of Florida
Gainesville, Florida

FREDERICK A. MURPHY
School of Veterinary Medicine
University of California, Davis
Davis, California

RUDOLF ROTT
Institut für Virologie
Justus-Liebig-Universität
Giessen, Germany

MICHAEL J. STUDDERT
School of Veterinary Science
University of Melbourne
Parkville, Victoria, Australia

DAVID O. WHITE
Department of Microbiology
University of Melbourne
Parkville, Victoria, Australia

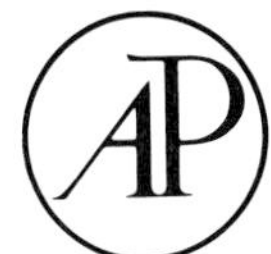

ACADEMIC PRESS, INC.
Harcourt Brace Jovanovich, Publishers
San Diego New York Boston
London Sydney Tokyo Toronto

This book is printed on acid-free paper. 

Academic Press, Inc.
1250 Sixth Avenue, San Diego, California 92101-4311

United Kingdom Edition published by
Academic Press Limited
24–28 Oval Road, London NW1 7DX

Library of Congress Cataloging-in-Publication Data

Veterinary virology / Frank J. Fenner . . . [et al.]. – 2nd ed.
p. cm.
Includes bibliographical references and index.
ISBN 0-12-253056-X
1. Veterinary virology. I. Fenner, Frank, date.
SF780.4V48 1993
636.089'64194–dc20 92-26706
CIP

PRINTED IN THE UNITED STATES OF AMERICA
93 94 95 96 97 98 MV 9 8 7 6 5 4 3 2 1

Contents

Preface

Animal virology has experienced explosive growth during the six years since the first edition of this book was published. Molecular biology is used to interpret viral structure and replication and, increasingly, the pathogenesis and epidemiology of viral diseases. Most changes have been in the Part I chapters and in the sections on viral structure and replication in the Part II chapters. A few new domestic animal viruses, notably the immunodeficiency viruses and the circoviruses, and a few new diseases, such as bovine spongiform encephalopathy, turkey rhinopneumonitis, and porcine epidemic abortion and respiratory syndrome, have been recognized. We hope that we have been able to incorporate this new knowledge without losing the balance that reviewers and users appreciated in the first edition.

As noted in the first edition, one of its authors, Peter Bachmann, died during its preparation. We have been fortunate in being able to maintain the European connection by persuading Professor Rudolf Rott to join our team.

We are indebted to Drs. G. L. Ada, A. Ardans, D. H. L. Bishop, R. V. Blanden, G. F. Browning, C. H. Calisher, M. S. Collett, L. Dalgarno, J. M. Dalrymple, J. den Boon, A. I. Donaldson, M. Fekadu, S. P. Fisher-Hoch, R. George, C. S. Goldsmith, R. Hinton, M. C. Horzinek, M. Koopmans, J. LeDuc, C. Lyerle, J. McCormick, S. Monroe, I. M. Parsonson, J. S. Smith, T. D. St George, M. K. Stoskopf, G. Wensvoort, E. G. Strauss, J. H. Strauss, H.-J. Thiel, D. W. Trent, T. Tsai, M. H. V. van Regenmortel, W. H. Wunner, and T. M. Yuill for reading the various chapters and assisting in other ways and to all those who assisted us with illustrations; they have been acknowledged in the figure legends.

We are grateful to Mr. Kevin Cowan for once again helping with the preparation of line drawings, to the Photographic Section of the John Curtin School of Medical Research for preparing the illustrations for publication, and to the staff of Academic Press for their assistance in the production of this book.

Frank Fenner
E. Paul J. Gibbs
Frederick A. Murphy
Rudolf Rott
Michael J. Studdert
David O. White

Preface
To First Edition

Diseases caused by viruses contribute significantly to animal morbidity and mortality and produce substantial economic losses. When the disease involves companion animals there is an additional sense of individual human loss. Much of this loss, even in developed countries, is due to acute diseases most commonly caused by viruses that are constantly present in the animal environment. Viruses that occur intermittently or are exotic in the animal environment of developed countries are the basis of additional costs to society because of the complexity of public programs that are necessary to prevent their introduction. Viruses that are zoonotic, i.e., viruses that are transmitted between animals and humans, add further to society's burden, both in terms of human suffering and in terms of demands on resources.

Losses due to acute viral diseases have been appreciated for many years, but through recent spectacular advances in our basic understanding of viral infections we now recognize additional, more subtle causes of morbidity and mortality. We have begun to appreciate the importance of losses due to virus-induced cancers, virus-induced immunosuppression and opportunistic infections, virus-induced slow central nervous system diseases, and virus-induced teratogenesis and reproductive failure. The rapidity with which advances are occurring in virology serves to emphasize the need for better understanding on the part of everyone involved in veterinary medicine, from the student to the teacher, and from the research worker in basic science to the veterinary practitioner. It is an exciting time in virology, especially veterinary virology, but it is also a demanding time.

Many books have appeared in recent years providing comprehensive information on basic, molecular biologic virology. In addition, many books have appeared for the clinical specialist, especially the single species clinical specialist. There is a need for each of these types of books, but we believe that there has been a growing need to bring the two poles of virology together—represented by basic biomedical virology and the clinical disciplines of infectious diseases, respectively. We believe that the underlying principles of virology hold the key to future improvements in the prevention and management of infectious diseases at the level of the individual animal, the herd or flock, and the animal population as a whole. This book has been written with such a purpose and perspective in mind, primarily for veterinary students and other graduate students interested in animal diseases, but we hope it will also prove useful to practicing veterinarians, animal scientists, biologists, microbiologists, and other allied professionals. We hope, for all readers, that our enthusiasm for the subject, our sense of excitement, is as infectious as some of the viral pathogens we describe.

The overall pattern follows that of "Medical Virology," written by two of the present authors and now in its third edition, to which this book is a companion volume. However, the detailed pattern differs in both structure and content. Part I, Principles of Animal Virology, consists of 16 chapters and uses examples drawn from studies of the viral diseases of domestic animals. Part II, Viruses of Domestic Animals, describes in 19 chapters the more important viral diseases of domestic animals according to viral family. In a series of tables in the last chapter, we have attempted to "cut the cake" in another way by listing disease syndromes found in various species of domestic animals, the viruses that cause them, their geographic distribution, and the availability of vaccines. The glossary comprises short definitions of words or terms that may not have been encountered before by students. Each entry is printed in italics when first used in the text.

We are grateful to Mrs. Marj Lee and Mr. Kevin Cowan, both of the Australian National University, for their devotion and skill in preparing the manuscript and line drawings, and to the staff of Academic Press for their assistance in the production of this book.

Frank Fenner
E. Paul J. Gibbs
Frederick A. Murphy
Michael J. Studdert
David O. White

PART I

Principles of Animal Virology

CHAPTER 1

Structure and Composition of Viruses

The unicellular microorganisms can be arranged in order of decreasing size and complexity: protozoa, fungi, bacteria, rickettsiae, mycoplasmas, and chlamydiae. These microorganisms, however small and simple, are cells. They always contain DNA as the repository of genetic information, they contain RNA, and they have their own machinery for producing energy and macromolecules. Unicellular microorganisms grow by synthesizing their own macromolecular constituents (nucleic acid, protein, carbohydrate, and lipid), and most multiply by binary fission.

Viruses, on the other hand, contain only one type of nucleic acid, either DNA or RNA, never both, and they differ from nonviral organisms in having two clearly defined phases in their life cycle. Outside a susceptible cell, the virus particle, or virion, is metabolically inert; it is the transmission phase of the virus. This extracellular transmission phase alternates with an intracellular reproductive phase, in which the virus consists of active viral genes that use the metabolic systems of the host to produce progeny genomes and viral proteins that assemble to form new virions. Further, unlike any unicellular microorganism, many viruses can reproduce themselves when only the nucleic acid of the viral *genome* enters the cell, that is, their nucleic acid is infectious. In contrast, in all stages of their life cycle nonviral organisms consist of cells that are bounded by cellular membranes and contain complete and largely independent metabolic systems that include mitochondria and ribosomes.

The key differences between viruses and unicellular microorganisms are listed in Table 1-1. Several important practical consequences flow from these differences. For example, some viruses can persist in cells by the integration of their DNA (or a DNA copy of their RNA) into the genome of the host cell, and they are not susceptible to antibiotics that act against specific steps in the metabolic pathways of bacteria.

The simplest conventional viruses consist of a nucleic acid genome and a protein coat. However, virologists also study *viroids,* which are infectious RNA molecules that lack a protein coat; so far viroids have been found only in plants. The so-called unconventional viruses, such as the scrapie agent, are thought by some to be devoid of nucleic acid, yet they exhibit characteristics like mutation that are associated with a genome of nucleic acid.

VIRAL MORPHOLOGY

Electron microscopy had as profound an effect on our knowledge of the morphology of viruses as light microscopy had on understanding of bacterial morphology. Early studies by Ruska in 1939–1941 were expanded during the 1950s to include thin sectioning of infected cells and metal shadowing of purified particles. Then in 1959 our knowledge of

TABLE 1-1

Contrasting Properties of Unicellular Microorganisms and Viruses

Property	Bacteria	Rickettsiae	Mycoplasmas	Chlamydiae	Viruses
>300 nm diameter	+	+	±	±	−
Growth on nonliving media	+	−	+	−	−
Binary fission	+	+	+	+	−
DNA and RNA	+	+	+	+	−
Nucleic acid infectious	−	−	−	−	+[a]
Ribosomes	+	+	+	+	−
Metabolism	+	+	+	+	−
Sensitivity to antibiotics	+	+	+	+	−[b]

[a] Some, among both DNA and RNA viruses.

[b] The antibiotic rifampicin inhibits poxvirus replication.

viral ultrastructure was transformed when *negative staining* was applied to the electron microscopy of viruses. A solution of potassium phosphotungstate (an electron-dense salt), when used to stain virus particles, fills the interstices of the viral surface, giving the resulting electron micrograph a degree of detail not previously possible. Electron micrographs of negatively stained preparations of virions representing all families of the viruses of vertebrates are shown in the relevant chapters of Part II of this book.

The *virion* (infectious virus particle) of the simplest viruses consists of a single molecule of nucleic acid surrounded by a protein coat, the *capsid.* In some of the more complex viruses the capsid surrounds a core, which consists of one or more proteins surrounding the viral nucleic acid; the capsid and associated nucleic acid then constitute the *nucleocapsid* (Fig. 1-2C). For some viruses the capsid is surrounded by a lipoprotein *envelope* (Figs. 1-1C,D and 1-2B).

The capsid is composed of a defined number of morphological units called *capsomers* (Figs. 1-1A and 1-2A), which are held together by noncovalent bonds. Within an infected cell, the capsomers self-assemble to form the capsid. The manner of assembly is strictly defined by the nature of the bonds formed between individual capsomers, which imparts symmetry to the capsid. Only two kinds of symmetry have been recognized, cubical (icosahedral) and helical (Fig. 1-1A,B).

Icosahedral Symmetry

The cubic symmetry found in viruses is invariably that of an icosahedron, one of the five classical "Platonic solids" of geometry; it has 12 vertices (corners), 30 edges, and 20 faces, each an equilateral triangle. It has axes of two-, three-, and fivefold rotational symmetry, passing through its edges, faces, and vertices, respectively (Fig. 1-3A,B,C). The icosahedron is the optimum solution to the problem of constructing, from repeating subunits, a strong structure to enclose a maximum volume. Before icosahedrons were discovered in viruses, the same principles were applied by the architect Buckminster Fuller to the construction of icosahedral buildings ("geodesic domes"). An object with icosahedral symmetry need not appear angular in outline; the virions of many animal viruses with *icosahedral symmetry* appear spherical with a bumpy surface.

Only certain arrangements of the capsomers can fit into the faces, edges, and vertices of the viral icosahedron. The capsomers on the faces and edges of adenovirus particles, for example, bond to six neighboring capsomers and are called *hexamers;* those at the vertices bond to five neighbors and are called *pentamers* (Fig. 1-1A). In virions of some viruses

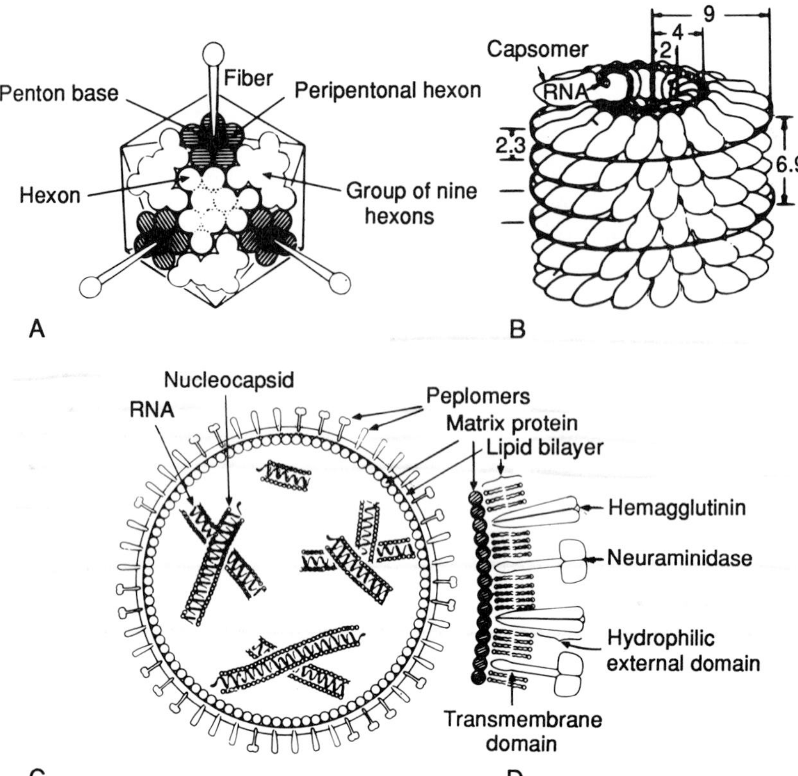

FIG. 1-1. *Features of virion structure, exemplified by adenovirus (A), tobacco mosaic virus (B), and influenza A virus (C, D). Not to scale. (A) Icosahedral structure of an adenovirus virion. All hexon capsomers are trimers of the same polypeptide, distinguished as "peripentonal" or "group of nine" by their location in the capsid. The penton base is a pentamer of another polypeptide; the fiber, a trimer of a third polypeptide. (B) The structure of helical nucleocapsids was first elucidated by studies of a nonenveloped plant virus, tobacco mosaic virus, but the principles apply to animal viruses with helical nucleocapsids, all of which are enveloped. In tobacco mosaic virus, a single polypeptide forms a capsomer. A total of 2130 capsomers assemble in a helix. The 6-kb ssRNA genome fits in a groove on the inner part of each capsomer and is wound to form a helix which extends the length of the virion. The virion is 300 nm long and 18 nm in diameter, with a hollow cylindrical core 4 nm in diameter. (C) Structure of a virion of influenza A virus. All animal viruses with a helical nucleocapsid and some of those with an icosahedral capsid are enveloped. The nucleocapsids with helical symmetry are long and thin (Fig. 1-2C) and in influenza A virus occur as eight segments, which may be loosely connected (not shown). The viral RNA is wound helically within the helically arranged capsomers, as shown for tobacco mosaic virus. (D) The envelope of influenza virus consists of a lipid bilayer in which are inserted several hundred glycoprotein peplomers or spikes; beneath the lipid bilayer there is a virus-specified matrix protein M1. The glycoprotein peplomers of influenza virus comprise two different proteins, hemagglutinin (a trimer) and neuraminidase (a mushroom-shaped tetramer), each of which consists of a hydrophilic cytoplasmic domain,*

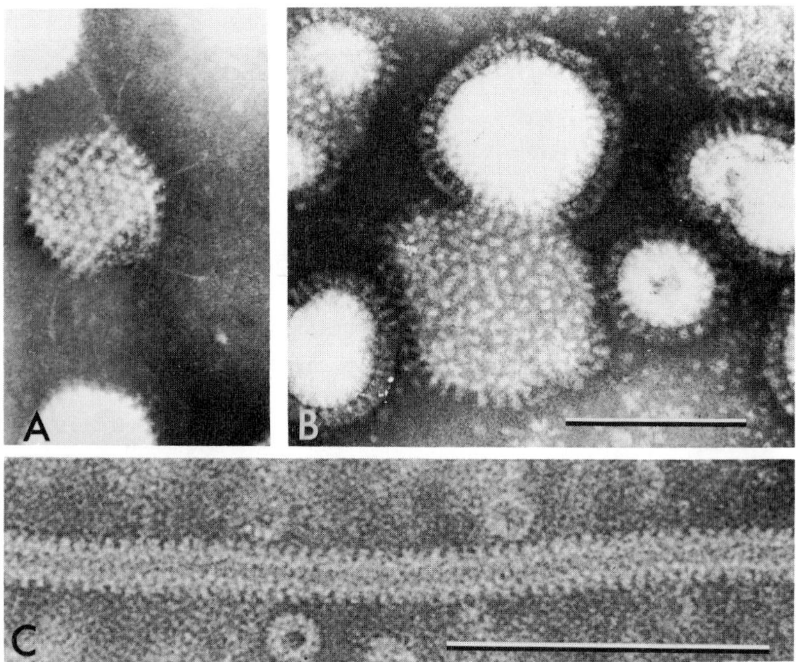

FIG. 1-2. *Morphological features of viral structure revealed by negative staining and electron microscopy (bars: 100 nm). (A) Virion of an adenovirus, showing icosahedral structure, hexons, and fibers projecting from vertices (compare with Fig. 1-1A). (B) Enveloped virion of influenza virus. The two types of peplomer, hemagglutinin and neuraminidase, are not distinguishable in the electron micrograph (compare with Fig. 1-1D), nor is the helical nucleocapsid usually visible (but see Fig. 29-1). (C) Nucleocapsid of parainfluenza virus. The RNA is wound within and protected by a helical capsid composed of thousands of identical capsomers (compare with Fig. 1-1B). The complete nucleocapsid is 1000 nm long, but in the intact virion it is folded within a roughly spherical envelope about 180 nm in diameter. (A and B, courtesy of Dr. N. G. Wrigley; C, courtesy Dr. A. J. Gibbs.)*

---

a hydrophobic transmembrane domain, and a hydrophilic external domain. Some 50 molecules of a fourth small membrane-associated protein, M2 (not shown), form a small number of "pores" in the lipid bilayer. [A, From S. Harrison, In *"Fields Virology" (B. N. Fields* et al.*, eds.), 2nd Ed., p. 55. Raven, New York, 1990; B, from C. F. T. Mattern,* In *"Molecular Biology of Animal Viruses" (D. P. Nayak, ed.), p. 5, Dekker, New York, 1977.]*

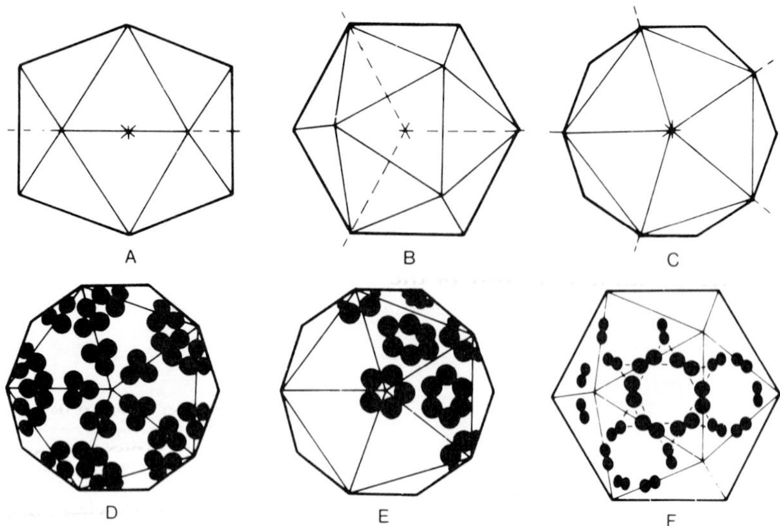

FIG. 1-3. *(Upper row) An icosahedron viewed along twofold (A), threefold (B), and fivefold (C) axes of symmetry. (Lower row) Various clusterings of capsid polypeptides are responsible for the characteristic appearances of particular viruses as seen by negative contrast electron micrography. For example, when capsid polypeptides are arranged as 60 trimers, capsomers themselves are difficult to define; this is the case with foot-and-mouth disease virus (D). When capsid polypeptides are grouped as 12 pentamers and 20 hexamers they form bulky capsomers, as is the case with parvoviruses (E). When capsid polypeptides form dimers on the faces they produce ringlike features on the virion surface, as is the case with caliciviruses (F).*

both hexamers and pentamers consist of the same polypeptide(s); in those of other viruses they are formed from different polypeptides. The arrangements of capsomers on the capsids of virions of three small icosahedral viruses are shown in Fig. 1-3D,E,F.

The examination by negative staining electron microscopy of quite crude preparations such as skin scrapings or clarified fecal samples can provide immediate morphologic identification of a virus, allowing assignment to a particular family. Combined with the clinical picture, electron microscopy is an important method of rapid diagnosis in diarrheal and skin diseases.

High-Resolution Structure. The recent demonstration by X-ray crystallography of the structure of the capsids of several picornaviruses (for example, foot-and-mouth disease virus), the canine parvovirus, and simian virus 40 (SV40) at near atomic resolution has provided a remarkable insight into capsid organization and assembly, the location of neutralizing epitopes, and aspects of virus attachment and penetration into cells. Among several picornaviruses examined, the amino acids of each of the three larger structural proteins are packaged so as to have a wedge-shaped eight-stranded antiparallel β-barrel domain (Fig. 1-4). The outer contour of the virion depends on the packing of these domains and on the way that the loops project from the framework. The capsomers of canine parvovirus consist of an unusually large wedge-shaped protein with a β-barrel core, hence the ability to form a 250-Å shell from only 60 subunits of a single protein. In virions of foot-and-mouth disease virus (see frontispiece) there are 60 large disordered protrusions at the surface, each corresponding to a copy of the major antigenic site.

Ultrastructural studies have also provided some insight into how virions bind to cell receptors. In this connection the words "receptor" and

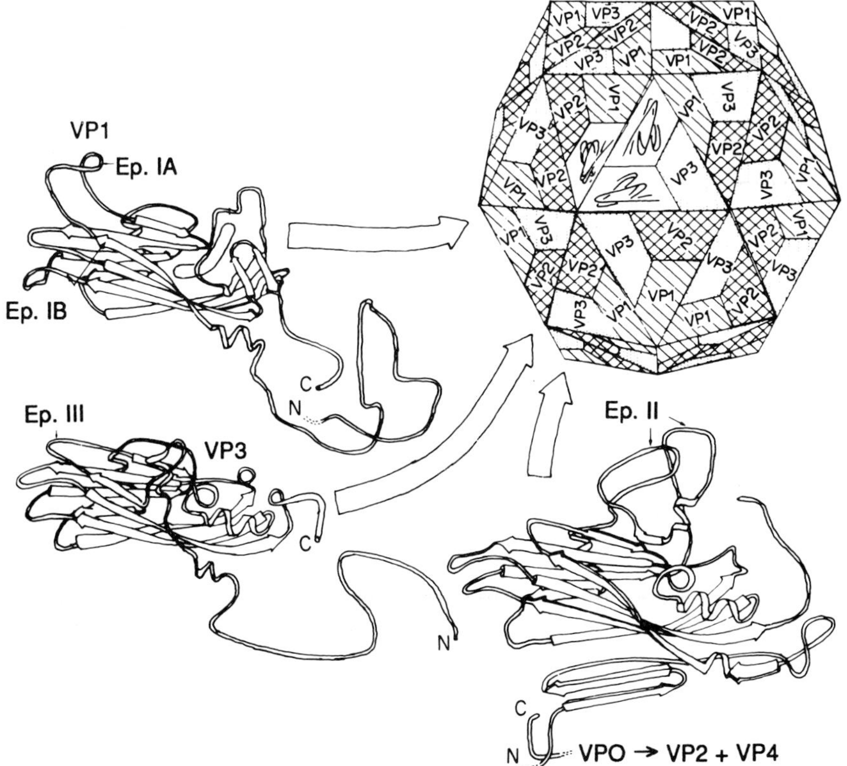

FIG. 1-4. *Structure of a picornavirus as determined by X-ray crystallography. Each of the viral structural proteins VP1, VP3, and VP0 (VP0 is cleaved during maturation to VP2 and VP4) has an eight-stranded antiparallel β-barrel structure. In the mature virion parts of VP1, VP2, and VP3 are intertwined to produce four neutralization epitopes, Ep. IA, Ep. IB, Ep. II, and Ep. III, the locations of which in the structural proteins and on the virion are indicated by these letters. [Modified from M. G. Rossmann and R. R. Rueckert,* Microbiol. Sci. **4,** *206 (1987).]*

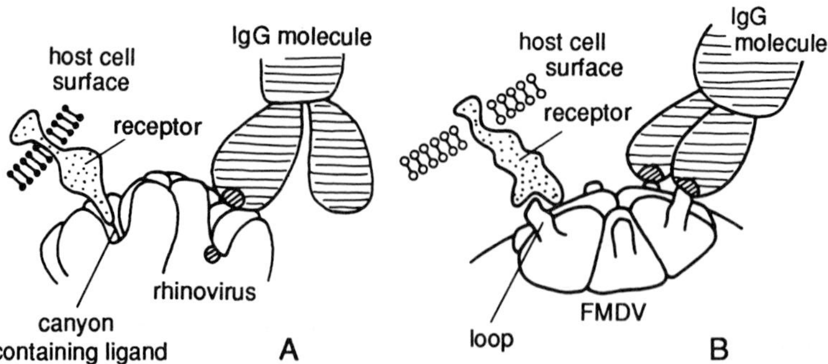

FIG. 1-5. *Models of the interactions between receptors on host cells and ligands on virions, using rhinovirus and foot-and-mouth disease virus as examples. (A) In the interaction of rhinovirus with its host cell, the ligands are situated within surface depressions ("canyons") near axes of fivefold symmetry. This location of the ligands serves to prevent antibody binding at those crucial sites. Antibodies specific for other antigenic sites on the surface of rhinoviruses do not necessarily block virion–cell receptor interaction. (B) In the interaction of foot-and-mouth disease virus with its host cell, the ligands are situated on flexible, sequence-variable "loops" extending from the surface of the virion. These loops are not protected from antibody binding, which does block virion–cell interaction. [Modified from M. G. Rossmann and R. R. Rueckert,* Microbiol. Sci. **4,** *206 (1987), and R. Acharya* et al., Vet. Microbiol. **23,** *21 (1990).]*

"ligand" are often used in imprecise ways. In this book we use the term *receptor* to designate the specific molecule or structure on the surface of the cell membrane that is recognized by a specific extracellular molecule or structure that binds to it. The *ligand* is the receptor-binding molecule of the virus. For example, the hemagglutinin of influenza virus is the ligand which binds to the cellular receptor, a glycoconjugate terminating in an *N*-acetylneuraminic acid. In some picornaviruses there is a deep canyon or pit encircling each fivefold axis (Fig. 1-5A). The amino acids within the canyon are far more conserved than residues elsewhere on the surface; it has been suggested that these conserved residues constitute at least part of the ligands that bind to the host cell receptors. Foot-and-mouth disease virus binds to the cell receptor via critical residues within highly flexible and sequence-variable superficial structures on the virion (Fig. 1-5B).

Helical Symmetry

The capsomers and nucleic acid genomes of several RNA viruses self-assemble as a cylindrical nucleocapsid which has *helical symmetry,* the viral RNA being coiled within the nucleocapsid (Figs. 1-1B,C and 1-2C). Each capsomer of such viruses consists of a single polypeptide molecule.

The plant viruses whose nucleocapsids have helical symmetry are rod-shaped and nonenveloped. However, in all animal viruses with helical nucleocapsids these are wound into a secondary coil and enclosed within a lipoprotein envelope.

Viral Envelopes

Virions acquire envelopes during maturation, by a process known as *budding* from cellular membranes. The lipids of the viral envelope are derived directly from the cell, but the proteins in the envelope are virus-coded. One kind of viral envelope protein structure is the glycoprotein *peplomer* (*peplos* = envelope) or *spike* (Fig. 1-1D), which can often be seen in electron micrographs as projections from the surface of the envelope (Fig. 1-2B). Another kind of envelope protein, *matrix protein,* is nonglycosylated and is found as a layer on the inside of the envelope of virions of several families; matrix protein provides added rigidity to the virion. For example, the envelope of rhabdoviruses with its projecting peplomers is closely applied to a layer of matrix protein which in turn interfaces with a helical nucleocapsid. Other enveloped viruses, including arenaviruses, bunyaviruses, and coronaviruses, have no matrix protein.

Envelopes are not restricted to viruses of helical symmetry; icosahedral viruses belonging to several families (African swine fever virus, herpesviruses, togaviruses, flaviviruses, and retroviruses) have envelopes. The infectivity of most enveloped viruses depends on the integrity of the envelope, but some poxviruses have an envelope which is not necessary for infectivity.

CHEMICAL COMPOSITION OF VIRIONS

Viruses are distinguished from all other forms of life by their simple chemical composition, which includes a genome comprising one or a few molecules of either DNA or RNA, a small number of proteins which form the capsid or are present within the virion as enzymes or regulatory proteins, and, in the case of enveloped viruses, a lipoprotein bilayer with associated glycoprotein peplomers and sometimes a matrix protein.

Viral Nucleic Acid

All viral genomes are *haploid,* that is, they contain only one copy of each gene, except for retrovirus genomes, which are *diploid.* Viral DNA or RNA can be *double-stranded* (*ds*) or *single-stranded* (*ss*). The genomes of representative members of most viral families have now been completely sequenced.

When carefully extracted from the virion, the nucleic acid of viruses of certain families of both DNA and RNA viruses is infectious, that is, when experimentally introduced into a cell it can initiate a complete cycle of viral replication, with the production of a normal yield of progeny virions. The essential features of the genomes of viruses of vertebrates are summarized in Table 1-2. Their remarkable variety is reflected in the diverse ways in which the information encoded in the viral genome is transcribed to RNA, then translated into proteins, and the ways in which the viral nucleic acid is replicated.

TABLE 1-2
Structures of Viral Genomes

Family or virus	Type and structure of virion nucleic acid
Circoviruses	Circular ssDNA, plus sense
Parvoviridae	Linear ssDNA, minus sense; with palindromic seqeunces at ends
Papovaviridae	Circular supercoiled dsDNA
Adenoviridae	Linear dsDNA with inverted terminal repeats and a covalently bound protein
Herpesviridae	Linear dsDNA; unique sequences flanked by repeat sequences; different isomers occur
Poxviridae	Linear dsDNA; both ends covalently closed, with inverted terminal repeats
African swine fever virus	Linear dsDNA; both ends covalently closed, with inverted terminal repeats
Hepadnaviridae	Circular dsDNA with ss region
Picornaviridae, *Caliciviridae*, *Togaviridae*, *Flaviviridae*, *Coronaviridae*, *Toroviridae*	Linear ssRNA, plus sense; serves as mRNA; 3′ end polyadenylated (except *Flaviviridae*); 5′ end capped, or protein covalently bound (*Picornaviridae, Caliciviridae*)
Paramyxoviridae, *Rhabdoviridae*, *Filoviridae*	Linear ssRNA, minus sense
Hepatitis D virus	Circular ssRNA, minus sense
Orthomyxoviridae	Segmented genome; 7 or 8 molecules of linear ssRNA, minus sense
Bunyaviridae	Segmented genome; 3 molecules of linear ssRNA, minus sense or ambisense; "sticky ends" allow circularization
Arenaviridae	Segmented genome; 2 molecules of linear ssRNA, minus sense or ambisense; "sticky ends" allow circularization
Reoviridae	Segmented genome; 10, 11, or 12 molecules of linear dsRNA
Birnaviridae	Segmented genome; 2 molecules of dsRNA
Retroviridae	Diploid genome, dimer of linear ssRNA, plus sense; hydrogen-bonded at 5′ ends; terminal redundancy; both 3′ termini polyadenylated, both 5′ ends capped

DNA. The genome of all DNA viruses consists of a single molecule, which is double-stranded except in the case of the parvoviruses and circoviruses, and may be linear or circular. The DNA of papovaviruses, hepadnaviruses, and circoviruses is circular; the circular DNA of hepadnaviruses is only partially double-stranded. Within the virion, the circular DNA of the papovaviruses is supercoiled.

Most of the linear viral DNAs have characteristics which enable them to adopt a circular configuration, which is a requirement for replication by what is called a rolling circle. The two strands of poxvirus DNA are covalently cross-linked at their termini, so that on denaturation the molecule becomes a large single-stranded circle. The linear dsDNA of several DNA viruses contains *repeat sequences* at the ends of the molecule that permit circularization. In adenovirus DNA there are inverted terminal repeats; these are also a feature of the ssDNA parvoviruses.

Another type of terminal structure occurs in adenoviruses, hepadnaviruses, parvoviruses, and some ssRNA viruses such as the picornaviruses and caliciviruses. In all of these a protein which has an essential function in replication of the genome is covalently linked to the 5′ terminus.

The size of viral DNA genomes ranges from 1.7 kilobases (kb) for the small ssDNA circoviruses to over 200 kilobase pairs (kbp) for the large dsDNA herpesviruses and poxviruses. As 1 kb or 1 kbp contains enough genetic information to code for about one average-sized protein, it follows that viral DNAs contain from about 2 to 200 genes and code for 2 to 200 proteins. However, the relationship between any particular nucleotide sequence and its protein product is not so straightforward. First, the DNA of most of the larger viruses, like that of cells, contains what appears to be redundant information, in the form of (1) repeat sequences and (2) *introns*, namely, regions which are noncoding and are *spliced* out from the primary RNA transcript to form the mRNA. On the other hand, a single such primary RNA transcript may be spliced or cleaved in several different ways to yield several distinct mRNAs, each of which may be translated into a different protein. Furthermore, a given DNA or mRNA sequence may be read in up to three different reading frames, giving rise to two or three proteins with different amino acid sequences. In different viruses, either or both strands of dsDNA are transcribed, in either a leftward or a rightward direction.

Viral DNAs contain several kinds of noncoding sequences, some of which are *consensus sequences* that tend to be conserved through evolution because they serve vital functions, including RNA polymerase recognition sites and promoters, enhancers, initiation codons for translation, termination codons, and RNA splice sites.

RNA. The genome of RNA viruses may be single-stranded or double-stranded. While some occur as a single molecule, others are segmented,

Arenavirus and birnavirus genomes consist of 2 segments, bunyavirus genomes of 3, orthomyxovirus of 7 or 8 (in different genera), and reovirus of 10, 11, or 12 (in different genera). Each of these molecules is unique (often a single "gene"). Except for the very small circular ssRNA of hepatitis D virus (the structure of which resembles that of viroids of plants), no animal virus RNA genome is a covalently linked circle. However, the ssRNAs of arenaviruses and bunyaviruses are "circular," by virtue of having hydrogen-bonded ends. The genomes of ssRNA viruses have considerable secondary structure, regions of base pairing causing the formation of loops, hairpins, etc., which probably serve as signals controlling nucleic acid replication, transcription, translation, and/or packaging into the capsid.

Single-stranded genomic RNA can be defined according to its *sense* (also known as *polarity*). If it is of the same sense as mRNA, it is said to be positive or plus sense. This is the case with the genomic RNA of picornaviruses, caliciviruses, togaviruses, flaviviruses, coronaviruses, toroviruses, and retroviruses. If, on the other hand, the genomic nucleotide sequence is complementary to that of mRNA, it is said to be negative or minus sense. Such is the case with the paramyxoviruses, rhabdoviruses, filoviruses, orthomyxoviruses, arenaviruses, and bunyaviruses, all of which have an RNA-dependent RNA polymerase (*transcriptase*) in the virion, which in the infected cell transcribes plus sense RNA, using the viral genome as template. With the arenaviruses and at least one genus of bunyaviruses, one of the RNA segments is *ambisense,* that is, both the genomic and complementary plus strand can act as mRNA.

Where the viral RNA is plus sense, it is usually *polyadenylated* at its 3′ end (in picornaviruses, caliciviruses, togaviruses, and coronaviruses, but not in flaviviruses) and *capped* at its 5′ end (togaviruses, flaviviruses, coronaviruses).

The size of ssRNA viral genomes varies from 1.7 to 33 kb and that of the dsRNA viruses from 7 to 27 kbp, a much smaller range than found among the dsDNA viruses. Accordingly most RNA viruses encode fewer than a dozen proteins. Most of the segments of the genomes of orthomyxoviruses and reoviruses are individual genes, each coding for one unique protein.

Other Features of Viral Genomes. Viral preparations often contain some particles with an atypical content of nucleic acid. Host cell DNA is found in some papovavirus particles, and cellular ribosomes are incorporated into arenaviruses. Part of the host cell 28 S rRNA has been found in the HA gene of influenza virus and ubiquitin-coding sequences in the genome of bovine viral diarrhea virus. Several copies of the complete viral genome may be enclosed within a single particle, or viral particles may be formed that contain no nucleic acid (empty particles) or that have an incomplete genome (*defective interfering particles*).

Viral Proteins

Some virus-coded proteins are *structural*, that is, they are part of the virion; some are *nonstructural* and are concerned with regulation of the replication cycle. An essential role for one class of structural proteins is to provide the viral nucleic acid with a protective coat; other structural proteins include ligands for binding to cell receptor molecules. The virions of all viruses of vertebrates contain several different proteins, the number ranging from 2 in the simplest viruses to over 100 in the most complex. For viruses with cubic symmetry, the structural proteins form an icosahedral capsid which sometimes encloses polypeptides that are intimately associated with the nucleic acid to form a core. In the orthomyxoviruses, paramyxoviruses, and some coronaviruses one of the glycoproteins of the envelope acts as a receptor-destroying enzyme.

The nonstructural proteins associated with virions are mainly enzymes, most of which are involved in nucleic acid transcription, regulation, processing, or replication. These include various types of transcriptases which transcribe mRNA from dsDNA or dsRNA viral genomes or from genomes of viruses with minus sense ssRNA. Reverse transcriptase, which transcribes DNA from RNA, is found in retroviruses and hepadnaviruses, and other enzymes found in retrovirus particles are involved in the integration of the transcribed DNA into the cellular DNA. Poxviruses, which replicate in the cytoplasm, carry a number of enzymes involved in processing RNA transcripts and replicating DNA.

Viral Lipids

Lipids constitute about 20–35% of the dry weight of enveloped viruses, the viral envelope being composed of cellular lipids and viral proteins. As a consequence, the composition of the lipids of particular viruses differs according to the composition of the membrane lipids of the host cells from which they came. Some 50–60% of the envelope lipid is phospholipid, and most of the remainder is cholesterol. Most lipid found in enveloped viruses is present as a typical lipid–protein bilayer, with most protein encoded by the virus and with virus-coded glycoprotein spikes embedded within the lipoprotein bilayer.

Viral Carbohydrates

Carbohydrates occur as oligosaccharide side chains of viral glycoproteins and glycolipids and as mucopolysaccharides. In the glycoproteins there is an N- or O-glycosidic linkage. In addition to the glycoprotein spikes of enveloped viruses, the virions of some of the more complex viruses also contain internal glycoproteins or glycosylated outer capsid proteins. Since these carbohydrates are usually synthesized by cellular transferases, their composition corresponds to that of the host cell.

PRESERVATION OF VIRAL INFECTIVITY

In general, viruses are more sensitive than bacteria or fungi to inactivation by physical and chemical agents. A knowledge of their sensitivity to environmental conditions is therefore important for ensuring the preservation of the infectivity of viruses as reference reagents, and in clinical specimens collected for diagnosis, as well as for their deliberate inactivation for sterilization, disinfection, and the production of inactivated vaccines. The principal environmental condition that may adversely affect the infectivity of viruses in clinical specimens is too high a temperature; other important conditions are high and low pH and the presence of lipid solvents and detergents.

Heat Stability

Animal viruses vary considerably in heat stability. Surface proteins are denatured within a few minutes at temperatures of 55°–60°C, with the result that the virion is no longer capable of normal cellular attachment and/or uncoating. At ambient temperature the rate of decay of infectivity is slower but usually significant. To preserve infectivity, viral preparations must therefore be stored at low temperature; 4°C (wet ice or a refrigerator) is usually satisfactory for a day or so, but longer term preservation requires much lower temperatures. Two convenient temperatures are −70°C, the temperature of frozen CO_2 ("dry ice") and of some mechanical freezers, or −196°C, the temperature of liquid nitrogen. As a rule of thumb, the half-lives of most viruses can be measured in seconds at 60°C, minutes at 37°C, hours at 20°C, days at 4°C, and years at −70°C or lower. The enveloped viruses are more heat-labile than nonenveloped viruses. The sensitivity of enveloped virions, notably those of bovine respiratory syncytial virus, also applies to repeated freezing and thawing, probably as a result of disruption of the virion by ice crystals. This poses problems in the collection and transportation of clinical specimens. The most practical way of avoiding such problems is to deliver specimens to the laboratory as rapidly as practicable, packed without freezing, on ice-cold gel packs.

In the laboratory, it is often necessary to preserve virus stocks for years. This is achieved in one of two ways: (1) rapid freezing of small aliquots of virus suspended in medium containing protective protein and/or dimethyl sulfoxide, followed by storage at −70° or −196°C; (2) freeze-drying (lyophilization), that is, dehydration of a frozen viral suspension under reduced pressure, followed by storage of the resultant powder at 4° or −20°C. Freeze-drying prolongs viability significantly even at ambient temperatures, and it is universally used in the manufacture of live-virus vaccines.

Ionic Environment and pH

On the whole, viruses are best preserved in an isotonic environment at physiological pH, but some tolerate a wide ionic and pH range. For example, whereas most enveloped viruses are inactivated at pH 5–6, rotaviruses and many picornaviruses survive the acidic pH of the stomach.

Lipid Solvents and Detergents

The infectivity of enveloped viruses is readily destroyed by lipid solvents such as ether or chloroform or detergents like sodium deoxycholate, so that these agents must be avoided in laboratory procedures concerned with maintaining the viability of viruses. On the other hand, detergents are commonly used by virologists to solubilize viral envelopes and liberate proteins for use as vaccines or for chemical analysis.

FURTHER READING

Acharya, R., Fry, E., Stuart, D., Fox, G., Rowlands, D., and Brown, F.(1990). The structure of foot-and-mouth disease virus: Implications for its physical and biological properties. *Vet. Microbiol.* **23,** 21.

Bishop, D. H. L. (1986). Ambisense RNA viruses: Positive and negative polarities combined in RNA virus genomes. *Microbiol. Sci.* **3,** 183.

Dubois-Dalco, M., Holmes, K. V., and Rentier, B. (1984). "Assembly of Enveloped RNA Viruses." Springer-Verlag, New York.

Harrison, S. C. (1990). Principles of virus structure. *In* "Fields Virology" (B. N. Fields, D. M. Knipe, R. M. Chanock, M. S. Hirsch, J. L. Melnick, T. P. Monath, and B. Roizman, eds.), 2nd Ed., p. 37. Raven, New York.

McGeogh, D. J. (1981). Structural analysis of animal virus genomes. *J. Gen. Virol.* **55,** 1.

Rossmann, M. G., and Johnson, J. E. (1989). Icosahedral RNA virus structure. *Annu. Rev. Biochem.* **58,** 533.

Rossmann, M. G., and Rueckert, R. R. (1987). What does the molecular structure of viruses tell us about viral functions? *Microbiol. Sci.* **4,** 206.

Tsao, J., Chapman, M. S., Agbandje, M., Keller, W., Smith, K., Luo, M., Smith, T. J., Rossman, M. G., Compans, R. W., and Parrish, C. R. (1991). The three-dimensional structure of canine parvovirus and its functional implications. *Science* **251,** 1456.

Wiley, D. C., and Skehel, J. J. (1990). Viral membranes. *In* "Fields Virology" (B. N. Fields, D. M. Knipe, R. M. Chanock, M. S. Hirsch, J. L. Melnick, T. P. Monath, and B. Roizman, eds.), 2nd Ed., p. 63. Raven, New York.

CHAPTER 2

Classification and Nomenclature of Viruses

There is good evidence to indicate that all organisms are infected with viruses: vertebrate and invertebrate animals, plants, algae, fungi, protozoa, and bacteria; and every species of animal, bacterium, and plant that has been intensively searched has yielded numerous different viruses belonging to several viral families. Since all viruses, whatever their hosts, share the features described in the previous chapter, viral taxonomists have developed a scheme of classification and nomenclature that is universal, but in this book we are concerned solely with the viruses of vertebrates, some of which (called arboviruses) also replicate in insects, ticks, or other arthropods.

Several hundred distinguishable viruses have been recovered from man, which is the best studied vertebrate host, and new ones are being discovered each year. Somewhat fewer have been recovered from each of the common species of farm and companion animals and from the commonly used laboratory animals. To simplify the study of this vast number of viruses we need to sort them into groups that share certain common properties.

CRITERIA FOR VIRAL CLASSIFICATION

Classification into major groups called families, and the subdivision families into genera, has now reached a position of substantial international agreement. Recently three families (*Paramyxoviridae, Rhabdoviridae, Filoviridae*) were grouped into a higher taxon, an order (*Mononegavirales*), on the basis of the similarity in genome structure and strategy of replication of the member viruses. It is likely that in the future other clusters of families with proven phylogenetic affinities will be grouped to form orders.

The primary criteria for delineation of families are (1) the kind of nucleic acid that constitutes the genome (see Table 1-2), (2) the strategy of viral replication, and (3) the morphology of the virion (Fig. 2-1). Subdivision of families into genera is based on criteria that vary for different families. Genera, usually defined by substantial differences in their genomes, contain from one to over a hundred species. The definition of species is more arbitrary, and virologists continue to argue about the criteria for the designation of species. In this book we will use the common vernacular names to distinguish viruses that cause different diseases.

Serology, more recently strengthened by the use of monoclonal antibodies, is of great value in the differentiation of viruses below the species level: types, subtypes, strains, and variants—terms that have no generally agreed taxonomic status. Characterization of the nucleic acid of the viral genome, as revealed by such techniques as nucleotide sequence analysis (partial or complete genome sequencing), restriction endonuclease mapping, electrophoresis in gels (especially useful for RNA viruses with segmented genomes), oligonucleotide fingerprinting, and molecular hybridization, is being used more and more to identify viruses and to distinguish differences between strains and variants.

NOMENCLATURE

Since 1966 the classification and nomenclature of viruses, at the higher taxonomic levels (families and genera), has been systematically organized by the International Committee on Taxonomy of Viruses. The highest taxon used is the order, named with the suffix *-virales*. Families are named with the suffix *-viridae*, subfamilies with the suffix *-virinae;* and genera with the suffix *-virus*. The prefix may be another latin word or may be a *sigla*, that is, an abbreviation derived from some initial letters. Order, family, subfamily, and generic names are capitalized and written in italics; vernacular terms derived from them are written in roman letters, without an initial capital letter. Currently, viral species are designated by vernacular terms, for example, rinderpest virus.

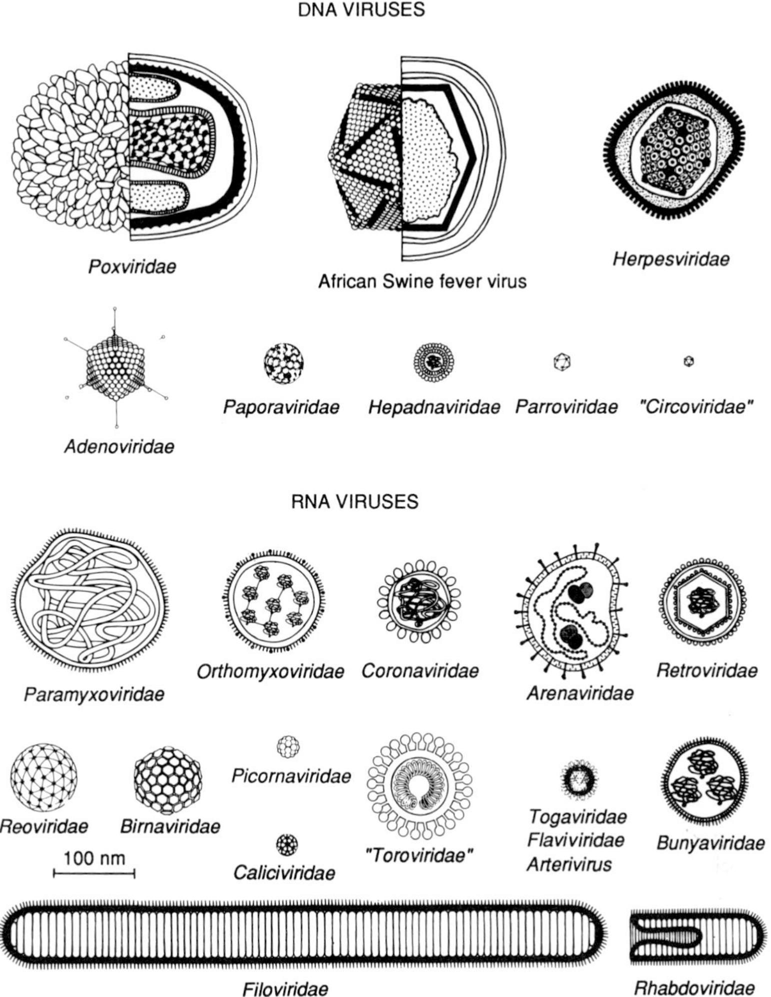

FIG. 2-1. *Diagram illustrating the shapes and sizes of animal viruses. The virions are drawn to scale, but artistic license has been used in representing their structure. In some, the cross-sectional structure of capsid and envelope are shown, with a representation of the genome; with the very small virions, only their size and symmetry is depicted.*

A brief description of each family of viruses of importance in veterinary medicine is given below, and their properties are summarized in Tables 2-1 and 2-2.

FAMILIES OF DNA VIRUSES

Provisional Family: "*Circoviridae*" (Circoviruses)

The prototype of a new family of DNA viruses, not yet officially named, was isolated from cultures of a pig kidney cell line in 1974, and later a high proportion of pigs in northern Germany were found to have antibodies to the virus. A similar virus produces beak and feather disease in psittacine birds. The isometric virion has a diameter of 16 nm; there are two structural proteins, and the genome is a covalently closed circle of plus sense ssDNA, 1.7 kb. Replication occurs only when the host cell is in the S phase of the cell cycle.

Family: *Parvoviridae* (Parvoviruses)

Genus: *Parvovirus* (parvoviruses of mammals and birds)
Genus: *Dependovirus* (adeno-associated viruses)

Parvoviruses (*parvus* = small) are about 20 nm in diameter, and they have icosahedral symmetry and a genome of ssDNA, 5 kb. The virions are relatively heat stable, and most species have a narrow host range. Animal pathogens of the genus *Parvovirus* include feline panleukopenia, mink enteritis, and Aleutian mink disease viruses, and canine, bovine, goose, human, porcine, murine, rat, and rabbit parvoviruses. Members of the genus *Dependovirus* are defective viruses, which depend on an adenovirus (or, experimentally, a herpesvirus) for replication. They occur in birds, cattle, horses, dogs, and humans but are not known to cause disease.

Family: *Hepadnaviridae* (Hepatitis B-like Viruses)

Genus: *Orthohepadnavirus* (mamalian hepatitis B-like viruses)
Genus: *Avihepadnavirus* (avian hepatitis B-like viruses)

Human hepatitis B virus and related viruses of other animals, all highly host-specific, comprise the family *Hepadnaviridae* (*hepa* = liver). The virions are spherical particles 42 nm in diameter, consisting of a 27-nm icosahedral core within a closely adherent outer capsid that contains cellular lipids, glycoproteins, and a virus-specific surface antigen

TABLE 2-1

Properties of Virions of Families of DNA Viruses

	Virion					Genome	
			Nucleocapsid				
Family or virus	Diameter (nm)	Envelope	Symmetry	Capsomers	Transcriptase	Nature[a, b]	Size (kb, kbp)
"Circoviridae"	16	−	Icosahedral	?	−	ss (+), circular	1.7
Hepadnaviridae	42	−	Icosahedral	?	+[c]	ds, circular[d]	3.2
Parvoviridae	20	−	Icosahedral	32	−	ss (−), linear	5
Papovaviridae	45, 55[e]	−	Icosahedral	72	−	ds, circular	5, 8[e]
Adenoviridae	70	−	Icosahedral	252	−	ds, linear	30–37
Herpesviridae	150	+	Icosahedral	162	−	ds, linear	120–220
Iridoviridae	125–300	+	Icosahedral	1892	+	ds, linear	150
African swine fever virus	220	+[f]	Icosahedral	1892	+	ds, linear	150
Poxviridae	260 × 160[g] 450 × 240[h]	+[f]	Complex	—	+	ds, linear	130–280

[a] All DNA virus genomes comprise a single molecule.

[b] ds, Double-stranded; ss, single-stranded; sense of single-stranded nucleic acid (+) or (−).

[c] Reverse transcriptase.

[d] Circular molecule is double-stranded for most of its length but contains a single-stranded region.

[e] Lower figures, *Polyomavirus;* higher figures, *Papillomavirus.*

[f] Not essential for infectivity.

[g] *Parapoxvirus.*

[h] All other genera.

(HBsAg). The genome is a small, circular, partially double-stranded DNA molecule, which consists of a long (3.2 kb) and a short (1.7–2.8 kb) strand.

The hepadnaviruses replicate in the nucleus of hepatocytes and cause hepatitis, which may progress to cirrhosis and primary hepatocellular carcinoma. The most important species is human hepatitis B virus, but other orthohepadnaviruses occur in woodchuck and ground squirrels and avihepadnaviruses in Pekin duck and heron.

Family: *Papovaviridae* (Papovaviruses)

Genus: *Papillomavirus* (papillomaviruses)
Genus: *Polyomavirus* (polyomaviruses)

The papovaviruses (sigla: *pa* = papilloma; *po* = polyoma; *va* = vacuolating agent) are small, nonenveloped icosahedral viruses which replicate in the nucleus and may transform infected cells. In the virion their nucleic acid occurs as a cyclic double-stranded molecule, which is infectious. There are two genera. *Papillomavirus* (wart viruses, 55 nm diameter) have a larger genome (8 kbp) which may persist in transformed cells in an *episomal* form. Viruses of the genus *Polyomavirus* (45 nm diameter) have a smaller genome (5 kbp) and may persist in cells via the integration of the genome into the host cell DNA.

Papillomaviruses occur in many species of mammals and birds. Individual papillomaviruses have a narrow host range. Bovine papillomaviruses, which cause cutaneous papillomas of cattle, and the virus of canine oral papillomatosis are among the most important; rabbit papilloma virus has been extensively used in studies of viral oncogenesis. Human papillomaviruses cause warts, and some types are associated with cancer of the cervix. The genus *Polyomavirus* includes SV40 (from rhesus monkeys) and mouse polyoma virus, both of which have been useful models for the study of viral oncogenesis, and an avian species, budgerigar fledgling disease virus, which is the only papovavirus that causes an acute disease.

Family: *Adenoviridae* (Adenoviruses)

Genus: *Mastadenovirus* (mammalian adenoviruses)
Genus: *Aviadenovirus* (avian adenoviruses)

The adenoviruses (*adeno* = gland) are nonenveloped icosahedral viruses 70 nm in diameter, with a single linear dsDNA genome of 30–37 kbp. They replicate in the nucleus. Human adenoviruses are usually associated with infection of the respiratory tract, and occasionally the eye and the intestinal tract. Many adenoviruses are characterized by prolonged subclinical infection.

Mastadenoviruses that are animal pathogens include equine adenovirus, bovine adenoviruses, infectious canine hepatitis virus, and canine adenovirus type 2. Pathogenic aviadenoviruses include those which cause egg drop syndrome and marble spleen disease. Some adenoviruses of other species of mammals and birds are also pathogenic. Some of the adenoviruses of man, cattle, and chickens cause tumors when inoculated into newborn hamsters and have been used in experimental studies on oncogenesis, but none causes tumors in its natural host.

Family: *Herpesviridae* (Herpesviruses)

- Subfamily: *Alphaherpesvirinae* (herpes simplex-like viruses)
  - Genus: *Simplexvirus* (herpes simplex-like viruses)
  - Genus: *Varicellovirus* (varicella-like viruses)
- Subfamily: *Betaherpesvirinae* (cytomegaloviruses)
  - Genus: *Cytomegalovirus* (human cytomegalovirus)
  - Genus: *Murocytomegalovirus* (mouse cytomegalovirus)
  - Proposed Genus: *Roseolovirus* (human herpesvirus 6)
- Subfamily: *Gammaherpesvirinae* (lymphoproliferative viruses)
  - Genus: *Lymphocryptovirus* (Epstein-Barr virus)
  - Genus: *Rhadinovirus* (ateline herpesviruses)

The herpesvirus (*herpes* = creeping) have enveloped virions about 150 nm in diameter, with icosahedral nucleocapsids about 100 nm in diameter. Their genome is a single linear molecule of dsDNA, 120–220 kbp. They replicate in the nucleus and mature by budding through the nuclear membrane, thus acquiring an envelope. This large family includes many important veterinary and human pathogens and has been subdivided into three subfamilies. *Alphaherpesvirinae* includes infectious bovine rhinotracheitis virus, bovine mammillitis virus, B-virus of monkeys, pseudorabies virus, equine rhinopneumonitis, abortion and coital exanthema viruses, feline rhinotracheitis virus, canine herpesvirus, avian infectious laryngotracheitis virus, and Marek's disease virus, as well as herpes simplex types 1 and 2 and varicella viruses of man. *Betaherpesvirinae* comprises the cytomegaloviruses, which are highly host-specific viruses of humans, cattle, pigs, horses, mice, guinea pigs, and other animals. The cytomegaloviruses of animals, like those of man, produce low-grade, chronic infections. All members of the subfamily *Gammaherpesvirinae* replicate in lymphoblastoid cells and cause latent infections; several of them are associated with tumors. They include baboon and chimpanzee herpesviruses, *Herpesvirus ateles* and *Herpesvirus saimiri* of monkeys, and Epstein-Barr (EB) virus in humans.

A feature of all herpesvirus infections is lifelong persistence of the virus in the body, usually in *latent* form. Excretion may occur continuously or intermittently without disease, or episodes of recurrent clinical disease and recurrent excretion may occur years after the initial infection.

Family: *Iridoviridae* (Icosahedral Cytoplasmic Deoxyviruses)

Genus: *Ranavirus* (frog viruses)
Genus: *Lymphocystivirus* (lymphocystis viruses of fish)

Unnamed Family: African Swine Fever Virus

Originally a number of large icosahedral DNA viruses that affect insects, nematodes, fish, and amphibians were grouped together with African swine fever virus into the family *Iridoviridae.* In 1984 African swine fever virus was removed from the family, but it has not yet been allocated to any other family. The family *Iridoviridae* (*irido* = iridescent) was defined on the characteristics of certain insect viruses, but it includes two genera that affect vertebrates. They are the largest icosahedral viruses (capsid, 125 nm in diameter), and those that affect vertebrates have enveloped virions 125–300 nm in diameter. The genome is a single linear molecule of dsDNA, 150 kbp. The host cell nucleus appears to be required for transcription and replication of DNA, but some DNA synthesis and assembly of virions take place in the cytoplasm.

The genus *Ranavirus* includes several members that affect amphibians, and a member of the genus *Lymphocystivirus* produces lymphocystis disease of fish. African swine fever virus is an important pathogen of swine, which can be transmitted by contact and also by ticks.

Family: *Poxviridae* (Poxviruses)

Subfamily: *Chordopoxvirinae* (poxviruses of vertebrates)
- Genus: *Orthopoxvirus* (vaccinia virus subgroup)
- Genus: *Parapoxvirus* (orf virus subgroup)
- Genus: *Avipoxvirus* (fowlpox virus subgroup)
- Genus: *Capripoxvirus* (sheeppox virus subgroup)
- Genus: *Leporipoxvirus* (myxoma virus subgroup)
- Genus: *Suipoxvirus* (swinepox virus subgroup)
- Genus: *Molluscipoxvirus* (molluscum virus subgroup)
- Genus: *Yatapoxvirus* (yaba/tanapox virus subgroup)

Subfamily: *Entomopoxvirinae* (poxviruses of insects)

The poxviruses (*pock* = pustule) are the largest and most complex viruses of vertebrates. The virions are brick-shaped, measuring 300–450 × 170–260 nm in all genera except *Parapoxvirus*, the virions of which are ovoid and measure 220–300 × 140–170 nm. All poxviruses have an inner core which contains a single linear molecule of dsDNA, 130–280 kbp. Unlike most other DNA viruses of vertebrates, poxviruses replicate in the cytoplasm, mRNA being transcribed by a virion-associated transcriptase. A large number of other virion-associated enzymes are involved in DNA synthesis.

The family is divided into two subfamilies, one of which, *Chordopoxvirinae,* comprises the poxviruses of vertebrates. This subfamily contains seven genera that include animal pathogens. The genus *Orthopoxvirus* includes cowpox, camelpox, ectromelia (mousepox), rabbitpox (a variant of vaccinia virus), and monkeypox viruses. Variola virus, which caused human smallpox, and vaccinia virus, used to control that disease, also belong to this genus. *Parapoxvirus* includes contagious pustular dermatitis, pseudocowpox (milker's nodes), and bovine papular stomatitis viruses. *Avipoxviruses* includes many bird-specific poxviruses; *Capripoxvirus* includes the viruses of sheeppox, goatpox, and lumpyskin disease of cattle. *Leporipoxvirus* includes myxoma and rabbit fibroma viruses, while the genus *Suipoxvirus* has only one member, swinepox virus, and the recently named genus *Yatapoxvirus* contains two viruses of African wildlife, yabapoxvirus and tanapoxvirus, both of which may infect humans.

FAMILIES OF RNA VIRUSES

Family: *Picornaviridae* (Picornaviruses)

Genus: *Enterovirus* (enteroviruses)
Genus: *Cardiovirus* (encephalomyocarditis-like viruses)
Genus: *Rhinovirus* (rhinoviruses)
Genus: *Aphthovirus* (foot-and-mouth disease viruses)
Genus: *Hepatovirus* (hepatitis A-like viruses)

The *Picornaviridae* (sigla: *pico* = small; *rna* = ribonucleic acid) comprise small nonenveloped icosahedral viruses 25–30 nm in diameter, which contain a single molecule of plus sense ssRNA (7.5–8.5 kb) and replicate in the cytoplasm. The genera *Enterovirus* and *Rhinovirus* include large numbers of species that affect domestic animals, usually without causing significant disease. An enterovirus causes swine vesicular disease, which may be confused with foot-and-mouth disease, and porcine enterovirus 1 causes polioencephalomyelitis. These two genera also include several important human pathogens, including the polioviruses. Foot-and-mouth disease virus, of the genus *Aphthovirus,* occurs as seven types and many antigenically distinct subtypes. It is among the most important of all viruses in veterinary medicine. The genus *Cardiovirus* includes

TABLE 2-2

Properties of Virions of Families of RNA Viruses

	Virion					Genome	
			Nucleocapsid				
Family or virus	Diameter[a] (*nm*)	Envelope	Symmetry	Capsomers	Transcriptase	Nature[b]	Size (kb, kbp)
Hepatitis D virus	36	+[c, d]	Icosahedral	?	−	ss (−), circular	1.7
Picornaviridae	25–30	−	Icosahedral	60	−	ss (+)	7.5–8.5
Caliciviridae	35–40	−	Icosahedral	32	−	ss (+)	8
Togaviridae	60–70	+[c]	Icosahedral	60	−	ss (+)	12
Flaviviridae	40–50	+[c]	Icosahedral	?	−	ss (+)	10
Coronaviridae	75–160	+[c]	Helical	?	−	ss (+)	27–33
"*Toroviridae*"	35 × 170	+[c]	Helical	?	−	ss (+)	20
Paramyxoviridae[e]	150–300	+	Helical	?	+	ss (−)	18–20
Rhabdoviridae[e]	180 × 75	+	Helical	?	+	ss (−)	13–16
Filoviridae[e]	790–970 × 80	+	Helical	?	+	ss (−)	12.7
Orthomyxoviridae	80–120	+	Helical	?	+	ss (−) 7, 8	13.6
Arenaviridae	110–130	+[c]	Helical	?	+	ss (−) 2	10–14
Bunyaviridae	90–120	+[c]	Helical	?	+	ss (−) 3	13.5–21
Reoviridae	60–80	−	Icosahedral	32, 92[f]	+	ds, 10, 11, 12[g]	18–27
Birnaviridae	60	−	Icosahedral	92	+	ds, 2	7
Retroviridae	80–100	+[c]	Icosahedral	?	+[h]	ss (+)	7–10[i]

[a] Some enveloped viruses are very pelomorphic and sometimes filamentous.

[b] All genomes except that of hepatitis D virus are linear; ss, single-stranded; ds, double-stranded; 2 to 12, number of segments in segmented genomes; (+) or (−), sense of single-stranded nucleic acid.

[c] No matrix protein.

[d] Envelope protein derived from hepatitis B virus.

[e] These three families are grouped in the order *Mononegavirales*.

[f] Inner capsid of *Orbivirus*, *Rotavirus*, and *Orthoreovirus*, 32; outer capsid of *Orthoreovirus*, 92.

[g] *Orthoreovirus* and *Oribivirus*, 10; *Rotavirus* and *Aquareovirus*, 11; *Coltivirus*, 12.

[h] Reverse transcriptase.

[i] Genome is diploid, two identical molecules being held together by hydrogen bonds at their 5′ ends.

encephalomyocarditis virus of swine and rodents, and the genus *Hepatovirus* includes human and simian hepatitis A viruses.

Family: *Caliciviridae* (Caliciviruses)

Genus: *Calicivirus* (caliciviruses)

The caliciviruses (*calix* = cup) are icosahedral viruses whose virions are 35–40 nm in diameter and have 32 cup-shaped depressions on the surface. The genome consists of one molecule of plus sense ssRNA, size 8 kb. Most species have a narrow host range. Several are of veterinary importance: vesicular exanthema virus of swine, San Miguel sea lion and related pinniped viruses, feline calicivirus, and the rabbit hemorrhagic disease virus. Caliciviruses have also been isolated from vesicular lesions of dogs, calves, and chimpanzees, and they have been demonstrated in the feces of humans, calves, pigs, and sheep with diarrhea.

Family: *Togaviridae* (Togaviruses)

Genus: *Alphavirus* (formerly "group A" arboviruses)
Genus: *Rubivirus* (rubella virus)

The togaviruses (*toga* = cloak) are small, spherical enveloped viruses 60–70 nm in diameter, containing plus sense ssRNA (12 kb) enclosed within an icosahedral core. They replicate in the cytoplasm and mature by budding from cell membranes. The genus *Alphavirus* contains many species, all of which are arthropod-transmitted. Important alphaviruses that infect both livestock and man include eastern, western, and Venezuelan equine encephalitis viruses; Ross River virus causes arthritis in humans. In nature the alphaviruses usually produce inapparent viremic infections of birds, some mammals, and reptiles, but in domestic animals and man generalized disease or encephalitis can sometimes result. Currently the only non-arthropod-borne togavirus is rubella virus, the only species in the genus *Rubivirus*.

Family: *Flaviviridae* (Flaviviruses)

Genus: *Flavivirus* (formerly "group B" arboviruses)
Genus: *Pestivirus* (hog cholera-like viruses)
Unnamed Genus: Hepatitis C virus

Flaviviruses (*flavi* = yellow; yellow fever virus) have an enveloped icosahedral virion 40–50 nm in diameter and a genome of 10 kb. Viruses of the largest genus, *Flavivirus*, are arthropod-borne, but those of the other two genera (*Pestivirus* and hepatitis C virus) are not. Flavivirus diseases of veterinary importance include louping ill, Wesselsbron disease, and turkey meningoencephalitis. Central European tick-borne encephalitis virus produces an inapparent infection in ruminants but may be excreted in the milk and cause disease in humans who drink contaminated milk. Important human pathogens include the viruses of yellow fever, dengue, and several arthropod-borne encephalitides. Pestiviruses include hog cholera virus, bovine virus diarrhea virus, and border disease virus of sheep. Hepatitis C virus is an important cause of hepatitis in humans.

Family: *Coronaviridae* (Coronaviruses)

Genus: *Coronavirus* (coronaviruses of mammals and birds)

The coronaviruses (*corona* = crown) are somewhat pleomorphic viruses 75–160 nm in diameter, with widely spaced, pear-shaped peplomers embedded in a lipoprotein envelope. The envelope lacks a matrix protein and encloses a core of helical symmetry with a single linear molecule of plus sense ssRNA, 27–33 kb. Some coronaviruses contain a receptor-destroying enzyme, neuraminate acetylesterase. Animal pathogens include calf coronavirus (neonatal diarrhea), transmissible gastroenteritis virus of swine, hemagglutinating encephalomyelitis virus of swine, feline infectious peritonitis virus, canine coronavirus, avian infectious bronchitis virus, murine hepatitis virus, and turkey bluecomb virus. Certain species of coronaviruses cause common colds in humans.

Family: *"Toroviridae"* (Toroviruses)

Genus: *Torovirus* (toroviruses)

The name *Torovirus* (*torus* = object shaped like a donut) has recently been adopted for viruses that are associated with diarrhea in horses (Berne virus) and calves (Breda virus). The virions are enveloped and disk-shaped (35 × 170 nm) and contain a nucleocapsid of helical symmetry; the genome is a single molecule of plus sense ssRNA, 20 kb. The genus has affinities with the coronaviruses and the genus *Arterivirus*.

Order: *Mononegavirales*

Because of basic similarities in the genome structure and mode of replication, three families of viruses with linear negative sense ssRNA genomes, *Paramyxoviridae, Rhabdoviridae,* and *Filoviridae,* have been grouped into an order, *Mononegavirales.*

Family: *Paramyxoviridae* (Paramyxoviruses)

Subfamily: *Paramyxovirinae*
  Genus: *Paramyxovirus* (paramyxoviruses)
  Genus: *Morbillivirus* (measleslike viruses)
Subfamily: *Pneumovirinae*
  Genus: *Pneumovirus* (respiratory syncytial viruses)

The paramyxoviruses have a large, roughly spherical enveloped virion 150–300 nm in diameter, with a helical nucleocapsid. Their genome consists of a single linear molecule of minus sense ssRNA (18–20 kb). The envelope contains two glycoproteins, a hemagglutinin (in most species with neuraminidase activity also) and a fusion protein.

The genus *Paramyxovirus* includes Newcastle disease virus, parainfluenza 1 virus (Sendai virus of mice), parainfluenza 3 virus of cattle, and other parainfluenza viruses of cattle and birds. Viruses of the genus *Morbillivirus* usually cause generalized infections: rinderpest of cattle, peste-des-petits-ruminants of sheep and goats, canine distemper and morbillivirus infection of seals, as well as measles in humans. The respiratory syncytial viruses (genus *Pneumovirus*), besides causing an important respiratory disease of human infants, cause respiratory diseases of cattle, sheep, and mice.

Family: *Rhabdoviridae* (Rhabdoviruses)

Genus: *Vesiculovirus* (vesicular stomatitis-like viruses)
Genus: *Lyssavirus* (rabieslike viruses)

The rhabdoviruses (*rhabdos* = rod) are bullet-shaped viruses, about 180 × 75 nm, containing a single molecule of minus sense ssRNA (13–16 kb). Their helical capsid is enclosed within a shell to which is closely applied an envelope with embedded peplomers. The virion matures at the plasma membrane. Animal pathogens in the genus *Vesiculovirus* include vesicular stomatitis, Chandipura, Piry, and Isfahan viruses (each of which is an occasional human pathogen), and the causative agents of several diseases of fish. The genus *Lyssavirus* includes rabies virus and several serologically related agents. Ungrouped rhabdoviruses that cause diseases in animals and that will probably eventually be allocated to several different genera include bovine ephemeral fever virus and several rhabdoviruses of fish.

Family: *Filoviridae* (Filoviruses)

Genus: *Filovirus* (Marburg and Ebola viruses)

Marburg virus was originally isolated in 1967 from monkeys imported into Germany from Africa and from humans infected when handling their tissues; Ebola virus was isolated from simultaneous outbreaks in hospitals in Zaire and Sudan in 1976–77. A related but less virulent virus was recently recovered from monkeys from the Philippines. The virions are pleomorphic and sometimes very long (*filum* = thread), maximum infectivity being associated with a particle 790–970 nm long and 80 nm wide. Their genome is a single molecule of minus sense ssRNA, 12.7 kb. They are known only by the sporadic infections and occasional nosocomial epidemics produced in humans in Africa and infections among monkeys imported from the Philippines. They cause hemorrhagic fever in humans and are Biosafety Level 4 pathogens, which may be worked with in the laboratory only under maximum biocontainment conditions. Following experimental inoculation, they cause disease in a variety of laboratory animals.

Family: *Orthomyxoviridae* (Influenza Viruses)

Genus: Influenza virus A and B (influenza A and influenza B viruses)
Genus: Influenza virus C (influenza C virus)

The orthomyxoviruses (*myxo* = mucus) are spherical RNA viruses 80–120 nm in diameter, with a helical nucleocapsid enclosed within an envelope acquired by budding from the plasma membrane. The genome consists of seven (influenza C virus) or eight (influenza A and B viruses) segments of minus sense ssRNA (total size, 13.6 kb). The envelope is studded with peplomers, which are of two kinds, a *hemagglutinin* and a neuraminidase, in influenza A and B viruses, and of one kind, hemagglutinin esterase, in influenza C virus.

Influenza A virus infects birds, horses, swine, mink, seals, and whales, as well as man; influenza B virus is a human pathogen only. Influenza C virus infects humans and swine, but rarely causes serious disease. Influenza A viruses of swine or birds and man undergo genetic reassortment in humans, pigs, or birds to generate novel subtypes ("antigenic shift") which cause major pandemics of influenza in man.

Family: *Arenaviridae* (Arenaviruses)

Genus: *Arenavirus* (arenaviruses)

Arenaviruses (*arena* = sand) are so named because of the presence of ribosome-like particles (resembling grains of sand in thin sections examined by electron microscopy) incorporated within pleomorphic enveloped virions 110–130 nm in diameter, which contain no matrix protein. The genome consists of two segments of minus sense or ambisense ss RNA (total size, 10–14 kb), each held in a circular configuration by hydrogen bonds. All cause natural inapparent infections of rodents.

Humans may develop serious generalized disease, for example, Lassa fever or lymphocytic choriomeningitis, following exposure to infected rodent urine. It has been found that lymphocytic choriomeningitis or a very closely related virus causes a severe hepatitis of marmosets (callitrichid arenavirus). Lassa, Machupo, and Junin viruses are Biosafety Level 4 pathogens.

Family: *Bunyaviridae* (Bunyaviruses)

Genus: *Bunyavirus* (Bunyamwera supergroup)
Genus: *Phlebovirus* (sandfly fever viruses)
Genus: *Nairovirus* (Nairobi sheep disease-like viruses)
Genus: *Uukuvirus* (Uukuniemi-like viruses)
Genus: *Hantavirus* (hemorrhagic fever with renal syndrome viruses)

Over 100 bunyaviruses (Bunyamwera is a locality in Africa) make up the largest single group of arboviruses. The enveloped virions are 90–120 nm in diameter, within which there are helical, circular nucleocapsids with a diameter of 2–2.5 nm. The genome consists of three molecules of minus sense or in *Phlebovirus* ambisense ssRNA (total size, 13.5–21 kb), each held in a circular configuration by hydrogen bonds. Virions replicate in the cytoplasm and bud from Golgi membranes. Because of their segmented genome, closely related bunyaviruses readly undergo genetic reassortment.

All except the hantaviruses are arboviruses that have wild animal reservoir hosts; some are transovarially transmitted in mosquitoes, with a high frequency. The hantaviruses, which are enzootic in rodents and cause hemorrhagic fever with renal syndrome in man, are not arthropod-transmitted. The genus *Phlebovirus* includes the important pathogen of sheep and man, Rift Valley fever virus, and the genus *Nairovirus* includes Nairobi sheep disease virus.

Family: *Reoviridae* (Reoviruses)

Genus: *Orthoreovirus* (reoviruses of animals)
Genus: *Orbivirus* (orbiviruses)
Genus: *Rotavirus* (rotaviruses)
Genus: *Coltivirus* (Colorado tick fever virus)
Genus: *Aquareovirus* (reoviruses of fish and shellfish)

The family name is a sigla, respiratory enteric orphan virus, reflecting the fact that members of the first discovered genus, *Orthoreovirus*, were found in both the respiratory and intestinal tract of man and most animals, but were not associated with any disease (orphan viruses were "viruses in search of a disease"). The distinctive feature of the family is that the virions contain dsRNA, in 10 (*Orthoreovirus* and *Orbivirus*), 11 (*Rotavirus* and *Aquareovirus*), or 12 segments (*Coltivirus*), with a total genome size for different viruses varying between 16 and 27 kbp. The virion is a nonenveloped icosahedron 60–80 nm in diameter. Orbiviruses (*orbi* = ring) are arboviruses that include bluetongue virus of sheep, epizootic hemorrhagic disease virus of deer, and African horsesickness virus. The rotaviruses (*rota* = wheel) include viruses that are important causes of diarrhea in domestic animals and humans, and the aquaviruses (*aqua* = water) cause diseases of fish and shellfish. The only known *Coltivirus* is the species that causes Colorado tick fever in humans.

Family: *Birnaviridae* (Birnaviruses)

Genus: *Birnavirus* (two-segment dsRNA viruses)

The family *Birnaviridae* (sigla: *bi* = two; *rna*) contains viruses with nonenveloped virions of icosahedral symmetry, 60 nm in diameter, which replicate in the cytoplasm. The genome consists of two segments of linear dsRNA (total size, 7 kbp). Animal pathogens include infectious bursal disease virus of chickens and infectious pancreatic necrosis virus of fish.

Family: *Retroviridae* (Retroviruses)

Genus: *Lentivirus* (HIV-like viruses; maedi/visna-like viruses)
Genus: *Spumavirus* (foamy viruses)
Unnamed Genus: Mammalian type B retroviruses
Unnamed Genus: Mammalian type C retroviruses
Unnamed Genus: Avian type C retroviruses
Unnamed Genus: Mammalian type D retroviruses
Unnamed Genus: HTLV/BLV-like viruses

The name *Retroviridae* (sigla: *re* = reverse; *tr* = transcriptase) is used for a large family of enveloped viruses 80–100 nm in diameter, with a complex structure and an unusual enzyme, reverse transcriptase. Uniquely among viruses, the genome is diploid, consisting of an inverted dimer of plus sense ssRNA, 7–10 kb in size. In the life cycle of the exogenous retroviruses the dsDNA copy of the viral genome transcribed by the viral *reverse transcriptase* is circularized and integrates into the cellular DNA as an essential part of the replication cycle. Proviral DNA of endogenous retroviruses is found in the DNA of all normal cells of many species of animals and may under certain circumstances be induced to produce virus.

This important family is subdivided into seven genera, only two of which have been given official generic names. The family contains many viruses of veterinary importance, including bovine leukemia virus, feline leukemia and sarcoma viruses, baboon, gibbon, and woolly monkey leukemia/sarcoma viruses, as well as avian reticuloendotheliosis, avian leukosis and sarcoma viruses, murine leukemia virus, and the mouse mammary tumor virus. The genus *Lentivirus* (*lenti* = slow) includes viruses responsible for several slowly developing but severe diseases: maedi/visna and progressive pneumonia of sheep, caprine arthritis–encephalitis, equine infectious anemia, human acquired immune deficiency syndrome (AIDS), and similar diseases in cats and some species of monkeys. The genus *Spumavirus* (*spuma* = foam) includes the "foamy viruses," which are a problem when they contaminate cultured cells but are not known to cause disease.

OTHER VIRUSES

There are a number of other viruses that belong to groups that are as yet unclassified, some of which cause diseases of veterinary importance.

Genus *Arterivirus*. The genus *Arterivirus* includes equine arteritis virus and possibly lactate dehydrogenase virus of mice and simian hemorrhagic fever virus. It was formerly classified with the *Togaviridae,* but its member viruses resemble coronaviruses more closely than togaviruses.

Hepatitis D Virus. Hepatitis D virus is a satellite virus dependent on the simultaneous replication of a hepadnavirus. The virion is about 38 nm in diameter and consists of a single protein, the 24-kDa delta antigen, surrounded by a hepadnavirus envelope. The genome of 1.7 kb of minus sense ssRNA contains regions of extensive base pairing and probably exists as a double-stranded rodlike structure similar to the viroids of plants. Hepatitis D virus is known only as a virus of humans who are simultaneously infected with hepatitis B virus, and it exacerbates the severity of the disease.

Astroviruses. Astrovirus (*astro* = star) is a name accorded unofficially to viruses with small spherical virions with a characteristic star-shaped surface pattern. These viruses have been found in the feces of calves, lambs, and man. The genome consists of one molecule of ssRNA about the same size as that of the picornaviruses, but they are probably a separate group.

Borna Disease Virus. An encephalomyelitis of horses and sheep, called Borna disease (Borna is a town in Germany where the disease was first observed), is caused by an unclassified enveloped RNA virus.

Subacute Spongiform Encephalopathies. The causative agents of the subacute spongiform encephalopathies remain enigmatic. Their infectivity is highly resistant to inactivation by physical and chemical agents, and they are nonimmunogenic. Nucleic acid has not been unequivocally detected. All produce slow infections with incubation periods measured in months or years, followed by progressive disease, which leads inexorably to death from a degenerative condition of the brain characterized by a spongiform appearance. The prototype is scrapie, a disease of sheep. Other members of veterinary importance are mink encephalopathy and "wasting disease" of mule deer and elk. Cattle in several European countries have been infected, possibly by feeding on material containing scrapie-infected sheep offal, and there has been a large outbreak of bovine spongiform encephalopathy (popularly known as "mad cow disease") in the United Kingdom.

GROUPINGS BASED ON EPIDEMIOLOGIC CRITERIA

In discussing the epidemiology and pathogenesis of viral infections it is often convenient to use groupings of viruses based on the routes of transmission.

Enteric viruses are acquired by ingestion of material contaminated with feces; they replicate primarily in the intestinal tract and remain localized. Enteric viruses important in veterinary medicine include the rotaviruses, coronaviruses, enteroviruses, and some adenoviruses.

Respiratory viruses are usually acquired by inhalation of droplets and replicate in the respiratory tract. The term is usually restricted to viruses that remain localized in the respiratory tract and includes the mammalian orthomyxoviruses and rhinoviruses, and some of the paramyxoviruses, coronaviruses, and adenoviruses.

Arboviruses (arthropod-borne viruses) infect arthropods that ingest vertebrate blood; they replicate in the tissues of the arthropod and can then be transmitted by bite to susceptible vertebrates. Viruses that belong to six families are included: all orbiviruses (a genus of the reoviruses), most bunyaviruses, flaviviruses, and togaviruses, some rhabdoviruses, and one DNA virus, African swine fever virus.

FURTHER READING

Fenner, F., and Gibbs, A. J., eds. (1988). "Portraits of Viruses." Karger, Basel.

Fraenkel-Conrat, H., and Wagner, R. R., eds. (1982–1984). "The Viruses," Vols. 1–19. Plenum, New York.

Francki, R. I. B., Fauquet, C. M., Knudsen, D., and Brown F., eds. (1991). "The Classification and Nomenclature of Viruses. Fifth Report of the International Committee on Taxonomy of Viruses." *Arch Virol. Suppl.* 2.

Matthews, R. E. F., ed. (1983). "A Critical Appraisal of Viral Taxonomy." CRC Press, Boca Raton, Florida.

CHAPTER 3

Viral Replication

Unraveling the complexities of viral replication is a central focus of much of experimental virology. Studies with bacteriophages in the 1940s and 1950s provided the first insights. With the development of mammalian cell culture procedures, the techniques used for the study of bacteriophages were adapted to animal viruses. Progress has been such that the basic mechanisms of transcription, translation, and nucleic acid replication have been characterized for all the major families of animal viruses and the strategy of gene expression and regulation clarified.

Our knowledge of viral replication is now very detailed and continues to grow in complexity. It was easier to generalize when we knew less, but now we know that every family of viruses is characterized by a unique replication strategy. In this chapter we present an overview of the subject, indicating similarities and differences in the replication strategies adopted by viruses of each family. Further information is provided in the viral replication sections of the chapters in Part II.

VIRAL REPLICATION CYCLE

One-Step Growth Curve

Most studies of the replication of animal viruses have been conducted using cultured mammalian cell lines growing either in suspension or as a monolayer adhering to a flat surface. Classic studies of this kind defined the "one-step growth curve," in which all cells in a culture are infected simultaneously by using a high *multiplicity of infection,* and the increase in infectious virus over time is followed by sequential sampling and titration (Fig. 3-1). Virus that is free in the medium can be titrated separately from virus that remains cell-associated. Shortly after infection, the inoculated virus "disappears"; infectious particles cannot be demonstrated, even intracellularly. This *eclipse period* continues until the first progeny virions become detectable some hours later. Nonenveloped

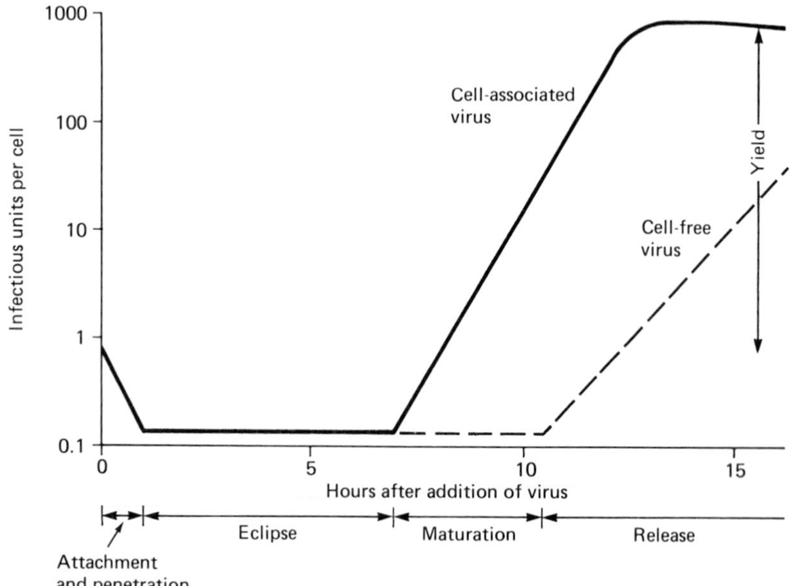

FIG. 3-1. *One-step growth curve of a nonenveloped virus. Attachment and penetration are followed by an eclipse period of 2–13 hours (see Table 3-1) during which cell-associated infectivity cannot be detected. This is followed by a period of several hours during which maturation occurs. Virions of nonenveloped viruses are often released late and incompletely, when the cell lyses. Release of enveloped virions occurs concurrently with maturation by budding from the plasma membrane.*

viruses mature within the cell and may be detectable for some time as infectious intracellular virions before they are released by cell lysis. Many enveloped viruses, on the other hand, mature by budding from the plasma membrane of the host cell (see Fig. 3-10) and are thus immediately released into the medium. The eclipse period generally ranges from 3 to 12 hours for viruses of different families (Table 3-1).

Early studies, relying on quantitative electron microscopy and assay of infectious virions, provided information about the early and the late events in the replication cycle (attachment, penetration, maturation, and release) but not about what happened during the eclipse period. Investigation of the expression and replication of the viral genome became possible only with the introduction of biochemical methods for the analysis of viral nucleic acids and proteins, and now all the sophisticated techniques of molecular biology are being applied to this problem.

TABLE 3-1

Characteristics of Replication of Viruses of Different Families

Family	Site of nucleic acid replication	Eclipse period (hours[a])	Budding (membrane)
Parvoviridae	Nucleus	6	None
Papovaviridae	Nucleus	13	None
Adenoviridae	Nucleus	10	None
Herpesviridae	Nucleus	4	Nuclear
Poxviridae	Cytoplasm	4	Golgi
African swine fever virus	Cytoplasm	5	Plasma
Picornaviridae	Cytoplasm	2	None
Caliciviridae	Cytoplasm	3	None
Togaviridae	Cytoplasm	2	Plasma
Flaviviridae	Cytoplasm	3	Endoplasmic
Coronaviridae	Cytoplasm	5	Golgi
Paramyxoviridae	Cytoplasm	4	Plasma
Rhabdoviridae	Cytoplasm	3	Plasma
Arenaviridae	Cytoplasm	5	Plasma
Bunyaviridae	Cytoplasm	4	Golgi
Orthomyxoviridae	Nucleus	4	Plasma
Reoviridae	Cytoplasm	5	None
Birnaviridae	Cytoplasm	4	None
Retroviridae	Nucleus	10	Plasma

[a] Differs with multiplicity of infection, strain of virus, cell type, and physiological condition.

Events during Eclipse Period

Figure 3-2 illustrates in a greatly simplified diagram the major steps that occur during the eclipse period, using adenovirus as an example. Following attachment, the virion is taken up by its host cell and is partially uncoated to expose the viral genome. Certain *early viral genes* are transcribed into RNA which may then be processed in a number of ways, including splicing. The early gene-products translated from this *messenger RNA (mRNA)* are of three main types: proteins that shut down

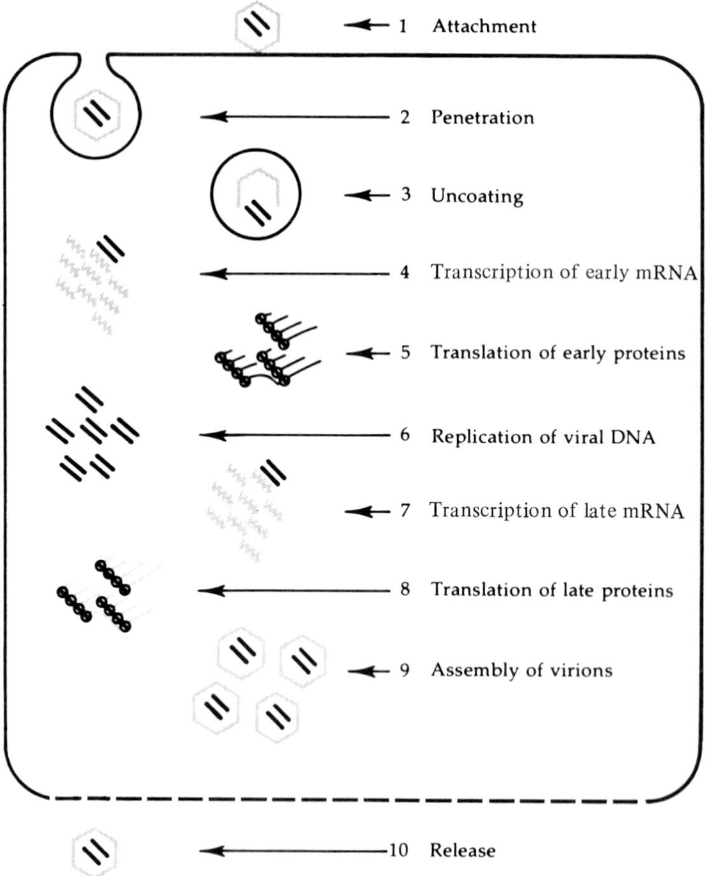

FIG. 3-2. *General features of the viral replication cycle, using adenovirus as a model. No topographic location for any step is implied. One step grades into the next such that, as the cycle progresses, several processes are proceeding simultaneously. Release usually occurs by cell lysis.*

cellular nucleic acid and protein synthesis, proteins that regulate the expression of the viral genome, and enzymes required for the replication of viral nucleic acid. Following viral nucleic acid replication, *late viral genes* are transcribed. The late proteins are principally viral structural proteins for assembly into new virions; some of these are subject to posttranslational modifications. Maturation occurs in the nucleus, and each infected cell yields thousands for new virions, which spread to infect other cells.

For most families of DNA viruses transcription and DNA replication take place in the cell nucleus, using the cellular RNA polymerase II and other cellular enzymes. Most RNA viruses replicate in the cytoplasm, and because cells lack the capacity to copy RNA from an RNA template, either the genome itself functions as mRNA or the viruses encode their own RNA polymerase to transcribe RNA from the RNA genome.

ATTACHMENT

To cause infection, virus particles must be able to bind to cells. Ligands on specific molecules on the surface of the virion bind to receptors on the plasma membrane of the cell (Table 3-2). For instance, X-ray crystallography reveals that the receptor for most orthomyxoviruses is the terminal sialic acid on an oligosaccharide side chain of a cellular glycoprotein (or glycolipid), while the ligand is in a cleft at the distal tip of each monomer of the trimeric viral hemagglutinin glycoprotein. The receptors for a number of other viruses are members of the immunoglobulin superfamily, such as ICAM-1 (intracellular adhesion molecule 1), which is the major receptor for most rhinoviruses, and CD4, the receptor for the human immunodeficiency viruses. Receptors for other viruses include hormone receptors and permeases. While there is a degree of specificity about the recognition of particular cellular receptors by particular viruses, quite different viruses (e.g., orthomyxoviruses and paramyxoviruses) may utilize the same receptor, and related viruses (e.g., human and mouse coronaviruses) may use quite different receptors. Viruses have evolved to make opportunistic use of a variety of membrane glycoproteins as their receptors, but the primary functions of these receptors have nothing to do with viruses.

UPTAKE (PENETRATION)

Following *attachment*, virions can enter cells by one of two main mechanisms: endocytosis or fusion.

TABLE 3-2

Examples of Viral Ligands and Cellular Receptors

Virus	Viral protein containing ligand	Target cell	Cell receptor
Pseudorabies virus	gIII	Various cell types	Heparan sulfate proteoglycans
Vaccinia virus	Epidermal growth factor	Various cell types	Epidermal growth factor receptor
Rhinovirus	VP1,2,3	Nasal epithelium	ICAM-1
Porcine polioencephalomyelitis virus	VP4	Intestinal epithelium	Member of IgG superfamily
Coronavirus	HE glycoprotein	Various cell types	Carcinoembryonic antigen family of glycoproteins
Rabies virus	Glycoprotein	Neuron	Acetyl cholinesterase receptor
Parainfluenza virus	H-N glycoprotein	Respiratory epithelium	Sialic acid-containing glycoproteins
Influenza A virus	Hemagglutinin	Respiratory epithelium	Sialic acid-containing glycoproteins
Rotavirus	VP7	Intestinal epithelium	Sialic acid-containing glycoproteins
Reovirus	σ1 (hemagglutinin)	T cell, neuron	β-Adrenergic receptor
Feline immunodeficiency virus	gp120	T cell, macrophage	?CD4
Gibbon leukemia virus	gp70	Lymphocyte	Permease

Endocytosis

The majority of mammalian cells are continuously engaged in *receptor-mediated endocytosis* for the uptake of macromolecules via specific receptors. Many enveloped and nonenveloped viruses use this essential cell function to initiate infection (Fig. 3-3). Attachment to receptors, which cluster at *clathrin-coated pits,* is followed by endocytosis into clathrin-coated vesicles that enter the cytoplasm and, after removal of the clathrin coat, fuse with endosomes (acidic prelysosomal vacuoles). Acidification within the vesicle triggers changes in the capsid protein VP4 of poliovirus, for example, leading to release of RNA from the virion into the cytosol. Likewise, at the acidic pH of the endosomes, the hemagglutinin molecule of influenza virus undergoes a conformational change, which enables fusion to occur between the viral envelope and the endosomal membrane, leading to release of the viral nucleocapsid into the cytoplasm. Many other nonenveloped and enveloped viruses undergo comparable changes.

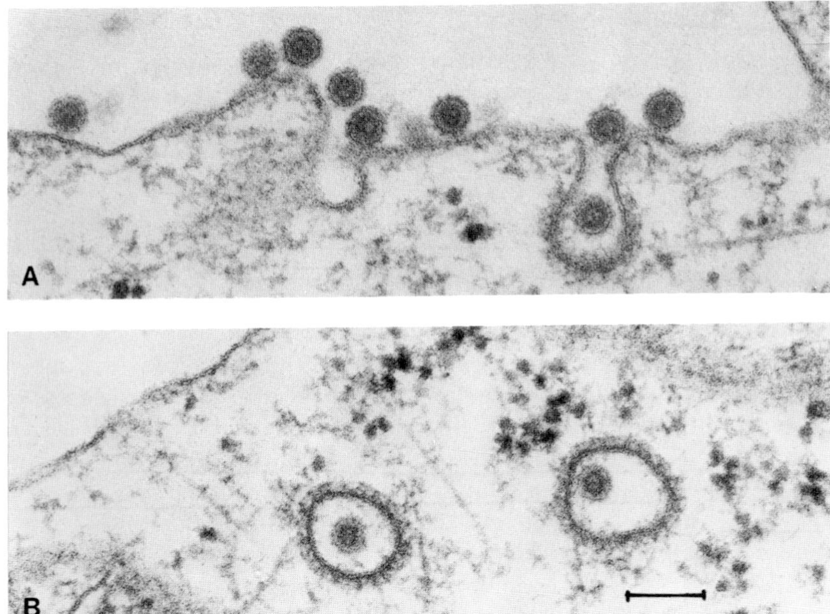

FIG. 3-3. *Receptor-mediated endocytosis: penetration by togavirus. (A) Attachment and movement into a clathrin-coated pit. (B) Endocytosis, producing a coated vesicle (bar: 100 nm). [A, From E. Fries and A. Helenius,* Eur. J. Biochem. **8,** *213 (1979); B, from K. Simons* et al., Sci. Am. **246,** *46 (1982), courtesy Dr. A. Helenius.]*

Fusion with Plasma Membrane

The F (fusion) glycoprotein of paramyxoviruses causes the envelope of these viruses to fuse directly with the plasma membrane of the cell, even at pH 7. This may allow the nucleocapsid to be released directly into the cytoplasm. A number of other enveloped viruses have the ability to fuse membranes, fusing host cell plasma membranes with their own envelope and thereby gaining entry of their nucleic acid.

UNCOATING

So that viral genes become available for transcription it is necessary that virions be at least partially uncoated. In the case of enveloped RNA viruses that enter by fusion of their envelope with either the plasma membrane or an endosomal membrane, the nucleocapsid is discharged directly into the cytoplasm, and transcription commences from viral nucleic acid still associated with this structure. With the nonenveloped icosahedral reoviruses only certain capsid proteins are removed, and the viral genome expresses all its functions without ever being released from the core. For most other viruses, however, uncoating proceeds to completion. For some viruses that replicate in the nucleus the later stages of uncoating occur there, rather than in the cytoplasm.

STRATEGIES OF REPLICATION

Replication of most DNA viruses involves mechanisms that are familiar in cell biology: transcription of mRNA from dsDNA and replication of DNA (Fig. 3-2). The situation is quite different for RNA viruses, which are unique in having their genetic information encoded in RNA. RNA viruses with different types of genomes (single-stranded or double-stranded, positive or negative sense, linear or segmented) have necessarily evolved different routes to the production of mRNA. In the case of ssRNA viruses of positive sense, the viral RNA itself functions as messenger, whereas all other types of viral RNA must first be transcribed to mRNA. Since eukaryotic cells contain no RNA-dependent RNA polymerase, negative sense ssRNA viruses and dsRNA viruses must carry an RNA-dependent RNA polymerase in the virion.

Further, eukaryotic cells are not equipped to translate *polycistronic* mRNA into several individual species of protein, because in general they cannot reinitiate translation part way along the mRNA. Whereas DNA viruses overcome this limitation by using the cellular mechanism of cleavage (and sometimes splicing) of their polycistronic RNA transcripts to yield monocistronic mRNA molecules. RNA viruses, most of which do not have access to the RNA processing and splicing enzymes of the nucleus, have developed a remarkable diversity of solutions to the problem, as outlined below.

The diverse strategies followed by viruses of different families for transcription and translation are illustrated diagrammatically in Fig. 3-4 (for DNA viruses) and Fig. 3-5 (for RNA viruses) and described below.

DNA Viruses

Papovaviruses, Adenoviruses, Herpesviruses. The papovaviruses, adenoviruses, and herpes viruses have in one respect the most straightforward strategy of replication, the viral DNA being transcribed within the nucleus by cellular DNA-dependent RNA polymerase II. There are two or more cycles of transcription, the various *transcription units* (groups of genes under the control of a single promoter) being transcribed in a given temporal sequence. Polycistronic but subgenomic RNA transcripts (corresponding to several genes but less than the whole genome) undergo cleavage and splicing to produce monocistronic mRNAs, introns being removed in the process.

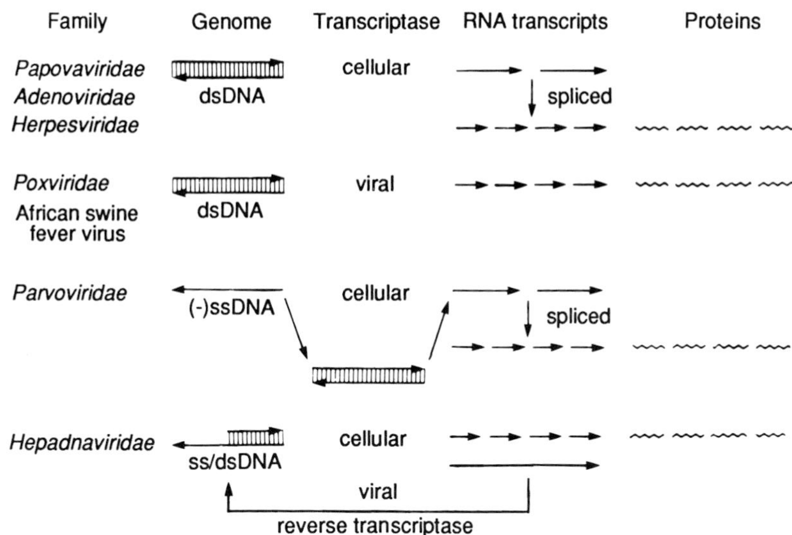

FIG. 3-4. *Simplified diagram showing essential features of the replication strategy of DNA viruses. The sense of each nucleic acid molecule is indicated by an arrow (plus, to the right; minus to the left). The number of mRNA and protein species for each virus has been arbitrarily shown as four. See text for details.*

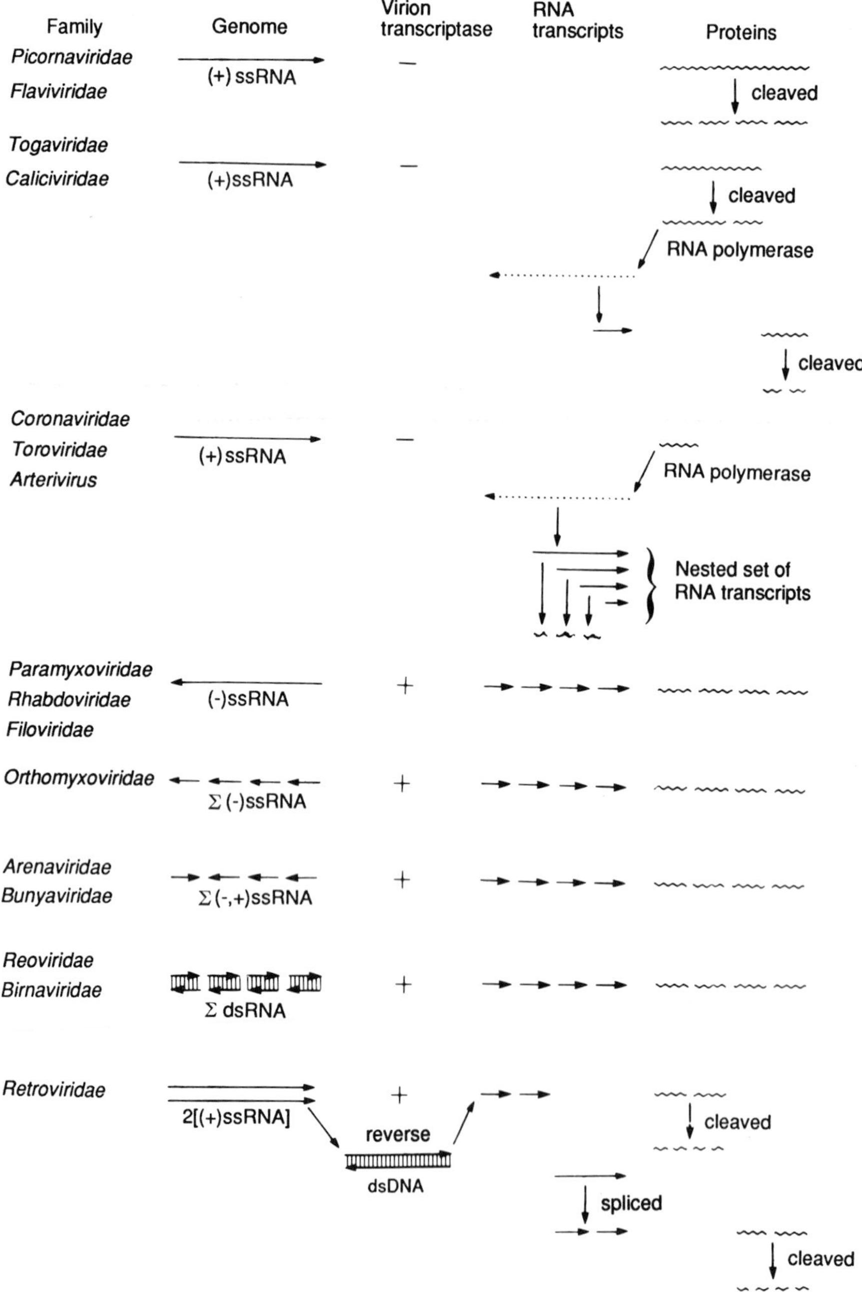
Family
Genome
Virion transcriptase
RNA transcripts
Proteins
Picornaviridae
Flaviviridae
(+) ssRNA
cleaved
Togaviridae
Caliciviridae
(+)ssRNA
cleaved
RNA polymerase
cleaved
Coronaviridae
Toroviridae
Arterivirus
(+) ssRNA
RNA polymerase
Nested set of RNA transcripts
Paramyxoviridae
Rhabdoviridae
Filoviridae
(-)ssRNA
Orthomyxoviridae
Σ (-)ssRNA
Arenaviridae
Bunyaviridae
Σ (-,+)ssRNA
Reoviridae
Birnaviridae
Σ dsRNA
Retroviridae
2[(+)ssRNA]
reverse
dsDNA
cleaved
spliced
cleaved

Poxviruses, African Swine Fever Virus. Poxviruses and African swine fever virus, which replicate in the cytoplasm, carry their own transcriptase in the virion. Their very large genomes encode numerous other enzymes that make them virtually independent of the cell nucleus. Monocistronic mRNAs are transcribed directly from the viral DNA.

Parvoviruses. The ssDNA of the parvoviruses uses cellular DNA polymerase to synthesize dsDNA, which is then transcribed in the nucleus and the transcripts processed by splicing to produce mRNAs.

Hepadnaviruses. The ssDNA portion of the partially dsDNA genome of hepadnaviruses is first completed by a virion-associated DNA polymerase, and the DNA converted to a supercoiled dsDNA. Transcription by cellular RNA polymerase II then occurs. Full-length plus sense RNA serves as a template for a viral reverse transcriptase and a minus sense DNA strand which in turn is the template for synthesis of the dsDNA. The mRNAs are transcribed from dsDNA starting from various promoters.

RNA Viruses

Picornaviruses, Togaviruses, Flaviviruses, Caliciviruses. The positive sense ssRNA viruses in the families *Picornaviridae, Togaviridae, Flaviviridae,* and *Caliciviridae* require no transcriptase in the virion, since the virion RNA itself functions as mRNA. The genome of the picornaviruses and flaviviruses, acting as a single polycistronic mRNA, is translated directly into a single *polyprotein* which is subsequently cleaved to give the individual viral polypeptides. One of these proteins is a RNA-dependent RNA polymerase, which replicates the viral genome, transcribing viral RNA into a complementary (minus sense) copy, which in turn serves as a template for the synthesis of plus strand (viral) RNA.

In togaviruses, only about two-thirds of the viral RNA (the 5′ end) is translated; the resulting polyprotein is cleaved into nonstructural proteins, all of which are required for RNA transcription and replication. Viral RNA polymerase makes a full-length minus strand, from which two species of plus strand are copied: full-length virion RNA, destined for encapsidation, and a one-third length RNA, which is colinear with

---

FIG. 3-5. *Simplified diagram showing essential features of the replication strategy of RNA viruses. The sense of each nucleic molecule is indicated by an arrow (+ to the right; − to the left; −, + for* Arenaviridae *and* Bunyaviridae *indicates ambisense RNA in one segment).* Σ, *Segmented genome; 2, diploid genome of* Retroviridae. *The number of mRNA molecules and protein molecules has been arbitrarily shown as four, as have the number of segments in viruses with segmented genomes (although less for* Arenaviridae, Bunyaviridae, *and* Birnaviridae). *See text for details.*

the 3′ terminus of the viral RNA and is translated into a polyprotein from which structural proteins are produced by cleavage. The caliciviruses have not been so extensively studied but also produce both genome-length and subgenomic mRNA species.

Coronaviruses, Toroviruses, Arteriviruses. The coronaviruses, toroviruses, and arteriviruses display a unique feature. Initially, part of the virion RNA acts as mRNA and is translated to produce an RNA polymerase, which then synthesizes a genome-length minus strand. From this, a *nested set* of overlapping subgenomic mRNAs with a common termination site is transcribed. Only the unique N-terminal sequence of each successive member of the set of overlapping transcripts is translated.

Paramyxoviruses, Rhabdoviruses, Filoviruses. The minus sense, nonsegmented ssRNA viruses of the families *Paramyxoviridae, Rhabdoviridae,* and *Filoviridae* carry an RNA-dependent RNA polymerase (transcriptase), which transcribes five subgenomic plus sense RNAs, each of which serves as a monocistronic mRNA. In contrast, transcription in the replication mode (by the replicase) produces a full-length plus strand which is used as the template for the synthesis of new viral RNA.

Orthomyxoviruses, Bunyaviruses, Arenaviruses. The minus sense RNA viruses of the families *Orthomyxoviridae, Bunyaviridae,* and *Arenaviridae* have segmented genomes, each segment of which is transcribed by a transcriptase carried in the virion to yield an mRNA which is translated into one or more proteins. In the case of the orthomyxoviruses, but not in the other two families, most of the segments encode single proteins. Furthermore, the S segment, at least, of arenaviruses and certain genera of bunyaviruses is ambisense, that is, part of the ssRNA molecule is plus sense and part minus sense. The replication strategy of ambisense RNA viruses, like the sense of their genomes, is mixed, with features of both plus sense and minus sense ssRNA viruses.

Reoviruses, Birnaviruses. Viruses of the families *Reoviridae* and *Birnaviridae* have segmented dsRNA genomes. The minus strand of each segment is separately transcribed in the cytoplasm by a virion-associated transcriptase to produce mRNA. These plus sense RNAs also serve as templates for replication. The resulting dsRNA in turn serves as the template for further mRNA transcription.

Retroviruses. In the retroviruses the viral RNA is plus sense, but instead of functioning as mRNA it is transcribed by a viral RNA-dependent DNA polymerase (reverse transcriptase) to produce first an RNA–DNA hybrid molecule, which is in turn converted to dsDNA (by another activity of the same enzyme) and inserted permanently into cellular DNA. This integrated viral DNA (*provirus*) is subsequently transcribed by cellular RNA polymerase II, followed by splicing of the RNA transcript as well as cleavage of the resulting proteins. Some full-length positive sense RNA transcripts associate in pairs to form the diploid genomes of new virions.

TRANSCRIPTION

Having outlined the several contrasting strategies of expression of the viral genome, we are now in a position to describe in more detail the processes of transcription, translation, and replication of viral nucleic acid, beginning with transcription. The viral RNA of plus sense ssRNA viruses binds directly to ribosomes and is translated in full or in part without the need for any prior transcriptional step. From all other classes of viral genomes, mRNA must be transcribed in order to begin the process of expression of the infecting viral genome. In the case of DNA viruses that replicate in the nucleus, the cellular DNA-dependent RNA polymerase II performs this function. All other viruses require a unique and specific transcriptase that is virus-coded and is an integral component of the virion. Cytoplasmic dsDNA viruses carry a DNA-dependent RNA polymerase, whereas dsRNA viruses have dsRNA-dependent RNA polymerase and minus sense ssRNA viruses carry a ssRNA-dependent RNA polymerase.

Regulation of Transcription from Viral DNA

In 1978 Fiers and colleagues presented the first complete description of the genome of an animal virus (Fig. 3-6). Analysis of the circular dsDNA molecule of the papovavirus SV40 and its transcription program revealed some remarkable facts, many of which can be generalized to other dsDNA viruses. First, the early genes and the late genes are transcribed in opposite directions, from different strands of the DNA. Second, certain genes overlap, so that their protein products have some amino acid sequences in common. Third, some regions of the viral DNA may be read in different reading frames, so that quite distinct amino acid sequences are translated from the same nucleotide sequence. Fourth, certain long stretches of the viral DNA consist of introns, which are transcribed but not translated into protein because they are excised from the primary RNA transcript.

For many years it has served us well to think of a one-to-one relationship between a gene and its gene-product (protein). Now that we are aware of overlapping reading frames, posttranscriptional cleavage, mul-

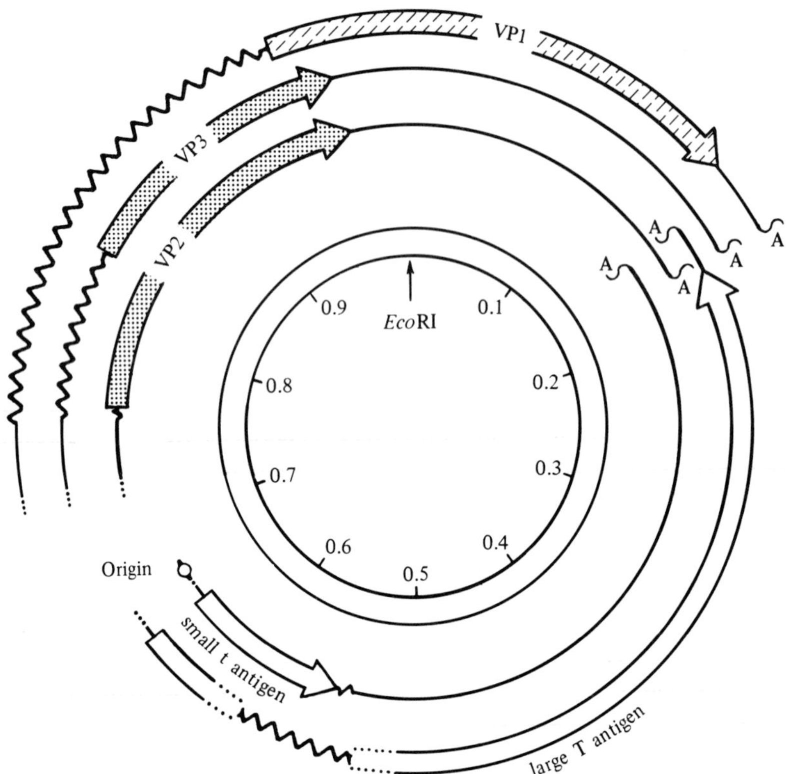

FIG. 3-6. *Transcription map of the DNA of the papovavirus SV40. The circular dsDNA is oriented with the* Eco*RI restriction endonuclease cleavage site at zero and the origin of DNA replication (origin) at map position 0.66. The direction of transcription of the early genes is counterclockwise on one DNA strand (open arrows), and that of the late genes is clockwise on the other strand (stippled and shaded arrows). The thin lines indicate regions of the primary RNA transcripts that are not translated into proteins, while the wavy lines indicate regions of the transcript that are spliced out (introns). The 3′-terminal poly(A) tail of each mRNA is labeled A. The coding regions of the primary transcript are shown as large arrows. The genes for the early proteins small t and large T overlap, as do those for the late proteins VP1, VP2, and VP3. Large T is coded by two noncontiguous regions of DNA. The amino acid sequence of VP3 corresponds with the C-terminal half of VP2. However, VP1 shares no part of its amino acid sequence with VP2 or VP3, even though the VP1 gene overlaps VP2 and VP3, because its mRNA is transcribed in a different reading frame. [Modified from W. Fiers* et al., Nature (London) **273,** *113 (1978).]*

tiple splicing patterns of RNA transcripts, and posttranslational cleavage of polyproteins, it is often too simplistic to designate a particular nucleotide sequence as a gene encoding a particular protein. It is more appropriate to talk in terms of the transcription unit, which is defined as a region of the genome beginning with the transcription initiation site and extending to the transcription termination site (including all introns and exons in between), the expression of which falls under the control of a particular promoter. "Simple" transcription units may be defined as those encoding only a single protein, whereas "complex" transcription units code for more than one.

Studies with adenoviruses have elucidated the nature of the mechanisms that regulate the expression of viral genomes, which operate principally, but not exclusively, at the level of transcription. There are several adenovirus transcription units. At different stages of the viral replication cycle, "pre-early," "early," "intermediate," and "late," the various transcription units are transcribed in a given temporal sequence. A product of the early region E1A induces transcription from the other early regions including E1B, but following viral DNA replication there is a 50-fold increase in the rate of transcription from the major late promoter relative to early promoters such as E1B, and a decrease in E1A mRNA levels. A second control operates at the point of termination of transcription. Transcripts that terminate at a particular point early in infection are read through this termination site later in infection to produce a range of longer transcripts with different polyadenylation sites.

Regulation of Transcription from Viral RNA

For RNA viruses, regulation of transcription is generally not as complex as for DNA viruses. In particular, the temporal separation into early genes transcribed before the replication of viral nucleic acid, and late genes thereafter, is not nearly so clear. In most families of viruses with plus sense genomic RNA, which serves as messenger, transcription is required only to make the minus strand needed for RNA replication.

Other mechanisms of regulation are required for viruses with nonsegmented minus sense RNA. Once the nucleocapsid is released into the cytoplasm, the RNA polymerase initiates transcription from the 3′ end of the genome. Since there is only a single promoter, one might imagine that only full-length plus-strand transcripts could be made. While some full-length plus strands are made as templates for RNA replication, mRNAs corresponding to each gene are also made, in the following fashion. The several genes in the viral RNA are each separated by a consensus sequence that includes termination and start signals as well as a short sequence of U residues which enables the transcriptase to generate a long poly(A) tail for each mRNA by a process of reiterative copying ("stuttering") (see Fig. 28-2). The complete mRNA is then cleaved off, but the enzyme continues on to transcribe the next gene, and so forth.

Paramyxovirus transcription also involves a process known as "editing." The P gene encodes two proteins, P and V, which share a common N-terminal amino acid sequence but differ completely in their C-terminal sequences because of a shift in the reading frame brought about by the insertion of two uncoded G residues into the RNA transcript by transcriptase stuttering.

Regulatory Genes and Responsive Elements

In analyzing viral genomes and RNA transcripts derived from them much attention has been given to identifying the open reading frames in order to derive the amino acid sequence of their gene products. More recently interest has also turned to the untranslated regions of the genome which contain numerous conserved (consensus) sequences, sometimes called motifs, which represent responsive elements in the regulatory region and play crucial roles in the expression of the genome. For example, each transcription unit in the viral genome has near its 3′ end an mRNA transcription initiation site (*start site*), designated as nucleotide +1. Within the hundred or so nucleotides upstream of the start site lies the *promoter,* which up-regulates the transcription of that gene (or genes). Upstream or downstream from the start site there may be a long sequence with several, maybe repeated, elements known as an *enhancer,* which enhances transcription even further. These regulatory regions are activated by the binding of viral or cellular DNA-binding proteins. Several such proteins may bind to adjacent responsive elements in such a way that they also bind to one another or otherwise interact, to facilitate attachment of the viral RNA polymerase. Viral regulatory genes that encode such regulatory proteins may act in *trans* as well as in *cis,* that is, they may *trans*-activate genes residing on a completely different molecule.

A description of the role of one of the six regulatory genes of the human immunodeficiency virus (HIV) will illustrate such regulatory mechanisms. When a DNA copy of the HIV genome is integrated into a chromosome of a resting T cell, it remains latent until a T-cell mitogen or a cytokine induces synthesis of the NF-κB family of DNA-binding proteins. NF-κB then binds to the enhancer present in the integrated HIV provirus, thereby triggering transcription of the six HIV regulatory genes. One of these, *tat,* encodes a protein which binds to a responsive element, TAR, within the HIV provirus, greatly augmenting (*trans-*

activating) the transcription of all HIV genes (including *tat* itself), and thereby establishing a positive feedback loop that enables the production of large numbers of progeny virions. Moreover, since TAR is present in all HIV mRNAs as well as in the proviral DNA, it is probable that *tat* enhances both transcription and translation.

Although the control of HIV transcription may be unusually complex because of its complicated replication cycle and requirement for the establishment of latency, HIV contains only nine genes, compared with up to one hundred in the case of some DNA viruses. Thus it may be anticipated that the regulation of expression of other viruses will turn out to be much more complex than had been thought.

Posttranscriptional Processing

Primary RNA transcripts from eukaryotic DNA are subject to a series of posttranscriptional alterations in the nucleus, known as *processing*, prior to export to the cytoplasm as mRNA. First, a cap, consisting of 7-methylguanosine (m^7Gppp), is added to the 5′ terminus of the primary transcript; the cap facilitates the formation of a stable complex with the 40 S ribosomal subunit, which is necessary for the initiation of translation. Second, a sequence of 50–200 adenylate residues is added to the 3′ terminus. This *poly(A) tail* may act as a recognition signal for processing and for transport of mRNA from the nucleus to the cytoplasm, and it may stabilize mRNA against degradation in the cytoplasm. Third, a methyl group is added to the 6 position to about 1% of the adenylate residues throughout the RNA (methylation). Fourth, introns are removed from the primary transcript and the *exons* are linked together in a process known as *splicing*. Splicing is an important mechanism for regulating gene expression in nuclear DNA viruses. A given RNA transcript can have two or more splicing sites and be spliced in several alternative ways to produce a variety of mRNA species coding for distinct proteins; both the preferred poly(A) site and the splicing pattern may change in a regulated fashion as infection proceeds.

Special mention should be made of an extraordinary phenomenon known as "cap-snatching." The transcriptase of influenza virus, which also carries endonuclease activity, steals the 5′ methylated caps from newly synthesized cellular RNA transcripts in the nucleus and uses them as primers for initiating transcription from the viral genome.

The rate of degradation of mRNA provides another possible level of regulation. Not only do different mRNA species have different half-lives,but the half-life of a given mRNA species may change as the replication cycle progresses.

TRANSLATION

Capped, polyadenylated, and processed monocistronic viral mRNAs bind to ribosomes and are translated into protein in the same fashion as cellular mRNAs. The sequence of events has been closely studied for reovirus. Each monocistronic mRNA molecule binds via its capped 5′ terminus to the 40 S ribosomal subunit, which then moves along the mRNA molecule until stopped at the initiation codon. The 60 S ribosomal subunit then binds, together with methionyl- tRNA and various initiation factors, after which translation proceeds.

In mammalian cells, mRNA molecules are *monocistronic* (encoding only one protein), and, with few exceptions, translation commences only at the 5′ initiation codon. However, with certain viruses polycistronic mRNA can be translated directly into its several gene-products as a result of initiation, or reinitiation, of translation at internal AUG start codons.

Where initiation of translation at an internal AUG is an option, a frameshift can occur. Another mechanism, known as ribosomal frameshifting, occurs fortuitously when a ribosome happens to slip one nucleotide forward or back along an RNA molecule. This phenomenon is exploited by retroviruses to access the reverse transcriptase reading frame hidden within the *gag* mRNA. Thus, considering also the phenomenon of RNA splicing and RNA editing described earlier, it can be seen that there are several mechanisms of exploiting overlapping reading frames to maximize the usage of the limited coding potential of the small genomes of viruses.

Most viral proteins undergo various posttranslational modifications such as phosphorylation (for nucleic acid binding), fatty acid acylation (for membrane insertion), glycosylation, or proteolytic cleavage (see below). Newly synthesized viral proteins must also be transported to the various sites in the cell where they are needed, for example, back into the nucleus in the case of viruses that replicate there. The sorting signals that direct this traffic are only beginning to be understood, as are the polypeptide chain binding proteins ("molecular chaperones") that regulate folding, translocation, and assembly of oligomers of viral as well as cellular proteins.

Glycosylation of Envelope Proteins

Viruses exploit cellular pathways normally used for the synthesis of membrane-inserted and exported secretory glycoproteins (Fig. 3-7). The programmed addition of sugars occurs sequentially as the protein moves in vesicles progressively from the rough endoplasmic reticulum to the Golgi complex and then to the plasma membrane. The side chains of

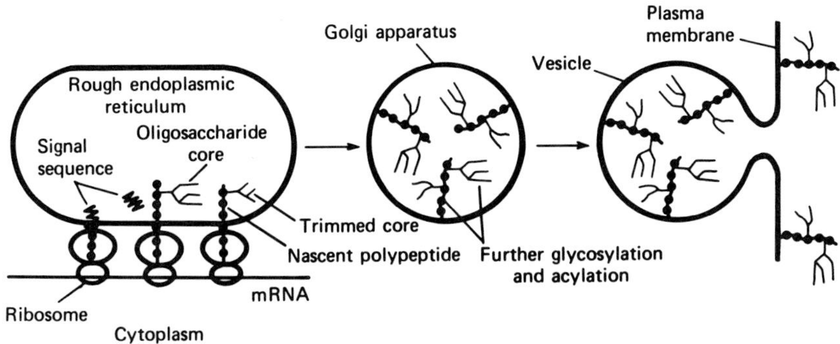

FIG. 3-7. *Glycosylation of viral protein. The amino terminus of viral envelope proteins initially contains a sequence of 15–30 hydrophobic amino acids, known as a signal sequence, which facilitates binding of the growing polypeptide chain (dotted) to a receptor site on the cytoplasmic side of the rough endoplasmic reticulum and its passage through the lipid bilayer to the luminal side. Oligosaccharides are then added in N-linkage to certain asparagine residues of the nascent polypeptide the* en bloc *transfer of a mannose-rich "core" of preformed oligosaccharides, and glucose residues are removed by glycosidases ("trimming"). The viral glycoprotein is then transported from the rough endoplasmic reticulum to the Golgi complex. Here the core carbohydrate is further modified by the removal of several mannose residues and the addition of further* N-*acetylglucosamine, galactose, and the terminal sugars sialic acid or fucose. The completed side chains are a mixture of simple ("high mannose") and complex oligosaccharides. A coated vesicle then transports the completed glycoprotein to the cellular membrane from which the particular virus buds.*

viral envelope glycoproteins are generally a mixture of simple ("high mannose") and complex oligosaccharides, which are usually N-linked (to asparagine) but less commonly O-linked to serine or threonine. The precise composition of the oligosaccharides is determined not only by the amino acid sequence and tertiary structure of the proteins concerned but more importantly by the particular cellular glycosyltransferases prevalent in the type of cell in which the virus happens to be growing at the time.

Posttranslational Cleavage of Proteins

In the case of the plus sense picornaviruses and flaviviruses, the polycistronic viral RNA is translated directly into a single polyprotein which carries protease activity that cleaves the polyprotein at defined recognition sites into smaller proteins. The first cleavage steps are carried out while the polyprotein is still associated with the ribosome. Some of the larger intermediates exist only fleetingly; others are functional for a short period but are subsequently cleaved by additional virus-coded proteases to smaller proteins with alternative functions. Posttranslational cleavage occurs in several other RNA virus families, for example, togaviruses and caliciviruses, in which polyproteins corresponding to large parts of the genome are cleaved. Some viruses encode several different proteases. Most are either trypsinlike (serine or cysteine proteases), pepsinlike (aspartyl proteases), or papainlike (thiol proteases).

Cellular proteases, present in particular organelles such as the Golgi complex or transport vesicles, are also vital to the maturation and assembly of many viruses. For example, cleavage of the hemagglutinin glycoprotein of orthomyxoviruses or the fusion glycoprotein of paramyxoviruses is essential for the production of infectious virions.

Classes of Viral Proteins

Table 3-3 lists the various classes of proteins encoded by the genomes of viruses. In general, the proteins translated from the early transcripts of DNA viruses include enzymes and other proteins required for the replication of viral nucleic acid, as well as proteins that suppress host

TABLE 3-3

Categories of Proteins Encoded by Viral Genomes

Structural proteins of the virion
Virion-associated enzymes, especially transcriptase[a]
Nonstructural proteins, mainly enzymes, required for transcription, replication of viral nucleic acid,[b] and cleavage of proteins
Regulatory proteins that control the temporal sequence of expression of the viral genome
Proteins down-regulating expression of cellular genes
Transactivators and oncogene products, e.g., growth factors or inactivators of cellular tumor suppressor proteins, that up-regulate expression of certain cellular genes[c]
Proteins influencing viral virulence, host range, tissue tropism, etc.[d]
Virokines[d] that act on noninfected cells to modulate the progress of infection in the body as a whole, e.g., by:
Negating the effects of interferons, tumor necrosis factor, etc.
Reducing the inflammatory response, complement activation, etc.
Subverting the immune response, e.g., by reducing *MHC proteins* on the infected cell surface

[a] RNA viruses of plus sense and nuclear DNA viruses do not encode a transcriptase.

[b] DNA viruses with large complex genomes, notably poxviruses and herpesviruses, also encode numerous enzymes needed for nucleotide synthesis.

[c] Herpeseviruses, adenoviruses, papovaviruses, and retroviruses.

[d] Recorded so far mainly in the more complex DNA viruses (poxviruses, herpesviruses, adenoviruses) but may be more widespread.

cell RNA and protein synthesis. The large DNA viruses (poxviruses and herpesviruses) also encode a number of enzymes involved in nucleotide metabolism.

The late viral proteins are translated from late mRNAs, most of which are transcribed from progeny viral nucleic acid molecules. Most of the late proteins are viral structural proteins, and they are often made in considerable excess.

Some viral proteins, including some with other important functions, serve as regulatory proteins, modulating the transcription or translation of cellular genes or of early viral genes. The large DNA viruses also encode numerous additional proteins, called *virokines,* which do not regulate the viral replication cycle itself but influence the host response to infection.

REPLICATION OF VIRAL NUCLEIC ACID

Replication of Viral DNA

Different mechanisms of DNA replication are employed by each family of DNA viruses. Since DNA polymerases cannot initiate synthesis of a new DNA strand but only extend synthesis from a short (RNA) primer, one end of the resulting product might be expected to remain single-stranded. Various DNA viruses have evolved different strategies for circumventing this problem. Viruses of some families have a circular DNA genome, others have a linear genome with complementary termini which serve as primers, while yet others have a protein primer covalently attached to each 5′ terminus.

Several virus-coded enzyme activities are generally required for replication of viral DNA: a helicase (with ATPase activity) to unwind the double helix; a helix-destablizing protein to keep the two separated strands apart until each has been copied; a DNA polymerase to copy each strand from the origin of replication in a 5′ to 3′ direction; an RNase to degrade the RNA primer after it has served its purpose; and a DNA ligase to join the Okazaki fragments together (see below). Often a single large enzyme carries two or more of these activities.

The papovavirus genome, with its associated cellular histones, morphologically and functionally resembles cellular DNA and utilizes host cell enzymes, including DNA polymerase α, for its replication. An early viral protein, large T, binds to site in the regulatory sequence of the viral genome, thereby initiating DNA replication. Replication of this circular dsDNA commences from a unique palindromic sequence and proceeds simultaneously in both directions. As in the replication of mammalian

DNA, both continuous and discontinuous DNA synthesis occurs (of "leading" and "lagging" strands, respectively) at the two growing forks. The discontinuous synthesis of the lagging strand involves repeated synthesis of short oligoribonucleotide primers, which in turn initiate short nascent strands of DNA (*Okazaki fragments*), which are then covalently joined by a DNA ligase to form one of the growing strands.

The replication of adenovirus DNA is quite different. Adenovirus DNA is linear, the 5′ end of each strand being a mirror image of the other (terminally repeated inverted sequences), and each strand is covalently linked to a protein, the precursor of which serves as the primer for adenoviral DNA synthesis. DNA replication proceeds from both ends, continuously but asynchronously, in a 5′ to 3′ direction, using a virus-coded DNA polymerase. It does not require the synthesis of Okazaki fragments.

Herpesviruses encode many or all of the "replication proteins" required for DNA replication, including a DNA polymerase, a helicase, a primase, a single-stranded DNA-binding protein, and a protein recognizing the origin of replication. Poxviruses and African swine fever virus, which replicate entirely within the cytoplasm, are self-sufficient in DNA replication. Hepadnaviruses, like the retroviruses, utilize plus sense ssRNA transcripts as intermediates for the production of DNA by reverse transcription. The ssDNA paroviruses use 3′ palindromic sequences that form a double-stranded hairpin structure as a primer for cellular DNA polymerase.

Replication of Viral RNA

The replication of RNA is a phenomenon unique to viruses. Transcription of RNA from an RNA template requires an RNA-dependent RNA polymerase, a virus-coded enzyme not found in uninfected cells. The replication of viral RNA requires first the synthesis of complementary RNA, which then serves as a template for making more viral RNA.

Where the viral RNA is of minus sense (orthomyxoviruses, paramyxoviruses, rhabdoviruses, filoviruses, arenaviruses, and bunyaviruses), the complementary RNA will be of plus sense, and the RNA polymerase involved resembles the virion-associated transcriptase used for primary transcription of mRNAs. However, whereas most transcripts from such minus sense viral RNA are subgenomic mRNA molecules, some full-length plus strands are also made, in order to serve as templates for viral RNA synthesis (replication). For some viruses there is good evidence that the RNA polymerases used for transcription and replication are distinct.

In the case of the plus sense RNA viruses (picornaviruses, caliciviruses, togaviruses, flaviviruses, and coronaviruses) the complementary RNA is minus sense. Several viral RNA molecules can be transcribed simultaneously from a single complementary RNA template, each RNA transcript being the product of a separately bound polymerase molecule. The resulting structure, known as the *replicative intermediate,* is therefore partially double-stranded, with single-stranded tails. Initiation of replication of picornavirus and calicivirus RNA, like that of adenovirus DNA, requires a protein, rather than an oligonucleotide, as primer. This small protein is covalently attached to the 5′ terminus of nascent plus and minus RNA strands, as well as to viral RNA, but not to mRNA. Little is known about what determines whether a given picornavirus plus sense RNA molecule will be directed (a) to a "replication complex," bound to smooth endoplasmic reticulum, where it serves as a template for transcription by RNA-dependent RNA polymerase into minus sense RNA; or (b) to a ribosome, where it serves as mRNA for translation into protein; or (c) to a procapsid, with which it associates to form a virion.

Retroviruses have a genome consisting of plus sense ssRNA. Unlike other RNA viruses, they replicate via a DNA intermediate. The virion-associated reverse transcriptase, using a *transfer RNA* (*tRNA*) molecule as a primer, makes a ssDNA copy. Then, functioning as a ribonuclease, the same enzyme removes the parental RNA molecule from the DNA–RNA hybrid. The free minus sense ssDNA strand is then copied to form a linear dsDNA, which contains an additional sequence know as the *long terminal repeat* (*LTR*) at each end. This dsDNA then circularizes and integrates into cellular DNA. Transcription of viral RNA occurs from this integrated (proviral) DNA.

ASSEMBLY AND RELEASE

Nonenveloped Viruses

All nonenveloped animal viruses have an icosahedral structure. The structural proteins of simple icosahedral viruses associate spontaneously to form capsomers, which self-assemble to form capsids into which viral nucleic acid is packaged. Completion of the virion often involves proteolytic cleavage of one or more species of capsid protein. The best studied example, that of poliovirus, is depicted in Fig. 3-8.

The mechanism of packaging viral nucleic acid into a preassembled empty procapsid has been elucidated for adneovirus. A particular protein binds to a nucleotide sequence at one end of the viral DNA known as the packaging sequence; this enables the DNA to enter the procapsid bound

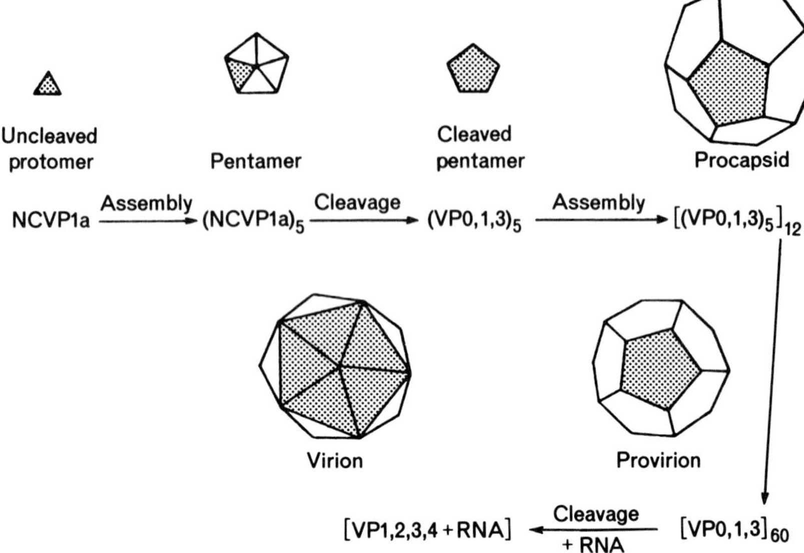

FIG. 3-8. *Overview of the assembly of a picornavirus. The capsomer precursor protein (NCVP1a) aggregates to form pentamers; each of the five NCVP1a molecules is then cleaved by viral protease into VP0, VP1, and VP3. Twelve such pentamers aggregate to form a procapsid. A final proteolytic event, which cleaves each VP0 molecule into VP2 and VP4, is required for RNA incorporation. The mature virion is a dodecahedron with 60 capsomers, each of which is made up of one molecule each of VP1, VP2, VP3, and VP4. X-Ray crystallography shows that the assembling units have extensions that reach across adjacent units to form second and third nearest neighbor relationships.*

to basic core proteins, after which some of the capsid proteins are cleaved to make the mature virion.

Most nonenveloped viruses accumulate within the cytoplasm or nucleus and are released only when the cell eventually lyses.

Maturation and Release of Enveloped Viruses

All mammalian viruses with helical nucleocapsids, as well as some of those with icosahedral nucleocapsids, for example, herpesviruses and togaviruses, mature by acquiring an envelope by budding through cellular membranes.

Budding from Plasma Membrane. Most enveloped viruses bud from the plasma membrane, although some bud on internal membranes and are then transported in vesicles to the cell surface. Insertion of the viral glycoprotein(s) into the lipid bilayer occurs by lateral displacement of cellular proteins from that patch of membrane (Fig. 3-9A). The monomeric cleaved viral glycoprotein molecules associate into oligomers to form the typical rod-shaped or club-shaped peplomer with a hydrophilic domain projecting from the external surface of the membrane, a hydrophobic transmembrane anchor domain, and a short hydrophilic domain projecting slightly into the cytoplasm. In the case of icosahedral viruses (e.g., togaviruses) each protein molecule of the nucleocapsid binds directly to the cytoplasmic domain of the membrane glycoprotein oligomer, thus molding the envelope around the nucleocapsid. In the more usual case of viruses with helical nucleocapsids, it is the matrix protein which attaches to the cytoplasmic domain of the glycoprotein peplomer; in turn the nucleocapsid protein recognizes the matrix protein, and this presumably initiates budding. Release of each enveloped virion does not breach the integrity of the plasma membrane; hence, thousands of virus particles can be shed over a period of several hours or days without significant cell damage (Fig. 3-10). Many but not all viruses that bud from the plasma membrane are noncytopathogenic and may be associated with persistent infections.

Epithelial cells display *polarity,* having an "apical" surface facing the

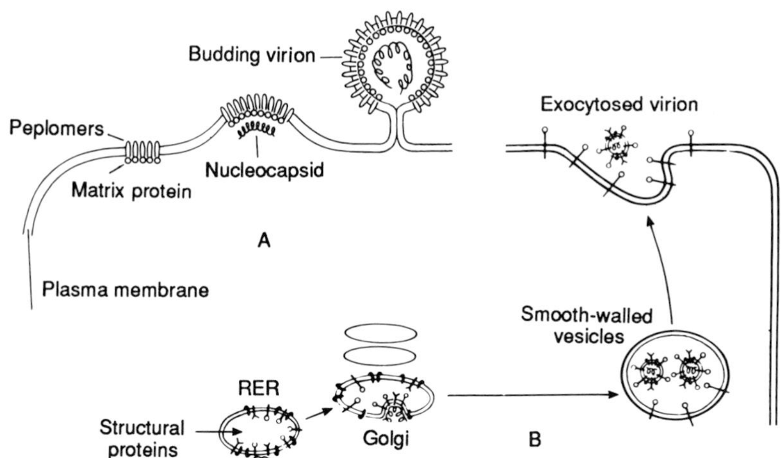

FIG. 3-9. *Maturation of enveloped viruses. (A) Viruses whose virion contains a matrix protein (and some viruses which do not) bud through a patch of the plasma membrane in which glycoprotein peplomers have accumulated over the patch of matrix protein. (B) Most enveloped viruses without a matrix protein bud into cytoplasmic vesicles [rough endoplasmic reticulum (RER) or Golgi], then pass through the cytoplasm in smooth-walled vesicles and are released by exocytosis. [B, Modified from K. V. Holmes,* In *"Fields Virology" (B. N. Fields* et al. *eds.), 2nd Ed., p. 847. Raven, New York, 1990.]*

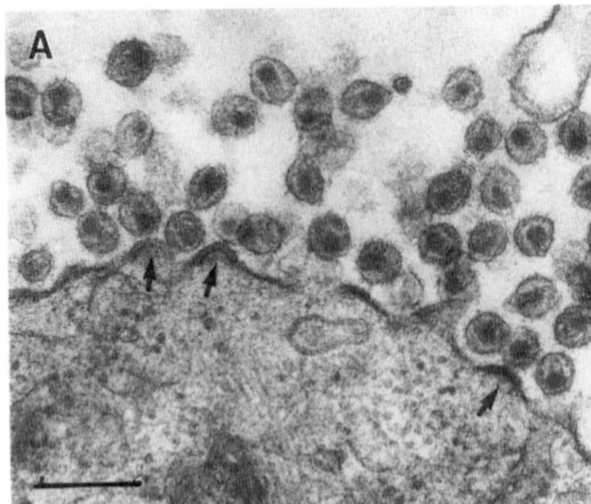

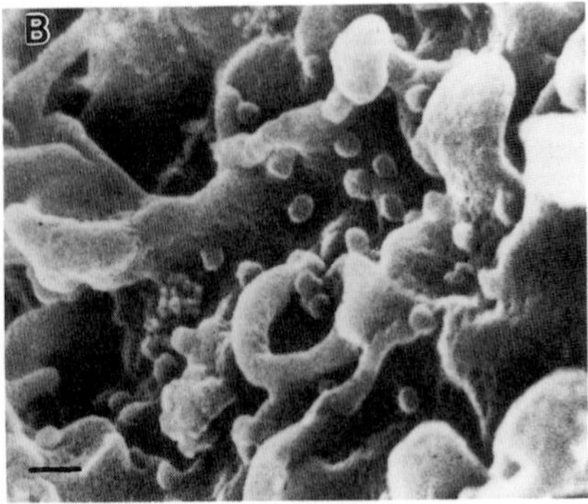

FIG. 3-10. *Virions of lentiviruses budding from the plasma membrane (bars: 100 nm). (A) Feline immunodeficiency virus budding from the plasma membrane of a feline T lymphocyte. Retroviruses have no matrix protein; the arrows indicate accumulations of patches of viral glycoprotein peplomers in the plasma membrane. (B) Scanning electron micrograph of human immunodeficiency virus budding from the plasma membrane of a human T lymphocyte. [A, From S. C. E. Friend* et al., Aust. Vet. J. **67,** *237 (1990), courtesy C. J. Birch and J. A. Marshall; B, courtesy Dr. C. S. Goldsmith.]*

outside world, which is separated by a tight junction from the "basolateral" surface. These surfaces are chemically and physiologically distinct. Viruses that are shed to the exterior, for example, influenza virus, tend to bud from the apical surface, whereas others, such as C-type retroviruses, bud through the basolateral membrane.

Exocytosis. Flaviviruses, coronaviruses, and bunyaviruses mature by budding through membranes of the Golgi complex or rough endoplasmic reticulum; vesicles containing the virus then migrate to the plasma membrane with which they fuse, thereby releasing the virions by *exocytosis* (Fig. 3-9B). Uniquely, the envelope of the herpesviruses is acquired by budding through the inner lamella of the nuclear membrane; the enveloped virions then pass directly from the space between the two lamellae of the nuclear membrane to the exterior of the cell via the cisternae of the endoplasmic reticulum.

FURTHER READING

Challberg, M. D., and Kelly, T. J. 1989). Animal virus DNA replication. *Annu. Rev. Biochem.* **58,** 671.

Crowell, R. L., and Lonberg-Holm, K., eds. (1986). "Virus Attachment and Entry into Cells." American Society for Microbiology, Washington, D.C.

Darnell, J., Lodish, H., and Baltimore, D. (1990). "Molecular Cell Biology," 2nd Ed. Scientific American Books, New York.

Fields, B. N., Knipe, D. M., Chanock, R. M., Hirsch, M. S., Melnick, J. L., Monath, T. P., and Roizman, B., eds. (1990). "Fields Virology," 2nd Ed. Raven, New York.
Krausslich, H. G., and Wimmer, E. (1988). Viral proteases. *Annu. Rev. Biochem* **57,** 701.
Marsh, M., and Helenius, A. (1989). Virus entry into cells. *Adv. Virus Res.* **36,** 107.
Rossmann, M. G., and Johnson, J. E. (1989). Icosahedral RNA virus structure. *Annu. Rev. Biochem.* **58,** 533.
Stephens, E. B., and Compans, R. W. (1988). Assembly of viruses at cellular membranes. *Annu. Rev. Microbiol.* **42,** 489.
Strauss, J. H. (1990). Viral proteases. *Semin. Virol.* **1,** 307.
Watson, J. D., Hopkins, N. H., Roberts, J. W., Steitz, J. A., and Weiner, A. M. (1987). "Molecular Biology of the Gene," Vol. 2, 4th Ed. Benjamin-Cummings, Menlo Park, California.

CHAPTER 4

Viral Genetics and Evolution

Viruses have a greater genetic diversity than any other group of organisms (see Table 1-2). This great variety has been produced by natural selection acting on viral genomes that are continuously changing as a result of mutation, recombination, and reassortment.

Our knowledge of virus genetics has been greatly expanded by the development during the 1970s of molecular cloning and nucleotide sequencing methods and the use of monoclonal antibodies, followed in the mid-1980s by the introduction of the polymerase chain reaction. One outcome of this work has been the realization that the same sequence may specify two or even three gene products, since mRNA may be transcribed in several different reading frames in each direction—so-called overlapping genes. The situation is further complicated by the fact that several mRNAs may be produced by different splicing patterns from the same reading frame or RNA transcript.

MUTATION

In every viral infection of an animal or a cell culture, one or a small number of virus particles replicates to produce millions of progeny. In such populations, errors in copying the nucleic acid inevitably occur; these are called *mutations.* Many mutations are lethal, because the mutated virus is unable to replicate. Whether a particular nonlethal mutation survives in the genotype depends on whether the resultant change in the gene-product is neutral or affords the mutant virus some selective advantage. In the laboratory, genetic variants are obtained by subjecting a virus population to some selective condition and isolating a *clone,* that is, a population of viral particles originating from a single virion, usually by growth from a single *plaque* in a cell monolayer, followed by replaquing.

Types of Mutations

Mutations can be classified either according to the kind of change in the nucleic acid or on the basis of their phenotypic expression.

Changes in Nucleic Acid. The most common mutations are single nucleotide substitutions (*point mutations*) or deletions and insertions, which may involve a single nucleotide although more commonly small blocks of nucleotides. Each point mutation has a characteristic frequency of reversion which can be accurately measured. The phenotypic expression of a mutation in one gene may be reversed not only by a back-mutation in the substituted nucleotide but, alternatively, by a *suppressor mutation* occurring elsewhere in the same gene, or even in a different gene. For example, some *temperature-sensitive* mutants of influenza virus developed as potential *attenuated* live-virus vaccines have reverted to virulence by virtue of an independent suppressor mutation in an apparently unrelated gene, which negates the effect of the original mutation. Deletion mutants rarely or never revert, so that nonrevertibility is used as a diagnostic criterion of this kind of mutation.

Classification of Mutants by Phenotypic Expression. Mutations that allow the production of progeny virions can also be classified by their phenotypic expression, such as the type of plaque they produce in a cell monolayer (plaque mutants) or their sensitivity to neutralization by antibody (escape mutants). Mutations affecting antigenic determinants of virion surface proteins may be strongly favored when viruses replicate in the presence of antibody, and they are of importance both in persistently infected animals (e.g., in visna/maedi and equine infectious anemia viruses and epidemiologically, as in vesicular exanthema of swine virus in sea lions and influenza viruses.

Conditional lethal mutants are produced by mutations that so affect a virus that it cannot grow under certain conditions that are determined by the experimenter, but can replicate under other, permissive, conditions. Their importance is that a single selective test can be used to obtain mutants in which mutations may be present in any one of several different genes. The conditional lethal mutants most commonly studied are those whose replication is blocked in certain host cells (*host range* mutants) or at certain defined temperatures (temperature-sensitive mutants). With the latter, the selective condition used is the temperature of incubation of infected cells. A point mutation in the genome, leading to an amino acid substitution in the translated polypeptide product, results in a structurally abnormal protein which although functional at the *permissive temperature* cannot maintain its structural integrity and functional conformation when the temperature is raised by a few degrees. Temperature-sensitive mutants, and the somewhat similar cold-adapted mutants, have been used extensively in attempts to produce attenuated live-virus vaccines.

Defective interfering (DI) mutants have been demonstrated in most families of viruses. The properties that define DI virus particles are that they cannot replicate alone, but can in the presence of a helper virus (usually parental wild-type virus), and that they interfere with and usually decrease the yield of wild-type virus.

All RNA DI particles that have been studied are deletion mutants. In the case of influenza viruses and reoviruses, which have segmented genomes, the defective virions lack one or more of the larger segments and contain instead smaller segments consisting of an incomplete portion of the encoded gene(s). In the case of viruses with a nonsegmented genome, DI particles contain RNA which is shortened—as little as one-third of the original genome may remain in the DI particles of vesicular stomatitis virus. Morphologically, DI particles usually resemble the parental virions, but the DI particles of vesicular stomatitis virus are smaller than wild-type virions. Sequencing studies of the RNA of DI particles reveal simple deletions and a great diversity of structural rearrangements.

Defective interfering particles increase preferentially with serial passage at high multiplicity in cultured cells because their shortened RNA genomes require less time to be replicated, are less often diverted to serve as templates for transcription of mRNA, and have enhanced affinity for the viral replicase, giving them a competitive advantage over their full-length infectious counterparts. These features also explain why on passage the DI particles interfere with the replication of full-length parental RNA with progressively greater efficiency.

The generation of defective genomes of DNA viruses can occur by any of a great variety of modes of DNA rearrangement. For example, papovavirus DI particles usually contain reiterated copies of the genomic origins of replication, which are sometimes interspersed with DNA of host cell origin.

Our knowledge of DI particles derives from studies in cultured cells, but they play a role in some disease conditions. By interference, they may attenuate the lethality of the parental infectious virus, and they may be involved in a variety of chronic animal diseases. However, because their defective and variable nature makes them difficult to detect in experiments with intact animals, much remains to be discovered about their role in disease.

Mutation Rates

Rates of mutation involving point mutations are probably the same in DNA viruses that replicate in the nucleus as they are in the DNAs of eukaryotic cells, since DNA replication is subject to the same "proofreading" exonuclease error-correction as operates in cells. Errors are estimated to occur at a rate of 10^{-8} to 10^{-11} per incorporated nucleotide (i.e., per base per replication cycle). Point mutations in the third nucleotide of a triplet often do not result in an altered amino acid, because of *coding redundancy*, and some point mutations are lethal because they produce nonfunctioning gene products or a stop codon or other aberrant regulatory sequences. Viable mutations that are neutral or deleterious in one host may provide a selection advantage in a different host.

The error rate in the replication of viral RNA is much higher than that of viral or cellular DNA, because there is no cellular proofreading mechanism for RNA. For example, the base substitution rate in the 11-kb genome of vesicular stomatitis virus is 10^{-3}–10^{-4} per base per replication cycle, so that nearly every progeny genome will be different from its parent and each other in at least one base. This rate of base substitution is about one million times higher than the average rate in eukaryotic DNA. Of course, most of the base substitutions are deleterious and the genomes containing them are lost. However, nonlethal mutations in the genome of RNA viruses accumulate very rapidly. For example, sequence analysis of the genome of two isolates of hepatitis C virus obtained from a chronically infected patient at an interval of 13 years showed that the mutation rate was about 2×10^{-3} base substitutions per genome site per year. These nucleotide changes were unevenly distributed throughout the genome, that is, different genes evolved at different rates. At the population level, outbreaks of human poliomyelitis type 1 in 1978–1979 were traced from the Netherlands to Canada and then to United States. Oligonucleotide mapping of the RNAs obtained from successive isolates of the virus from different people showed that over a period of 13 months of epidemic transmission there were about 100 base changes in a genome of 7441 bases.

It is important to recognize that every virus, as defined by its conventional phenotypic markers, is a genetically complex population that comprises multiple mutants, a minority of which will be dominant under defined conditions of replication. Nevertheless, in nature some viruses, even RNA viruses such as measles virus, appear to be remarkably stable in their virulence and antigenicity. This appears to be due to a combination of selective pressures and the small size of the inocula involved in aerosol transmission.

Mutagenesis

Spontaneous mutations occur because of chance errors during replication. Mutation frequency can be enhanced by treatment of virions or isolated viral nucleic acid with physical agents such as UV- or X-irradiation or with chemicals such as nitrous acid or nitrosoguanidine. Base analogs, such as 5-fluorouracil, are mutagenic only when virus is grown in their presence because they act after incorporation into the viral nucleic acid.

Site-Directed Mutagenesis. Instead of relying on change mutations anywhere in the genome, genetic engineering makes it possible to produce mutations at any site of interest. *Site-directed mutagenesis* enables the experimenter to introduce mutations at a selected site in a DNA molecule [a DNA genome or *complementary DNA* (*cDNA*) transcribed from an RNA genome]. Several techniques to achieve this are available, most of which rely on the sequence specificity of restriction endonucleases. For example, the purified ssDNA, which has been transferred to an appropriate vector such as bacteriophage M13, is annealed to a short oligonucleotide that is homologous to the relevant region but contains the desired nucleotide. Progeny phages containing the mutated genome are selected by hybridization with the oligonucleotide probe, and marker rescue is used to recover the mutated gene in infectious virus. The polymerase chain reaction can be used to verify the location of the genetic lesions.

Until recently, site-directed mutagenesis and other types of genetic engineering were restricted to DNA viruses and plus strand RNA viruses, from which cDNA could be produced by reverse transcription. However, it has become possible to apply these methods of *reverse genetics* to minus strand viruses, including those with segmented genomes. Site-directed mutagenesis has opened up new research areas; for example, the function of individual genes and the proteins for which they code, or of particular regions of these genes and proteins, can be dissected. At a practical level, mutations can be introduced into particular genes, such as those concerned with viral virulence, to produce mutants suitable for use as attenuated live-virus vaccines.

Adaptation to Cell Culture or Laboratory Animals

Although much experimentation with viruses of veterinary importance can be carried out in natural hosts, major advances usually depend on the growth of the viruses in cultured cells or in a laboratory animal. Such adaptation depends on a series of empirically generated mutations and progressive selection of the best growing mutant.

Some viruses produce clinical signs of disease the first time that they are inoculated into an experimental animal, for instance, eastern equine encephalitis virus in suckling mice. In other cases miminal signs of infection are observed initially, but after serial passage, sometimes prolonged, clinical disease is regularly produced, as, for example, in the adaptation of bluetongue and bovine ephemeral fever viruses to mice. Likewise, newly isolated viruses at first often fail to grow in certain kinds of cultured cells, but can be adapted by serial passage (e.g., street rabies virus adapted to neuroblastoma cells). Most modern virologic research is performed with strains of virus adapted to grow rapidly to high yield and to produce plaques or cytopathic changes in continuous cell lines. A frequent by-product of such adaptation to a new experimental host is the coincident attenuation of the virus for its original host; for example, after adaptation to pig kidney cell cultures, infectious canine hepatitis virus (an adenovirus) is attenuated for the dog.

Genetic Analysis of Viruses That Cannot Be Cultured. Growth in cell culture is not essential for the study of viral nucleic acids and proteins, since the introduction of the polymerase chain reaction has made it possible to produce virtually unlimited quantities of any required nucleic acid. Remarkable progress has been made in the genetic analysis of some noncultivable viruses, such as the bovine papillomaviruses, by using DNA extracted directly from papillomas collected at the abattoirs, and the complete nucleotide sequences of rabbit hemorrhagic fever calicivirus and of hepatitis C virus genomes have been determined without either virus having been cultured.

GENETIC RECOMBINATION BETWEEN VIRUSES

When two different viruses simultaneously infect the same cell, genetic recombination may occur between the newly synthesized nucleic acid molecules. This may be categorized as *intramolecular recombination, reassortment,* and *reactivation* (if one of the viruses has been inactivated).

Intramolecular Recombination

Intramolecular recombination involves the exchange of nucleic acid sequences between different but usually closely related viruses during viral replication (Fig. 4-1A). It occurs with all dsDNA viruses, presumably because of strand-switching by the viral DNA polymerase. Among RNA viruses, intramolecular recombination has been demonstrated for picornaviruses, coronaviruses, a togavirus, and an arterivirus. It may be more widespread, because detection has relied on the recovery of viable recombinants; the use of the polymerase chain reaction following reverse transcription may overcome this lack of sensitivity. For some viruses recombination can also occur between viral and cellular RNA and DNA.

There is evidence that Western equine encephalitis virus arose as a result of intramolecular recombination between a Sindbis-like virus and Eastern equine encephalitis virus. In experimental situations, intramolecular recombination may occur between viruses belonging to different families; the best example is between SV40 (a papovavirus) and adenoviruses. Both SV40 and adenovirus DNAs become integrated into cellular DNA, so it is perhaps not surprising to find that when rhesus monkey cells which harbor a persistent SV40 infection are superinfected with an adenovirus, not only does *complementation* occur, the SV40 acting as a helper in an otherwise abortive adneovirus infection, but recombination occurs between SV40 DNA and adenovirus DNA to yield hybrid (recombinant) DNA which is packaged into adenovirus capsids. Integration of viral DNA into cellular DNA by intramolecular recombination occurs in cells transformed by adenoviruses, hepadnaviruses, and polyomaviruses, but not always in cells transformed by papillomaviruses or certain herpesviruses, in which transformation may occur although the viral DNA usually remains episomal (see Chapter 11).

Unlike other RNA viruses, retroviruses have no replicating pool of viral RNA. Although the genome of retroviruses is plus sense ssRNA, replication does not occur until the genomic RNA is transcribed into DNA by the virion-associated reverse transcriptase and the resultant dsDNA integrated into the DNA of the host cell. However, both minus strand and plus strand recombination occur between the two DNA copies

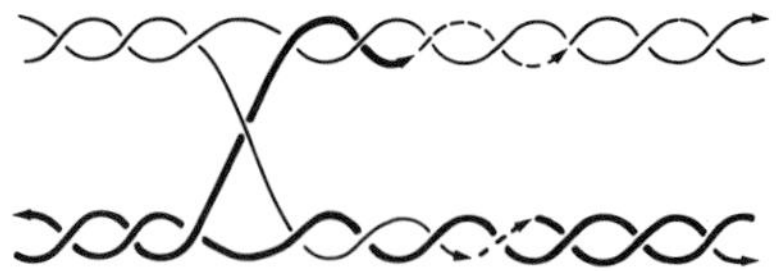

A. Intramolecular recombination

B. Genetic reassortment

C. Polyploidy

D. Heteropolyploidy

E. Phenotypic mixing

genome "a"
capsid "A"

genome "a"
mixed capsid

F. Phenotypic mixing

or

genome "b"
capsid "B"

genome "a"
capsid "B"

G. Transcapsidation

FIG. 4-1. *Genetic recombination, polyploidy, phenotypic mixing, and transcapsidation. (A) Intramolecular recombination, as in a dsDNA virus. (B) Reassortment of genome fragments, as in reoviruses and orthomyxoviruses. (C) Polyploidy, as seen in unmixed infections with paramyxoviruses. (D) Heteropolyploidy, as may occur in mixed infections with paramyxoviruses and other enveloped RNA viruses. (E–G) Phenotypic mixing: (E) enveloped viruses; (F) viruses with icosahedral capsids; (G) extreme case of transcapsidation or genomic masking.*

of the diploid genome, as well as between the DNA provirus and cell DNA. In the latter instance, a retrovirus may pick up a *cellular oncogene;* such oncogenes are incorporated into the viral genome to become *viral oncogenes,* which confer the property of rapid oncogenicity on the retrovirus concerned (see Chapter 11).

Reassortment

A variety of recombination called *reassortment* occurs with viruses that have segmented genomes, whether these are ssRNA or dsRNA and consist of 2 (*Arenaviridae, Birnaviridae*), 3 (*Bunyaviridae*), 8 (influenza A virus), 10 (*Reovirus, Orbivirus*), or 11 (*Rotavirus*) segments (Fig. 4-1B). In a single cell infected with two related viruses of each of these groups, there is an exchange of segments with the production of various stable reassortants. Reassortment occurs in nature and is an important source of genetic variability.

Reactivation

The term *multiplicity reactivation* is applied to the production of infectious virus by a cell infected with two or more viruses of the same strain, each of which has suffered a lethal mutation in a different gene. Multiplicity reactivation could theoretically lead to the production of infectious virus if animals were to be inoculated with vaccines produced by UV-irradiation or treatment with certain chemicals; accordingly these methods of inactivation are not used for vaccine production. *Cross-reactivation* or *marker rescue* are terms used to describe genetic recombination between an infectious virus and an inactivated virus of a related but distinguishable genotype, or a fragment of DNA from such a virus; they are useful techniques for the experimental virologist.

INTERACTIONS BETWEEN VIRAL GENE-PRODUCTS

In addition to interactions between viral nucleic acids, viral gene products, namely, proteins, can interact in various ways that affect the phenotype. For the most part such interactions are a laboratory phenomenon, but some are useful for genetic analysis.

Complementation

Complementation is the term used to describe all cases in which interaction between viral gene-products (structural proteins, enzymes, etc.) in doubly infected cells results in the yield, or an increased yield, of one or both viruses. Complementation reflects the fact that one virus provides a gene-product which the other cannot make, thus enabling the latter to replicate in the mixedly infected cell. Mutants can be allocated to specific genes by complementation analysis, which depends on nonidentity of function. Complementation can also occur between unrelated viruses, for example, between an adenovirus and adeno-associated virus (a parvovirus) or between SV40 and an adenovirus in monkey cells.

Phenotypic Mixing

Following mixed infection by two viruses which share certain common features, some of the progeny may acquire phenotypic characteristics from both parents, although their genotype remains unchanged. For example, when cells are coinfected with influenza virus and a paramyxovirus, the envelopes of some of the progeny particles contain viral antigens derived from each parent. However, each virion contains the nucleic acid of only one parent, and hence on passage it produces only virions resembling that parent (Fig. 4-1E,F). Phenotypic mixing is an essential part of the life cycle of envelope-defective retroviruses, progeny virions being called *pseudotypes* and having the genome of the defective parental virus but the envelope glycoproteins of the helper retrovirus, in whose company it will always be found.

Experimentally, and in nature with some plant viruses, phenotypic mixing of nonenveloped viruses can take the form of transcapsidation (Fig. 4-1G), in which there is partial or usually complete exchange of capsids. For example, poliovirus nucleic acid may be enclosed within a coxsackievirus capsid, or the adenovirus 7 genome may be enclosed within an adenovirus 2 capsid. Since the viral ligands that govern cell attachment reside in the capsid, transcapsidation can change cell tropisms.

Polyploidy

With the exception of the retroviruses, which are diploid, all viruses of vertebrates are haploid, that is, they contain only a single copy of each gene. Even with the retroviruses, diploidy is in no sense comparable to that seen in eukaryotic cells, since both copies of the genome are essentially identical and derived from the same parental virus. Among viruses that mature by budding from the plasma membrane, for example, paramyxoviruses, it is sometimes found that several nucleocapsids (and thus genomes) are enclosed within a single envelope (*polyploid* or *heteropolyploid,* Fig. 4-1C,D).

MAPPING VIRAL GENOMES

Viral genomes can be mapped in a variety of ways. Restriction endonuclease mapping of the viral DNA is a convenient way of recognizing and classifying some viruses. Since the early 1980s methods of nucleotide sequencing have been continually improved, and the complete sequence has now been determined for at least one representative of every viral family. These methods have to a large extent replaced recombination and oligonucleotide mapping.

Restriction Maps

Several hundred specific bacterial endonucleases, called *restriction endonucleases,* have been identified and purified from various bacteria. Each recognizes a unique short, *palindromic sequence* of nucleotides (a sequence that reads the same backward as forward), four to nine nucleotide pairs long. Depending on the location and frequency of the particular palindromic sequence in a DNA molecule, a restriction endonuclease cleaves the DNA into a precise number of fragments of precise sizes. Other endonucleases, recognizing different sequences, cleave the same DNA into different numbers and sizes of fragments. The DNA fragments may be separated by gel electrophoresis. Different viruses, often even very closely related strains of the same virus, yield characteristically different restriction endonuclease fragment patterns, sometimes called fingerprints or restriction fragment length polymorphisms (RFLPs). These have been invaluable for distinguishing between different species or strains of viruses with large genomes, such as orthopoxviruses or herpesviruses. The order of the fragments from left to right can be determined to provide a physical map of the genome. Restriction enzymes can also be used to analyze the molecularly cloned cDNA copies of genes or genomes from RNA viruses, and to locate the specific physical locations on the viral chromosome of various genetic markers.

Sequence Analysis

A great deal of information can be gleaned from the sequence of nucleotides in a viral genome. *Open reading frames* (*ORF*) are translatable sequences starting with methionine (AUG) and uninterrupted by stop codons (UAA, UAG, UGA). The function of the predicted protein can sometimes be surmised by the similarity of its sequence to that of a protein of known function. Such comparisons are carried out by searching international computer databases of nucleotide and amino acid sequences. It is also possible from an examination of the sequence to find characteristic groups of amino acids, or motifs, that indicate which parts will have particular functions, such as *signal sequences* for targeting proteins to the endoplasmic reticulum or the plasma membrane, transmembrane sequences, glycosylation sites, and nucleotide binding sites. Short sequence motifs can also be identified which serve as signals in gene expression. The methionine codons (AUG), which initiate translation at the beginning of all open reading frames, are usually embedded in a consensus sequence GCCGCC/GCCAUGG. Sites of mRNA cleavage and polyadenylation are often signaled by AAUAAA followed by certain other signals. The start sites for transcription by RNA polymerase II are usually 25–30 base pairs downstream from an A + T-rich sequence, the *TATA box.*

Oligonucleotide Mapping

Before restriction endonuclease mapping and sequencing were widely used, oligonucleotide fingerprinting (mapping) techniques using T1 ribonuclease provided a fast and powerful procedure for differentiating between different isolates of RNA viruses.

Recombination Maps

Among viruses that undergo intramolecular recombination, the probability of recombination occurring between two markers reflects the distance between them, and recombination frequencies in adjacent intervals are approximately additive. Two-factor crosses are used to determine recombination frequencies between pairs of mutants, and for very close or distant markers three-factor crosses are used to resolve ambiguities. Recombination maps have been constructed for several DNA viruses and for poliovirus.

RECOMBINANT DNA TECHNOLOGY

The discovery of restriction endonucleases, and the recognition of other enzymes involved in DNA synthesis (polymerases, ligases, transferases), opened up the possibility of deliberately introducing specific foreign DNA sequences into DNA molecules. When the recombinant molecules replicate, there is a corresponding amplification of the foreign DNA. The process is called *molecular cloning*. When the inserted DNA is placed in frame with appropriate upstream and downstream regulatory sequences, it is expressed, that is, the polypeptide specified by the foreign DNA is produced. Expression is usually achieved by incorporating the foreign DNA into a *bacteriophage* or a bacterial *plasmid* (Fig. 4-2), which serves as a *cloning and expression vector* when introduced into the appropriate bacterial or other cells. Vectors are available that replicate in bacteria, yeasts, insect and animal cells, and in intact animals. For animal cells, a variety of animal viruses are used as vectors, notably SV40, bovine papilloma virus, retroviruses, and vaccinia virus. The cluster of techniques used is often called recombinant DNA technology or "genetic engineering."

Uses of Genetic Engineering

In addition to its great value for experimental virology, practical applications of genetic engineering to animal viruses include the development of nucleic acid probes for diagnosis by nucleic acid hybridization (see Chapter 12) and novel methods for the production of vaccines, including the use of vaccinia or fowlpox virus as vectors (see Chapter 13).

Combined with the polymerase chain reaction and the availability of simple and fast methods of nucleotide sequencing, genetic engineering has also led to studies of animal virus genomes that could not be previously contemplated. Among the achievements so far are the following:

1. Complete sequencing of the genome of viruses representing all DNA virus families.
2. Complete sequencing of cDNA corresponding to the entire genome of viruses representing all RNA virus families.
3. Recognition of the number and sequence of viral or proviral DNAs that are integrated into the DNA of transformed cells.
4. Marker rescue by transfection with gene fragments, as a method of genetic mapping.
5. Production of proteins coded by specific viral genes using bacterial, yeast, insect, and animal cell expression systems, or by cell-free translation.
6. Synthesis of peptides based on DNA sequence data.

TRANSGENIC ANIMALS

Transgenic animals provide a new tool for investigating many problems in virology, immunology, and biology in general. In experimental biology transgenic animals have been most commonly produced with mice, either by using retrovirus vectors or more commonly by injecting selected fragments of DNA into the nuclei of fertilized eggs washed out of the mouse oviduct, but the same techniques are also used for other animals. After replacement, some ova develop normally to form the base

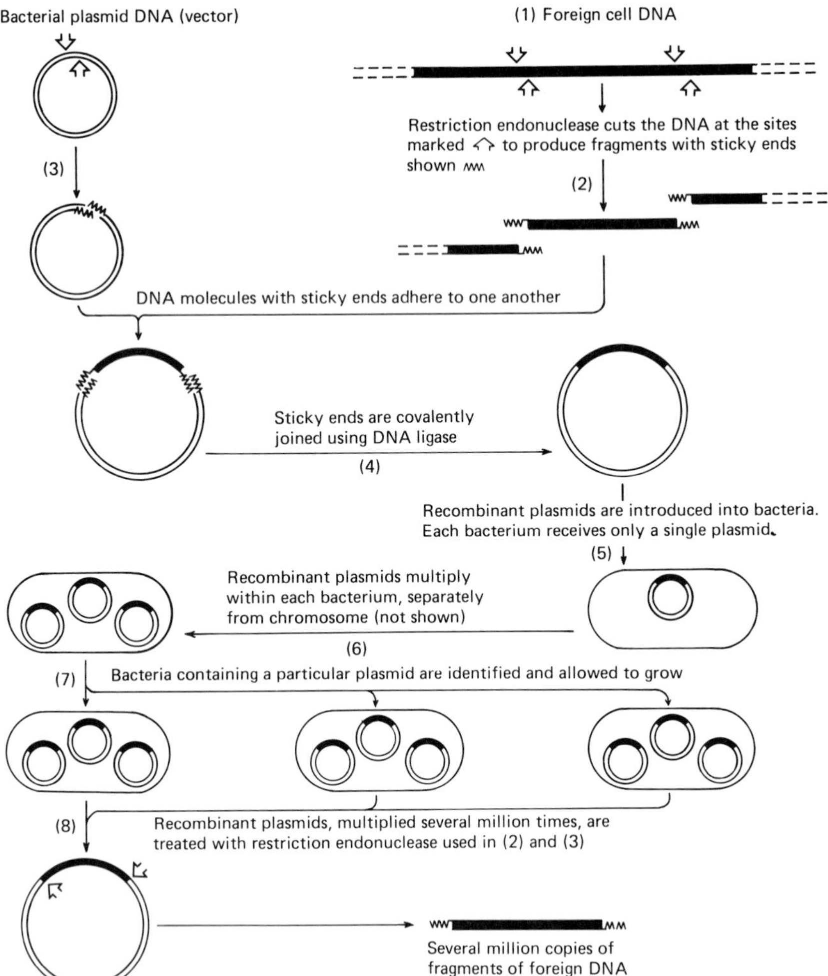

FIG. 4-2. *Steps in obtaining recombinant DNA. In parallel, DNA (genome DNA or cDNA from virion RNA or mRNA) from a virus (1) is cut into fragments by a selected restriction endonuclease (2), and the circular DNA molecule of the plasmid vector is cut with the same endonuclease (3). The viral DNA is inserted and ligated into the plasmid DNA, which is thus circularized again (4). The plasmid is then introduced into the host bacterium by transformation (5). Replication of the plasmid as an episome (6) may produce many copies per bacterial cell (for small plasmids), or there may be only one copy (for large plasmids). Bacteria containing the desired plasmid are identified, cloned, and allowed to grow (7). The plasmids are isolated from the bacteria, and the viral DNA insert is excised (8) using the same restriction endonuclease employed in steps (2) and (3). In this way a specified gene may be replicated several millionfold. With appropriate genetic engineering including the use of regulatory and termination sequences, the protein product of the inserted gene may be expressed in prokaryotic or eukaryotic cells.*

of a colony of transgenic animals. The technique has enormous potential for enlarging our understanding of viral biology, for it provides insights into the potential role in viral pathogenesis of individual viral gene products in the context of the intact animal. Using genes from other animals (human, domestic animal) will provide the opportunity to investigate in laboratory animals the role of products of particular genes of those hosts. For example, transgenic mice containing the DNA for the early region of bovine papillomavirus developed skin tumors at 8–9 months of age. Extrachromosomal viral DNA was detected in tumor cells and integrated viral DNA in normal tissues.

GENETIC VARIATION AND VIRAL EVOLUTION

The genetic mechanisms described, operating under the pressure of Darwinian selection, have been responsible for viral evolution (Table 4-1). We will discuss in more detail how one DNA virus, myxoma virus, and one RNA virus, influenza A virus, have evolved over the past few decades, the one in rabbits and the other in humans, birds, and horses.

Genetic Changes in Virus and Host in Myxomatosis

Myxomatosis, caused by the leporipoxvirus myxoma virus, occurs naturally as a mild infection of rabbits in South America and California

TABLE 4-1
Examples of Genetic Mechanisms That Have Affected Viral Evolution[a]

Mechanism	Example
Point mutation	Lethal chicken influenza due to a single point mutation
Intramolecular recombination	Western equine encephalitis virus produced by recombination between Eastern equine encephalitis virus and a Sindbis-like alphavirus
Genetic reassortment	Pandemic human influenza A subtypes H2N2 (1957) and H3N2 (1968)
Recombination and mutation	Changes in poliovaccine following vaccination
Biased hypermutation[b] (uridine to cytosine transitions)	Evolution of subacute sclerosing panencephalitis virus from measles virus
Genetic rearrangement[c]	Evolution of rubella virus

[a] Based on E. D. Kilbourne, *Curr. Opin. Immunol.* **3**, 518 (1991).
[b] Missense mutations of M gene.
[c] Compared with alphavirus genome, the order of helicase and NS P3 region is reversed in rubella virus.

(*Sylvilagus* spp.), in which it produces a skin tumor from which virus is transmitted mechanically by biting insects. However, in laboratory (European) rabbits (*Oryctolagus cuniculus*), myxoma virus causes a lethal infection, a finding that led to its use for biological control of wild European rabbits in Australia.

The wild European rabbit was introduced into Australia in 1859 for sporting purposes and rapidly spread over the southern part of the continent, where it became the major animal pest of the agricultural and pastoral industries. Myxoma virus from South America was successfully introduced into the rabbit population in 1950; when originally liberated the virus produced case–fatality rates of over 99%. This highly virulent virus was readily transmitted by mosquitoes. Farmers operated "inoculation campaigns" to introduce virulent myxoma virus into wild rabbit populations.

It might have been predicted that the disease and with it the virus would disappear at the end of each summer, owing to the greatly diminished numbers of susceptible rabbits and the greatly lowered opportunity for transmission by mosquitoes during the winter. This must often have occurred in localized areas, but it did not happen over the continent as a whole. The capacity of virus to survive the winter conferred a great selective advantage on viral mutants of reduced lethality, since during this period, when mosquito numbers were low, rabbits infected by such mutants survived in an infectious condition for weeks instead of a few days. Within three years such "attenuated" mutants became the dominant strains throughout Australia. Some inoculation campaigns with the virulent virus produced localized highly lethal outbreaks, but in general the viruses that spread through the rabbit populations each year were the "attenuated" strains, which because of the prolonged illness in their hosts provided a greater opportunity for mosquito transmission. Thus the original highly lethal virus was progressively replaced by a heterogeneous collection of strains of lower virulence, but most of them still virulent enough to kill 70–90% of genetically unselected rabbits.

Rabbits that recover from myxomatosis are immune to reinfection. However, since most wild rabbits have a life span of less than 1 year, herd immunity is not so critically important in the epidemiology of myxomatosis as it is in infections of longer lived species. Selection for genetically more resistant animals operated from the outset. In areas where repeated outbreaks occurred, the genetic resistance of surviving rabbits increased progressively. The early appearance of viral strains of lower virulence, which allowed 10% of genetically unselected rabbits to recover, was an important factor in allowing the number of genetically resistant rabbits to increase. In areas where annual outbreaks occurred, the genetic resistance of the rabbits changed such that the case–fatality rate after infection under laboratory conditions with a particular strain of virus fell from 90% to 25% within 7 years. Subsequently, in areas where there were frequent outbreaks of myxomatosis, somewhat more virulent strains of myxoma virus became dominant, because they produced the kind of disease that was best transmitted in populations of genetically resistant rabbits. Thus, the ultimate balance struck between myxoma virus and Australian rabbits involved adaptations of virus and host populations, reaching a dynamic equilibrium which finds rabbits still greatly reduced compared with their premyxomatosis numbers, but too numerous for the wishes of farmers and conservationists.

Genetic Changes in Influenza A Virus

Influenza A viruses produce important diseases in birds, man, swine, horses, and mink. Because of the significance of human influenza and the longevity of man, the most detailed long-term study of the evolution of influenza viruses has been carried out with influenza A virus in man. Human influenza virus was first isolated in 1933. Since that time viruses have been recovered from all parts of the world, and their antigenic properties have been studied in considerable detail, thus providing an opportunity for observing continuing evolutionary changes.

Influenza A virus periodically causes epidemics in man, swine, horses, birds, and occasionally in other animals such as seals. Subtypes are classified according to the two envelope antigens, the hemagglutinin (H) and neuraminidase (N). All of the fourteen subtypes of the H molecule have been found in birds, three of them also in man, two in pigs, horses, seals, and whales, and one in mink. The nine N subtypes show a similar distribution.

The outstanding feature of influenza virus is the antigenic variability of the envelope glycoproteins, H and N, which undergo two types of changes, known as *antigenic drift* and *antigenic shift*. Antigenic drift occurs within a subtype and involves a series of point mutations; those affecting neutralizing epitopes produce strains each antigenically slightly different from its predecessor. Antigenic shift involves the acquisition of a gene for a completely new H or N.

Antigenic Shift. Influenza A virus was first isolated in 1933, but the prevalent human subtype was suddenly replaced with a new subtype in 1957 (H1N1 to H2N2) and in 1968 (H2N2 to H3N2). After the H2N2 strain ("Asian flu") first appeared in China in 1957, it rapidly spread round the world, as did the H3N2 strain ("Hong Kong flu") after 1968, each displacing the then prevalent subtype. In 1977 the H1N1 subtype mysteriously reappeared, and since then the two subtypes H3N2 and H1N1 have cocirculated, and viruses that are reassortments between the two subtypes have been occasionally isolated.

The H glycoprotein molecules of different subtypes are, by definition, quite distinct serologically. Further information about their degree of relatedness, and thus possibly their evolutionary history, has been derived from sequencing, which shows that the 14 known subtypes found in birds evolved from a common ancestor and share a common basic structure. However, there is only about 30% homology between the amino acid sequences of human H3 and H2, whereas the homology between strains within each subtype is usually over 90%. In other words, the many strains that emerged by antigenic drift within the H2 subtype between 1957 and 1968 are closely related genetically, and within the H3 subtype, strains which have become prevalent since 1968 are also closely related to one another; however, there are major differences between the two groups. Clearly, sharp discontinuities in the evolutionary pattern occurred with the emergence of the new subtype H2 in 1957 and again with the appearance of H3 in 1968.

What is the mechanism of this abrupt change in subtypes, which is referred to as antigenic shift? The answer has come from comparing the sequences of H genes from human influenza subtypes with those of influenza A viruses isolated from other mammals and birds. Such studies reveal much closer homology between human H3 and an avian influenza H3 than between human H3 and human H2 viruses. As laboratory studies have clearly demonstrated the ease with which genetic reassortment can occur in mammals and birds, it seems reasonable to suppose that new subtypes of human influenza virus are derived by naturally occurring genetic reassortment between influenza viruses infecting man and other animals. Study of all eight genome segments of human H2 and H3 viruses shows that the H3 gene and PB1 gene (one of the polymerase genes) of the Hong Kong strain were almost certainly derived from an avian host, presumably by reassortment, whereas the N gene and the other five genes are similar to those of the H2N2 virus.

However, not all "new" influenza viruses in mammals arise by reassortment between a preexisting mammalian strain and an avian virus. For example, the H1N1 swine influenza virus strain that appeared in Europe in 1979 was derived directly from birds, and the equine H3N8 influenza virus that appeared in north China in 1989 was very different from the H3N8 equine influenza virus currently found elsewhere in the world, but was very similar to an avian H3N8 influenza A virus.

Antigenic Drift. After antigenic shift introduces a new pandemic strain, antigenic drift begins as point mutations accumulate in all the

RNA segments of the strain. Mutations in the gene that codes for the hemagglutinin include some which alter its antigenic sites. When antiserum against the previously prevalent strain no longer neutralizes the variant, a new strain has emerged. Most of the significant changes in the hemagglutinin are clustered in five regions of the molecule which are thought to be important antigenic sites. Substitution of a single amino acid in a critical antigenic site may totally abolish the capacity of the existing antibody to bind to that site. On the other hand, some regions of the H protein are conserved in all human and avian strains, presumably because they are essential for the maintenance of the structure and function of the molecule. The important feature of antigenic drift in human influenza viruses is that in immune populations the new strains have a selective advantage over their predecessors and tend to displace them. Although minor variants can cocirculate, the general rule is that one novel strain supplants previous strains of that subtype in a particular region.

Avian Influenza in Pennsylvania in 1983. In April 1983 an avian influenza virus appeared in chickens in Pennsylvania, producing a mortality of less than 10%. Its serotype was H5N2, and comparison of the genome segments of this isolate with other influenza A isolates by RNA hybridization indicated that all its genes were closely related to the genes of H5N2 isolates from wild birds in the eastern United States at the time. In October 1983 a change occurred in its virulence, such that the mortality rate in infected chickens suddenly rose to over 80%.

Comparison of individual RNA segments of the April and October isolates by oligonucleotide mapping showed that genetic reassortment had not occurred, suggesting that the change in virulence had been due to a small number of point mutations (i.e., genetic drift). Previous studies of reassortants between virulent avian influenza virus (fowl plague virus) and avirulent avian or human influenza viruses had shown that virulence for birds is polygenic but that the H gene is of major importance. For example, the virulence of another virulent avian serotype, H7 virus, has been shown to be linked to the ease of cleavage of the H protein in cultured cells. Sequencing of the H genes from the mild and virulent H5N2 strains revealed seven nucleotide differences which resulted in four amino acid changes in the H protein. One of these changes affects a glycosylation site near the site of cleavage between the H1 and H2 subunits of the H molecule. Cleavage of the H molecule occurs more readily in the virulent strain. The two strains also differ in the extent to which they produce defective interfering particles, which are much more frequent in the original, less virulent strain. The practical significance of the critical single base change in the RNA of the H genome segment of the H5N2 avian influenza virus that occurred in October 1983 is underlined by the fact that control measures, which involved the slaughter of millions of chickens because of the threat posed to the poultry industry of the United States, cost more than $60 million.

FURTHER READING

Coen, D. M. (1990). Molecular genetics of animal viruses. *In* "Fields Virology" (B. N. Fields, D. M. Knipe, R. M. Chanock, M. S. Hirsch, J. L. Melnick, T. P. Monath, and B. Roizman, eds.), 2nd Ed., p. 123. Raven, New York.

Fenner, F., and Ross, J. (1993). Myxomatosis. *In* "The Rabbit in Britain, France and Australasia: The Ecology of a Successful Colonizer," (in press). Oxford Univ. Press, Oxford.

Holland, J. J. (1990). Defective viral genomes. *In* "Fields Virology" (B. N. Fields, D. M. Knipe, R. M. Chanock, M. S. Hirsch, J. L. Melnick, T. P. Monath, and B. Roizman, eds.), 2nd Ed., p. 151. Raven, New York.

Jarvis, T. C., and Kirkegaard, K. (1991). The polymerase in its labyrinth: Mechanisms and implications of RNA recombination. *Trends Genet.* **7,** 186.

Klenk, H.-D., and Rott, R. (1989). The molecular biology of influenza virus pathogenecity. *Adv. Virus Res.* **34,** 247.

Murphy, B. R., and Webster, R. G. (1990). Orthomyxoviruses. *In* "Fields Virology" (B. N. Fields, D. M. Knipe, R. M. Chanock, M. S. Hirsch, J. L. Melnick, T. P. Monath, and B. Roizman, eds.), 2nd Ed., p. 1091. Raven, New York.

Notkins, A. L., and Oldstone, M. B. A., eds. (1989). Transgenic mice: Expression of viral genes. *In* "Concepts in Viral Pathogenesis III," p. 158. Springer-Verlag, New York.

Pringle, C. R. (1990). The genetics of viruses. *In* "Topley and Wilson's Principles of Bacteriology, Virology and Immunity" (L. H. Collier and M. C. Timbury, eds.), 8th Ed., Vol. 4, p. 69. Arnold, London.

Ramig, R. F. (1990). Principles of animal virus genetics. *In* "Fields Virology" (B. N. Fields, D. M. Knipe, R. M. Chanock, M. S. Hirsch, J. L. Melnick, T. P. Monath, and B. Roizman, eds.), 2nd Ed., p. 95. Raven, New York.

Roux, L., Simon, A. E., and Holland, J. J. (1991). Effects of defective interfering viruses on virus replication and pathogenesis *in vitro* and *in vivo*. *Adv. Virus Res.* **40,** 181.

Sambrook, J., Fritsch, E. F., and Maniatis, T. (1989). "Molecular Cloning: A Laboratory Manual," 2nd Ed. Cold Spring Harbor Laboratory, New York.

CHAPTER 5

Virus-Induced Changes in Cells

Virus-induced changes at the cellular, subcellular, and molecular levels are most easily studied in cultured cells; the results of such observations can then be extrapolated to the *in vivo* situation. The various types of interactions that can occur between virus and cell are summarized in Table 5-1. Viral infections may be categorized as *cytocidal (lytic)* or *noncytocidal (nonlytic)*. Not all viral infections are *productive,* that is, lead to the production of new virions. Cell changes of a profound nature, leading to cell death in some cases and cell transformation in others, may also occur in *nonproductive infections.* Looked at from the point of view of the cell rather than the virus, certain kinds of cells are permissive, namely, they support complete replication of a particular virus, while others are nonpermissive, with replication being blocked at some point. Cytopathic changes can occur in both productive and nonproductive infections and in permissive and nonpermissive cells. Cellular *transformation,* produced by oncogenic viruses, is described in Chapter 11.

CYTOPATHIC EFFECTS OF VIRUS INFECTIONS

Many viruses kill the cells in which they replicate, so that when infection of cells in monolayer cultures is initiated by a small dose of virus, progressive damage is seen as the infection spreads, and under suitable

TABLE 5-1
Types of Virus–Cell Interaction

Type of infection	Effects on cell	Production of infectious virions	Examples
Cytocidal (lytic)	Morphological changes in cells (cytopathic effects); inhibition of protein, RNA, and DNA synthesis; cell death	+	Alphaherpesviruses, enteroviruses, reoviruses
Persistent noncytocidal	No cytopathic effect; little metabolic disturbance; cells continue to divide; possible loss of special functions of some differentiated cells	+	Arenaviruses, rabies virus, most retroviruses
Persistent noncytocidal (nonproductive)	Usually nil	Normally −, but virus may be induced[a]	Distemper and bovine paramyxoviruses in brain cells
Transformation	Alteration in cell morphology; cells can be passaged indefinitely; may produce tumors when transplanted to experimental animals	−, oncogenic DNA viruses; +, oncogenic retroviruses	See Chapter 11

[a] By cocultivation, irradiation, or chemical mutagens.

conditions plaques are produced. When infection is initiated by a large amount of virus, damage may occur across the whole monolayer at the same time. Virus-induced cell damage is known as the *cytopathic effect* (CPE) of the virus, and it can often be observed by low-power light microscopy is unstained cell cultures (Figs. 5-1 and 5-2A,B,C). Fixation and staining of the cell monolayer may reveal further diagnostic details, notably *inclusion bodies* and *synctia*. The nature and speed of development of the cytopathic effect are characteristic of the particular virus involved and therefore represent important early criteria for the identification of clinical isolates (see Chapter 12).

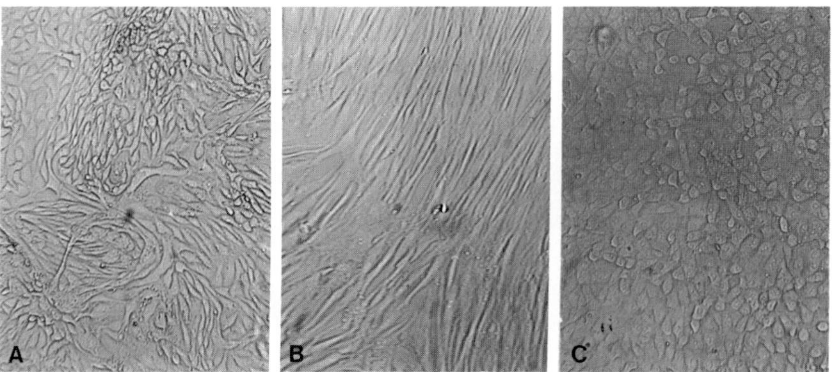

FIG. 5-1. *Unstained confluent monolayers of the three main types of cell cultures, as they appear by low-power light microscopy, through the wall of the tissue culture vessel. Magnification:* ×50. *(A) Primary monkey kidney epithelium. (B) Diploid strain of fetal fibroblasts. (C) Continuous line of epithelial cells. (Courtesy I. Jack.)*

Inclusion Bodies

A characteristic morphological change in cells infected by certain viruses is the formation of inclusion bodies, which are recognized by light microscopy following fixation and staining (Fig. 5-3). Depending on the virus, inclusion bodies may be single or multiple, large or small, intranuclear or intracytoplasmic, round or irregular in shape, and acidophilic or basophilic when stained.

The most striking viral inclusion bodies are the intracytoplasmic inclusions found in cells infected with poxviruses, paramyxoviruses, reoviruses, and rabies virus and the intranuclear inclusion bodies found in cells infected with herpesviruses, adenoviruses, parvoviruses, and Borna disease virus. Some viruses, for example, canine distemper and rinderpest viruses, may produce both nuclear and cytoplasmic inclusion bodies in the same cell. Many inclusions have been shown to be accumulations of viral structural components; for example, the intracytoplasmic inclusions in cells infected with paramyxoviruses and rabies virus are masses of viral nucleocapsids. The basophilic intracytoplasmic inclusions invariably found in cells infected with poxviruses are sites of viral synthesis (viral "factories") made up of masses of viral protein and nucleic acid. Other very prominent inclusion bodies, found in the cytoplasm of cells infected with fowlpox, ectromelia, and cowpox viruses, are acidophilic and consist of an accumulation of one particular viral protein; such inclusions may or may not also contain numerous mature virions. In a few instances, for example, adenoviruses in the nucleus and reoviruses in the cytoplasm, electron microscopy shows that inclusion bodies are

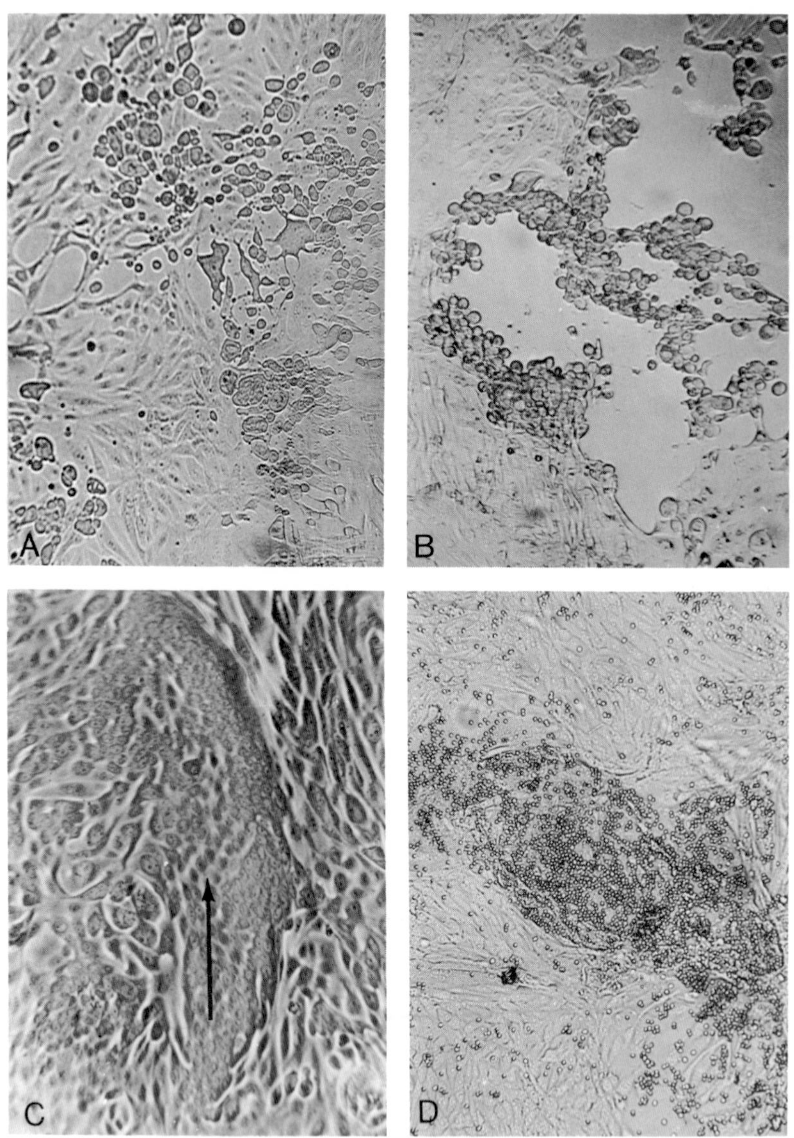

FIG. 5-2. *Cytopathic effects produced by different viruses. The cell monolayers are shown as they would normally be viewed in the laboratory, unfixed and unstained. Magnification: ×45. (A) Enterovirus: rapid rounding of cells, progressing to complete cell lysis. (B) Herpesvirus: focal areas of swollen, rounded cells. (C) Paramyxovirus: focal areas of cells are fused to form syncytia. (D) Hemadsorption: erythrocytes adsorb to infected cells that incorporate hemagglutinin into the plasma membrane. (Courtesy I. Jack.)*

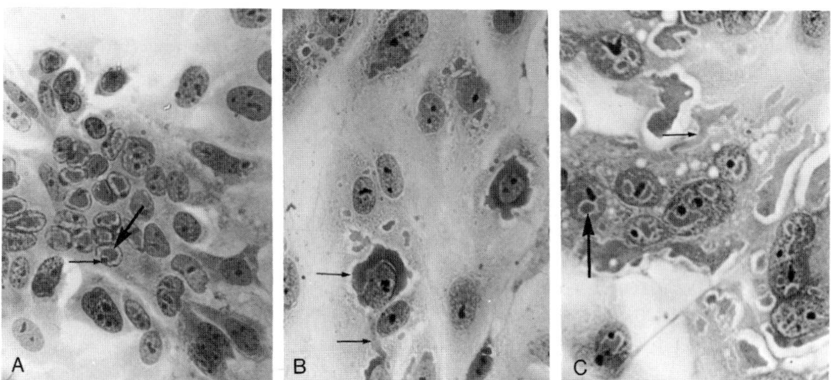

FIG. 5-3. *Types of viral inclusion bodies (hematoxylin and eosin stain). Magnification: ×200. (A) Intranuclear inclusions and syncytium (herpesvirus). Small arrow, nucleolus; large arrow, inclusion body. Note margination of chromatin, separated from the inclusion body by a halo. (B) Intracytoplasmic inclusions (reovirus). Arrows indicate inclusion bodies in perinuclear locations. (C) Intranuclear and intracytoplasmic inclusions and syncytia (morbilliviruses). Small arrow, intracytoplasmic inclusion body; large arrow, intranuclear inclusion body. (Courtesy I. Jack).*

aggregates of virions. Other nuclear inclusion bodies, such as those found in cells infected with herpesviruses, are the result of late degenerative changes and condensation and margination of chromatin, and they are made obvious by the presence of an unstained halo which is a shrinkage artifact produced by fixation.

Effects of Viruses on Plasma Membrane

In the course of their replication, viruses belonging to several families cause changes in the plasma membrane of the cell by insertion of viral glycoproteins. As discussed in Chapter 3, viral glycoproteins are not inserted at random in the plasma membrane. Viruses that mature at the apical surface of glandular epithelial cells are shed into the environment, whereas those maturing at the basolateral surface move to other sites in the body, sometimes entering the bloodstream and establishing systemic infection. For example, wild-type Sendai virus, which causes a localized respiratory infection, buds apically, whereas a pantropic variant buds basolaterally.

Viral glycoproteins inserted into the plasma membrane may produce cell fusion and/or allow hemadsorption. In addition, virus-coded antigens in the plasma membrane constitute a target for specific immune mechanisms, both humoral and cellular, which may result in lysis of the cell before significant numbers of new virions are produced, thus slowing the progress of infection and hastening recovery. In some cases the immune response may precipitate immunopathologic disease. Some viral antigens incorporated in the cell membrane, found in cells that are transformed by viruses (see Chapter 11), behave as *tumor-associated transplantation antigens.*

Cell Fusion. A conspicuous feature of the infection of cell monolayers by lentiviruses, paramyxoviruses, some herpesviruses, and some other viruses is the production of syncytia, also called *polykaryocytes* or giant cells (see Figs. 5-2C and 5-3C), which result from the fusion of the infected cell with neighboring infected or uninfected cells. Such syncytia are often seen in the tissues of animals infected with these viruses.

At high multiplicity of infection, paramyxoviruses may cause rapid fusion of cultured cells, as a consequence of adsorption of input virus to the plasma membrane. Cell biologists have used this phenomenon to produce functional heterokaryons by fusing different types of cells. For example, in the pioneering experiments by Milstein and Kohler that produced the first *monoclonal antibodies,* UV-inactivated parainfluenza virus was used to produce *hybridoma* cells by fusion of antibody-producing B lymphocytes with non-antibody-producing myeloma cells.

Hemadsorption by Virus-Infected Cells. Cells in monolayer culture infected with orthomyxoviruses, paramyxoviruses, and togaviruses, all of which bud from the plasma membrane, acquire the ability to adsorb erythrocytes. This phenomenon, known as *hemadsorption* (see Fig. 5-2D), is due to the incorporation into the plasma membrane of viral glycoproteins assembled into peplomers. On the envelope of the virion, the same glycoprotein peplomers are responsible for *hemagglutination.* Hemadsorption and hemagglutination can be used to demonstrate infection with noncytopathogenic as well as cytocidal viruses, and they can be demonstrated quite early in the replication cycle. The technique is used in the diagnosis of diseases caused by these viruses (see Chapter 12). Hemadsorption–inhibition assays, in which infected cells are first exposed to antibody, can also be used.

Effects of Viruses on Cytoskeleton

Infection by many viruses leads to a disruption of cytoskeletal fiber systems by a depolymerization of microfilaments and/or microtubules. On the other hand, the cytoplasmic cytoskeleton and the nuclear matrix, which provide the physical site for many metabolic activities of the cell, are also used for the subcellular compartmentalization of viral replicative processes.

Other Histologic Changes in Virus-Infected Cells

In addition to changes directly attributable to viral replication, most virus-infected cells also show nonspecific changes, very much like those induced by physical or chemical insults. The most common early and potentially reversible change is what pathologists call "cloudy swelling"; this change is associated with increasing permeability of the plasma membrane. Electron microscopic study of such cells reveals diffuse swelling of the nucleus, distention of the endoplasmic reticulum and mitochondria, and rarefaction of the cytoplasm. Later in the course of many viral infections the nucleus becomes condensed and shrunken and cytoplasmic density increases. Cell destruction can be the consequence of further loss of osmotic integrity and leakage of lysosomal enzymes into the cytoplasm. This progression, overall, is called by pathologists "the common terminal pathway to cell death."

As seen with the electron microscope, these specific and nonspecific changes in virus-infected cells are dramatic and varied. Early changes in cell structure often involve proliferation of various components of the cell; for example, herpesviruses cause increased synthesis of the nuclear membranes, flaviviruses cause proliferation of endoplasmic reticulum, picornaviruses and caliciviruses cause a distinctive synthesis of microvesicles in the cytoplasm, and many retroviruses cause peculiar fusions of cytoplasmic membranes. Later in the course of infection, many lytic viruses cause nuclear, organelle, and cytoplasmic disintegration and/or condensation, with terminal loss of cell membrane integrity. In many cases the inevitability of cell death is obvious, but in other cases host cell functional loss is subtle and cannot be associated easily with particular ultrastructural pathologic changes. In nonlytic infections most functional losses cannot be easily attributable to damage that is morphologically evident. Specific examples reflecting the range of host cell changes occurring in virus-infected cells are included in many of the chapters in Part II.

MECHANISMS OF CELL DAMAGE

The genomes of viruses vary greatly in size, and those of the larger viruses encode many proteins that have a variety of efects (Table 5-2). Some of the proteins encoded by viral genomes are essential for viral replication; others affect cellular genes and are responsible for the morphological changes just described.

So many biochemical changes occur in cells infected with cytocidal viruses that the eventual death of the cell cannot readily be ascribed to

TABLE 5-2

Viral Proteins That Contribute to Pathogenesis by Affecting Host Responses

Structural proteins of the virion, e.g., adenovirus penton and fiber proteins
Proteins down-regulating expression of cellular genes
Transactivators, which up-regulate expression of certain cellular genes
Oncogene products, e.g., growth factors or inactivators of cellular tumor suppressor proteins, which up-regulate the cell[a]
Proteins influencing viral virulence, host range, tissue tropism, etc.
Virokines,[b] which act on noninfected cells to influence the progress of infection in the body as a whole, e.g., by:
Negating the effects of interferons, tumor necrosis factor, etc.
Reducing the inflammatory response, complement activation, etc.
Subverting the immune response, e.g., by reducing MHC proteins on infected cell surfaces

[a] Oncogenic viruses (see Chapter 11).

[b] Recorded so far mainly in the more complex DNA viruses (poxviruses, herpesviruses, adenoviruses) but may be more widespread (see Chapter 7).

one particular event; rather it will be a consequence of the cumulative action of several such insults. Cell damage by certain viruses can occur even without replication of the virus, for example, when late stages of the expression of the viral genome are blocked experimentally or in certain natural abortive infections.

Interactions with Cellular Transcription Mechanisms

Especially with viruses that use host cell polymerase II to synthesize viral mRNA, specific mechanisms are sometimes found that alter host cell transcription so as to promote the synthesis of viral mRNA. Thus, infection with most DNA viruses inhibits transcription of cellular protein-coding genes by RNA polymerase II, thus decreasing competition for nucleotide precursors. A similar inhibition by some RNA viruses that do not use the host cell RNA polymerase presumably provides higher precursor pools in the cytoplasm for viral RNA synthesis.

A variety of mechanisms have been described whereby viral infection stimulates cellular RNA polymerase activity. For example, herpes simplex virus transcribes its five immediate early genes by releasing a virion tegument protein that binds to a host cell, sequence-specific DNA-binding protein; the virion–host cell protein complex binds to the five immediate early viral gene promoters containing the specific sequence. On the other hand, adenovirus infection increases the activity of host cell RNA polymerases via the E1A gene product, which increases the activity of several transcription factors, thus increasing the level of transcription of the viral genes.

Interactions with RNA Processing Pathways

The first evidence for RNA splicing, a common and important event in the production of eukaryotic cell mRNAs, came from studies with adenovirus mRNAs. Some viruses are able to regulate the assembly of splicing complexes or the processing pathway into which a transcript enters. Influenza virus uses a novel mechanism to promote viral transcription. Host cell nascent RNA transcripts are cleaved by a viral endonuclease, and the capped 5′ end of the host transcript is used for completing the synthesis of viral mRNA, a phenomenon described as "cap-snatching."

Interactions with Translational Apparatus

A number of mechanisms operate to inhibit host cell mRNA translation after viral infection, thus providing the viral mRNA with increased availability of ribosomal subunits, translation factors, tRNAs, and amino acid precursors. One such change seen after poliovirus infection is the replacement of cellular polyribosomes by a new class of very large polyribosomes produced by the binding of the 8-kb virion RNA to ribosomes.

Interactions with Cellular DNA Replication

Both RNA and DNA viruses inhibit host cell DNA synthesis, thus providing precursors and host cell structures or replication proteins for viral DNA synthesis. A variety of mechanisms operate. Inhibition of cellular DNA synthesis may be secondary to the inhibition of cellular protein synthesis. More specific mechanisms include the displacement of cellular DNA from its normal site of replication, seen with herpesviruses, the action of a poxvirus DNase on nuclear DNA, the insertion of viral proteins into the host cell replicase complex, and the redirection of the host cell DNA polymerase to replicate viral DNA.

With some viruses the viral DNA is stably maintained within the host cell, either integrated into the cellular DNA, as with retroviruses, or as an extrachromosomal element or episome, as with bovine papilloma virus. In both situations host cell genes operate to define the range of cells in which integration occurs or to control the episome copy number.

Shutdown of Cellular Protein Synthesis

Most cytocidal viruses code for proteins that shut down the synthesis of cellular proteins. The shutdown is particularly rapid and severe in infections of cultured cells by picornaviruses and some poxviruses and herpesviruses. With some other viruses (e.g., adenoviruses), the shutdown occurs later and is more gradual, whereas with noncytocidal viruses such as arenaviruses and retroviruses there is no shutdown and no cell death. Some viruses (e.g., flaviviruses) are cytocidal even though they do not shut down cellular protein synthesis very well.

The mechanisms are varied, and not all are clearly understood. In cases where the inhibition of cellular protein synthesis develops gradually and late in the replication cycle, it is possibly due to competition for ribosome subunits by the large excess of viral mRNA. When viral mRNA is not in excess, the shutdown may provide a selective advantage by allowing the viral message to bind to ribosomes and initiate translation. The adenovirus E1b protein inhibits the transport of cellular mRNAs from nucleus to cytoplasm, and the protease 2A protein of picornaviruses inactivates the cap-binding protein that is required for the binding of cellular mRNAs to ribosomes. As a final example, certain herpesviruses bring about selective degradation of cellular mRNA.

Cytopathic Effects of Viral Proteins

Large numbers of viral components accumulate in the cell late in the replication cycle. Some of these, particularly certain capsid proteins (e.g., adenovirus penton and fiber proteins), are toxic to cells. Viral proteins that are inserted into the plasma membrane may cause cell fusion, as well as providing a target for the immune response *in vivo*. Insertion of viral proteins into the plasma membrane can also change membrane permeability, leading directly to loss of osmotic integrity, cell swelling, and death.

NONCYTOCIDAL INFECTIONS

Noncytocidal viruses usually do not kill the cells in which they replicate, but often produce *persistent infection,* in which the infected cells produce and release virions but overall cellular metabolism is little affected, with the infected cells continuing to grow and divide. This type of cell–virus interaction is found in cells infected with several kinds of RNA viruses: arenaviruses, retroviruses, and some paramyxoviruses, for example, in all of which virions are released by budding from the plasma membrane. Although such virus-yielding cells may grow and divide in culture for long periods, there are slow, progressive changes that with some exceptions (e.g., some retroviruses) ultimately lead to cell death. In the intact animal, cell replacement occurs so rapidly in most organs and tissues that, at least in the short term, the slow fallout of cells due to persistent infection may have no effect on overall function. However, persistently infected differentiated cells may lose their capacity to carry out specialized functions, and if neurons are destroyed they are not replaced. Also, antigenic changes produced in the cell membrane of persistently infected cells provoke immune responses, which can rapidly lead to destruction of the infected cells and often nearby uninfected cells (see Chapter 9).

Effects on Functions of Specialized Cells

Although they do not immediately kill cells, infections with noncytocidal viruses often interfere with the specialized functions of differentiated cells. For example, lymphocytic choriomeningitis (LCM) virus replicating in somatotropic cells of the pituitary gland of the persistently infected mouse lowers the production of the mRNA for growth hormone in the infected cells, thus impeding the growth and development of the animal. Similarly, LCM virus replicating in β cells of the islets of Langerhans in the pancreas can induce hyperglycemia in the mouse, not dissimilar to insulin-dependent diabetes in man. β-Adrenergic receptors and opiate receptors are impaired in brain cells persistently infected with measles or rabies viruses. Viruses that infect lymphocytes may induce a generalized immunosuppression. Rhinovirus infection of the nasal epithelium results in cilial stasis and later the destruction of cilia, although the cells are often not killed. This effect can be demonstrated in organ culture (Fig. 5-4), and it is important in lowering the resistance of the respiratory tract to secondary bacterial infection.

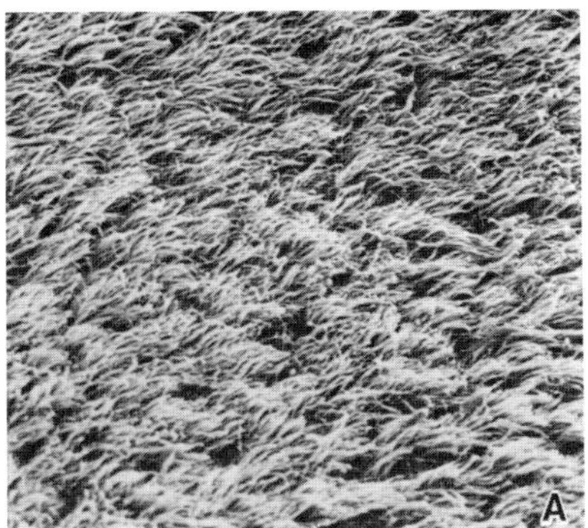

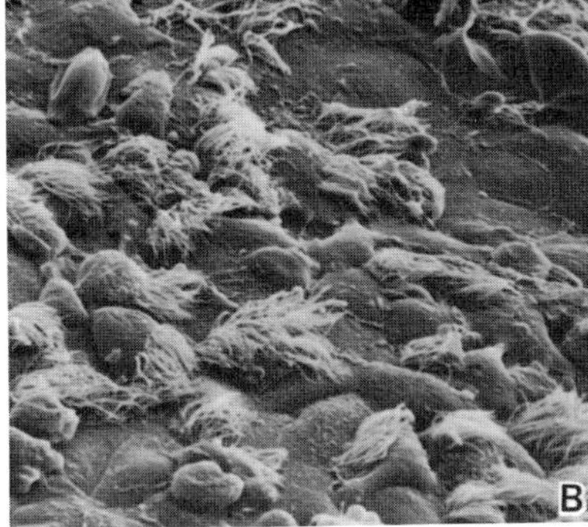

FIG. 5-4. *Effect of rhinovirus on bovine epithelium grown* in vitro *as an explant culture, as shown by scanning electron microscopy. (A) Normal appearance of ciliated cells. (B) Six days after infection many cells are rounded up or detached. [From S. E. Reed and A. Boyde,* Infect. Immun. **6,** *68 (1972).]*

INTERFERENCE AND INTERFERONS

Viral *interference* is said to occur when a virus-infected cell population resists superinfection with the same or a different virus. The interfering virus does not necessarily have to replicate to induce interference, and the ability of the challenge virus to replicate may be completely or only partially inhibited. Two main mechanisms have been demonstrated: (1) interference mediated by defective interfering mutants and operating only against the homologous virus (see Chapter 4) and (2) interference mediated by *interferon.*

Interferons

In 1957 Isaacs and Lindenmann found that cells of the chorioallantois of the embryonated hen's egg infected with influenza virus released into the medium a nonviral protein which protected uninfected cells against infection with the same or unrelated viruses. This discovery encouraged the view that safe, nontoxic specific antiviral agents could be developed. Despite an enormous amount of work on this group of proteins, the availability of interferon as a therapeutic agent for the treatment of virus diseases of man and domestic animals remains an unfulfilled dream. The discovery in the early 1980s that interferon had anticancer effects stimulated further research which showed that the interferons were typical members of a large family of normal cellular regulatory proteins called *cytokines.* Much work has been done on human and mouse interferons, and we now know that in these species there are more than a dozen interferons, falling into three chemically distinct types, known as interferon α, interferon β, and interferon γ. All mammalian species have complex families of genes encoding different subtypes of interferon α and one interferon β gene, but cattle, horses, and pigs have multiple interferon β genes. Nonmammalian vertebrates have interferon β genes but no interferon α genes.

The 1980s witnessed the discovery and cloning by recombinant DNA technology of the genes for several human and bovine interferons, and the corresponding proteins have been purified. Interferons β and γ, but generally not α, are glycosylated, and most of the human interferons occur as multimers of a monomer of M_r about 20,000.

Interferons α and β are not made constitutively in significant amounts, but their synthesis is induced by virus infection—any virus, multiplying in virtually any type of cell, in any vertebrate species. Interferon γ is made only by T lymphocytes and only following antigen-specific or mitogenic stimulation; it is a *lymphokine,* with immunoregulatory functions. Some interferons, especially β and γ, display a certain degree of host species specificity; for instance, mouse interferons are ineffective in humans and vice versa. However, there is no viral specificity, in that interferon α, β, or γ induced by, say, a paramyxovirus is fully effective against a togavirus, but certain cloned interferon subtypes may be much more effective against some viruses than against others.

Antiviral Action of Interferons

Following its induction by viral infection, interferon is released from the infected cell and binds to a specific receptor on the plasma membrane of other cells. There appears to be a common receptor for interferon α and β, and another for interferon γ. Binding triggers a cascade of biochemical events. The ligand–receptor complex is internalized by endocytosis, and a cytoplasmic DNA-binding protein known as E factor becomes activated and migrates to the nucleus, where it binds to a 14-base pair nucleotide consensus motif which is present in the 5′-regulatory region of most interferon-inducible genes. These events up-regulate the expression of over 20 other cellular genes. Many of the induced protein products directly or indirectly inhibit the replication of virus, each in a different way. Furthermore, it has recently become apparent that, although the interferon-treated cell becomes resistant to most or all viruses, individual interferon-induced proteins are effective only against a limited range of viruses. Two well-studied examples illustrate the range of possibilities.

P1 Kinase. The P1 protein kinase, which is made constitutively at low levels in untreated cells, is up-regulated by interferon α, β, or γ. Its induction is mediated by dsRNA, which is an intermediate or by-product formed in the course of RNA virus replication. Following induction, P1 kinase first phosphorylates itself, then the initiation factor eIF-2, inactivating it. Because eIF-2 is required to initiate synthesis of all polypeptides, interferon-induced P1 kinase can inhibit synthesis of all proteins of any virus.

Many viruses, however, have developed strategies for circumventing this universal antiviral defense mechanism. For example, adenoviruses encode low-M_r RNAs which bind to P1 kinase, preventing its activation. Reoviruses, which might be expected to be exceptionally susceptible to interferons because they have a dsRNA genome, are not, because their capsid protein $\sigma 3$ binds much more strongly to its own dsRNA than does P1 kinase, and influenza virus infection activates a cellular regulator that inhibits the induction of P1 kinase.

2-5A Synthetase. The enzyme 2-5A synthetase, which also requires dsRNA for its induction, catalyzes the synthesis from ATP of an unusual family of short-lived oligonucleotides known as (2′–5′)pppA(pA)$_n$, or 2-

5A for short. In turn, 2-5A activates a cellular endonuclease, RNase L, which destroys mRNA, thereby inhibiting host cell protein synthesis. The 2-5A synthetase/RNase L system is known to be effective against picornaviruses, but its wider relevance has yet to be established.

Mx Protein. A team of Swiss virologists has conducted elegant studies on a family of GTP-binding proteins known as Mx proteins which are induced by interferon α and β and determine the susceptibility of mice to influenza virus infection. Only strains of mice carrying the Mx gene survived challenge with influenza virus; congenic mice with a deletion mutation in the Mx gene died. Dual fluorescent antibody staining of infected tissues revealed that the circle of uninfected cells surrounding a zone of virus-infected cells was synthesizing large amounts of Mx protein that had diffused out from the infected locus. Interferon itself, in the absence of virus infection, similarly induced production of the Mx protein, *in vitro* or *in vivo*. Transfection of cultured Mx^- cell lines with the Mx gene converted them permanently to a state of resistance to influenza virus. Finally, transgenic mice produced by transfecting the Mx gene into Mx^-, influenza-susceptible mice were shown to be resistant to challenge with influenza virus (but not other viruses) and to make the Mx protein following infection with influenza virus or the administration of interferon.

Interferons as Cytokines

Interferons were discovered as antiviral agents, defined accordingly, and generally regarded as such by virologists for many years. However, interferons exert a wide range of other effects on cells, acting as cytokines which bind to specific receptors on the cell surface and initiate a cascade of events including inhibition of cell division, changes in the plasma membrane, and modulation of the immune system.

Role of Interferons in Recovery from Viral Infection

Most cells in the body are capable of producing interferons in response to viral infection; interferons can be found in the mucus bathing epithelial surfaces and are produced by most cells of mesenchymal origin. Lymphocytes, especially T cells and *natural killer (NK) cells,* as well as macrophages, produce large amounts of interferon α and γ, and these cells probably constitute the principle source of circulating interferon in systemic viral infections. Further information on the role of interferons in recovery from viral infections is presented in Chapter 7.

FURTHER READING

Carrasco, L. (1987). "Mechanisms of Viral Toxicity in Animal Cells." CRC Press, Boca Raton, Florida.

de Maeyer, E., and de Maeyer-Guignard, J. (1988). "Interferons and Other Regulatory Cytokines." Wiley, New York.

Fraenkel-Conrat, H., and Wagner, R. R., eds. (1984). Viral cytopathology. "Comprehensive Virology," Vol. 19, Plenum, New York.

Kaariainen, L., and Ranki, M. (1984). Inhibition of cell functions by RNA-virus infections. *Annu. Rev. Microbiol.* **38,** 91.

Kozak, M. (1986). Regulation of protein synthesis in virus-infected animal cells. *Adv. Virus Res.* **31,** 229.

Moller, G., ed. (1987). Gamma interferon. *Immunol. Rev.* **97.**

Oldstone, M. B. A. (1984). Virus can alter cell function without causing cell pathology: Disordered function leads to imbalance of homeostasis and disease. *In* "Concepts in Viral Pathogenesis I" (A. L. Notkins and M. B. A. Oldstone, eds.), p. 269. Springer-Verlag, New York.

Pestka, S., Langer, J. A., Zoon, K. C., and Samuel, C. E. (1987). Interferons and their actions. *Annu. Rev. Biochem.* **56,** 727.

Russell, W. C., and Almond, J. W., eds. (1987). "Molecular Basis of Virus Disease." *Soc. Gen. Microbiol. Symp.* **40,** Cambridge Univ. Press, London and New York.

Schneider, R. J., and Shenk, T. (1987). Impact of virus infection on host cell protein synthesis. *Annu. Rev. Biochem.* **56,** 317.

Schrom, M., and Bablanian, R. (1981). Altered cellular morphology resulting from cytocidal virus infection. *Arch. Virol.* **70,** 173.

Staeheli, P. (1990). Interferon-induced proteins and the antiviral state. *Adv. Virus Res.* **38,** 147.

CHAPTER 6

Mechanisms of Infection and Viral Spread through the Body

Although viruses replicate quite differently from unicellular microorganisms, this distinction disappears to some extent if viruses are considered at the levels of the whole animal and animal populations. To cause infection, viruses, like other infectious agents, must gain entry to the body, multiply, and spread, either locally or systemically, and in systemic infections localize in the appropriate target organ. To be maintained in nature, infectious virions must be shed across a body surface (so that infection of other animals can occur by direct contact or from the environment), or be taken up directly from the blood by an arthropod vector or a needle, or be passed congenitally.

ROUTES OF ENTRY

To infect its host, a virus must first infect cells of one of the body surfaces, or the body surface may be bypassed via parenteral inoculation, by either a wound, needle, or the bite of an arthropod or vertebrate. The major routes of infection are summarized in Fig. 6-1, in which the body is represented as a set of surfaces, each of which consists of a sheet of

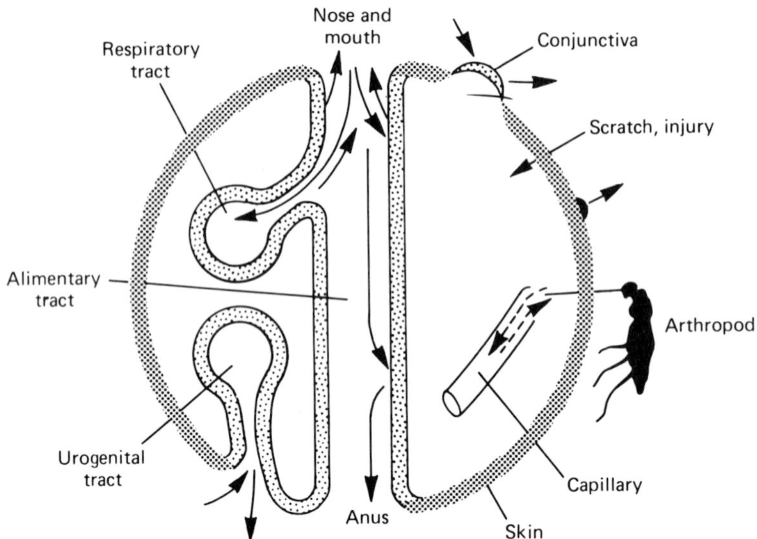

FIG. 6-1. *Surfaces of the body in relation to the entry and shedding of viruses. (Modified from C. A. Mims and D. O. White, "Viral Pathogenesis and Immunology." Blackwell, Oxford, 1984.)*

epithelial cells that separates the internal tissues of the host from the outside world.

Skin

The skin is the largest organ in the body, and since its outer layer consists of keratinized cells it provides a tough and usually impermeable barrier to the entry of viruses. However, after entry through minor abrasions or by artifical puncture, some viruses replicate in the skin to produce local lesions, for example, cowpox, orf and fowlpox viruses, many herpesviruses, and the papillomaviruses (Table 6-1). The most efficient way by which viruses are introduced through the skin is by the bite of an arthropod vector, such as a mosquito, tick, sandfly, or midge. Such insects may be mechanical vectors (e.g., for myxomatosis and fowlpox viruses), but most viruses introduced in this way replicate in the vector. Viruses that are transmitted by and replicate in arthropod vectors are called arboviruses. Infection can be acquired through the bite of an animal, as in rabies. Finally, introduction of a virus by skin penetration may be *iatrogenic,* or by the hand of veterinarian, for example, transmission of equine infectious anemia virus by a contaminated needle or orf or papillomavirus by ear tagging or tattooing. Generalized infection of the skin, producing an exanthem such as is found in lumpyskin disease,

TABLE 6-1
Example of Viruses That Initiate Infection of Skin, Oral Mucosa, Genital Tract, or Eye

Route	Family or genus	Viruses
Minor abrasion (skin or oral mucosa)	*Papillomavirus*	All species
	Herpesviridae	All species
	Poxviridae	Cowpox, swinepox, orf, bovine papular stomatitis, pseudo-cowpox, fowlpox viruses
	Picornaviridae	Swine vesicular disease virus
	Rhabdoviridae	Vesicular stomatitis virus
Arthropod bite		
Mechanical	*Poxviridae*	Fowlpox, swinepox, myxoma viruses
	Rhabdoviridae	Vesicular stomatitis virus
	Retroviridae	Equine infectious anemia virus
Biological	Unclassified	African swine fever virus
	Alphavirus	All species
	Flaviviridae	Many species
	Rhabdoviridae	Bovine ephemeral fever, vesicular stomatitis viruses
	Bunyaviridae	Rift Valley fever, Nairobi sheep disease viruses
	Orbivirus	Bluetongue, African horse sickness viruses
Bite of vertebrate	*Rhabdoviridae*	Rabies virus
	Retroviridae	Feline immunodeficiency virus
Contaminated needle or equipment	All viruses causing systemic infection, e.g.,	
	Papillomavirus	All species
	Togaviridae	Hog cholera, bovine virus diarrhea viruses
	Retroviridae	Equine infectious anemia, bovine leukemia viruses
Genital tract	*Papillomavirus*	Bovine papilloma virus
	Herpesviridae	Many species
	Togaviridae	Equine arteritis virus
Conjunctiva	*Herpesviridae*	Infectious bovine rhinotracheitis virus, equine herpesvirus 1
	Adenoviridae	Canine herpesviruses 1 and 2

sheeppox, and swine vesicular disease, for example, is due to viral spread via the bloodstream.

Respiratory Tract

Although lined by cells that are susceptible to infection by many viruses, the respiratory tract is ordinarily protected by effective cleansing mechanisms. A mucus blanket and ciliated cells line the upper and much of the lower respiratory tract. Inhaled virions deposited on these surfaces are trapped in mucus, carried by ciliary action to the pharynx, and then swallowed or coughed out. Particles 10 μm or more in diameter are usually trapped on the nasal mucosa. Particles 5–10 μm in diameter are often carried to the trachea and bronchioles, where they are usually trapped in the mucus blanket. Particles of 5 μm or less are often inhaled directly into the lungs, and some may reach the alveoli. In the lungs viruses may be destroyed by alveolar macrophages, or they may infect alveolar epithelial cells.

Despite these protective mechanisms, the respiratory tract is, overall, the most common portal of entry of viruses into the body (Table 6-2). All viruses that infect the host via the respiratory tract probably do so by attaching to specific receptors on epithelial cells. Following respiratory infection, many viruses remain localized, for instance, rhinoviruses, adenoviruses, and influenza virus in mammals, while others become systemic, for example, foot-and-mouth disease, canine distemper, rinderpest, hog cholera, and Newcastle disease viruses.

Oropharynx and Intestinal Tract

Many viruses are acquired by ingestion. They may either be swallowed directly or infect cells in the oropharynx and then be carried to the intestinal tract. The esophagus is rarely infected, probably because of its

TABLE 6-2
Viruses of Animals That Initiate Infection of Respiratory Tract

Family	Viruses
Producing respiratory disease	
Adenoviridae	Most species
Herpesviridae	Most species
Picornaviridae	Rhinoviruses, aphthoviruses
Caliciviridae	Feline calicivirus
Coronaviridae	Infectious bronchitis virus of chickens
Paramyxoviridae	Parainfluenza, respiratory syncytial viruses
Orthomyxoviridae	Influenza viruses of swine and horses
Producing systemic disease, usually without initial respiratory signs	
Parvoviridae	Feline panleukopenia virus, canine parvovirus
Herpesviridae	Pseudorabies, bovine malignant catarrhal fever, Marek's disease viruses
Togaviridae	Hog cholera virus
Paramyxoviridae	Canine distemper, rinderpest viruses
Orthomyxoviridae	Fowl plague virus
Arenaviridae	Lymphocytic choriomeningitis virus

tough stratified squamous epithelium and the rapid passage of swallowed material over its surface. The intestinal tract is partially protected by mucus, which may contain specific secretory antibodies (IgA), but the constant movement of its contents provides opportunities for virions to attach to specific receptors. Virions may also be taken up by specialized M cells that overlie Peyer's patches in the ileum, from where they may be passed to adjacent mononuclear cells in which they may replicate.

There are other protective substances in the intestinal tract: from the stomach caudally, acid, bile, and proteolytic enzymes may destroy viruses. In general, viruses that cause intestinal infection, such as enteroviruses, rotaviruses, caliciviruses, and parvoviruses (Table 6-3), are acid- and bile-resistant. However, there are examples of acid- and bile-labile viruses that cause important intestinal infections; for example, bovine, porcine, and murine coronaviruses are protected during passage through the stomach of young animals by the buffering capacity of milk.

Coronaviruses, rotaviruses, parvoviruses, and certain unclassified small RNA viruses are now recognized as the major causes of viral diarrhea; the majority of intestinal infections caused by enteroviruses and adenoviruses are asymptomatic. Some enteroviruses (e.g., porcine, avian, and murine encephalomyelitis viruses) are important causes of generalized infection but do not produce signs referable to the intestinal tract. Parvoviruses cause diarrhea after reaching cells of the intestinal tract via viremic spread.

Infection by Other Routes

The genital tract is the route of entry of several important pathogens, for example, bovine herpesvirus 1, equine herpesvirus 3, and porcine

TABLE 6-3

Viruses of Animals That Intitiate Infection of Intestinal Tract

Family/Genus	Viruses
Producing diarrhea	
Coronaviridae	Some coronaviruses
Toroviridae	Breda and Bern viruses
Pestivirus	Bovine virus diarrhea virus
Reoviridae	Rotaviruses
Unclassified	Astroviruses
Producing systemic disease, usually without diarrhea	
Adenoviridae	Some adenoviruses
Caliciviridae	Vesicular exanthema of swine virus
Picornaviridae	Some enteroviruses

papillomavirus. The conjunctiva, although much less resistant to viral invasion than the skin, is constantly cleansed by the flow of secretion (tears) and is wiped by the eyelids. The conjunctiva may be infected locally and may sometimes be a portal of entry for systemic infections; experimentally, infection with a wide range of viruses can be achieved via this route.

HOST SPECIFICITY AND TISSUE TROPISMS

All viruses exhibit some degree of host and tissue specificity. The first requirement for infection of a cell is a correspondence between viral attachment molecules (ligands) and cellular receptors. Following penetration and uncoating, viral replication may be dependent on the activity of regulatory elements in the viral genome: enhancers, promoters, and transcriptional activators, as well as factors that govern the permissiveness of the cell for complete viral replication.

Receptors

At the level of the individual virion and the cell, infection is preceded by an interaction between viral surface proteins containing appropriate ligands and specific receptors on the plasa membrane of the susceptible cell (see Table 3-2). Although ligand–receptor interactions are simplest to study in cultured cells, the results so obtained may not reflect the situation *in vivo*. For example, human amnion cells do not become susceptible to poliovirus until they have been cultivated for some 7 days *in vitro*. If the receptors are removed, as, for example, by treating mice with neuraminidase intranasally, there is substantial protection against intranasal infection with influenza virus until the receptors regenerate. Receptors for particular viruses are frequently restricted to certain types of cells; infection occurs only in these cells, thus accounting for both the cell and organ tropism of the virus and accordingly its pathogenic action.

Viral Enhancers

Enhancers are short sequences of nucleotides, often repeated in tandem, that increase transcription from other genes on the same DNA molecule, perhaps by serving as a binding site for the cellular RNA polymerase II, and thus regulate transcription in a cell- or tissue-specific fashion. The DNA of papillomaviruses contains an enhancer that is specifically active only in keratinocytes, and indeed only in a subset of these cells. Further evidence for the tissue specificity of papovavirus enhancers comes from studies of transgenic mice containing the early gene region of JC papovavirus, a common human virus which very occasionally causes the neurologic disease progressive multifocal leukoencephalopathy. The offspring of transgenic mice with early genes from the JC virus develop a neurologic disease characterized pathologically by dysfunction of myelin-producing oligodendrogliacytes which mimics the naturally occurring disease.

Enhancer regions have also been defined in the genomes of retroviruses, several herpesviruses, and hepatitis B virus, all of which appear to influence the tropism of the relevant viruses by regulating the expression of viral genes in specific types of cells. For example, certain strains of avian leukosis virus induce lymphomas, whereas other strains produce osteoporosis. The disease pattern appears to be determined by enhancer regions in the LTR region of the viral genome, although non-LTR sequences may also play a role.

MECHANISMS OF SPREAD IN THE BODY

Viruses may remain localized in cells of the body surface through which they entered: skin, respiratory tract, intestine, genital tract, or conjunctiva. Alternatively, they may cause generalized infections, which are usually associated with lymphatic spread and viremia and subsequent localization in particular organs.

Local Spread on Epithelial Surfaces

Many viruses replicate in epithelial cells at the site of entry, produce a localized or spreading infection in the epithelium, and are then shed directly into the environment. Infection spreads by sequential infection of neighboring cells. In the skin, papillomaviruses initiate infection in the basal layer of the epidermis, but maturation, with the production of virions, occurs only when the cells become keratinized as they move toward the skin surface. Many poxviruses produce infection via the skin, but in addition to spreading from cell to cell, there is also local subepithelial and lymphatic spread.

Viruses that enter the body via the mouth or respiratory tract can spread rapidly in the layer of fluid on these moist epithelial surfaces. After infections of the mammalian respiratory tract by paramyxoviruses and influenza virus, or the intestinal tract by rotaviruses or coronaviruses, there is little or no invasion of subepithelial tissues. Although these viruses usually enter lymphatics and thus have the potential to spread, they do not appear to replicate in deeper tissues, possibly because appropriate virus receptors or other permissive cellular factors, such as cleavage-activating proteases, are restricted to epithelial cells or because the temperature of deeper tissues is higher than the optimal temperature for viral replication.

Restriction of infection to an epithelial surface cannot be equated with lack of severity of clinical disease. Large areas of intestinal epithelium may be damaged by rotaviruses and coronaviruses, for example, causing severe diarrhea. The severity of localized infections of the upper respiratory tract depends on their location: infections of the upper respiratory tract may produce severe rhinitis but few other signs, infection of the bronchioles or alveoli produces more severe respiratory distress, and viral infections of both the upper and lower respiratory tract may predispose to secondary bacterial invasion.

Subepithelial Invasion and Lymphatic Spread

After traversing the epithelium and its basement membrane to reach the subepithelial tissues, virions are immediately exposed to tissue macrophages and can enter the lymphatics that form a network beneath the skin and all mucosal epithelia (Fig. 6-2). Virions that enter lymphatics

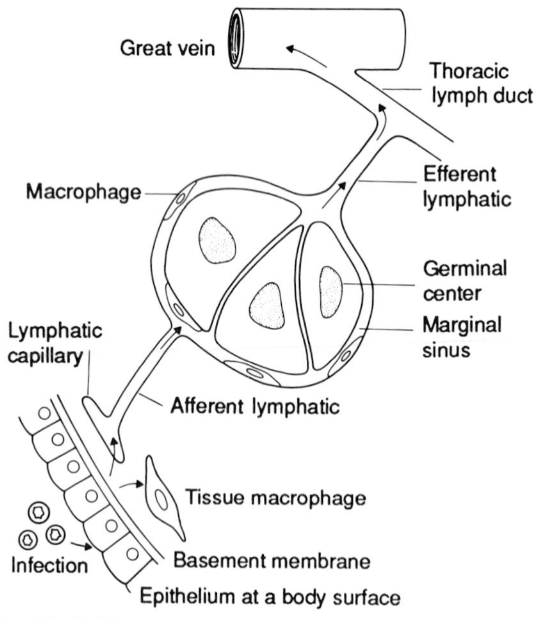

FIG. 6-2. *Subepithelial invasion and lymphatic spread of viruses. (From C. A. Mims and D. O. White, "Viral Pathogenesis and Immunology," Blackwell, Oxford, 1984.)*

are carried to local lymph nodes. As they enter, they are exposed to macrophages and may be engulfed. Such virions may be inactivated and processed and their component antigens (epitopes) presented to lymphocytes in such a way that an immune response is initiated (see Chapter 8). Some viruses, however, replicate in macrophages (e.g., many retroviruses, canine distemper virus, some adenoviruses, and some herpesviruses); others infect lymphocytes or dendritic cells. Some virions may pass straight through lymph nodes to enter the bloodstream. Monocytes and lymphocytes circulate through the body, and there is a constant movement of lymphocytes directly from the blood into the lymph nodes.

There is often a local inflammatory response, the extent of which depends on the extent of tissue damage. Local blood vessels are dilated and rendered more permeable, so that monocytes and lymphocytes, lymphokines, immunoglobulins, and complement components can be delivered directly to the site of infection, with a consequent increase in host resistance, especially after the immune response has been initiated.

Spread by the Bloodstream: Viremia

The blood is the most effective and rapid vehicle for the spread of virus through the body. Once a virus has reached the bloodstream, usually via the lymphatic system (Fig. 6-2), it can localize in any part of the body within minutes. The first entry of virus into the blood is called primary viremia. This early viremia may be clinically silent, known to have taken place only because of the invasion of distant organs. Further virus replication leads to the sustained liberation of much higher concentrations of virus, producing a later secondary viremia (Fig. 6-3), which can in turn lead to the establishment of infection in yet other parts of the body.

In the blood, virions may be free in the plasma or may be associated with leukocytes, platelets, or erythrocytes. Viruses carried in leukocytes, generally lymphocytes or monocytes, are not cleared so readily or in the same way as viruses circulating free in the plasma. Being protected from antibodies and other plasma components, they can be carried to distant tissues. Monocyte-associated viremia is a feature of canine distemper, bluetongue, feline leukemia, and beta- and gammaherpesvirus infections, and lymphocyte-associated viremia is a feature of Marek's disease, LCM, and feline immunodeficiency virus infections. Rarely, as in African swine fever and bluetongue, virions may be associated with erythrocytes. Certain mouse leukemia viruses infect megakaryocytes; the circulating platelets derived from them are infected, but they do not appear to be important in the pathogenesis of viral infections. Neutrophils have a very short life span and powerful antimicrobial mechanisms; they are rarely infected, although they may contain phagocytosed virions. Par-

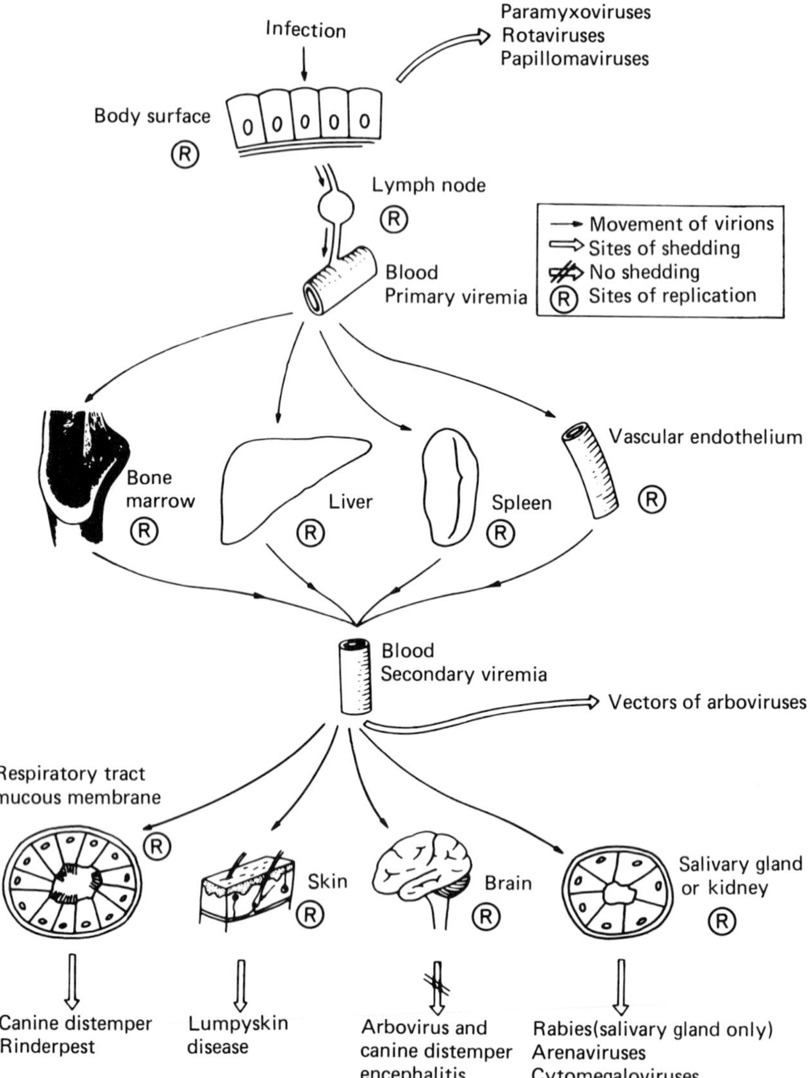

FIG. 6-3. *Spread of virions through the body, indicating sites of replication and important routes of shedding of various viruses. (Modified from C. A. Mims and D. O. White, "Viral Pathogenesis and Immunology." Blackwell, Oxford, 1984.)*

voviruses, hepadnaviruses, enteroviruses, togaviruses, and flaviviruses circulate free in the plasma.

Virions circulating in the plasma encounter many kinds of cells, but two kinds play a special role in determining their subsequent fate: tissue macrophages and vascular endothelial cells.

Role of Macrophages. Macrophages are very efficient phagocytes and are present in all compartments of the body: in alveoli, subepithelial tissues, sinusoids of the lymph nodes, free in plasma, and above all in the sinusoids of the liver, spleen, and bone marrow. Together with dendritic cells and B lymphocytes, macrophages are antigen processing and presenting cells and therefore play a pivotal role in initiation of the primary immune response (see Chapter 8). A direct antiviral action of macrophages depends on the age of the host and the site of their origin in the body; indeed, even in a given site there are subpopulations of macrophages that differ in susceptibility. Their state of activation is also important. The kinds of interactions that may occur between macrophages and virions are described in relation to those found in the sinusoids of the liver, the Kupffer cells, in Fig. 6-4.

Differences in virus–macrophage interactions may account for differences in the virulence of virus strains and differences in host resistance. Besides being efficient phagocytes, macrophages have Fc and C3 receptors in their plasma membrane, which enhance their ability to ingest virions, especially when these are coated with antibody or complement. If macrophages are susceptible, however, as with the immunodeficiency retroviruses, this can lead to infection rather than inactivation, and the antibody may enhance rather than prevent infection.

Vascular Endothelial Cells. The vascular endothelium with its basement membrane and tight cell junctions constitutes the blood–tissue interface and, for particles such as virions, often a barrier. Parenchymal invasion by circulating virions depends on localization in the endothelial cells of capillaries and venules, where blood flow is slowest and the barrier thinnest. Virions may move passively between or through endothelial cells and basement membranes, or they may infect endothelial cells and "grow" through this barrier. This subject has been most intensively studied in relation to viral invasion of the central nervous system (see below), but it also applies to secondary invasion of the skin, pulmonary epithelium, salivary gland epithelium, intestinal epithelium, kidney, and placenta.

Maintenance of Viremia. Because virions circulating in the blood are continuously removed by macrophages, viremia can be maintained only if there is a continuing introduction of virus into the blood from infected

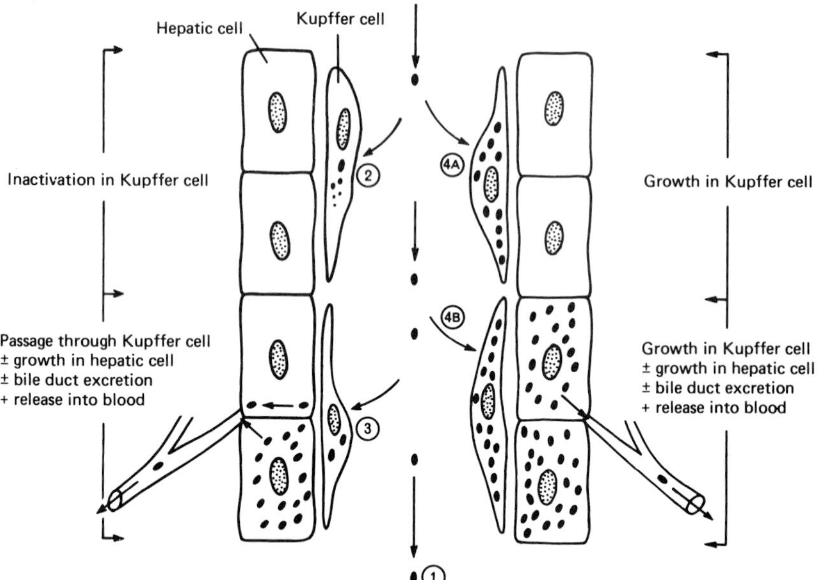

FIG. 6-4. *Types of interactions between viruses and macrophages, exemplified by the Kupffer cells lining a sinusoid in the liver. (1) Macrophages may fail to phagocytose virions; for example, in Venezuelan equine encephalitis virus infection this is an important factor favoring prolonged viremia. (2) Virions may be phagocytosed and destroyed. Because the macrophage system is so efficient, viremia with such viruses can be maintained only if virions enter the blood as fast as they are removed. (3) Virions may be phagocytosed and then passively transferred to adjacent cells (hepatocytes in the liver). If, like Rift Valley fever virus, the virus replicates in these cells it can cause clinical hepatitis, and the virus produced in the liver can sustain a high level of viremia. (4) Virions may be phagocytosed by macrophages and then replicate in them. With some viruses, such as lactate dehydrogenase virus in mice, only macrophages are infected (4A), and progeny virions enhance the viremia, which reaches an extremely high level. More commonly (4B), as in infectious canine hepatitis, virus replicates in both macrophages and hepatic cells, producing severe hepatitis. (Modified from C. A. Mims and D. O. White, ''Viral Pathogenesis and Immunology.'' Blackwell, Oxford, 1984).*

tissues, or if there is impairment of the macrophages. Circulating leukocytes can themselves constitute a site for viral replication, but viremia is usually maintained by infection of the parenchymal cells of target organs like the liver, spleen, lymph nodes, and bone marrow. In some infections, for example, hog cholera, the viremia is partly maintained by infection of endothelial cells. Striated and smooth muscle cells may be an important site of replication of some enteroviruses, togaviruses, and rhabdoviruses; virions are transferred to the blood via the lymph.

Invasion of Skin

As well as being a site of initial infection, the skin may be invaded via the bloodstream, producing erythema, which may be generalized but more often localized and readily seen on exposed, hairless, nonpigmented areas such as the snout, ears, paws, scrotum, and udder. Primary involvement of the epidermis or separation of epidermis from dermis by fluid pressure results in vesiculation. Erosion or sloughing of the epithelium results in ulceration and scabbing, but prior to ulceration a vesicle may be converted to a pustule by polymorphonuclear cell infiltration. More severe involvement of the dermal vessels may lead to petechial or hemorrhagic lesions, although coagulation defects and thrombocytopenia may also be important in the production of such lesions.

Invasion of Respiratory and Intestinal Tracts

The respiratory and intestinal tracts are usually infected directly by inspired or ingested virions. Sometimes viremic infections reach the respiratory epithelium, causing bronchitis and pneumonia; such infections, like airway-derived infections, may cause an interstitial pneumonia. Among intestinal infections, parvoviruses circulating in the blood infect the dividing intestinal epithelial cells in the crypts of Lieberkuhn, so that the epithelial cells that are continuously lost from the tips of the villi are not replaced.

Central Nervous System

Because of the critical physiologic importance of the central nervous system and its vulnerability to damage by any process that harms neurons directly or via increased intracranial pressure, viral invasion of the central nervous system is always a serious matter. Viruses can spread from the blood to the brain either after localizing in blood vessels in meninges and choroid plexus, with invasion of the neurons then occurring from the cerebrospinal fluid, or more directly after localizing in blood vessels of the brain and spinal cord (Fig. 6-5). Although the cerebral capillaries represent a morphological blood–brain barrier, most viruses that invade the central nervous system cross these vessels. Some viruses infect the vascular endothelial cells prior to infection of the cells of the brain parenchyma; others appear to be transported across the capillary walls without endothelial cell infection. Rarely, virus may be carried across capillary walls into the brain parenchyma via infected leukocytes. Subsequent spread in the central nervous system can take place via the cerebrospinal fluid or by sequential infection of neural cells.

Viruses, such as some enteroviruses, that cause meningitis rather than encephalitis may traverse the blood–cerebrospinal fluid junction in the

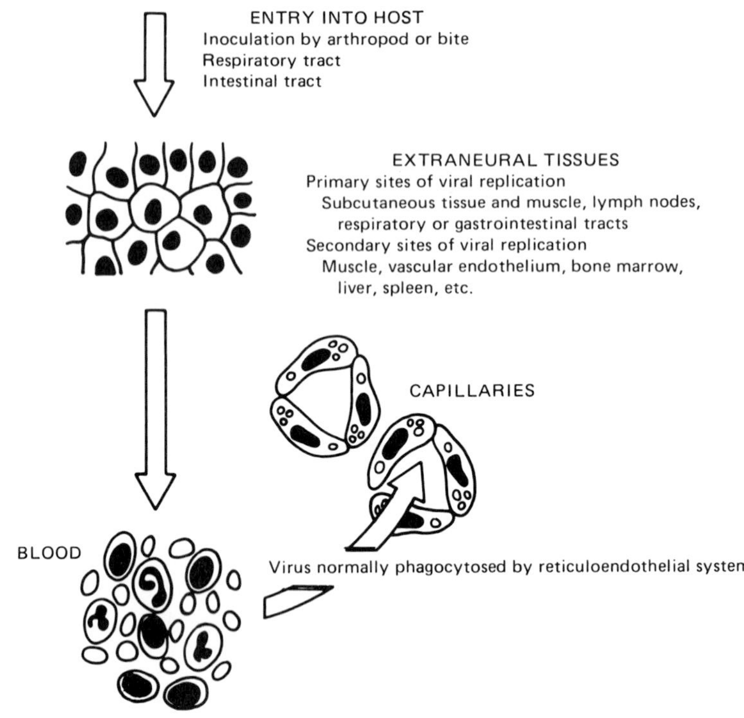

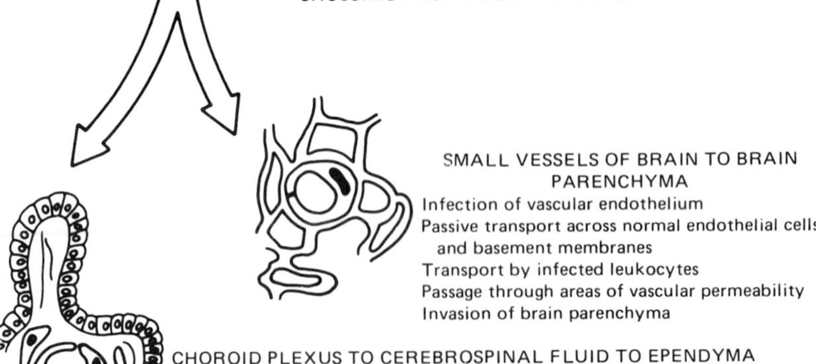

FIG. 6-5. *Steps in the hematogenous spread of virus into the central nervous system. (From R. T. Johnson, "Viral Infections of the Nervous System." Raven, New York, 1982.)*

meninges or may grow in the epithelium of the choroid plexus. Characteristically, they are found in the cerebrospinal fluid.

The other important route of infection of the central nervous system is via the peripheral nerves, as seen, for example, in rabies, herpes B virus encephalitis, pseudorabies, and bovine herpesvirus 1 encephalitis. Viruses may pass either centripetally from the body surface to the central nervous system or sensory ganglia, or centrifugally from the center to the periphery, as in the reactivation of bovine herpesvirus 1 in ganglia. The relevant subviral moieties travel quite slowly, at up to 10 mm per hour. Herpesvirus capsids travel to the central nervous system in axon cytoplasm, and while doing so also sequentially infect the Schwann cells of the nerve sheath. Rabies virus and Borna disease virus also travel to the central nervous system in axon cytoplasm, but they usually do not infect the nerve sheath. Sensory, motor, and autonomic nerves may be involved in the neural spread of these viruses. Rabies virus, Borna disease virus, and some togaviruses are able to use the olfactory nerve for movement to the central nervous system; they can infect olfactory neuroepithelial cells, which are exposed in the epithelium of the nares and have their axonal endings in the olfactory bulb of the brain.

Lytic infections of neurons, whether due to togaviruses, herpesviruses, or other viruses, lead to the three histologic hallmarks of encephalitis: neuronal necrosis, phagocytosis of neurons by microglial cells (neuronophagia), and perivascular infiltration by mononuclear cells (perivascular *cuffing*), the latter an immune response (see Chapter 8). The cause of clinical neurologic signs in other central nervous system infections is more obscure. Rabies virus infection is noncytocidal; it evokes little of the inflammatory reaction or cell necrosis found in many other viral encephalitides, yet it is highly lethal for most mammalian species. Still other pathologic changes are produced by some of the viruses that cause slowly progressive diseases of the central nervous system (see Chapter 10). In bovine spongiform encephalopathy and scrapie of sheep, for example, there is slow neuronal degeneration and vacuolization; in visna virus infections changes in glial cell membranes lead to demyelination.

Invasion of Other Organs

Almost any organ may be infected via the bloodstream with one or another kind of virus, but most viruses have well-defined organ and tissue tropisms. The clinical importance of infection of various organs and tissues depends in part on their role in the economy of the body. The critical importance of the brain, heart, and lungs is self-evident, and invasion of the liver, causing severe hepatitis, as in Rift Valley fever and infectious canine hepatitis, is a life-threatening situation.

Delivery of circulating virus to the salivary glands or mammary glands may lead to lesions in those organs and excretion of virions in the saliva or milk. Infection of muscle cells occurs with several togaviruses and coxsackieviruses, while infection of the synovial cells of goats by caprine arthritis–encephalomyelitis virus produces arthritis.

Infection of Fetus

Most viral infections of the dam have no harmful effect on the fetus, but some blood-borne viruses cross the placenta to reach the fetal circulation, sometimes after establishing foci of infection in the placenta. Severe cytolytic infections of the fetus cause fetal death and resorption or abortion, outcomes which are common, for example, in pseudorabies and parvovirus infections in swine. Also important are the teratogenic effects of less lethal viruses such as bovine virus diarrhea virus and Akabane virus infections in cattle and sheep (Table 6-4).

The outcome of infections of pregnant animals with teratogenic viruses is influenced by gestational age. Generally, infection in the early period of gestation is most damaging. Little is known of the pathogenesis of most fetal infections, but experimental studies of bluetongue virus and Akabane virus infections in bovine fetuses and parvovirus infections in swine fetuses have led to some insight. The source of the virus is most often maternal infection, which is often subclinical but is associated with viremia and transplacental passage. Infections early in pregnancy usually lead to fetal death and abortion. Later in pregnancy the course of most fetal infections is influenced by the developing fetal immune response. For example, infections with porcine parvovirus after day 65–70 of gestation result not in fetal death, but in fetal antibody production and recovery. When bovine virus diarrhea virus infects the fetus in the first half of gestation, immune tolerance is established, leading to lifelong persistent infection and chronic disease. When the infection occurs late in gestation there is usually an effective immune response resulting in elimination of the virus and no disease. When viral replication in the fetus is rapid, as in alphaherpesvirus infections of the horse, cow, pig, and dog, fetal death and abortion can occur, often during the last third.

VIRUS SHEDDING

The shedding of infectious virions maintains infection in animal populations (see Chapter 14), and it usually occurs via one of the body openings or surfaces involved in the entry of viruses. With localized infections the same openings are involved in both entry and exit (see Fig. 6-1); in

TABLE 6-4

Viral Infections of Fetus or Embryo

Animal	Family	Virus	Syndrome
Cattle	*Herpesviridae*	Infectious bovine rhinotracheitis virus	Fetal death, abortion
	Togaviridae	Bovine virus diarrhea virus	Fetal death, abortion, congenital defects, inapparent infection with lifelong carrier state and shedding
	Bunyaviridae	Akabane virus	Fetal death, abortion, stillbirth, congenital defects
	Retroviridae	Bovine leukemia virus	Inapparent infection, leukemia
	Reoviridae	Bluetongue virus	Fetal death, abortion, congenital defects
Horse	*Herpesviridae*	Equine herpesvirus 1	Fetal death, abortion, neonatal disease
	Togaviridae	Equine arteritis virus	Fetal death, abortion
Swine	*Parvoviridae*	Parvovivus	Fetal death, abortion, mummification, stillbirth, infertility
	Herpesviridae	Pseudorabies virus	Fetal death, abortion
	Flaviviridae	Japanese encephalitis virus	Fetal death, abortion
	Togaviridae	Hog cholera virus	Fetal death, abortion, congenital defects, inapparent infection with lifelong carrier state and shedding
Sheep	*Togaviridae*	Border disease virus	Congenital defects
	Bunyaviridae	Rift Valley fever virus	Fetal death, abortion
		Nairobi sheep disease virus	Fetal death, abortion
	Reoviridae	Bluetongue virus	Fetal death, abortion, congenital defects
Dog	*Herpesviridae*	Herpesvirus	Perinatal death
Cat	*Parvoviridae*	Feline panleukopenia virus	Cerebellar hypoplasia
	Retroviridae	Feline leukemia virus	Inapparent infection, leukemia, fetal death
Mouse	*Parvoviridae*	Rat virus	Fetal death
	Arenaviridae	Lymphocytic choriomeningitis virus	Inapparent infection with lifelong carrier state and shedding
Chicken	*Picornaviridae*	Avian encephalomyelitis virus	Congenital defects, fetal death
	Retroviridae	Avian leukosis/sarcoma viruses	Inapparent infection, leukemia, other diseases

generalized infections a greater variety of modes of shedding is recognized (see Fig. 6-3), and some viruses are shed from multiple sites. The amount of virus shed in an excretion or secretion is important in relation to transmisson. Very low concentrations may be irrelevant unless very large volumes of infected material are transferred; on the other hand, some viruses occur in such high concentrations that a minute quantity of material, for example, less than 5 μl, can transmit infection.

Skin

The skin is an important source of virus in diseases in which transmission occurs by direct contact via small abrasions, for example, papillomatosis. Although skin lesions are produced in several generalized diseases, in only a few of these are viruses shed from skin lesions. However, foot-and-mouth disease virus, vesicular stomatitis virus, poxvirus, and some herpesvirus infections produce vesicular or pustular lesions in which there are large amounts of virus. Even here, however, virus shed in saliva and aerosols is more important, as far as transmission is concerned, than that shed via the skin lesions. Localization of virus in the feather follicles is important in providing a mechanism for the shedding of Marek's disease virus by infected chickens.

Respiratory Secretions

Many different viruses that cause either localized disease of the respiratory tract or generalized infections are shed in fluid expelled from the respiratory tract. Respiratory viruses, such as infectious bovine rhinotracheitis virus, paramyxoviruses, some coronaviruses, and bovine respiratory syncytial virus, are excreted in both nasal and oral secretions. Shedding may continue to occur during convalescence or recurrently after that time, especially with herpesviruses.

Saliva

A few viruses are shed into the oral cavity, often from infected salivary glands or from the lung or nasal mucosa. Salivary spread depends on activities such as licking, nuzzling, grooming, or biting. For feline immunodeficiency virus saliva and biting appear to be the major mode of transmission.

Feces

Enteric viruses are shed in the feces, and the more voluminous the fluid output the greater is the environmental contamination they cause. Viruses excreted in the feces are in general more resistant to inactivation by environmental conditions than are the respiratory viruses, especially when suspended in water.

Other Routes of Shedding

Genital Secretions. Several viruses that cause important diseases of cattle, horses, and sheep are excreted in the semen and transmitted during coitus.

Urine. Urine, like feces, tends to contaminate food supplies and the environment. A number of viruses, for example, rinderpest, infectious canine hepatitis, and foot-and-mouth disease viruses, replicate in tubular epithelial cells in the kidney and are shed in the urine. Viruria is lifelong in arenavirus infections of rodents and constitutes the principal mode of contamination of the environment by these viruses.

Milk. Several species of viruses replicate in the mammary gland and are excreted in milk, which may serve as a route of transmission of caprine arthritis–encephalitis virus, mouse mammary tumor virus, and some of the tick-borne flaviviruses.

Blood and Internal Organs. Blood is the usual source from which arthropods acquire viruses, and blood may also be the source of viruses transferred to the ovum or fetus. Arthropod transmission may be either biological, with a phase of viral replication in the vector before it can infect another animal (such viruses are called arboviruses), or mechanical, with no replication in the vector. Equine infectious anemia virus and bovine leukemia virus may be transmitted mechanically by arthropods or more commonly by needles and other equipment contaminated with blood. Carnivores and omnivores may be infected by consuming virus-containing meat; for example, hog cholera, African swine fever, and vesicular exanthema of swine viruses are often transmitted to swine that eat garbage containing contaminated pork scraps. Bovine spongiform encephalopathy was probably spread to cattle in feed containing scrapie-infected sheep offal.

No Shedding

Many sites of viral replication are nonproductive from the point of view of virus shedding. Sometimes these are necessary during the stepwise invasion of the host during generalized infections; others are dead-end sites of viral replication which are the cause of major disease in the host, as with arthropod-borne virus infection of the central nervous system. Many retroviruses are not shed, but are transmitted directly in the germ plasm or by infection of the egg or developing embryo.

FURTHER READING

Johnson, R. T. (1982). "Viral Infections of the Nervous System" Raven, New York.

Lentz, T. L. (1990). The recognition event between virus and host cell receptor: A target for antiviral agents. *J. Gen. Virol.* **71,** 751.

Mims, C. A. (1989). The pathogenetic basis of viral tropism. *Am. J. Pathol.* **135,** 447

Mims, C. A., and White, D. O. (1984). "Viral Pathogenesis and Immunology." Blackwell, Oxford.

Notkins, A. L., and Oldstone, M. B. A., eds. (1984, 1986, 1989). "Concepts in Viral Pathogenesis," Vols. 1, 2, and 3. Springer-Verlag, New York.

Sweet, C., and Smith, H. (1990). The pathogenicity of viruses. *In* "Topley and Wilson's Principles of Bacteriology, Virology and Immunity" (L. H. Collier and M. C. Timbury, eds.), 8th Ed., Vol. 4, p. 105. Arnold, London.

Tyrrell, D. A. J. (1983). How do viruses invade mucous surfaces? *Philos. Trans. R. Soc. London Sec. B* **303,** 75.

CHAPTER 7

Determinants of Viral Virulence and Host Resistance

The development of live-virus vaccines depends on the observation that virus strains may differ greatly in their *virulence,* namely, their capacity to produce disease or death. Conversely, within a susceptible host species infected with a particular strain of virus there are often striking differences between individual animals in their levels of resistance. The determinants of viral virulence are usually multigenic, and the determinants of host susceptibility/resistance are multifactorial. Within a susceptible species, the resistance of individual animals varies not only with the genetic constitution of the host (which may affect, among other things, the capacity to mount an immune response), but also with age, nutritional status, stress, and many other factors. Together, these genetic and physiologic factors determine what is called the "nonspecific" or "innate" resistance of the host, in contrast to acquired, immunologically specific resistance to reinfection that results from the operation of the immune response, as described in the next chapter.

VIRAL VIRULENCE AND HOST RESISTANCE

The word virulence is used in this book as a measure of pathogenicity, that is, the ability of a virus to cause disease in the infected host animal, rather than, as sometimes, as a measure of infectiousness or transmissibility, a different property that is discussed in Chapter 14. The virulence of a particular strain of a given virus administered by a particular route of inoculation to a particular strain of a laboratory animal can be measured by determining the dose of virus required to cause death in 50% of animals of that strain (*lethal dose 50, LD_{50}*). For example, with the susceptible BALB/c strain of mouse, the LD_{50} of a virulent strain of ectromelia virus was 5 virions, compared with 5000 for a moderately attenuated strain and about 1 million for a highly attenuated strain.

In viral infections occurring in nature, virulence may vary over a wide range, from strains that almost always cause inapparent infections to others where infection is usually associated with disease. Among the latter, some virus strains cause death more frequently than others, factors such as dose and host resistance being equal.

Susceptibility to infection or disease, or its reciprocal, resistance, can be measured by keeping the strain of virus constant and determining the ratio of the *infectious dose 50* (*ID_{50}*) to the LD_{50}. Thus with a virulent strain of ectromelia virus tested in highly susceptible BALB/c mice, the ID_{50} was 1–2 virions and the LD_{50} about 5, whereas for the resistant C57BL strain the ID_{50} was 1–2 virions but the LD_{50} was 1 million. The severity of an infection therefore depends on the interplay between the virulence of the virus and the resistance of the host. One can regard an acute infection as a race between the ability of the virus to replicate, spread in the body, and cause disease and the ability of the host to curtail and control these events.

Variability in the response of individual animals to infection with a given virus is regularly observed during epidemics; for example, during an outbreak of Venezuelan equine encephalitis, one horse may die, another may merely develop a febrile disease, and a third may have a completely subclinical infection, the only evidence of which is a sharp rise in antibody and lifelong immunity to reinfection. The dose of infecting virus may be influential, but this is by no means the only factor. Both genetic and physiologic factors can influence the outcome of exposure to a virus.

GENETIC DETERMINANTS OF VIRULENCE

Unraveling the genetic basis of virulence has long been one of the major goals of animal virology, and also one of the most difficult to achieve, since many genes, both viral and host, are involved in the outcome of each infection. With advances in molecular genetics it has been possible to dissect the problem in a more precise way.

The most detailed studies have been those carried out with retroviruses and oncogenic DNA viruses to determine the genetic basis of cellular transformation and oncogenicity (see Chapter 11). Experiments with herpesviruses are beginning to reveal the genetic basis of latency with these viruses (see Chapter 10). With viruses causing acute infections, those with segmented genomes have provided a more easily manipulated experimental model, since each segment of the genome of influenza viruses and reoviruses, for example, is in most cases equivalent to one gene and reassortants can be readily obtained. Study of a number of reassortants involving different genome segments enables the functions that relate to virulence to be assigned to particular genes. In addition, a detailed understanding of the basis of virulence at the molecular level has been obtained with human poliovirus, and to a lesser extent with foot-and-mouth disease virus, where it has been possible to compare the sequences of the genomes of strains of high and low virulence, including vaccine strains. Investigations with vaccinia virus have revealed the complexity of the armamentarium of viral gene products directed against various components of host resistance.

Influenza Virus

Experiments with influenza virus in mice have confirmed the view advanced by the pioneer in the field, F. M. Burnet, that virulence is multigenic. Recent studies show that one essential requirement for virulence in the chicken and neurovirulence in the mouse is that the hemagglutinin protein (HA) must be cleaved. In nonpathogenic strains of avian influenza virus, the HA1 and HA2 moieties of the hemagglutinin are linked by a single arginine, whereas in virulent strains the linker is a sequence of several basic amino acids and is more readily cleaved. Virulent strains thus contain HA which is activated (cleaved) in a wide spectrum of different types of cell; hence they can replicate and spread throughout the host. Nonpathogenic strains, on the other hand, soon reach a barrier of cells which lack appropriate HA-cleaving enzymes.

Perhaps the most striking demonstration of how a minor single nucleotide change in the HA gene can make all the difference between relative avirulence and high virulence was the finding that a single amino acid substitution in the HA protein of influenza A, subtype H5, in 1983 led to a devastating outbreak of fowl plague on poultry farms in Pennsylvania (described in Chapter 4). The point mutation abolished a glycosylation site, thus exposing to proteolysis the cleavage site previously concealed by an oligopolysaccharide side chain.

However, virulence is only partly explained by this factor, for when reassortants were made between highly virulent and avirulent strains of avian influenza virus, exchange of any one of the eight RNA segments could modify the virulence. Studies with a variety of reassortants showed that, for each reassortant, an optimal combination of genes (the optimal "gene constellation") was selected which favored survival in nature and determined virulence.

Reovirus

Although reoviruses are not major pathogens of domestic animals, a highly illuminating analysis of the virulence of reoviruses for mice has been carried out with reassortant viruses. The fact that the protein product of each of the ten genome segments has been isolated and characterized has allowed determination of their functions and effects on virulence (Table 7-1). Four genes (S1, M2, L2, and S4) encode the four polypeptides that are found on the outer capsid (Fig. 7-1). Each plays a role in determining virulence. Gene S1 specifies the hemagglutinin (protein σ1), which is located on the vertices of the icosahedron and is responsible for cellular and tissue tropism. With reovirus 3, but not reovirus 1, the σ1 protein is responsible for binding to neurons, whose sequential infection leads to fatal encephalitis, and it is also responsible for viral spread from foot pad to the spinal cord via peripheral nerves. Gene M2 specifies polypeptide

TABLE 7-1

Genetic Analysis of Virulence of Reoviruses, Based on Studies with Mutants and Reassortants

Gene	Protein	Properties	Significance in infections of mice
S1	σ1	Reovirus 3: binds to neurons	Neural spread, encephalitis
		Reovirus 1: binds to ependymal cells	Hydrocephalus
		Binds to T and B cells	Infection of lymphocytes
		Recognized by T cells and neutralizing antibodies	Protective antigen
		Reovirus 1: binds to enterocytes	Reovirus 1 more pathogenic than reovirus 3 after oral infection
		Reovirus 3: does not bind to enterocytes	
M2	μ1C	Reovirus 3: inactivated by intestinal proteases	Nonvirulent by mouth
		Reovirus 1: not inactivated by intestinal proteases	Virulent by mouth
S4	σ3	Inhibits RNA and protein synthesis	Role in persistent infection
L2	λ2	Role in RNA transcription	Affects level of replication in gut, hence role in transmissibility

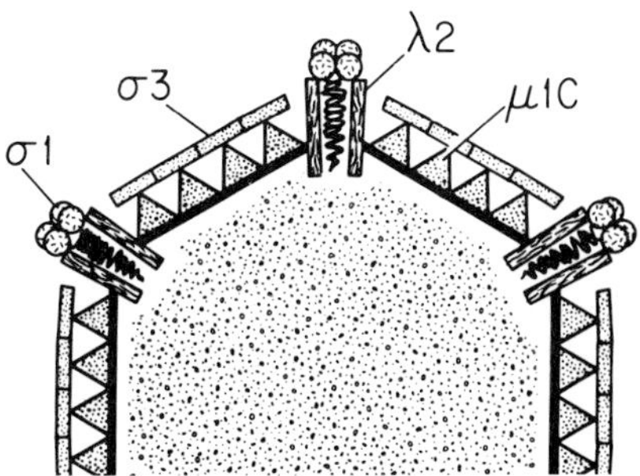

FIG. 7-1. *Schematic diagram of part of the reovirus outer capsid, showing the location of the polypeptides that play a major role in virulence. σ1 is located at the vertices of the icosahedron and consists of two components: a globular dimer at the surface, which is responsible for hemagglutination and cell attachment, and an α-helical region which anchors the hemagglutinin by interaction with the λ2 spike protein. The polypeptides μ1C and σ3 are associated with each other, in a ratio of one molecule of μ1C to two molecules of σ3, on the surfaces of the icosahedral capsid. [Modified from L. A. Schiff and B. N. Fields,* In *"Fields Virology" (B. N. Fields* et al., *eds.), 2nd Ed., p. 1277. Raven, New York, 1990.]*

μ1C, which determines sensitivity of the virion to chymotrypsin and hence affects the capacity of the virus to grow in the intestine. Thus μ1C of reovirus 3 is protease-sensitive, and reovirus 3 is avirulent by mouth; μ1C of reovirus 1 is protease-resistant, and the virus is infectious by mouth. A reassortant with the M2 gene from reovirus 1 and the S1 gene from reovirus 3 was infectious orally and caused fatal encephalitis. Gene L2 specifies the λ2 spike protein, which is primarily a core protein but surrounds σ1; it is a guanylyltransferase and plays a role in RNA transcription. The ability of reovirus to reach high titers in the gut and be efficiently transmitted via feces is associated with the λ2 spike protein. Gene S4 specifies polypeptide σ3, which inhibits protein and RNA synthesis in infected cells; mutations in the S4 gene play a role in establishing persistent infection in cultured cells.

This sort of structure–function analysis serves as an important model for the study other dsRNA viruses, such as the orbiviruses, rotaviruses, and birnaviruses, and ssRNA viruses with segmented genomes such as bunyaviruses and arenaviruses. Preliminary studies with rotaviruses suggest that the products of genome segment 4, which specifies the outer capsid protein VP4, are associated with hemagglutination, neutralization, restriction of growth in some tissue culture cells, and mouse virulence.

Poliovirus

Although useful sequencing studies have been carried out with vaccine strains of foot-and-mouth disease virus, the best analyzed example of the determinants of virulence in a picornavirus is human poliovirus. Its genome is a single molecule of ssRNA, and the entire nucleotide sequence of several strains has been determined. Because vaccine strains are required to be infectious by mouth but not cause central nervous system disease, the virulence of polioviruses is narrowly defined as the ability to replicate and cause lesions after introduction into the central nervous system of primates.

Comparison of the nucleotide sequence of the poliovirus vaccine strains with that of the virulent parental strains shows that there are a number of base substitutions scattered along the entire genome. Here, too, virulence results from a nonpredictable multigenic constellation.

Vaccinia and Cowpox Viruses

The poxviruses are much larger and more complex viruses than any yet discussed, and the genetic control of virulence is correspondingly more complex. Interest in its virulence has been stimulated by proposals to use vaccinia virus as a vector for human and veterinary vaccines. Recent work has shown that many of the large number of genes that affect virulence have effects on the defense mechanisms of the host.

The first poxvirus gene to be shown to affect virulence was the gene for vaccinia virus thymidine kinase (TK), which is not required for replication in cultured cells. However, TK^- mutants are much less virulent than wild type in animals. The envelope of vaccinia virus, which contains at least seven virus-coded polypeptides, is not essential for infection of either cultured cells or animals, but enveloped forms are much more virulent because they spread around the animal body more effectively.

Cowpox virus replicates in a wide range of cells, but three open reading frames have been identified which affect its replication in the nonpermissive Chinese hamster ovary (CHO) cell. In animals these genes are probably important in determining host range and tissue tropisms. Deletion analysis of vaccinia virus has shown that 56 of a total of 198 open reading frames are not required for replication in cells. Many of these are located at the ends of the genome and affect virulence in animals (Table 7-2). The vaccinia growth factor (VGF) has homologies with epidermal growth factor and appears to induce localized hyperplasia of uninfected cells around foci of infection. A 35-kDa protein, which has been called the vaccinia virus complement-binding protein, blocks the classical complement pathway by binding to C4b. Then there are at least three distinct

TABLE 7-2

Gene-Products of Vaccinia Virus and Cowpox Virus That Influence Pathogenesis[a]

Designation	Virus[b]	Gene product	Putative function
VGF	VV	Secreted growth factor	Stimulates proliferation of surrounding uninfected cells
TK	VV	Thymidine kinase	Affects growth *in vivo*
SPI-1	VV	40K serpin	Unknown
Red pock gene	CPV	38K serpin	Inhibitor of blood coagulation
35K gene	VV	35K protein	Binds to C4b (complement)
CHO host range gene	CPV	77K protein	Affects host range
A-type inclusion gene	CPV	160K protein	Major component of inclusion body; prolongs virus survival
HA gene	VV	Hemagglutinin	Promotes cell-to-cell spread
14K gene	VV	14K envelope protein	Affects penetration and viral spread
ORF NIL	VV	13.8K secreted protein	Role in neurovirulence

[a] Based on P. C. Turner and R. W. Moyer, *Curr. Top. Microb. Immunol.* **163,** 125 (1990).
[b] VV, Vaccinia virus; CPV, cowpox virus.

serum protease inhibitor (serpin) genes in vaccinia virus. Serpins exert a control over a number of critical events associated with connective tissue turnover, coagulation, complement activation, and inflammatory reactions. The presence of the 38K gene of cowpox virus, which encodes a serpinlike protein, is associated with the bright red pock produced on the chorioallantoic membrane and higher virulence for a number of experimental animals. It has been suggested that the serpin delays the onset or decreases the magnitude of the inflammatory response.

GENETIC DETERMINANTS OF RESISTANCE

Genetic differences in susceptibility are most obvious when different animal species are compared. Common viral infections often tend to be less pathogenic in their natural host species than in certain exotic or introduced species. For instance, foot-and-mouth disease virus causes a severe disease in European cattle, but none in the African buffalo. Donkeys are more resistant to African horsesickness than are horses or mules, while zebras are refractory. An even more stiking example is myxoma virus, which produces a small benign fibroma in its natural host, *Sylvila-*

gus brasiliensis, but an almost invariably fatal generalized infection in European rabbits (*Oryctolagus cuniculus*).

Accurate genetic data on resistance to infection are almost unobtainable in many species, because genetic, physiologic, and environmental differences are generally confounded. With inbred strains of mice, however, it has been possible to study the genetics of resistance to viral infection in some detail. For example, the susceptibility of mice to certain flaviviruses and to mouse hepatitis virus (a coronavirus) is under the control of a single gene which determines the capacity of macrophages to support the growth of virus. Likewise, the resistance of certain mice to influenza virus infection is controlled by the Mx gene, whose gene product is induced by interferons α/β (see Chapter 5).

Cellular Receptors

The presence or absence of receptors on the plasma membrane is a fundamental determinant of susceptibility (see Table 3-2). In the late 1940s it was shown that pretreatment of mice with neuraminidase intranasally conferred substantial protection against intranasal challenge with influenza virus, which was transient because there was rapid regeneration of receptors. The resistance of certain strains of chickens to avian retroviruses is attributable to a single gene that codes for a cellular receptor.

Human polioviruses provide an example of the importance of cellular receptors at the species level. These viruses ordinarily infect only primates; mice and other nonprimates are insusceptible because their cells lack appropriate receptors. However, poliovirus RNA, when introduced into mouse cells *in vivo* or in culture, can undergo a single cycle of replication. Since progeny virions from such an artificial infection face mouse cells lacking receptors, they are unable to initiate a second cycle of replication. Transfer of the human poliovirus receptor gene into mouse L cells or into transgenic mice makes either the cells or the mice susceptible to infection with polioviruses.

Immune Response Genes

Immunologic responses are determined and controlled by a large number of different genes usually located in clusters but on different chromosomes. A range of primary, that is, inherited, defects of these genes is recognized; they range from the absence of a single immunoglobulin class such as IgA, the commonest primary defect in humans, to agammaglobulinemia, where the number of functional B cells is greatly reduced or absent, to severe combined immunodeficiency as recognized in certain Arabian foals in which there is a total absence of functional B and T lymphocytes. These "experiments of nature" are of interest in understanding the significance of particular immunologic functions in particular virus infections.

Immune responsiveness to particular antigens differs greatly from one strain of mouse to another, being under the control of specific *immune response (Ir) genes.* There are many of these genes, most of them situated in the region known as the *major histocompatibility complex (MHC).* Most other genetic determinants of virus susceptibility are not directly related to the immune response and map outside the MHC locus. Individuals with a genetically determined poor immune response to neutralizing epitopes on the surface proteins of a given virus would presumably have difficulty in controlling infection with that particular virus. In the mouse at least, absence of a specific response is generally recessive. Susceptibility of mice to infection with cytomegaloviruses, retroviruses, and lymphocytic choriomeningitis virus has been shown to be linked to particular MHC genotypes. Some breeds of domestic animals (e.g., sheep) are so inbred that particular viral susceptibility and resistance patterns have been found to be associated with specific immune responsiveness patterns.

Macrophages

Macrophages play a central role as determinants of resistance, in part because of their role in processing and presenting antigens and in part because of their intrinsic susceptibility to infection, which is independent of antibodies or the action of lymphokines, although it is often influenced by these immune factors. Many viruses multiply in macrophages, and in some diseases, such as equine infectious anemia and Aleutian disease of mink, they appear to be the only susceptible cells. Often viral replication is abortive (Table 7-3), but sometimes the apparent insusceptibility of macrophages is due to endogenous interferon production. Production of interleukin inhibitors and other immunosuppressive factors by macrophages is important in pathogenesis, and tumor necrosis factor from infected macrophages has both antiviral and pathogenic effects.

PHYSIOLOGIC FACTORS AFFECTING RESISTANCE

A great variety of physiologic factors affect resistance, the most important being the immune response, which is described in detail in Chapter 8. Among the many nonspecific factors in resistance the following are important.

TABLE 7-3
Susceptibility of Macrophages to Viral Infection

Virus	Host	Type of macrophage	Viral growth
Mouse cytomegalovirus	Mouse	Peritoneal	Defective
Pig cytomegalovirus	Pig	Alveolar	Normal
African swine fever virus	Pig	Liver and other	Normal
Aleutian disease parvovirus	Mink	Most	Normal
Mouse hepatitis coronavirus	Mouse	Peritoneal, liver	Normal
Sendai parainfluenza virus	Mouse	Alveolar, peritoneal	Defective
Visna lentivirus	Sheep	Most	Normal

Age

Virus infections tend to be most serious at the extremes of life—in the very young and the very old. The high susceptibility of newborn animals to many viral infections is of considerable importance in livestock production. It can also be exploited for the laboratory diagnosis of viral diseases. Before cell culture techniques became available, foot-and-mouth disease virus isolation, titration, and neutralizing antibody assays were carried out in suckling mice. Infant mice are still useful for the isolation of togaviruses, flaviviruses, bunyaviruses, and rhabdoviruses.

In laboratory animals the first few weeks of life are a period of very rapid physiologic change. For example, during this time mice pass from a stage of immunologic nonreactivity (to many antigens) to immunological maturity. This change profoundly affects their reaction to viruses like lymphocytic choriomeningitis virus, which induces a persistent tolerated infection when inoculated into newborn mice but an immune response in mice infected when over 1 week old. Most domestic animals are reasonably mature immunologically at the time of birth but are still very susceptible to infection with viruses against which their dam has no antibody—an unusual circumstance unless the particular virus has been recently introduced. If the umbrella of maternal antibody usually provided in mammals through colostrum or transplacental transfer is missing, the newborn animal is particularly vulnerable to infections with viruses such as canine distemper virus, canine parvovirus, hog cholera virus, bovine virus diarrhea virus, enterpathogenic coronaviruses, rotaviruses, and various herpesviruses during the first few weeks of life.

In man, there are viruses that tend to produce more severe disease in adults than in children. For example, varicella virus, usually the cause of an uncomplicated disease in children, may produce severe pneumonia in adults; mumps in adults may be complicated by orchitis. There are few parallels in domestic animals, but one example is bovine virus diarrhea virus, which generally infects calves subclinically, whereas older animals have a higher probability of developing clinical disease (see Chapter 25).

Finally, not all age-related changes in virus susceptibility are immune-mediated. For example, porcine rotavirus infects enterocytes in the upper part of the small intestine of newborn piglets, but within 2 days after birth these cells are resistant to infection. This may be due to a loss of receptors or to a loss of the capacity to transport but not internalize macromolecules. The age-dependent resistance of mice to herpes simplex virus appears to be closely correlated with changes in macrophage susceptibility.

Cell Differentiation

The state of differentiation of the cell often exerts a major effect on its reaction to viral infection. The warts produced by papillomaviruses in many species of animals provides a classic example. Productive infection is not seen in the deeper layers of the epidermal tumor but occurs only when the cells become keratinized as they move to the surface layers. Basal cells contain 50–200 copies of viral DNA, but viral antigens and finally viral particles are produced only as the cells differentiate as they approach the surface of the skin. Other examples involve cells of the immune system. For example, vesicular stomatitis and distemper viruses, which do not replicate in normal (resting) peripheral blood lymphocyte cultures, do so when cells differentiate after activation by mitogen. Likewise, visna virus infects monocytes abortively, with low levels of transcription of viral RNA, but the infection becomes productive as the cells differentiate into macrophages.

Other cellular physiologic factors, such as the stage of the mitotic cycle, may affect susceptibility. Autonomously replicating parvoviruses replicate only in cells that are in the S phase of the cell cycle. In young cats feline panleukopenia virus infects rapidly dividing cells in the bone marrow and intestinal epithelium to produce leukopenia and diarrhea, while in the cat fetus the rapidly dividing cells of the germinal layer of the cerebellum are destroyed, resulting in cerebellar hypoplasia.

Nutrition

Malnutrition can interfere with any of the mechanisms that act as barriers to the entry, replication, or progress of viruses through the body. It has been repeatedly demonstrated that severe nutritional deficiencies will interfere with the production of antibody and cell-mediated immune responses, with the activity of phagocytes, and with the integrity of skin and mucous membranes. However, often it is impossible to disentangle adverse nutritional effects from other factors such as poor husbandry and hygiene. Moreover, just as malnutrition can exacerbate viral infections, so viral infections can exacerbate malnutrition, thus creating a vicious cycle.

For all domestic mammals, maternal IgG in colostrum plays an important role in providing protection against a wide range of microorganisms, from day one to several months after birth. The protection provided by IgG is reinforced for enteric infections by maternal IgA and nonspecific factors such as fatty acids produced by lipase. In primates early protection of the newborn is provided by a more fail-safe mechanism, namely, *in utero* transfer of IgG.

Hormones, Pregnancy, and Stress

There are few striking differences in the susceptibility of males and females to viral infections (except in the obvious instances of viruses with a predilection for tissues such as testis, ovaries, or mammary glands). Pregnancy significantly increases the likelihood of severe disease following infection with certain viruses, for example, Rift Valley fever virus in sheep. Herpesvirus infections may be reactivated during pregnancy, leading to abortion or perinatal infection.

The immunosuppressive effects of therapeutic doses of corticosteroids exacerbates many viral infections, such as infectious bovine rhinotracheitis and pseudorabies. The precise mechanism is not understood, but corticosteroids reduce inflammatory and immune responses and depress interferon synthesis. It is also clear that adequate levels of these hormones are vital for the maintenance of normal resistance to infection. The stress of overcrowding and long-distance transport is believed to contribute to shipping fever in cattle via adrenocortical immunosuppression.

Fever

Almost all viral infections in domestic animals are accompanied by fever. The principal mediator of the febrile response appears to be a peptide regulatory factor (cytokine), interleukin 1 (previously known as endogenous pyrogen). Interleukin 1 is produced in macrophages and is induced during immune responses. It is found in inflammatory exudates and acts on the temperature-regulating center in the anterior hypothalamus. Interferons are also pyrogenic when present in sufficiently high concentration; their antiviral effects are discussed below.

Fever profoundly disturbs bodily functions. The increased metabolic rate, achieved by increasing the metabolic activity of phagocytic cells and the rate at which inflammatory responses are induced, might be expected to exert antiviral effects. *In vitro* experiments have shown that antibody production and T-cell proliferation induced by interleukin 1 are greatly increased when cells are cultured at 39°C rather than at 37°C. On the other hand, when fever was prevented in animals experimentally infected with vaccinia virus or influenza virus, the ensuing disease was more severe and much more virus was excreted.

Exposing rabbits to high temperatures greatly diminishes the severity of their response to myxoma virus; lowered temperatures increase the severity of the disease. Local effects may also occur. When the skin was kept cool after intradermal inoculation of bovine herpesvirus 2, the local lesions appeared earlier, were larger, contained more virus, and lasted longer. On the other hand, temperature-sensitive *(ts)* mutants are usually less virulent than wild-type strains.

Role of Interferons in Recovery from Viral Infection

Interferons are proteins that are induced in virus-infected cells and interfere with the replication of viruses. Their properties and mode of action were described in Chapter 5; here we consider their role in the animal. It is difficult to determine which cell types, or even which tissues and organs, are responsible for most interferon production *in vivo*, but, extrapolating from findings with cultured cells, one can probably assume that most cells in the body are capable of producing interferons in response to viral infection. Certainly, interferons can be found in the mucus bathing epithelial surfaces such as the respiratory tract, and interferon is produced by most or all cells of mesenchymal origin. Lymphocytes, especially T cells, NK cells, and *killer (K) cells*, as well as macrophages, produce large amounts of interferon α and γ, and they are probably the principal source of circulating interferon in viral infections characterized by a viremic stage.

There are experimental data supporting a central role for interferons in recovery following at least some viral infections. For example, in the early 1970s Gresser and colleagues showed that mice infected with any of several nonlethal viruses, or with sublethal doses of more virulent viruses, die if anti-interferon serum is administered. Perhaps the most persuasive evidence, however, comes from a more recent study with transgenic mice. Mice transgenic for the human IFN-β gene showed enhanced resistance to pseudorabies virus, in proportion to the resulting concentration of circulating interferon. Serum from the transgenic mice also protected mice against the unrelated vesicular stomatitis virus, and this protection was abrogated by anti-interferon serum.

Although it is widely thought that interferons constitute a first line of defense in the process of recovery from viral infections, it is not the most important factor in recovery. If this were so one might expect that a systemic infection with any virus, or immunization with a live vaccine, might, through interferon, protect an animal against challenge with an unrelated virus for a short period, yet this cannot be demonstrated experimentally. The evidence is somewhat stronger that infection of the upper respiratory tract with one virus will provide temporary and strictly local protection against others. Perhaps this distinction provides the clue that the direct antiviral effect of interferons is limited in both time and space. Its main antiviral role may be to protect cells in the immediate vicinity of the initial focus of infection for at most a few days.

Multiple Infections

Multiple infections with viruses and bacteria are important in infections of the respiratory and intestinal tracts. Viral infections of the respiratory tract often lower resistance to bacterial superinfection; for example, shipping fever is initiated by a variety of respiratory viruses, but the serious signs are due to infection with *Pasteurella multocida* (see Chapter 9). There is a synergism between influenza virus and *Staphylococcus aureus,* such that after double infection of mice, pneumonia develops only if the staphlococcus produces a protease that cleaves the hemagglutinin. In mice, simultaneous administration of a rotavirus and an enterotoxigenic strain of *Escherichia coli* leads to more severe diarrhea and a higher mortality rate. Under intensive management systems, such as cattle feedlots or broiler chicken houses, multiple infections are common, and it can be difficult to establish which is the primary infection and what is synergistic in these situations.

FURTHER READING

Brinton, M. A., and Nathanson, N. (1981). Genetic determinants of virus susceptibility: Epidemiologic implications of murine models. *Epidemiol. Rev.* **3,** 115.

Buller, R. M. L., and Palumbo, G. J. (1991). Poxvirus pathogenesis. *Microbiol. Rev.* **55,** 80.

Chandra, R. K. (1979). Nutritional deficiency and susceptibility to infection. *Bull. WHO* **57,** 167.

Klenk, H.-D., and Rott, R. (1989). The molecular biology of influenza virus pathogenicity. *Adv. Virus Res.* **34,** 247.

Mims, C. A., and White, D. O. (1984). "Viral Pathogenesis and Immunology." Blackwell, Oxford and London.

Turner, P. C., and Moyer, R. W. (1990). The molecular pathogenesis of poxviruses. *Curr. Top. Microbiol. Immunol.* **163,** 125.

Tyler, K. L., and Fields, B. N. (1990). Pathogenesis of viral infections. *In* "Fields Virology" (B. N. Fields, D. M. Knipe, R. M. Chanock, M. S. Hirsch, J. L. Melnick, T. P. Monath, and B. Roizman, eds.), 2nd Ed., p. 213. Raven, New York.

CHAPTER 8

Immune Response to Viral Infections

In response to the constant threat of invasion by microorganisms and viruses, vertebrates have evolved an elaborate set of defensive measures, called, collectively, the immune system. During the initial encounter with a virus, the immune system of the host recognizes as foreign certain viral macromolecules (proteins, carbohydrates) called *antigens,* which elicit several kinds of responses to eliminate the virus and to prevent reinfection. Cells of the *humoral immune system* (B lymphocytes) respond to an antigenic stimulus by producing and secreting specific immunoglobulins called *antibodies;* cells of the *cell-mediated immune system* (T lymphocytes) respond by the activation of several kinds of T lymphocytes and the production and secretion of several kinds of lymphokines. In each case the immune system carries out highly specific recognition processes wherein effector cells interface with small discrete sites on the invading virus particle that are called *antigenic determinants* or *epitopes.* The immune system then triggers more generalized effector processes that attack and remove the invading virus and virus-infected cells. The recognition processes also drive an amplification cascade, so that the scale of the immune response matches the scale of the virus infection, and a memory cascade, so that reinfection at a later time can be dealt with very quickly.

The immune response terminates many viral infections before much damage has been done, resulting in mild or even subclinical infection; this chapter deals with the role of the immune response in recovery from viral infection and resistance to reinfection. Later chapters address situations where the immune system does not function so effectively: where the immune response is actually harmful, causing tissue damage in vital organs (Chapter 9), and where the virus evades the immune system and establishes a persistent infection (Chapter 10).

COMPONENTS OF THE IMMUNE SYSTEM

The immune system comprises several kinds of lymphocytes as well as cells of the monocyte/macrophage lineage, dendritic cells, and NK cells. Lymphocytes, with their specific surface receptors, are the key to immunologic specificity. Any given T or B lymphocyte possesses receptors with specificty for a particular epitope. When T or B lymphocytes bind antigen they respond by dividing to form an expanded clone of cells (clonal expansion). B lymphocytes differentiate into plasma cells, which secrete specific antibody. T lymphocytes secrete soluble factors known as *lymphokines* or *interleukins,* which are representatives of a large family of hormones, known generically as *cytokines,* that modulate the activities of other cells involved in the immune response. Some of the T and B cells revert to small lymphocytes, which are long-lived and are responsible for *immunologic memory.* Whereas antibodies and the receptors on B cells recognize areas of foreign antigens in their original conformation, T-cell receptors recognize short peptides in association with certain of the individual host's own membrane glycoproteins known as *MHC proteins.*

Antigen-Presenting Cells

Cells of the monocyte/macrophage and *dendritic cell* lineages play a central role in the immune response to viruses, notably in antigen processing and presentation (Fig. 8-1). As a class, cells with these functions are called *antigen-presenting cells.* The most efficient antigen-presenting cells are MHC class II-rich dendritic cells, including Langerhans cells of the skin and the interdigitating dendritic cells of lymph nodes, so named because they interdigitate with CD4^{+}T cells to which they present antigen. Unlike dendritic cells, macrophages are phagocytic; they express little class II MHC protein while resting, but are stimulated to do so following activation. After priming and activation, B lympho-

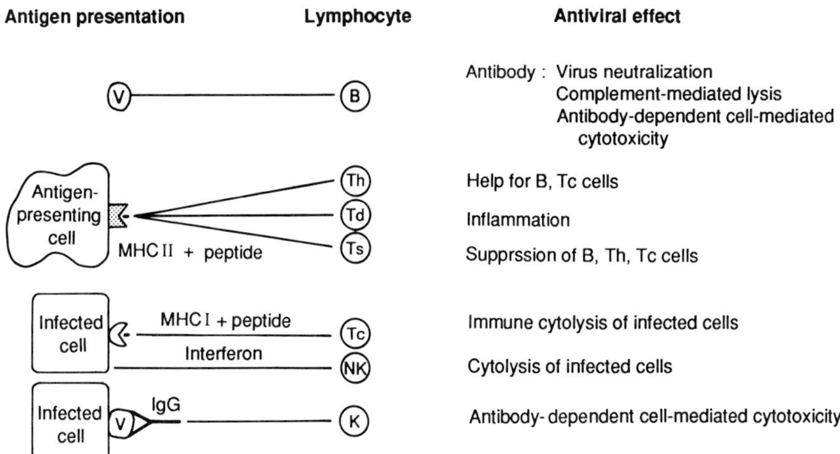

FIG. 8-1. *Cells involved in antiviral immune responses. V, Virus or viral antigen; MHC-I, MHC-II, MHC proteins of class I and II, respectively, with viral peptide bound in groove. Ts, Suppressor, Th, helper, Td, delayed hypersensitivity, Tc, cytotoxic T lymphocytes; NK, natural killer cell; K, killer cell. Antigen-presenting cells process inactivated virus or viral proteins via the endosomal pathway, and the peptides associate with class II MHC proteins. Some viral proteins produced during viral replication undergo proteolysis through the cytosolic pathway, and the resulting peptides associate with class I MHC proteins. (Modified from C. A. Mims and D. O. White, "Viral Pathogenesis and Immunology." Blackwell, Oxford, 1984.)*

cytes also serve as antigen-presenting cells; they are important during the latter stages of the primary response and during the secondary response (see below). To understand the intricacies of antigen processing and presentation, one must know something about the structure and intracellular trafficking of MHC proteins.

The *major histocompatibility complex (MHC)* is a genetic locus encoding several MHC class I proteins and several MHC class II proteins, each of which occurs in many allelic forms. Class I glycoproteins are found in the plasma membrane of most types of cells; class II glycoproteins are confined principally to antigen-presenting cells. At the distal tip of each class of MHC protein there is a groove (Fig. 8-2), within which variable residues provide a degree of specificity for the particular range of short peptides that can occupy it. Peptides recovered from class I molecules are usually 8 or 9 amino acids long; peptides binding to class II proteins range from 13 to 17 amino acids. The peptide–MHC complex is in turn recognized, with a considerably higher degree of specificity, by the

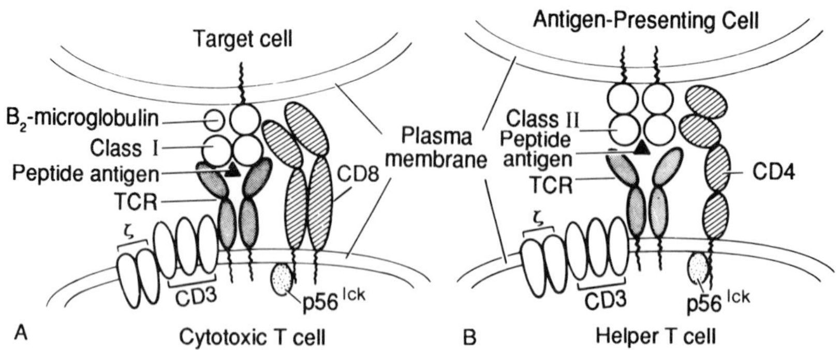

FIG. 8-2. *Model for the interaction between CD4 or CD8 and MHC proteins. (A) CD8 on a cytotoxic T cell binds to a class I MHC protein on a target cell and interacts with a T-cell receptor (TCR) molecule that is binding to the same class I protein and to a peptide. (B) CD4 on a helper T cell binds to a class II MHC protein on an antigen-presenting cell and interacts with a TCR molecule that is binding both to the same class II MHC protein and to a peptide. The TCR is shown (heavy shading) as a heterodimer of two polypeptide chains, α and β, each with a constant domain spanning the membrane and a variable region containing the antigen-binding groove; the TCR is associated with the accessory molecule CD3, a complex of three polypeptides (γ, δ, ε) plus a homodimer of ζ, which is thought to serve as a signal transducer for the TCR, being phosphorylated by the tyrosine kinase* $p56^{lck}$ *(stippled) which is associated with the accessory molecules CD4 and CD8 (striped). The class I MHC protein is shown as a polypeptide chain with extracellular domains, associated with* β_2*-microglobulin; the class II MHC is depicted as comprising two polypeptide chains, each having two extracellular domains. [From J. R. Parnes,* In *"Encyclopedia of Human Biology" (R. Dulbecco, ed.), Vol. 2, p. 225. Academic Press, San Diego, 1991.]*

T-cell receptor (TCR) of the appropriate clone of T cells. During ontogeny, positive selection of developing T cells in the thymus by "self" MHC molecules results in mature T cells that can recognize foreign peptides only if they are in the groove of "self" MHC protein, not foreign MHC molecules. This phenomenon, which has been extensively investigated in laboratory experimentation, is known as *MHC restriction.*

Noninfectious virus or viral proteins taken up by antigen-presenting cells pass progressively through early endosomes to late (acidic) endosomes and prelysosomes, where they degraded by proteolytic enzymes (the *endosomal pathway*). Certain of the resulting viral peptides are able to bind to the class II MHC molecules which continually recycle between the plasma membrane and these acidic endosomes. Viral proteins found in cells supporting viral replication are also subject to proteolysis, but in this case the degradation occurs in the *cytosol* (the *cytosolic pathway*).

These peptides assemble with class I MHC molecules in the endoplasmic reticulum to form a stable complex, which is then exported to the cell surface. Thus in general, peptides derived from endogenously synthesized viral proteins in infected cells associate with MHC class I protein and the complex is recognized by $CD8^+$ T cells, thus eliciting a Tc cell response, whereas peptides derived from exogenous viral proteins endocytosed by antigen-presenting cells associate with class II MHC protein and the complex is recognized by $CD4^+$ T cells, leading to a Th cell response.

Any individual animal has only a certain number of MHC alleles, and antigenic peptides bind only certain MHC molecules. If the peptide–MHC complex is important in eliciting a protective immune response to a serious viral infection, animals lacking suitable MHC proteins will be genetically more susceptible to that disease. A further cause of increased susceptibility lies in the possible absence, from the T cell repertoire of an individual animal, of lymphocytes bearing receptors for a particular MHC–peptide complex.

T Lymphocytes

There are two principal classes of lymphocytes: *T lymphocytes,* so named because of their dependence on the thymus for their maturation from pluripotent hemopoietic stem cells, and *B lymphocytes,* derived from the bursa of Fabricius in birds or its equivalent, the bone marrow, in mammals. These differ not only in their different antigen-receptors, but also in surface markers and function. Functionally, T lymphocytes are classified into four subsets: *helper (Th)* and *suppressor (Ts)* lymphocytes are regulator cells; *cytotoxic (Tc)* and *delayed hypersensitivity (Td)* lymphocytes are effector cells (Table 8-1). Close examination of T-cell clones indicates that a single cell type can discharge more than one of these functions and secrete a range of different lymphokines, but it may recognize a particular determinant only in association with a particular class of MHC molecule on the surface of the cell.

TABLE 8-1
Subsets of T Lymphocytes

Subset	Marker	MHC restriction	Function
Helper (Th)	CD4	Class II	Th_2: help for B or Tc cells Th_1: inflammation
Cytotoxic (Tc)	CD8	Class I, usually	Cytolysis of virus-infected cells
Suppressor (Ts)	CD8	?	Suppression of B, Th, or Tc cells

Helper T Cells. Th cells carry a surface marker known as CD4. They recognize viral peptides in association with class II MHC protein, usually on the surface of an antigen-presenting cell. They then secrete cytokines which in turn activate the Th cells themselves and subsequently activate other types of lymphocytes, such as B cells, helping them to produce antibody, or Tc cells, helping them to acquire cytotoxicity.

Cytotoxic T Cells. Tc cells carry the CD8 surface marker and generally recognize viral peptides in association with class I MHC molecules. Following activation, they lyse cells which have that particular viral peptide bound to that MHC class I protein on their surface.

Delayed Hypersensitivity T Cells. Td cells are generally $CD4^+$ (but may be $CD8^+$) and recognize peptides in association with class II (or sometimes class I) MHC protein. Td cells secrete a variety of lymphokines which set up an inflammatory response and greatly augment the immune response by attracting both monocytes/macrophages and other T cells to the site, and also activating them to proliferate, differentiate, and secrete additional cytokines themselves. Td cells are generally considered to be a subpopulation of Th cells. Two major classes of $CD4^+$ cells have been described. Th_1 ("inflammatory" T cells) are defined as typically secreting the cytokines interleukin 2 (IL-2), interferon γ (IFN-γ), and tumor necrosis factor β (TNF-β) [plus granulocyte–macrophage colony-stimulating factor (GM-CSF) and IL-3], mediating delayed hypersensitivity (DTH) *in vivo* and promoting IgG2a production, whereas Th_2 ("helper" T cells) are defined as typically secreting IL-4, IL-5, and IL-6 (plus GM-CSF and IL-3), providing help but not DTH and promoting a switch to the IgG1 isotype. However, individual CD^+ T-cell clones vary widely in the particular combinations of cytokines they produce; the two dominant patterns described above tend to emerge only in chronic persisting infections, best studied in leishmaniasis, and after long-term culture.

Suppressor T Cells. Ts cells are the least well-characterized class of T cells. Functionally, there is no doubt that certain populations of $CD4^-$, CD^+, I-J^+ T cells can be demonstrated to down-regulate other T-cell and/or B-cell-mediated immune responses. However, it has proved difficult to clone the T cells that display this property, and some immunologists remain skeptical about the existence of a unique Ts cell type with a unique suppressor function. Currently, it appears likely that T cells may, under particular circumstances, suppress various arms of the immune response in a variety of ways, for example, (1) by direct cognate interaction with an effector B or Tc cell, or (2) indirectly, by suppression of a helper T cell, or (3) via antigen-specific soluble factors or antigen-nonspecific cytokines.

The effector response of T cells is generally transient; for instance, in certain acute infections Tc and Td activities peak about 1 week after the onset of a viral infection, and disappear by 2–3 weeks. In rare cases this may be attributable to the destruction of infected cells and removal of the antigenic stimulus, or it may be a function of Ts cells.

γ/δ T Lymphocytes. A second class of T cells with a different type of receptor composed of polypeptide chains designated γ and δ is found principally in epithelia such as the skin, gut, and lungs. They display a relatively limited immunologic repertoire, reflecting a highly restricted V (variable) gene usage, and there is emerging evidence that these T cells are sometimes involved in the immune response to viral infections.

Cytokines

Cytokines are secretory proteins which regulate the proliferation, differentiation, and/or maturation of nearby cells. Many are produced by T lymphocytes (lymphokines) or monocytes/macrophages (monokines) and serve to regulate the immune response by coordinating the activities of the various cell types involved. Thus, while cytokines are not antigen-specific, their production and actions are often antigen-driven.

Cytokines affect cells in the immediate vicinity, particularly at cell–cell interfaces where directional secretion may occur. Target cells carry receptors for particular cytokines. A single cytokine may exert a multiplicity of biological effects, often acting on more than one type of cell. Moreover, different cytokines may exert similar effects, though perhaps via distinct postreceptor signal transduction pathways, resulting in synergism.

Cytokines up-regulate or down-regulate the target cell, and different cytokines can antagonize one another. Typically, a cytokine secreted by a particular type of cell activates another type of cell to secrete a different cytokine or to express receptors for a particular cytokine, and so on in a sort of chain reaction. Because of the intricacy of the cytokine cascade it is rarely possible to attribute a given biological event *in vivo* to a single cytokine.

Cytokines (Table 8-2) can influence viral pathogenesis in a number of ways: (1) augmentation of the immune response, for example, of cytotoxic T cells by tumor necrosis factor or by interferon γ which up-regulates MHC protein expression; (2) regulation of the immune response, for example, antibody isotype switching by interleukin 4, 5, 6, or interferon γ; (3) suppression of the immune response, for example, interleukin 10 inhibits the synthesis of interferon γ; (4) inhibition of viral replication by interferons; (5) up-regulation of viral gene expression, for example, TNF-α and interleukin 6, binding to their receptors on T cells, induce the

TABLE 8-2

Cytokines and Their Sources, Targets, and Effects[a]

Cytokine	Principal source	Principal targets/effects
IL-1	Monocytes/macrophages	Proliferation of T cells; IL-2 receptor expression; antibody; fever
IL-2	T cells	Proliferation and differentiation of T cells
IL-3	T cells	Hematopoiesis, stem cells and mast cells
IL-4	Th cells, bone marrow stromal cells	Proliferation and differentiation of B, T, M; switch to IgG1, IgE
IL-5	Th cells	Proliferation and differentiation of B, E; switch to IgA
IL-6	T cells, macrophages, other	Proliferation and differentiation of lymphocytes; antibody; fever
IL-7	Bone marrow stromal cells	Proliferation of pre-B and pre-T cells
IL-8	Various	Chemotaxis, neutrophils and T cells
TNF-α, β	Monocytes, other	Proliferation and differentiation of T, B, M, N, F; fever, cachexia
TGF-β	Various	Inhibits proliferation of T, B, and stem cells
IFN-α, β	Leukocytes, other	Antiviral; fever
IFN-γ	Th cells	Antiviral; activation of Tc, M, NK; IgG2a switch; up-regulates MHC and Fc receptors
GM-CSF	T, M, F, endothelium	Hematopoiesis, granulocytes, monocytes

[a] IL, Interleukin; TNF, tumor necrosis factor; TGF, transforming growth factor; IFN, interferon; CSF, colony-stimulating factor; T, T lymphocyte; B, B lymphocyte; M, monocyte/macrophage; NK, natural killer cell; E, eosinophil; N, neutrophil; F, fibroblast. Cytokines are pleiotropic in their action. Only certain important cytokines are listed.

synthesis of the DNA-binding protein NFκB, which in turn binds to the regulatory region of the integrated HIV provirus and promotes HIV gene transcription.

B Lymphocytes

Some of the pluripotent hemopoietic stem cells originating from fetal liver and later from bone marrow differentiate into B lymphocytes, which are characterized by the presence on their surface of specific antigen-binding receptors, receptors for complement (C3), and receptors for the Fc portion of immunoglobulin. During ontogeny, complex DNA rearrangements occur involving recombination between hundreds of inherited V immunoglobulin gene segments to yield potentially millions of combinations. Each individual B lymphocyte and its progeny expresses only one of these immunoglobulin genes; hence by the time an animal is born there is a vast number of B lymphocytes expressing different monomeric IgM molecules as surface receptor proteins. Such cells have three possible fates: they may react with a self-antigen (many but not all such cells are eliminated); they may react with a foreign antigen, undergo clonal expansion, and secrete antibody to that antigen; or, like other effector cells, they may be short-lived and soon die. In contrast to T cells, the receptors of B cells are antibody-like molecules that recognize antigens in their native state, rather than as peptides bound to MHC protein, hence B cells react directly with viral proteins, or even virions. When the particular clones of B cells bearing receptors complementary to any one of the several epitopes on an antigen bind that antigen, they respond, after receiving the appropriate signals from Th cells, by division and differentiation into antibody-secreting plasma cells.

Each *plasma cell* secretes antibody of only a single specificity, corresponding to the particular V (variable) domains of the immunoglobulin (Ig) receptor it expresses. Initially this antibody is of the IgM class, but an antigen-induced gene translocation brings about a class switch by associating the V gene segments with a different H (heavy) chain constant domain. Thus, after a few days IgG, IgA, and sometimes IgE antibodies of the same specificity begin to dominate the immune response. Early in the immune response, when large amounts of antigen are present, there is an opportunity for antigen-reactive B cells to be triggered even if their receptors fit the epitope with relatively poor *affinity;* the result is the production of antibody which binds the antigen with low *avidity.* Later on, when only small amounts of antigen remain, B cells that have evolved by hypermutation in their V_H genes to produce receptors that bind the antigen with high affinity are selected (*affinity maturation*), hence the avidity of the antibody secreted increases correspondingly.

Immunologic Memory

Following priming by antigen and clonal expansion of lymphocytes, a population of long-lived *memory cells* arises which persists indefinitely. Memory T cells are characterized by particular surface markers (notably CD45RO) and adhesion (homing) molecules that are associated with a distinct recirculation pathway. When reexposed to the same antigen, even many years later, they respond more rapidly and more vigorously than in the primary encounter. Memory B cells, on reexposure to antigen, also display an *anamnestic (secondary) response,* with production of larger amounts of specific antibody.

Little is known about the mechanism of the longevity of immunologic memory in T or B lymphocytes in the absence of demonstrable chronic infection. The cells are periodically restimulated by the original antigen retained indefinitely as antigen–antibody complexes on follicular dendritic cells in lymphoid follicles, or by surrogate antigen in the form of either fortuitously cross-reactive antigens or anti-idiotypic antibodies. However, there is evidence that in some cases memory T and B lymphocytes may survive for a many years without dividing, until restimulated following reinfection.

B Cells as Antigen-Presenting Cells. Memory B cells serve as very efficient antigen-presenting cells. Viral antigen, or the virion itself, binds to the specific immunoglobulin receptors on the B lymphocyte and is endocytosed then cleaved into peptides, which are in turn re-presented on the surface of the B cell. These peptides, which generally represent different epitopes from those recognized (on the same antigen) by the B cell, associate with class II MHC proteins on the B-cell plasma membrane and are presented to the corresponding, already activated $CD4^+$ T cells, which respond by secreting cytokines that provide help for the B cell to make antibody. Such cognate interaction, involving close physical association of T and B cells, ensures efficient delivery of "helper factors" (cytokines) from the Th cell to the relevant primed B cell.

Antibodies

The end result of activation and maturation of B cells is the production of antibodies, which react specifically with the epitope identified initially by their receptors. Antibodies fall into four main classes: two monomers, IgG and IgE, and two polymers, IgM and IgA. All immunoglobulins of a particular class have a similar structure, but they differ widely in the amino acid sequences comprising the antigen-binding site, which determines their specificity for a given antigenic determinant.

The commonest immunoglobulin found in serum, IgG, consists of two "heavy" and two "light" chains, and each chain consists of a "constant" and a "variable" domain. The chains are held together by disulfide bonds. Papain cleavage separates the molecules into two identical *Fab fragments,* which contain the antigen-binding sites, and an *Fc fragment,* which carries the sites for various effector functions such as complement fixation, attachment to phagocytic cells, and placental transfer.

The immunologic specificity of an antibody molecule is determined by its ability to bind specifically to a particular epitope. The binding site is located at the amino-terminal end of the molecule and is composed of certain hypervariable sequences within the "variable" domains of both light and heavy chains. Of the approximately 220 amino acids of the variable domain of a heavy chain–light chain pair, between 15 and 30 appear to make up the binding site. Antibody specificity is a function of both the amino acid sequence at these sites and their three-dimensional configuration.

The major class of antibody in the blood is immunoglobulin G (IgG), which occurs as IgG1, IgG2, IgG3, and IgG4 subclasses. Following systemic viral infections, IgG continues to be synthesized for many years and is the principal mediator of protection against reinfection. The subclasses of IgG differ in the "constant" region of their heavy chains and consequently in biological properties such as complement fixation, binding to phagocytes, and transfer into colostrum and milk. In cattle and sheep, IgG1 is the major immunoglobulin in the colostrum (Table 8-3) and plays a major role in protecting newborn animals against infections.

IgM is a particularly avid class of antibody, being a pentamer of 5 IgG equivalents, with 10 Fab fragments and therefore 10 antigen-binding sites. Because IgM is formed early in the immune response and is later replaced by IgG, specific antibodies of the IgM class are diagnostic of recent (or chronic) infection. IgM antibodies are also the first to be found in the fetus as it develops immunologic competence in the second half of pregnancy. Since IgM does not cross the placenta from dam to fetus in any species, the presence of IgM antibodies against a particular virus in a newborn animal is diagnostic of intrauterine infection.

IgA is a dimer, with four Fab fragments. Passing through epithelial cells, IgA acquires a secretory component to become secretory IgA, which is secreted through mucosae into the respiratory, intestinal, and urogenital tracts. Secretory IgA is more resistant to proteases than other immunoglobulins, and it is the principal immunoglobulin on mucosal surfaces and, in some species of animals, in milk and colostrum (Table 8-3). For this reason IgA antibodies are important in resistance to infection of the respiratory, intestinal, and urogenital tracts, and IgA antibody responses are much more effectively elicited by oral or respiratory than by systemic

TABLE 8-3

Concentrations of Immunoglobulin Classes in Colostrum and Milk of Mammalian Species

	Immunoglobulin concentration (g/liter)					
	Colostrum			Milk		
Species	IgG	IgA	IgM	IgG	IgA	IgM
Human	0.3	**120**[a]	1.2	0.1	**1.5**	0.01
Cattle	**36–77**	4–5	3.2–4.9	**1.0–1.8**	0.2	0.04
Swine	**62**	10	3.2	1.4	**3.0**	1.9
Horse	**80**	9	4	0.35	**0.8**	0.04
Dog	2.0	**13.5**	0.3	0.01	**3.6**	0.06

[a] Bold-face type indicates major components.

administration of antigen, a matter of importance in the design and route of delivery of some vaccines (see Chapter 13).

Antibodies directed against certain epitopes on the surface of virions neutralize infectivity; they may also act as opsonins, facilitating the uptake and destruction of virions by macrophages. In addition, antibody may attach to viral antigens on the surface of infected cells, leading to their destruction following activation of the classical or alternate complement pathways or by arming and activating Fc receptor-bearing cells such as K cells, polymorphonuclear leukocytes, and macrophages (antibody-dependent cell-mediated cytotoxicity).

Complement

The *complement system* consists of a series of serum components which can be activated to "complement" the immune response (Fig. 8-3). As well as the *classical complement activation pathway,* which is dependent on the presence of an antigen–antibody complex, there is also an *alternate,* antibody-independent pathway. Both are important in viral infections.

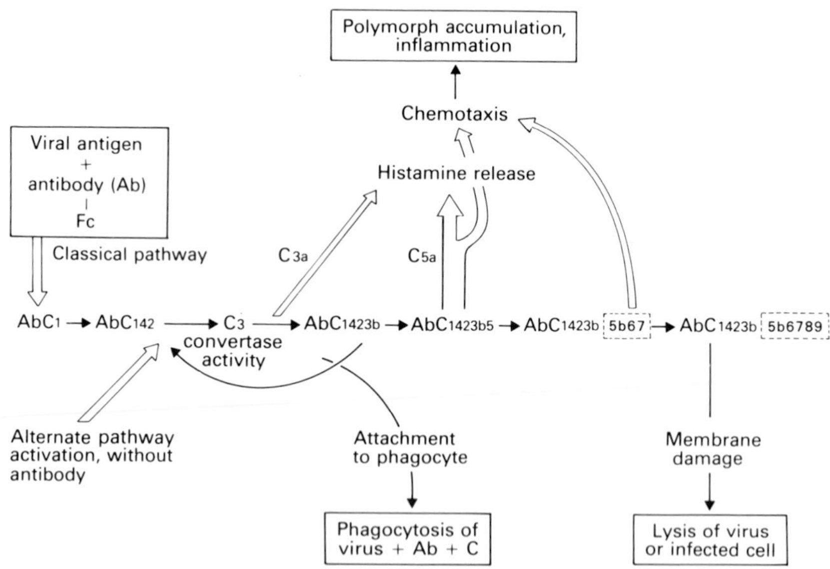

FIG. 8-3. *Diagram of the complement activation sequence by the classical and alternate pathways and the antiviral action of complement. The numbers of the complement components are not sequential because they were assigned before the sequence of action was elucidated. (From C. A. Mims and D. O. White, "Viral Pathogenesis and Immunology." Blackwell, Oxford, 1984.)*

Activation of complement by the classical pathway may lead to the destruction of virions or virus-infected cells, as well as to inflammation. Virions are destroyed as a result of opsonization, enhancement of neutralization, or lysis of the viral envelope. Complement activation following interaction of antibody with viral antigens in tissues leads to inflammation and the accumulation of leukocytes. Activation of complement via the alternate pathway appears to occur mainly after infections with enveloped viruses that mature by budding through the plasma membrane; since it does not require antibody, the alternate pathway can occur immediately after viral invasion.

Natural Killer Cells

Natural killer (NK) cells are a heterogeneous group of $CD3^-$, $CD16^+$, $CD56^+$ large granular lymphocytes of uncertain lineage which have the capacity to kill virus-infected cells and tumor cells. The basis for their selectivity for virus-infected cells is not known. They display no immunologic specificity for particular viral antigens, no memory, no MHC restriction, and no dependence on antibody. They may be an important early defense mechanism, since their activity is greatly enhanced within 1 or 2 days of viral infection. Virus-induced activation of NK cells is mediated by interferon, acting synergistically with IL-2, and NK cells themselves secrete several cytokines including IFN-γ and TNF-α.

IMMUNE RESPONSES TO VIRAL INFECTION

The major features of the *primary immune response* to a typical acute viralinfection are illustrated in Fig. 8-4. The large boxes highlight three crucially important phenomena which contribute to recovery from infection: (1) destruction of infected cells, (2) production of interferon, and (3) neutralization of the infectivity of progeny virions produced during the infectious process. The flowchart illustrates, in a simplified fashion, the interactions of the various cell types that participate in these events. Shortly after infection, some virus particles are phagocytosed by macrophages. Except in the case of certain viruses that are capable of growing in macrophages, the engulfed virions are destroyed. Their proteins are cleaved into shorter peptides which are presented on the surface of the macrophage in association with class II MHC protein. This combination is recognized by the appropriate clones of $CD4^+$ lymphocytes.

Td (mainly Th_1) lymphocytes respond by clonal proliferation and release of lymphokines, which attract blood monocytes to the site and induce them to proliferate and to differentiate into activated macro-

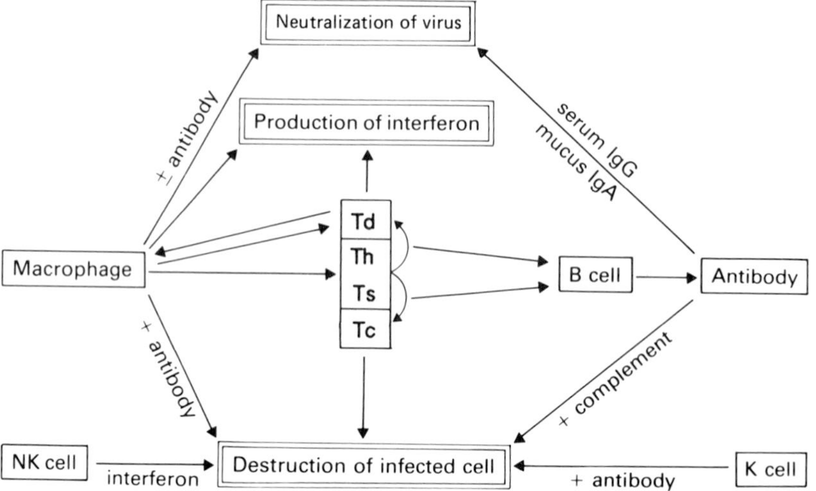

FIG. 8-4. *Immune responses to viral infection. For explanation see text. (From C. A. Mims and D. O. White, "Viral Pathogenesis and Immunology." Blackwell, Oxford, 1984.)*

phages, the basis of the inflammatory response. Th_2 lymphocytes respond by secreting a different set of lymphokines that assist the appropriate clones of B cells, following binding of viral antigen, to divide and differentiate into plasma cells. Tc cells are activated following recognition of viral peptides in association with MHC class I on the surface of infected cells. The Tc response usually peaks at about 1 week after infection, compared with the antibody response which peaks later (2–3 weeks). NK cell activity is maximal by 2 days, and interferon activity peaks in concert with the peak titer of virus.

Antibody synthesis takes place principally in the spleen, lymph nodes, gut-associated lymphoid tissues, and bronchus-associated lymphoid tissues. The spleen and lymph nodes receive viral antigens via the blood or lymphatics and synthesize antibodies mainly restricted to the IgM class early in the response and IgG subclasses subsequently. On the other hand, the submucosal lymphoid tissues of the respiratory and digestive tracts, such as the tonsils and Peyer's patches, receive antigens directly from overlying epithelial cells, and they make antibodies mainly of the IgA class.

Immune Cytolysis of Virus-Infected Cells

Destruction of infected cells is an essential feature of recovery from viral infections, and it results from any of four different processes: cytotoxic T cells, antibody–complement-mediated cytotoxicity, antibody-dependent cell-mediated cytotoxicity, and NK cells. Since some viral proteins, or peptides derived therefrom, appear in the plasma membrane before any virions have been produced, lysis of the cell at this stage brings viral replication to a halt before significant numbers of progeny virions are released.

Cytolysis by cytotoxic T cells occurs by a complex mechanism involving the secretion of perforin, which forms ion channels through the plasma membrane of the target cell. *Antibody–complement-mediated cytoxicity* is readily demonstrable *in vitro* even at very low concentrations of antibody. The alternate complement activation pathway (see Fig. 8-3) appears to be particularly important in this phenomenon. *Antibody-dependent cell-mediated cytoxicity* is mediated by leukocytes that carry *Fc receptors:* macrophages, polymorphonuclear leukocytes, and other kinds of killer (K) cells. NK cells, on the other hand, are activated by interferon, or directly by viral glycoproteins. They demonstrate almost no immunologic specificity, but preferentially lyse virus-infected cells. Finally, in the presence of antibody, macrophages can phagocytose and digest virus-infected cells.

Neutralization of Viral Infectivity

In contrast to T cells, B cells and antibody generally recognize epitopes that are *conformational,* that is, the critical residues that make contact with the antigen-binding site of the antibody molecule are not necessarily contiguous in the primary amino acid sequence but may be brought into close apposition as a result of the folding of the polypeptide chain(s) to produce the native conformation. Such B-cell epitopes are generally located on the surface of the protein, often on prominent protuberances or loops, and particularly with RNA viruses represent relatively variable regions of the molecule, differing between strains of that species of virus.

While specific antibody of any class can bind to any accessible epitope on a surface protein of a virion, only those antibodies that bind with reasonably high avidity to particular epitopes on a particular protein of the outer capsid or envelope of the virion are capable of neutralizing viral infectivity. The key protein is usually the one containing the ligand by which the virion attaches to receptors on the host cell.

Neutralization is not simply a matter of coating the virion with antibody, nor indeed of blocking attachment to the host cell. Except in the presence of such high concentrations of antibody that most or all accessible antigenic sites on the surface of the virion are saturated, neutralized virions may still attach to susceptible cells. In such cases the neutralizing block occurs at some point following adsorption and entry. One hypothesis is that, whereas the virion is normally uncoated intracellularly in a controlled way that preserves its infectivity, a virion–antibody complex may be destroyed by cellular enzymes. In the case of picornaviruses, neutralizing antibody appears to distort the capsid, leading to loss of a particular capsid protein and rendering the virion vulnerable to enzymatic attack.

RECOVERY FROM VIRAL INFECTION

Cell-mediated immunity, antibody, complement, phagocytes, and interferons and other cytokines are all involved in the response to viral infections and may alone or in concert be responsible for recovery, depending on the particular host–virus combination (see Fig. 8-4).

Role of T Lymphocytes

T-cell depletion by neonatal thymectomy or antilymphocyte serum treatment increases the susceptibility of experimental animals to most viral infections; for example, T-cell-depleted mice infected with ectromelia virus fail to show the usual inflammatory mononuclear cell infiltration in the liver, develop extensive liver necrosis, and die, in spite of the production of antiviral antibodies and interferon. Virus titers in the liver and spleen of infected mice can be greatly reduced by adoptive transfer of immune T cells taken from recovered donors; this process is class I MHC restricted, implicating Tc cells, and is lifesaving.

Another experimental approach is to ablate completely all immune potential, then add back one or more of the separate components of the immune system. With mice treated in this way, virus-primed Tc lymphocytes of defined function and specificity, cloned in culture then transferred to infected mice, have been shown to save the lives of mice infected with lymphocytic choriomeningitis virus, influenza virus, and several other viruses.

Although T-cell determinants and B-cell epitopes on surface proteins of viruses sometimes overlap, the immunodominant Tc determinants can be situated on the relatively conserved proteins located in the interior of the virion, or on nonstructural virus-coded proteins that occur only in virus-infected cells. Hence T-cell responses are generally of broader specificity than neutralizing antibody responses and display cross-reactivity between strains and serotypes. When the gene encoding a protein that fails to elicit any neutralizing antibody (e.g., N or M proteins of influenza virus) is incorporated in the genome of vaccinia virus, the T cells elicited following infection with this construct can adoptively transfer to naive mice complete protection against challenge.

Congenital Immunodeficiencies. The approach least subject to laboratory artifact is simple clinical observation of viral infections in animals or children suffering from primary immunodeficiencies. For example, athymic or *nude mice,* which are congenitally deficient in T cells, are highly susceptible to many viral infections. In certain families of Arabian horses there is a total or near total absence of both B and T lymphocytes. Characteristic findings are a lymphophenia and a hypogammaglobulinemia, which render foals unusually susceptible to infections, especially with equine adenoviruses. There are also several types of B-lymphocyte deficiencies which predispose newborns of various domestic animals to severe infections. Among these are a primary agammaglobulinemia of thoroughbred horses, a selective deficiency in foals of IgM-producing B cells, a deficiency of IgG2-synthesizing cells in some breeds of cattle, and a dysgammaglobulinemia in certain lines of white leghorn chickens. Furthermore, there are conditions characterized by a T-cell deficiency due to thymic hypoplasia. Of different origin and signficance, but of great practical importance, are secondary agammaglobulinemias and hypogammaglobulinemias in foals, piglets, lambs, and especially calves that are associated with the failure of antibody transfer via colostrum (see below).

The data obtained from these clinical conditions and experimental approaches indicate a key role for T lymphocytes in recovery from generalized viral infections. Lymphocytes and macrophages normally predominate in the cellular infiltration of virus-infected tissues; in contrast with bacterial infections, polymorphonuclear leukocytes are not at all plentiful. Animals or humans with severe T-cell deficiencies due to thymic aplasia, lymphoreticular neoplasms, or chemical immunosuppression show increased susceptibility to herpesviruses and to certain other viral infections. Perhaps the most informative example is that of measles in infants with thymic aplasia. In these T-cell-deficient infants there is no sign of the usual measles rash but an uncontrolled and progressive growth of virus in the respiratory tract, leading to fatal pneumonia. This reveals two aspects of the role of T cells. Evidently, in the normal child, the T-cell-mediated immune response controls infection in the lung and also plays a vital role in the development of the characteristic skin rash.

Role of Natural Killer Cells

The role of NK cells in recovery from viral infection is not yet certain. "Beige" mice, which have substantially reduced NK cell activity, or normal mice depleted of NK cells by treatment with NK-specific antiserum show increased replication of some viruses but not others. Athymic mice have normal numbers of NK cells but usually die if infected with viruses that produce generalized viral infections. NK cells probably represent a nonspecific defense mechanism of particular relevance in the early stage of primary virus infections, but they are less crucial than either T cells or antibody in clearing the infection and play no role in the establishment of immunologic memory.

Role of Antibody

In generalized diseases characterized by a viremia in which virions circulate free in the plasma, circulating antibody plays an additional role. Because no instances of severe pure B-cell deficiency have been identified in animals, we need to turn to human examples to help elucidate the situation. Unlike those with a T-cell deficit, children with severe primary agammaglobulinemia recover normally from measles or varicella but are about 10,000 times more likely than normal individuals to develop paralytic disease after vaccination with live attenuated poliovirus vaccine. They have normal cell-mediated immune and interferon responses, normal phagocytic cells, and complement, but cannot produce antibody, which is essential if poliovirus spread to the central nervous system via the bloodstream is to be prevented.

Although there is reasonably good evidence that antibody plays a key role in recovery from picornavirus, togavirus, flavivirus, and parvovirus infections, it does not necessarily follow that the antibody is acting solely by neutralizing virions. Indeed it has been shown that certain nonneutralizing monoclonal antibodies can save the lives of mice, presumably by antibody-dependent cell-mediated cytotoxicity or antibody–complement-mediated lysis of infected cells, or by opsonizination of virions for macrophages.

IMMUNITY TO REINFECTION

Whereas a large number of interacting phenomena contribute to recovery from viral infection, the mechanism of acquired immunity to reinfection with the same agent appears to be much simpler. The first line of defense is antibody, which, if acquired by active infection with a virus that causes systemic infections, continues to be synthesized and protects against reinfection for many years. The solidity of acquired immunity generally correlates well with the titer of antibody in the serum. Further, passive transfer of antibody alone, whether by passive immunization or by maternal transfer from dam to fetus or newborn, provides excellent protection against many viral infections. If the antibody defenses are inadequate, the mechanisms that contribute to recovery are called into play again, the principal differences on this occasion being that the dose of infecting virus is reduced by antibody and that preprimed memory T and B lymphocytes generate a more rapid secondary response.

As a general rule the secretory IgA antibody response is short-lived compared to the serum IgG response. Accordingly, resistance to reinfection with respiratory viruses and some enteric viruses tends to be of limited duration. Thus reinfection with the same serotype of parainfluenza virus or respiratory syncytial virus is not uncommon.

The immune response to the first infection with a virus can have a dominating influence on subsequent immune responses to antigenically related viruses, in that the second virus often induces a response that is directed mainly against the antigens of the original viral strain. For example, the antibody response of humans to sequential infections with different strains of influenza A virus is largely directed to antigens characterizing the particular strain of virus with which a particular individual was first infected. This phenomenon has been called "original antigenic sin" and is also seen in infections with enteroviruses, reoviruses, paramyxoviruses, and togaviruses. Original antigenic sin has important implications for interpretation of seroepidemiologic data, for understanding immunopathologic phenomena, and particularly for the development of efficacious vaccination strategies.

PASSIVE IMMUNITY

There is abundant evidence for the efficacy of antibody in preventing infection. For example, artificial *passive immunization* (injection of antibodies) temporarily protects against infection with canine distemper, feline panleukopenia, hog cholera, and many other viral infections (see Chapter 13). Furthermore, natural passive immunization, namely, the transfer of maternal antibody from dam to fetus or newborn, protects the newborn for the first few months of life against most of the infections that the dam has experienced.

Natural Passive Immunity

Natural passive immunity is important for two major reasons: (1) it is essential for the protection of young animals, during the first weeks or months of life, from the myriad of microorganisms, including viruses, that are present in the environment into which animals are born; (2) maternally derived antibody interferes with active immunization of the newborn and must therefore be taken into account when designing vaccination schedules (see Chapter 13).

Transfer of Maternal Antibodies. Maternal antibodies may be transmitted in the egg yolk in birds or across the placenta or via colostrum and/or milk in mammals. Different species of mammals differ strikingly in the predominant route of transfer of maternal antibodies, depending on the structure of the placenta of the species (Table 8-4). In species in which the maternal and fetal circulations are separated by relatively few (1–3) placental layers, antibody of the IgG (but not IgM) class is able to cross the placenta, and maternal immunity is transmitted mainly by this route. However, the placenta of most domestic animals is more complex (5–6 layers) and acts as a barrier even to IgG; in these species maternal immunity is transmitted to the newborn via colostrum and, to a much lesser extent, via milk.

Different species differ in regard to the particular class or subclass of immunoglobulin that is preferentially transferred to the newborn in colostrum (see Table 8-3), but in most domestic animals it is mainly IgG. In cattle there is a selective transfer of IgG1 from the serum across the alveolar epithelium of the mammary gland during the last few weeks of pregnancy, such that the level of IgG1 in colostrum may reach 40 g/liter compared with about 13 g/liter in serum.

The selective transfer of IgG from the maternal circulation across the mammary alveolar epithelium is a function of the Fc fragment of the molecule. The large amounts of IgG present in colostrum are ingested and *translocated* in large intracytoplasmic vesicles by specialized cells present in the small intestine, to reach the circulation of the newborn in an undegraded form. Small amounts of other antibodies (IgM, IgA) present in colostrum or milk may in some species also be translocated across the gut, but they quickly disappear from the circulation of the young animal. The period after birth during which antibody, ingested as colostrum, is translocated is sharply defined and very brief (about 48 hours) in most domestic animals (see Table 8-4). The mechanism of *translocation cutoff* is not known.

In birds there is a selective transfer of IgG from the maternal circulation; the level of IgG in chicken egg yolk is 25 g/liter compared with 6 g/liter in the maternal circulation. A laying hen produces about 100 g of IgG per year for transfer to yolk, which is about as much as she synthesizes for her own needs. IgG enters the vitelline circulation and hence that of the chick from day 12 of incubation. Some IgG is also transferred to the amniotic fluid and swallowed by the chick. Close to the time of hatching, the yolk sac with the remaining maternal immunoglobulin is completely taken into the abdominal cavity and incorporated into the wall of the small intestine of the chick.

Maternal antibody in the bloodstream of the newborn mammal or

TABLE 8-4
Transfer of Natural Passive Immunity in Mammals

Species	Type of placentation	Number of placental layers		Prenatal transfer (via placenta)	Postnatal transfer (via gut)	Translocation cutoff time (days)
		Maternal	Fetal			
Cow, swine, horse	Epitheliochorial	3	3	0	+++	2
Sheep, goat	Syndesmochorial	2 or 3	3	0	+++	2
Dog, cat	Endotheliochorial	1	2 or 3	±	+++	2
Mouse, rat	Hemochorial	0	3	++	+	16–20

newly hatched chick is destroyed quite rapidly, with first-order kinetics. The half-life, which is somewhat longer than in adult animals, ranges from about 21 days in the cow and horse to 8 or 9 days in the dog and cat to only 2 days in the mouse. Of course, the newborn animal will be protected against infection with any particular virus only if the IgG of the dam contains specific antibodies, and protection may last much longer than one IgG half-life if the initial titer against that virus is high.

Although the levels of IgA transferred via colostrum to the gut of the newborn animal are considerably lower than those of IgG, the IgA helps to protect the neonate against enteric viruses against which the dam has developed immunity. Moreover, there is evidence that after translocation cutoff immunoglobulins present in ordinary milk, principally IgA but also IgG and IgM, may continue to provide some protective immunity against gut infections. Often the newborn encounters viruses while still partially protected. Under these circumstances the virus replicates, but only to a limited extent, stimulating an immune response without causing significant disease. The newborn thus acquires active immunity while partially protected by maternal immunity.

Failure of Maternal Antibody Transfer. The failure or partial failure of maternal antibody transfer is the most common immunodeficiency disease of domestic animals. For example, between 10% and 40% of dairy calves and up to 20% of foals fail to receive adequate levels of maternal antibody. Mortality during the neonatal and early adolescent period, particularly from respiratory and enteric diseases, is higher than at any other time of life, and there is a strong correlation with failure of antibody transfer. Biological reasons for failure are birth of weak or deformed animals, delay to first suckle, death of the dam, poor colostrum production, low antibody levels in maternal serum and thus in colostrum, poor maternal instinct particularly in primiparous dams, premature lactation, too many in the litter, and bulling of the weak in the litter by the strong. Of these, the most critical factors are the amount of colostrum available and the delay between birth and first suckling. Poor management may also play a role, by the imposition of unnatural conditions on parturition and early suckling.

The transfer of maternal antibody to the newborn and its persistence are of paramount importance for the control of infectious diseases of domestic animals, and maternal immunization to protect the newborn is an important strategy in veterinary medicine (see Chapter 13).

FURTHER READING

Bjorkman, P. J., and Parham, P. (1990). Structure, function and diversity of class I major histocompatibility complex molecules. *Annu. Rev. Biochem.* **59,** 253.

Bloom, B. R., and Oldstone, M. B. A., eds. (1991). Immunity to infection. *Curr. Opin. Immunol.* **3,** 453.

Brandtzaeg, P. (1989). Overview of the mucosal immune system. *Curr. Top. Microbiol. Immunol.* **146,** 13.

Davis, M. M. (1990). T cell receptor gene diversity and selection. *Annu. Rev. Biochem.* **59,** 475.

Dimmock, N. J. (1984). Mechanisms of neutralization of animal viruses. *J. Gen. Virol.* **65,** 1015.

Notkins, A. L., and Oldstone, M. B. A., eds. (1984, 1986, 1989). "Concepts in Viral Pathogenesis," Vols. 1, 2, and 3. Springer-Verlag, New York.

Paul, W. D., ed. (1989). "Fundamental Immunology," 2nd Ed. Raven, New York.

Roitt, I. M., Brostoff, J., and Male, D. K. (1989). "Immunology," 2nd Ed. Churchill Livingstone, London.

Rothbard, J. B., and Gefter, M. L. (1991). Interactions between immunogenic peptides and MHC proteins. *Annu. Rev. Immunol.* **9,** 572.

Sercarz, E., and Berzofsky, J., eds. (1988). "Immunogenicity of Protein Antigens," Vols. 1 and 2. CRC Press, Boca Raton, Florida.

Steinman, R. M. (1991). The dendritic cell system and its role in immunogenicity. *Annu. Rev. Immunol.* **9,** 271.

Thomas, D. B., ed. (1991). "Viruses and the Immune Response." Dekker, New York.

Trinchieri, G. (1989). Biology of natural killer cells. *Adv. Immunol.* **47,** 187.

van Regenmortel, M. H. V., and Neurath, A. R., eds. (1991). "Viruses and the Immune Response," Vols. 1 and 2. Elsevier, Amsterdam.

CHAPTER 9

Mechanisms of Disease Production

In the previous four chapters we have analyzed various aspects of viral infections of animals, exploring how viruses affect cells, how infection of animals occurs, how viruses spread to various parts of the body, and how the host animal responds to infection by immunologic and other mechanisms. This chapter and the next two are concerned with the clinical consequences of these interactions, namely, disease. The first part of this chapter covers the ways in which viral replication damages tissues and organs and the ways in which the body's own responses may cause damage. In the second part of the chapter the pathogenesis of acute viral infections which produce respiratory, intestinal, generalized, and neurologic disease are presented as examples.

VIRAL DAMAGE TO TISSUES AND ORGANS

The mechanisms by which viruses damage cells were discussed at the subcellular and cellular levels in Chapter 5. Here we apply these concepts at the level of tissues and organs. The severity of disease in the animal is not necessarily correlated with the degree of cytopathology produced by the virus *in vitro*. Many viruses that are cytocidal in cultured cells do not produce clinical disease (e.g., many enteroviruses), whereas some that are noncytocidal *in vitro* cause a lethal disease *in vivo* (e.g., rabies virus). Depending on the organ affected, considerable cell and tissue damage can occur without producing signs of disease, for example, a large number of liver cells can be destroyed without significant clinical signs. When damage to cells does impair the function of an organ or tissue, this may be of minor importance in one part of the body, such as muscle or subcutaneous tissue, but of great importance in the heart or the brain. Likewise, edema of a tissue may be unimportant in most sites in the body but may have serious consequences in the brain, because of the resulting increase in intracranial pressure, the lung, where it may interfere with gaseous exchange, and the heart, where it may interfere with conduction.

Sometimes the whole pathologic picture in an animal may be explained by the direct damage to cells caused by a highly cytocidal virus. Mice inoculated intravenously with a large dose of Rift Valley fever virus, for example, develop overwhelming hepatic necrosis within 4 hours of injection, because the virions pass quickly through the Kupffer cells to infect the hepatic cells, which are rapidly lysed. In this experimental model, the defense mechanisms of the host are quite unable to cope with the rapid lethal damage to a vital organ.

In other situations infected cells may show no obvious damage, but specialized cells may carry out their functions less effectively. For example, lymphocytic choriomeningitis virus infection of hybridoma cells appears harmless, but less antibody is produced by infected than by uninfected cells. In mice, the same virus infects cells of the anterior pituitary that produce growth hormone without cytopathic effect; however, the output of growth hormone is reduced and as a result the mice are runted, and persistent infection of islet cells in the pancreas may result in a lifelong elevation of blood glucose levels (diabetes). Viruses may alter the expression of cell surface markers by an indirect mechanism; thus changes in class II MHC expression after infection of glial cells by mouse hepatitis virus may be due to the production of interferon γ.

Epithelial Damage Predisposing to Secondary Bacterial Infection

As well as having direct adverse effects, viral infections of the respiratory or digestive tracts often predispose animals to secondary bacterial infections. Viral infection increases the susceptibility of the respiratory tract to bacteria that are normal commensals in the nose and throat. For example, in cattle, parainfluenza virus 3 or other viruses may destroy ciliated epithelia and cause exudation, allowing *Pasteurella haemolytica* and other bacteria to invade the lungs and cause secondary bacterial pneumonia ("shipping fever," see below). Rhinoviruses and respiratory syncytial viruses damage the mucosa in the nasopharynx and sinuses, predisposing to bacterial superinfection which commonly leads to purulent rhinitis, pharyngitis, and sinusitis. Similarly, in the intestinal tract, rotavirus and coronavirus infections may lead to an increase in susceptibility to enteropathogenic *Escherichia coli,* and the synergistic effect leads to severe diarrhea. Conversely, proteases secreted by bacteria may activate influenza virus infectivity by proteolytic cleavage of the hemagglutinin.

Veterinary pathologists are particularly conscious of the potentiating effect on viral diseases of coinfection with parasites. Domestic animals are almost universally infected with protozoa and helminths, and a high parasitic load generally lowers host resistance to viruses and bacteria.

DAMAGE TO THE IMMUNE SYSTEM

Because the immune system plays a key role in protection against infections, viral damage to its components can exacerbate the severity of disease or predispose to superinfection with other infectious agents. In addition, both specific acquired immunodeficiency and generalized immunosuppression can occur in viral infections.

Infection of the *bursa of Fabricius* in chickens (the site of B-cell differentiation) with infectious bursal disease virus (a birnavirus) leads to atrophy of the bursa and a severe deficiency of B lymphocytes, with an increase in susceptibility to bacteria, particularly *Salmonella* and *E. coli,* and Marek's disease, Newcastle disease, infectious bronchitis, and infectious laryngotracheitis viruses. Similarly immune deficiency caused by feline leukemia and feline immunodeficiency viruses predisposes to a wide range of secondary infections.

Since the discovery in 1983 of the human immunodeficiency virus (HIV), the agent that causes the acquired immunodeficiency syndrome (AIDS) in man, similar viruses have been discovered in monkeys (simian immunodeficiency viruses, SIVs) and cats (feline immunodeficiency virus, FIV). All these viruses are members of the genus *Lentivirus,* and each has a similar though not identical genome structure. In susceptible animals each of these viruses probably acts in a similar way, namely, by destroying helper T cells, thus causing profound immunosuppression, which, after a prolonged clinical course, leads to death from opportunistic infections.

Infections with certain other viruses (e.g., hog cholera, bovine virus diarrhea, canine distemper viruses, feline and canine parvoviruses) may temporarily suppress humoral and/or cell-mediated immune responses. The immune response to unrelated antigens is reduced or abrogated in such animals, and the situation is thus distinct from suppression of the immune response to a specific virus by immune tolerance. The mechanisms involved in such general immunosuppression are not fully understood but may result from the replication of virus in lymphocytes and/or macrophages. Many viruses are capable of replication in macrophages, and several have been shown to grow in T cells, especially activated T cells. Some herpesviruses replicate nonproductively in B cells, transforming them and altering their function.

Although viral infection can induce immunosuppression, conversely immunosuppression allows enhanced viral replication. When the immune system is suppressed by endogenous or exogenous factors, latent herpesvirus, adenovirus, or papovavirus infections can be reactivated. Such situations are frequently encountered following the use of cytotoxic drugs or irradiation for organ transplantation in humans, and are also a feature of AIDS. Immunosuppression, usually of unknown origin, is probably responsible, at least in part, for reactivation of herpesviruses in animals.

IMMUNOPATHOLOGY AS A CAUSE OF DISEASE

Aspects of the immune response to viral infection are an essential part of the pathogenesis of most virus diseases. Infiltration of lymphocytes and macrophages, with accompanying release of cytokines and inflammation, is a regular feature of viral infection. Such common signs as fever, erythema, edema, and enlargement of lymph nodes have an immunologic basis. However, there are viral diseases in which the cardinal manifestations are caused by the body's immune response. When pathologic changes are made less severe by immunosuppressive treatment, it is assumed that immunopathology makes an important contribution to the disease.

Immunopathologic (hypersensitivity) reactions are traditionally classified into types I, II, III, and IV (Table 9-1). Although advances in cellular immunology have blurred some of the distinctions, the classification is still convenient. For most viral infections it is not known whether immunopathology makes a significant contribution to disease, and, if so, which of the four classical "hypersensitivity reactions" is implicated. Nevertheless, it is instructive to discuss the possible involvement of different kinds of hypersensitivity reactions in viral diseases.

TABLE 9-1

Basic Types of Hypersensitivity Reactions

Item	Hypersentivity type			
	I Anaphylactic	II Antibody-dependent cytotoxic	III Immune complex	IV Delayed (cell-mediated)
Time course				
Initiation	Minutes	Minutes	3–6 hours	18–24 hours
Persistence	Minutes	Dependent on antigen and antibody	Dependent on antigen and antibody	Weeks
Transfer with	IgE	IgM, IgG	IgG	T lymphocytes
Complement required	No	Usually	Yes	No
Histamine-dependent	Yes	No	Yes	No
Histology	Edema, congestion, eosinophils	Cell destruction, phagocytosis	Necrosis, neutrophils, later plasma cells	Lymphocytes, macrophages, necrosis
Viral immunopathology	Minor, ?some erythema	Minor, ?some erythema	Major Acute: fever Chronic: immune complex disease	Major in brain, lung

Hypersensitivity Reactions: Type I (Anaphylactic)

Type I hypersensitivity reactions depend on the interaction of antigens with IgE bound to the surface of mast cells via an Fc receptor, resulting in the release of histamine and heparin and the activation of serotonin and plasma kinins. Except for its possible contribution to some types of erythema and possibly in some acute respiratory infections, anaphylaxis is probably not important in viral immunopathology, but it is responsible for some adverse reactions to viral vaccines, owing to the presence of impurities such as egg proteins.

Hypersensitivity Reactions: Type II (Antibody-Dependent Cytotoxic)

Originally applied to cytotoxic reactions attributable to antibodies to autologous antigens, as in blood transfusion reactions, the type II cytolytic reactions also occur when antibody, having combined with viral antigen on the cell surface, activates the complement system, leading to cell lysis. Alternatively, antibodies can sensitize virus-infected cells to destruction by cytotoxic T lymphocytes, natural killer cells, polymorphonuclear leukocytes, or macrophages, via antibody-dependent cell-mediated cytotoxicity. While it has been clearly demonstrated that virus-infected cells are readily lysed by all of these mechanisms *in vitro*, their relative role in viral diseases *in vivo* is unclear, although there is some evidence that they may be operative in certain herpesvirus infections. Uninfected cells can be targets for type II reactions, as when complement-mediated lysis occurs after equine infectious anemia virus binds to horse erythrocytes and contributes to the anemia seen in this disease.

Hypersensitivity Reactions: Type III (Immune Complex Mediated)

Antigen–antibody reactions cause inflammation and cell damage by a variety of mechanisms. If the reaction occurs in extravascular tissues there is edema, inflammation, and infiltration of polymorphonuclear leukocytes, which may later be replaced by mononuclear cells. This is a common cause of mild inflammatory reactions. These immune complex reactions constitute the classical Arthus response and are of major importance, especially in persistent viral infections. If they occur in the blood, they produce circulating *immune complexes,* which are found in most viral infections. The fate of the immune complexes depends on the ratio of antibody to antigen. If there is a large excess of antibody, each antigen molecule is covered with antibody and removed by macrophages, which have receptors for the Fc component of the antibody molecule. If the amounts of antigen and antibody are about equal, lattice structures which develop into large aggregates are formed and removed rapidly by the reticuloendothelial system.

In some persistent infections, however, viral antigens or virions themselves are continuously released into the blood, but the antibody response is weak and antibodies are of low avidity. Complexes continue to be deposited in glomeruli over periods of weeks, months, or even years, leading to impairment of glomerular filtration and eventually to chronic glomerulonephritis. A classic example is lymphocytic choriomeningitis infection in mice infected *in utero* or as neonates. Viral antigens are present in the blood, and small amounts of nonneutralizing antibody are formed, giving rise to immune complexes which are progressively deposited on renal glomerular membranes. Depending on the strain of mouse, the end result may be glomerulonephritis, uremia, and death. Circulating immune complexes may also be deposited in the walls of the small blood vessels in skin, joints, and choroid plexus, where they attract macrophages and activate complement. Prodromal rashes, seen commonly in exanthems in humans but rarely in domestic animals, are probably caused in this way.

In addition to these local effects, antigen–antibody complexes generate systemic reactions, such as the fever which marks the end of the incubation period in generalized viral infections. Fever is mediated by interleukin 1, which is liberated from macrophages and polymorphonuclear leukocytes.

Rarely, systemic immune complex reactions may activate the enzymes of the coagulation cascade, leading to histamine release and increased vascular permeability. Fibrin is deposited in the kidneys, lungs, adrenals, and pituitary gland, causing multiple thromboses with infarcts and scattered hemorrhages, a condition known as disseminated intravascular coagulation. This is seen in hemorrhagic fevers in man, many of which are zoonoses caused by arenaviruses, bunyaviruses, filoviruses, or flaviviruses. Kittens infected with feline infectious peritonitis virus, a coronavirus, display this phenomenon, and it also occurs in fowl plague and hog cholera.

Hypersensitivity Reactions: Type IV (Cell-Mediated)

Unlike all the previous types, the type IV or "delayed hypersensitivity" reactions are mediated by cells rather than antibody. They are T-lymphocyte-mediated immune reactions, involving inflammation, lymphocytic infiltration, macrophage accumulation, and activation by lymphokines secreted by Td cells. Once again, the classic virological model is lymphocytic choriomeningitis virus infection, this time primary infection of adult mice. After intracerebral inoculation this noncytocidal virus replicates harmlessly in the meninges, ependyma, and choroid plexus epithelium until about the seventh day, when a Tc-lymphocyte-mediated immune response occurs, causing severe meningitis, cerebral edema, and death. Elsewhere than in the central nervous system, Tc cells help to control infection; within the rigid confines of the skull these changes are fatal. The death of mice infected in this way can be completely prevented by chemical immunosuppression, by X-irradiation, or by antilymphocyte serum. Type IV hypersensitivity reactions are important in the pathogenesis of Borna disease and may also contribute to consolidation of the lung, probably mediated by Td cells, in various severe lower respiratory tract diseases.

Although occasionally the cause of immunopathology, cell-mediated immune responses are generally an important component of the process of recovery from viral infections (see Chapter 8), as becomes evident if they are abrogated by cytotoxic drugs or are absent, as in some immunodeficiency diseases.

Autoimmune Diseases

The sharing of structurally similar regions in viral proteins with similar structures in host proteins has been called *molecular mimicry.* If viral and host determinants are similar enough to cross-react, yet different enough to break immunologic tolerance, epitope mimicry may be important in the induction of various autoimmune diseases. For example, a monoclonal antibody directed against the neutralizing domain of coxsackie B4 virus also reacts against heart muscle; this virus is suspected to have a role in myocarditis in humans. There is also suggestive evidence for matches of amino acid sequence between myelin basic protein (MBP) and viral proteins (Table 9-2). Such molecular mimicry may be involved in the neurologic disorders associated with the lentivirus infections, visna, and caprine arthritis–encephalitis, and in the rare occurrence of postvaccinial encephalitis in humans. Inoculation of a neuritogenic epitope in the P2 protein in peripheral nerve myelin will cause the experimental equivalent of Guillain-Barré syndrome. There is mimicry between this epitope and a sequence in the influenza virus NS2 protein. Ordinarily, this protein is removed from influenza virus vaccine during its purification. Failure to do this in some batches of swine influenza vaccine used in the crisis program mounted in the United States in 1976–1977 may account for the apparent increase in incidence of the syndrome at that time.

Enveloped viruses can incorporate cellular antigens, such as Forssman antigen, blood group antigens, and the "mononucleosis antigen," into

TABLE 9-2
Epitope Mimicry between Basic Myelin Protein and Viruses Causing Diseases of Myelin[a]

Virus	Disease		Epitope mimicry
Visna	Demyelination	Virus	T G K I P W I L L P G R
		MBP	S G K V P W — L K P G R
Caprine arthritis–encephalitis	Encephalitis	Virus	T G K I P W I L L P G K
		MBP	S G K V P W — L K P G R
Vaccinia	Postinfection encephalitis	Virus	S I N R G F K G V D R G
		MBP	S A H K G F K G D V A Q
Influenza	Guillain-Barré syndrome	Virus	Q L G Q K F E E
		P2[b]	K L G Q E F E E

[a] From P. R. Carnegie and M. A. Lawson, *Today's Life Sci.* **3**(2), 14 (1991).
[b] P2, Protein of peripheral nerves.

their envelope if these antigens are present in the host cell, with the potential for the production of autoantibodies.

OTHER PHYSIOLOGIC DISTURBANCES

Some pathologic changes found in viral infections cannot be attributed to direct cell destruction by the virus, nor to inflammation, nor to immunopathology. Perhaps the most important of these effects relate to alterations in the function of various endocrine glands, notably the adrenals, in response to the stress of the infectious disease. Sometimes endocrine epithelial cells affected by noncytocidal viruses are not killed, but their secretory functions are damaged; for example, infection of mice with encephalomyocarditis virus (a picornavirus) may lead to diabetes because of the action of the virus on the β cells of the islets of Langerhans. Some effects of lymphocytic choriomeningitis virus have already been mentioned. These examples come from well-studied experimental animal models; similar changes probably occur in natural infections but have not yet been documented.

Most viral diseases are accompanied by a number of vague general clinical signs, such as fever, malaise, anorexia, and lassitude. Little is known about the causes of these signs, which collectively can significantly reduce the performance of the animal and impede recovery. Fever can be attributed to interleukin 1 and possibly to interferons. These and other soluble mediators produced by leukocytes, or released from virus-infected cells, may be responsible for the other clinical signs also.

REPRESENTATIVE MODELS OF ACUTE VIRAL INFECTIONS

We are now in a position to examine in some detail the pathogenesis of selected examples of each of the four main categories of acute infections: respiratory, intestinal, generalized, and those affecting the central nervous system. We begin with two prototypes of viral respiratory diseases: influenza, about which a great deal is known from experimental studies, and the complex respiratory infections of cattle known as shipping fever, as an example of synergistic viral/bacterial infection.

Respiratory Infections

The sequence of events in respiratory infections is rather similar no matter what kind of virus is involved. Acute respiratory infections are exemplified by influenza in horses and swine.

Influenza. Virus particles in aerosolized droplets or on fomites are inhaled and alight on the film of mucus that covers the epithelium of the upper respiratory tract. Droplets of different sizes alight at different levels of the respiratory tree, and infection may accordingly be initiated at particular levels; however, in general the upper respiratory tract is the site of initial infection. Immediately on alighting, the virus is met by host defense mechanisms; if the animal has previously been infected with the same or a very similar strain of influenza virus, antibody (mainly IgA) present in the mucus may neutralize it. Mucus also contains glycoproteins similar to the receptor molecules on respiratory epithelial cells, which may combine with virions and prevent them from attaching to epithelial cells. In turn, the viral neuraminidase may destroy enough glycoprotein to allow virions to attach to and infect an epithelial cell.

If the initial host defenses fail, the virus moves deeper into the airways, where it faces another physiologic barrier mechanism, namely, the cleansing action of beating cilia. Inhaled particles, including virions, are normally carried via the mucous flow generated by cilial beating action to the pharynx, where they are swallowed. However, it has been shown with influenza viruses and other respiratory viruses that initial invasion and destruction of just a few epithelial cells can initiate a lesion which can progressively damage the protective layer of mucus and lay bare more and more epithelial cells. Viral replication progresses, and large numbers of progeny virions are budded into the lumen of the airway. Early in infection, cilial beating helps to move released progeny virus along the airway, thereby spreading the infection. As secretions become more profuse and viscous, the cilial beating becomes less effective and ceases as epithelial cells are destroyed.

In studies in experimental animals, the spread of the infection via contiguous expansion from initial foci often does not stop until virtually every columnar epithelial cell at that airway level is infected. The result is complete denuding of large areas of epithelial surface (Fig. 9-1) and the accumulation in the airways of large amounts of transudates, exudates containing inflammatory cells, and necrotic epithelial cell debris. The consequent respiratory distress is made worse by forced movement of animals. Where infection of the epithelium of the nasal passages, trachea, and bronchi proceeds to a fatal outcome, there are usually one or more of three complications: bacterial superinfection (nurtured by the accumulation of fluid and necrotic debris in the airways), infection and destruction of the lung parenchyma and the alveolar epithelium, and/or blockage of airways that are so small in diameter that mucous plugs cannot be opened by forced air movements. Blockage of the airways is of most significance in the newborn. In all of these complications there is hypoxia and a pathophysiologic cascade that leads to acidosis and uncontrollable fluid exudation into airways.

Degeneration of respiratory tract epithelial surfaces during influenza infection is extremely rapid, but so is regeneration. In studies of influenza in ferrets, for example, it has been shown that the development of a complete new columnar epithelial surface via hyperplasia of remaining transitional cells may be complete in a few days. The transitional epithelium and the newly differentiated columnar epithelium that arises from

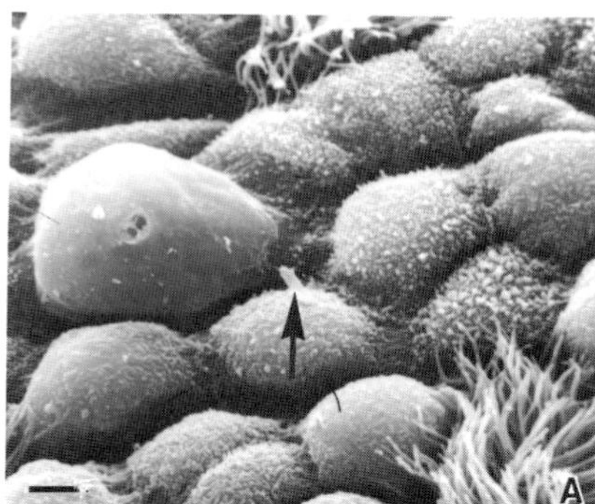

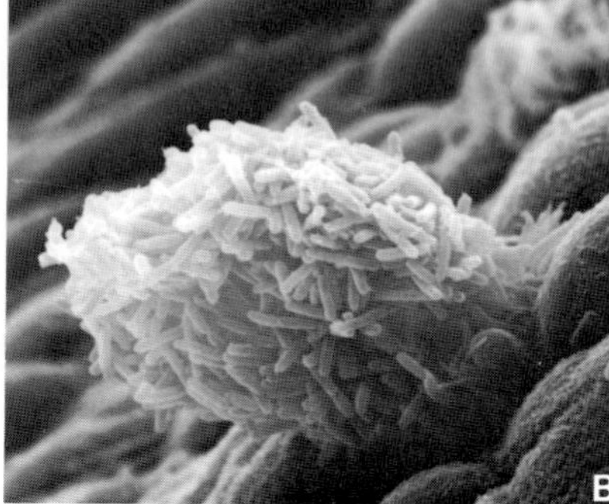

FIG. 9-1. *Scanning electron micrographs showing the adherence of* Pseudomonas aeruginosa *to the mouse trachea. (bar: 2 μm). (A) Normal mouse trachea, showing a single bacterium (arrow) on a serous cell. (B) Microcolony adhering to desquamating cells in an influenza virus-infected trachea. [From R. Ramphal* et al., Infect. Immun. **27,** *614 (1980); courtesy Dr. P. A. Small, Jr.]*

it are resistant to infection, probably by virtue of interferon production. Other host defenses, including antibody- and cell-mediated immune mechanisms, also play a part in terminating the infection.

Whereas influenza virus infection in mammals, as described, is generally restricted to the cells of the respiratory tract, in birds influenza viruses often cause an inapparent infection of the digestive tract. However, viremia and spread to other organs including the brain occur with virulent strains of avian influenza virus, in which the hemagglutinin is activated in a broad range of cell types.

Viral–Bacterial Synergistic Respiratory Infections (Shipping Fever). In cattle there is a seasonal incidence of bronchopneumonia that corresponds with the extra stress of harsh climatic conditions and husbandry practices in fall and early winter, as well as the extra activity of respiratory viruses and mycoplasmas at that time of year. This syndrome of bronchopneumonia, often extending to a true fibrinous pleuropneumonia, is called shipping fever in many countries. In the United States and Canada the syndrome represents the most economically important health problem in cattle, especially feedlot cattle. The syndrome, despite having diverse initial causes, has a common terminal pathway and etiology, the terminal manifestations being caused by overwhelming infection by *Pasteurella haemolytica* and to a lesser extent *P. multocida*.

Respiratory virus infections, augmented by the pathophysiologic effects of stress, alter the susceptibility of cattle to *Pasteurella* species that are normally present in the upper respiratory tract by a number of independent and interdependent mechanisms. The influence of respiratory epithelial tissue damage and fluid exudation into airways, as described above for influenza, is a major factor favoring bacterial growth following all respiratory virus infections. Viral infections can also alter bovine host defense mechanisms in other ways: (1) they can be directly immunosuppressive or can damage macrophage and neutrophil function in the lungs and airways; (2) they may induce such an exuberant inflammatory response that the delicate epithelial surfaces of the alveoli are destroyed; and (3) they can alter the surface properties of respiratory epithelial cells so as to favor bacterial adherence and the growth of bacterial microcolonies. These microcolonies in turn resist phagocytosis and the effects of antibodies and antibiotics, and they can more readily enter the lower respiratory tract. Another effect of viral damage to epithelial cells is the release of iron, which enhances bacterial growth and colonization. The complex of interactions between various factors during the development of respiratory disease is represented diagrammatically in Fig. 9-2.

Control of the viral infections that initiate shipping fever appears to be more important than control of the terminal bacterial pneumonia. The

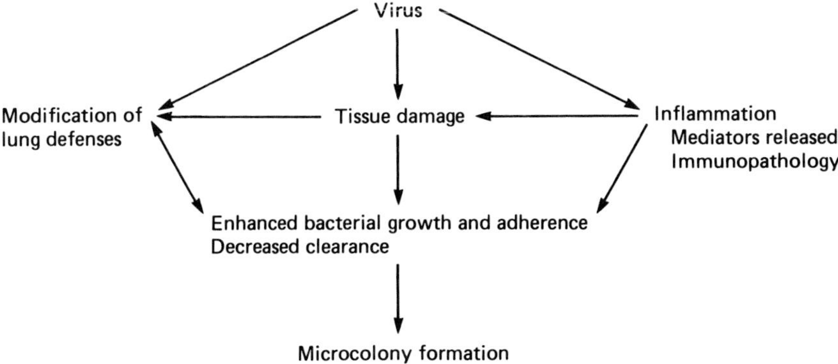

FIG. 9-2. *Interactions between events associated with viral and bacterial infections in the development of respiratory disease ("shipping fever") in cattle. [From L. A. Babiuk,* In *"Applied Virology" (E. Kurstak, ed.), p. 431. Academic Press, Orlando, Florida, 1984.]*

Pasteurella species involved are always present in the upper respiratory tract of cattle, and it is not likely that they could be eliminated. Likewise, species of *Pasteurella* have proved less amenable to control by vaccines. The speed with which antibiotic therapy is initiated does influence the eventual outcome, but in many cases extensive damage has already been done by the time of diagnosis. If microcolonies have been established and have progressed to abscess formation, there is added difficulty in delivering effective antibiotic levels so as to reach the bacteria. Even when the animal does not die, it is prone to further debilitating diseases. Viral vaccine programs, aimed at preventing the pathogenetic cascade, must be measured and justified indirectly, by the overall effect they have on the prevalence of the multifactorial pneumonia.

Intestinal Diseases

Diarrhea in animals is often multifactorial, and interactions of infectious agents with immunologic, environmental, and nutritional factors can often exacerbate the disease. The principal causes of viral diarrhea in domestic animals are rotaviruses and coronaviruses; other viruses involved are pestiviruses, caliciviruses, astroviruses, and parvoviruses. Infection occurs by ingestion of virus. Except with parvoviruses, in which infection of the intestinal tract is part of a systemic infection, the incubation period is very short.

Different viruses characteristically infect different parts of the villi of the intestinal tract, with rotaviruses and coronaviruses infecting cells at the tip and parvoviruses cells in the crypts. All cause marked shortening and occasional fusion of adjacent villi (Fig. 9-3), so that the absorptive surface of the intestine is reduced, resulting in fluid accumulation in the lumen of the gut and diarrhea. Infection generally begins in the proximal part of the small intestine and spreads progressively to the jejunum and ileum and sometimes to the colon. The extent of such spread depends on the initial dose, the virulence of the virus, and the immunologic status of the host. In the presence of maternal antibody, infection can occur, but the degree of viral replication is limited and diarrhea is mild or does not occur.

With rotaviruses and coronaviruses, which infect cells at the tips of the villi, as infection progresses the absorptive cells are replaced by immature cuboidal epithelial cells whose absorptive capacity and enzymatic activity are greatly reduced. These cells are relatively resistant to viral infection, so that the disease is often self-limiting if dehydration is not so severe as to be lethal. The rate of recovery is rapid, since the crypt cells are not damaged. In contrast, recovery is slow after infections with parvoviruses, which destroy cells of the crypts.

The mechanism of fluid loss in viral infections is different from that in bacterial infections, but the net loss may be of the same magnitude. In viral infections fluid loss is mainly a loss of extracellular fluid due to impaired absorption, and osmotic loss due primarily to the presence of undigested lactose in the lumen (in sucking animals), rather than active secretion. As virus destroys the absorptive cells there is a loss of those enzymes responsible for the digestion of disaccharides, and the loss of differentiated cells diminishes glucose carrier, sodium carrier, and Na^+, K^+-ATPase activities. This leads to a loss of sodium, potassium, chloride, bicarbonate, and water, and the development of acidosis. Another cause of acidosis is increased microbial activity associated with the fermentation of undigested milk. Acidosis can create a K^+ ion exchange across the cellular membrane, affecting cellular functions that maintain the normal potassium concentration. Hypoglycemia due to decreased intestinal absorption, inhibited glyconeogenesis, and increased glycolysis follows, completing a complex of pathophysiologic changes that if not promptly corrected results in death of the animal. Effective management of viral diarrheas in young animals requires prompt action to prevent continued loss of fluids and electrolytes.

In many cases of diarrhea in animals more than one virus is active; if two viruses have different sites of replication their combined effect may be severe. Furthermore, many bacterial infections, for example, with enterotoxic *E. coli*, are more severe if combined with a viral infection.

The viral diarrheas are essentially diseases of the first few weeks or

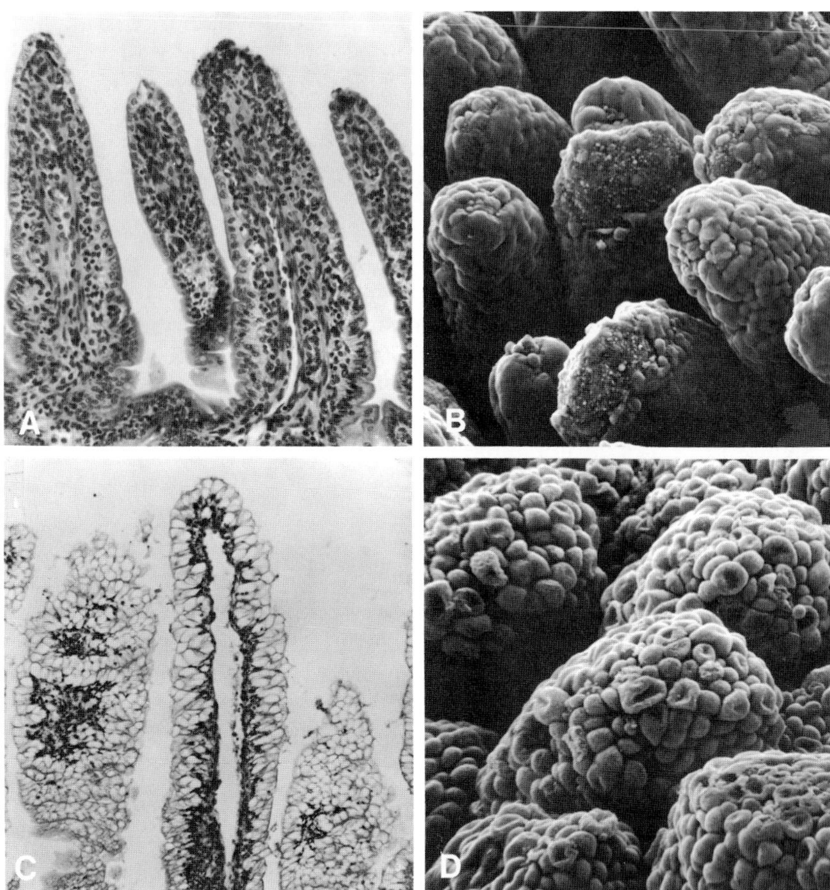

FIG. 9-3. *Scanning electron and light micrographs of intestinal tissues from a gnotobiotic calf sacrificed 30 minutes after onset of rotavirus diarrhea. (A) Proximal small intestine with shortened villi and a denuded villus tip (second from right). Hematoxylin and eosin stain; magnification: ×120. (B) Appearance of the same level of intestine as in (A) depicting denuded villi by scanning electron microscopy. Magnification: ×180. (C) Distal small intestine with normal vacuolated epithelial cells and normal villi. Hamatoxylin and eosin stain; magnification: ×75. (D) Same area as in (C) seen by scanning electron microscopy. Epithelial cells appear round and protruding. Magnification: ×210. [From C. A. Mebus* et al., Vet. Pathol. **14,** *273 (1977); and R. G. Wyatt and A. Z. Kapikian,* In *"Textbook of Pediatric Infectious Diseases" (R. D. Feigin and J. D. Cherry, eds.), Saunders, Philadelphia, Pennsylvania, 1981; courtesy A. Z. Kapikian.]*

months of life, and susceptibility decreases rapidly with increasing age. To prevent infection of newborn animals, antibody must be present continuously in the lumen of the gut. This does not occur for more than about 7 days unless the dam is hyperimmunized against the common etiologic agents. Since local immunization of the newborn is often not practical, further emphasis on this strategy of prevention should be encouraged (see Chapter 13).

Generalized Diseases

Canine Distemper. Canine distemper, caused by a virus of the genus *Morbillivirus* (family *Paramyxoviridae*), is a good model for studying the pathogenesis of generalized viral infections. It is an acute, self-limited, systemic disease, but in some dogs virus invades the central nervous system and causes encephalitis. In a minority of dogs the virus persists in the brain and may cause the late neurological disease known as old dog encephalitis (Fig. 9-4).

Infection occurs via virus inhalation into the respiratory tract. Following initial infection of the respiratory epithelium and alveolar macrophages, virus is transferred within 2 days into mononuclear cells in the bronchial lymph nodes and tonsils. During the first week, before the onset of signs, cell-associated virus spreads via the bloodstream to the bone marrow, spleen, thymus, cervical and mesenteric lymph nodes, and macrophages in the lamina propria of the stomach and small intestine.

The rate of spread and the distribution of virus after the eighth to ninth day vary and appear to depend on the rate of development of neutralizing antibody, although the role of cell-mediated immunity has not been adequately studied. No antibody is found on the seventh day, but in some dogs the titer reaches 1:100 or higher on the eighth or ninth day. In such animals there is no further spread of virus; virus disappears rapidly from the lymphatic tissues, and the infection remains subclinical. If measurable antibody is not present on the ninth day or if a titer of 1:100 has not been attained by the fourteenth day, virus spreads throughout the body. As well as continued infection of mononuclear cells in the lymphatic system, extensive infection of the epithelium in the intestinal, respiratory, and urogenital tracts, skin, and exocrine and endocrine glands occurs. Infection of the gastrointestinal tract causes vomiting and diarrhea, infection of the respiratory tract causes bronchitis and sometimes pneumonia, and infection of the skin is associated with dermatitis.

The brain is sometimes infected, usually after infection in visceral organs has come to an end. The virus appears first in meningeal macrophages and mononuclear cells in perivascular adventitia and later in

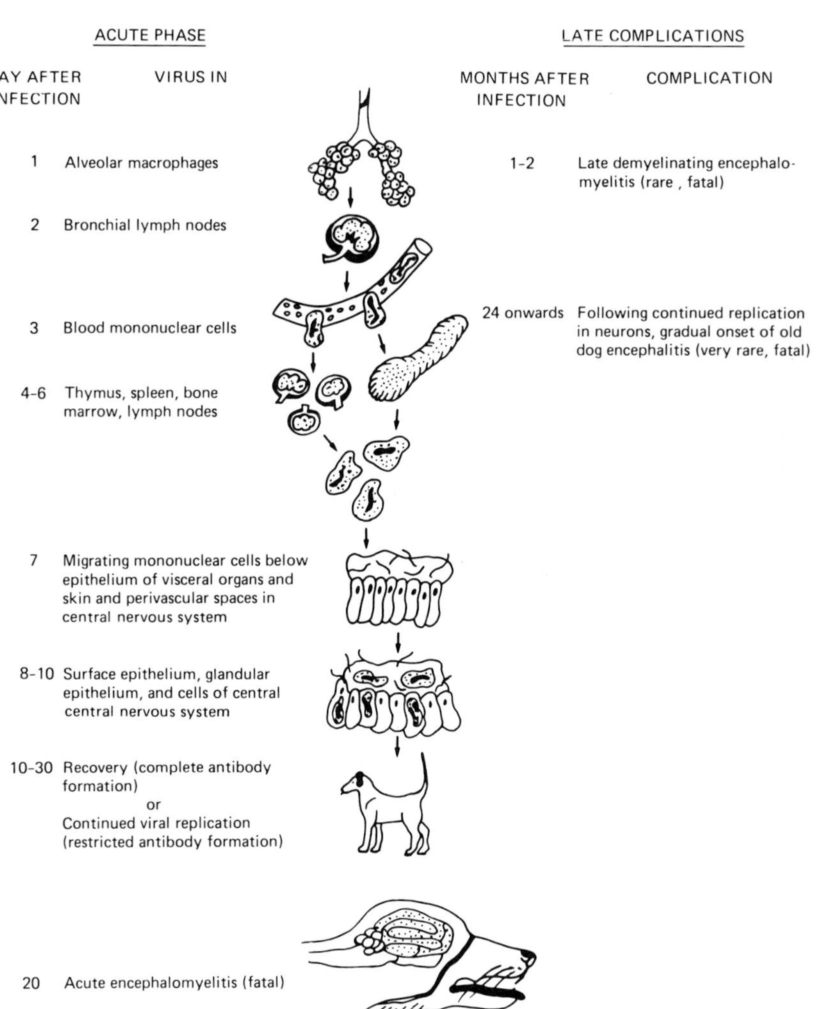

FIG. 9-4. *Diagram illustrating the pathogenesis of canine distemper. (Based on the work of Dr. M. J. G. Appel.)*

ependymal cells, glial cells, and neurons. The infection of neurons is associated with behavioral changes, local myoclony, tonic–clonic spasms, and paresis, which often persist after recovery. Forty to sixty days after apparent recovery, some dogs suffer from postinfection encephalitis, with characteristic demyelination, often leading to death. In these dogs, high titers of neutralizing antibody occur in both blood and cerebrospinal fluid. In addition, very occasionally dogs that have recovered from distemper suffer from encephalitis years later, "old dog encephalitis." Like subacute sclerosing panencephalitis in humans who have recovered from measles, this appears to be due to the very slow replication and spread of distemper virus in the brain. This complication, like acute canine distemper itself, has become rare as distemper vaccination has become more general.

The course of acute canine distemper is affected by the extent of secondary bacterial infection, but this factor does not affect the central nervous system diseases. Recovery from canine distemper is followed by prolonged immunity, probably lifelong.

Neurologic Diseases

Rabies. The pathogenesis of rabies is remarkable in that invasion, spread to the central nervous system, and the development of signs occur with minimal immunologic responses, yet, even after infection has occurred, early administration of antibody and/or vaccine can often prevent disease. Infection by the bite of a rabid animal usually results in deposition of rabies-infected saliva deep in the striated muscles, but rabies can occur, albeit with less certainty, after superficial abrasion of the skin. Initially virus replicates in the muscle cells or cells of the subepithelial tissues until it has reached a sufficient concentration to reach motor or sensory nerve endings in the muscle or skin. Here it binds specifically to the acetylcholine receptor or other receptors and enters nerve endings. This begins the second phase of infection, in which neuronal infection and centripetal passive movement within axons leads to involvement of the central nervous system. The *incubation period,* namely, the time between the infective bite and the development of signs of central nervous system involvement, is usually between 14 and 90 days but may occasionally be as long as 4 years, possibly because virus remains sequestered in striated muscle cells before entering peripheral nerves and ascending to the brain.

Although rabies proteins are highly antigenic, neither humoral nor cell-mediated responses can be detected during the stage of movement of virus from the site of the bite to the central nervous system, probably because very little antigen is delivered to the immune system; most antigen is sequestered in muscle cells or within nerve axons. However, this early stage of infection is accessible to antibody, hence the efficacy of the classical Pasteurian postinfection vaccination, especially if combined with the administration of hyperimmune immunoglobulin. Immunologic intervention is effective during the long incubation period because of the delay between the initial viral replication in muscle cells and the entry of virus into the protected environment of the nervous system.

Movement along the nerves eventually delivers virus to the central

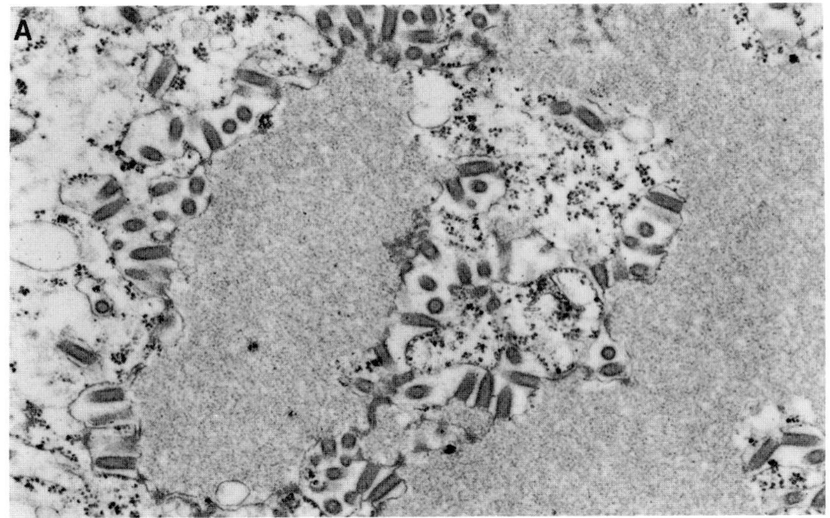

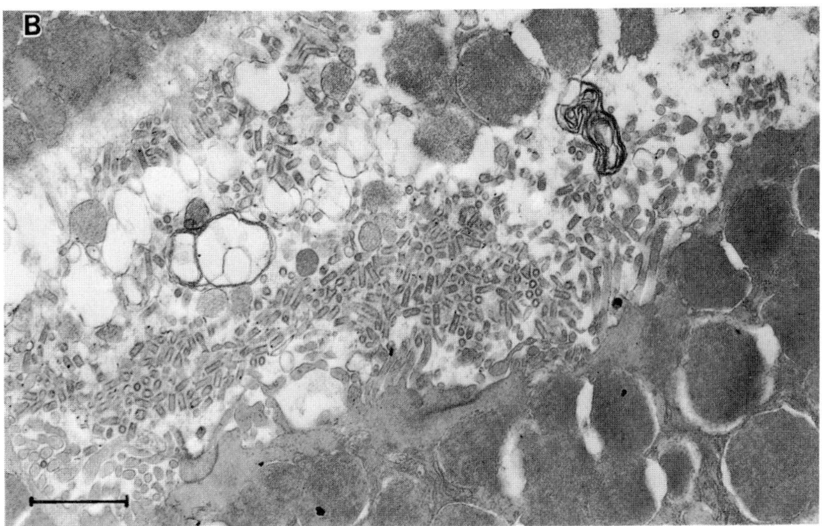

FIG. 9-5. *Electron micrographs of rabies virus infection in the brain (A) and salivary gland (B) (bar: 500 nm). In both organs the infection is noncytopathic; however, in the brain nearly all virus is formed by budding on internal membranes of neurons and so is trapped, while in the salivary gland nearly all virus is formed by budding on the apical plasma membrane of mucous epithelial cells, where virions become free to enter the salivary duct. Some reservoir host species can have 10^6 ID_{50} of rabies virus per milliliter of saliva at the time of peak transmissibility. (A) Street rabies virus from a dog in the cytoplasm of a neuron of a mouse 10 days after infection. Bullet-shaped virions are budding on internal cellular membranes; the granular material is excess viral nucleocapsids forming an inclusion body which by light microscopy is seen as a Negri body. (B) Street rabies virus in the saliva of a fox. Bullet-shaped virions, having budded from mucuous epithelial cells, are accumulating in the salivary duct where they are free to be transmitted in salive injected during a bite.*

nervous system, usually the spinal cord initially. An ascending wave of neuronal infection and neuronal dysfunction then occurs. Virus reaches the limbic system, where it replicates extensively, and the release of cortical control of behavior leads to "furious" rabies. Spread within the central nervous system continues, and when replication occurs in the neocortex the clinical picture changes to "dumb" rabies. Depression, coma, and death from respiratory arrest follow.

However, before this—and indeed coincidentally with its replication in the limbic system that leads to fury—virus moves centrifugally from the central nervous system down peripheral nerves to a variety of organs: adrenal cortex, pancreas, and, most importantly, the salivary glands. In the nervous system most virus is assembled on cytoplasmic membranes within cells; the cells are not lysed, so that little viral antigen is released to stimulate host defense mechanisms. In the salivary gland, however, virions bud almost exclusively from plasma membranes at the lumenal surface of mucous cells and are released in high concentrations into the saliva (Fig. 9-5). Thus, at the time when viral replication within the central nervous system causes the infected animal to become furious and bite indiscriminately, the saliva is highly infectious.

On histopathologic examination there is little evidence of brain damage, yet electron microscopic or fluorescent antibody studies show that almost all neurons are infected. There is minimal cellular destruction to match the extensive neurologic dysfunction seen in the disease.

FURTHER READING

Babiuk, L. A. (1984). Virus-induced gastroenteritis in animals. *In* "Applied Virology" (E. Kurstak, ed.), p. 349. Academic Press, Orlando, Florida.

Babiuk, L. A., Lawman, M. P. J. and Bielefeldt, O. H. (1988). Viral–bacterial synergistic interaction in respiratory disease. *Adv. Virus Res.* **35,** 219.

Lawman, M. J. I., Campos, M., Ohmann, H. B., Griebel, P., and Babiuk, L. A. (1989). Recombinant cytokines and their therapeutic value in veterinary medicine. *In* "Animal Biotechnology" (L. A. Babiuk and J. P. Phillips, eds.), *Comprehensive Biotechnology* series. Pergamon, Oxford.

Lehmann-Grube, F. (1989). Diseases of the nervous system caused by lymphocytic choriomeningitis virus and other arenaviruses. *In* "Handbook of Clinical Neurology" (R. R. McKendall, ed.), p. 355. Elsevier, Amsterdam.

Mims, C. A., and White, D. O. (1984). "Viral Pathogenesis and Immunology." Blackwell, Oxford.

Notkins, A. L., and Oldstone, M. B. A., eds. (1984, 1986, 1989). "Concepts in Viral Pathogenesis," Vols. 1, 2, and 3. Springer-Verlag, New York.

Oldstone M. B. A., ed. (1989). Molecular mimicry. Cross-reactivity between microbes and host proteins as a cause of autoimmunity. *Curr. Top. Microbiol. Immunol.* **145,** 1.

Russell, W. C., and Almond, J. W. (1987). "Molecular Basis of Virus Disease," Fortieth Symp. Soc. Gen. Microbiol. Cambridge Univ. Press, Cambridge.

CHAPTER 10

Persistent Infections

The features of the pathogenesis of viral infections described in Chapter 6, namely, the establishment of infection followed by spread of the virus, either locally or systemically, are found in all viral infections. With many viruses, especially those that produce infections localized in the respiratory tract or the intestinal tract, the sequel to the establishment and spread of the virus is an acute disease, which results in either death (rarely) or recovery with elimination of the virus from the body. The pathogenesis of several such acute infections is described in Chapter 9. However, even in some of these acute infections, such as canine distemper, there is a minority of cases in which virus is not eliminated, but may persist for months or years, causing late pathologic manifestions. More importantly, viruses of some families, notably the herpesviruses, cause infections that persist for the life of the animal, although episodes of clinical disease might occur infrequently and at long intervals. In addition, viruses have been found to be responsible for many chronic diseases, in which virus persists for months or for life and causes continuing, often subtle, pathologic effects. These persistent viral infections are important for four reasons. (1) They are often of epidemiologic importance, since they create carrier animals that serve as a source of infection for other animals, thereby enabling the virus to persist in the population even if its infectivity is low. (2) They may be reactivated and cause recurrent acute episodes of disease. (3) They may lead to immunopathologic disease. (4) They are sometimes associated with neoplasms.

Persistent infections of one type or another are produced by a wide range of viruses; indeed, in veterinary medicine acute self-limiting infections seem to be the exception rather than the rule, apart from most viral diarrheas and respiratory infections. As in cultured cells, such infections may be characterized by the continuous or intermittent production of infectious virus or by the persistence of the viral genome either as provirus or as an episome. Some viruses, characteristically the alphaherpesviruses, produce cytocidal infections in cell cultures but persistent as well as cytocidal infections *in vivo*, the different types of infection often occurring in different cell populations.

CATEGORIES OF PERSISTENT INFECTIONS

For convenience, persistent infections may be subdivided into three categories: (1) *latent infections,* in which infectious virus is not demonstrable except when reactivation occurs, episodes that are sometimes but not always associated with recurrent disease (see Table 10-1); (2) *chronic infections,* in which infectious virus is always demonstrable and often shed and disease may be absent, chronic, or may develop late, often with an immunopathologic basis (see Table 10-2); and (3) *slow infections,* in which infectious virus gradually increases during a very long preclinical phase, leading to a slowly progressive lethal disease (see Table 10-3).

The key distinctions between the three groups of persistent infections are illustrated diagrammatically in Fig. 10-1. It may be noted that these three categories are defined primarily in terms of the extent of viral replication in the body during the long period of persistence; the presence or absence of shedding and of disease are secondary issues as far as categorization is concerned. Some persistent infections in all three categories are associated with disease, some are not, but the "carrier" status of all such animals makes them a potential source of infection for others. While there are some persistent infections that possess features of more than one of these categories, it is useful to retain the terms so as to focus attention on the vital question, namely, what is the virus doing during its lifelong sojourn in the body?

LATENT INFECTIONS

Latency following recovery from a primary acute infection is a general feature of infections with herpesviruses (Table 10-1). The mechanisms of latency and reactivation are assumed to be comparable for all herpesvi-

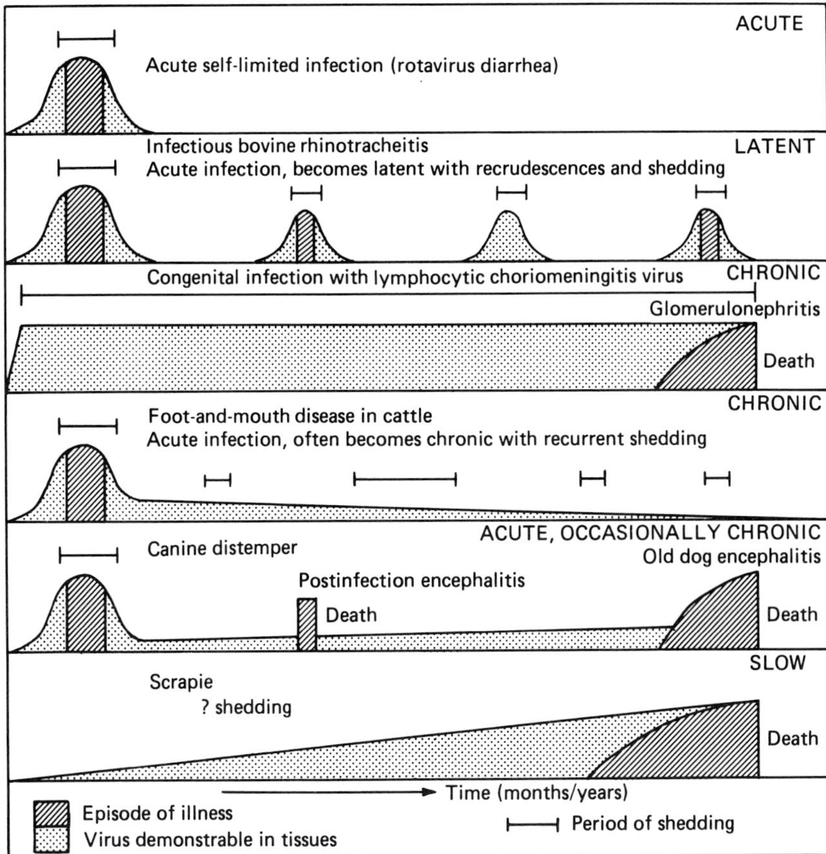

FIG. 10-1. *Diagram depicting the presence and shedding of virus and the occurrence of clinical signs in acute self-limited infections and various kinds of persistent infections, as exemplified by the diseases indicated. The time scale is notional and the duration of various events approximate.*

ruses but have been described in greatest detail in herpes simplex, varicella–zoster, and EB virus infection in humans and to a lesser extent in pseudorabies in swine and infectious bovine rhinotracheitis. During a primary infection with infectious bovine rhinotracheitis virus (an alphaherpesvirus), virions move to the cranial or spinal ganglia along the axons of sensory nerves. The genome of the virus persists latently in neurons in these ganglia, probably as an episome. Periodically it is reactivated, and infectious virus is produced and moves down the sensory nerves again until it reaches the nasal mucous membranes or the skin, where further proliferation occurs in epithelial cells, with virus shedding.

TABLE 10-1

Latent Infections: Persistent Infections with Viral Latency and Reactivation, with or without Recurrent Clinical Episodes

		Sites of infection			
Virus	Disease	During disease episodes	Between disease episodes	Virus shedding	Neutralizing antibodies
Bovine herpesvirus 1	Infectious bovine rhinotracheitis	Respiratory and genital mucosa	As episomal DNA, in cerebral or dorsal root ganglion neurons	During disease episodes, in saliva and genital secretions	+
Cytomegalovirus (several host-specific viruses)	Usually subclinical	Various epithelial cells	As episomal DNA, in salivary gland and bladder epithelial cells and leukocytes	Sporadically throughout life in saliva and urine	+

There is debate as to whether intermittent reactivation of latent virus is always associated with the development of lesions or clinical disease, but reactivation and shedding of virus constitute the mechanism whereby virus is maintained from generation to generation in the bovine population.

Betaherpesviruses (cytomegaloviruses) establish latent infections, probably in salivary gland and bladder epithelia as well as in monocytes and/or lymphocytes. Virus is shed, intermittently or continuously, particularly into the oropharynx, from which it may be transmitted via saliva, and into the urine, from which it may be transmitted directly. Aside from the observation that cytomegalovirus infection may occur after organ transplantation in humans using organs apparently free of infectious virus or viral antigen, little is known of the molecular biology of cytomegalovirus latency.

Molecular Basis of Alphaherpesvirus Latency

The alphaherpesviruses are always cytocidal in cultured cells, so elucidation of the molecular basis of latency has had to be derived from experiments with herpesvirus infections of mice and rabbits. Such studies have established a number of interesting facts. In the ganglia, the viral DNA occurs as *episomes,* namely, extrachromosomal plasmids, in about 1% of the neurons in a ganglion, with 20–100 copies per cell. During latency, two or three "latency-associated" transcripts are produced, but no viral antigen is synthesized from these transcripts. However, experiments with mutants show that production of these transcripts is not essential for the establishment or maintenance of latent infection. If the neurons are cultured *in vitro,* reactivation occurs and mature infectious virions are produced, with cell lysis. *In vivo,* such cell lysis would be incompatible with continuing latency. Perhaps a subviral form, possibly only the viral DNA, is replicated and passes within the axon to neuroepidermal junctions, then producing infectious virus in the epithelial cells. It is possible that maintenance of latency requires that, after each reactivation event, some viral genomes return via axons to reside in additional neurons.

CHRONIC INFECTIONS

A large number and variety of viral infections fall into the category of chronic persistent infections (Table 10-2), which is marked by continuous virus production. There may be no disease (e.g., chronic foot-and-mouth disease infections), chronic disease (e.g., African swine fever), or disease

TABLE 10-2

Chronic Infections: Persistent Infections with Virus Demonstrable for Long Periods, with or without Disease

Virus (genus)	Host	Sites of persistent infection	Virus shedding	Antibodies	Chronic disease
Aleutian disease (*Parvovirus*)	Mink	Macrophages	Continuous	++ (Nonneutralizing)	Late: vasculitis, glomerulonephritis, fatal
African swine fever virus	Swine	Hemopoietic system	Variable	+ (Nonneutralizing)	Intermittent fever
Foot-and-mouth disease virus (*Aphthovirus*)	Cattle, buffalo	Soft palate and pharynx	Intermittent and prolonged	+	No signs
Feline calicivirus (*Calicivirus*)	Cat	Oropharynx	Intermittent and prolonged	+	No signs
Canine distemper virus (*Morbillivirus*)	Dog	Brain	Nil	++ (Serum)	Rarely: old dog encephalitis
				+ (Cerebrospinal fluid)	
Hog cholera virus (*Pestivirus*)	Swine (congenital infection)	Widespread	Continuous	+ (Nonneutralizing)	Systemic, progressive, fatal
Lymphocytic choriomeningitis virus (*Arenavirus*)	Mouse	Widespread	Continuous	+ (Nonneutralizing)	Sometimes late glomerulonephritis
Borna disease virus	Horse, sheep	Neural cells	Nil	+ (Nonneutralizing)	Polioencephalitis

occurring only as a later complication (e.g., old dog encephalitis after canine distemper). Virus may be shed for years (e.g., foot-and-mouth disease in cattle) or not at all (e.g., old dog encephalitis). Some of the infections listed in Table 10-2 are described more fully in the appropriate chapters of Part II; here we present three illustrative examples: lymphocytic choriomeningitis in congenitally infected mice, chronic foot-and-mouth disease infection in cattle, and old dog encephalitis.

Lymphocytic Choriomeningitis

Lymphocytic choriomeningitis, caused by an arenavirus, is the classic persistent viral infection, consideration of which was important for the formulation by Burnet of the concept of *immunological tolerance.* Lymphocytic choriomeningitis virus is transmitted horizontally and *in utero,* such that every mouse in a colony may become infected. Infected mice are normal at birth and appear normal for most of their lives, although careful study of the physiologic activity of some endocrine glands shows that certain specialized functions may be impaired. Almost every cell in the mouse is infected and remains so throughout life, and the infected mice have persistent viremia and viruria. Circulating free antibody cannot be detected, but immunological tolerance is not complete, since some antibody is formed and circulates as virion–IgG–complement complexes, which are infectious. However, there is no cell-mediated immune response to the virus. Late in life inbred mice (but not wild house mice) may exhibit "late disease" due to the deposition of viral antigen–antibody complexes, for example, in the renal glomeruli. Other members of the family *Arenaviridae* cause similar persistent infections of wild rodents in Africa and South America and produce severe disease, with hemorrhagic signs, when man is accidentally infected (Lassa fever, Bolivian and Argentine hemorrhagic fevers).

Foot-and-Mouth Disease

Although convalescence after foot-and-mouth disease in cattle is often protracted, it used to be thought that recovery was complete, with elimination of the virus. However, it now known that foot-and-mouth disease viruses can cause a persistent infection of the pharynx in cattle, sheep, goats, and other ruminants. Not all infected animals become carriers, nor is there any correlation between antibody levels and the carrier state. Cattle vaccinated with inactivated vaccine may become carriers if subsequently infected.

The recovery of virus from pharyngeal fluids is often intermittent, possibly because of variability in sampling technique, but isolations have been made from cattle and buffalo for up to 2 years after infection. The mechanism of persistence is unknown, and its epidemiologic significance is difficult to assess. Pharyngeal fluids may contain large amounts of virus, which may be aerosolized by cattle when they cough, but attempts to demonstrate transmission from carrier to susceptible cattle have given equivocal results, although transfer of infection from persistently infected African buffalo to cattle is known to occur.

Old Dog Encephalitis

Canine distemper is an acute systemic infection in which the majority of dogs recover completely within 1 month of the onset of signs (see Chapter 9). In a minority of cases dogs that have recovered from canine distemper continue to harbor the virus in brain cells, where it replicates slowly and eventually produces old dog encephalitis. The situation is analogous to that of subacute sclerosing panencephalitis in the corresponding human infection, measles.

In subacute sclerosing panencephalitis, at the time of death, certain nerve cells contain large masses of viral nucleocapsids, but complete virions are not made, apparently because a mutant virus has been selected *in vivo* which is defective in the production of matrix protein and other envelope components. Nevertheless, the complete viral genome must be present, as measles virus can be isolated *in vitro* by cocultivation of brain cells with permissive cells. The situation is similar in old dog encephalitis, but virus can be cultivated directly from the brains of affected dogs.

SLOW INFECTIONS

The term *slow infections* was originally used to describe slowly progressive lentiviral diseases found in sheep in Iceland. The term is now used to categorize several viral infections that have a very long preclinical phase (incubation period) and then cause a slowly progressive, invariably lethal disease. Slow infections are persistent infections in that the infectious agent can be recovered from infected animals during the preclinical phase and also after clinical signs have appeared. There are two groups of slow infections (Table 10-3), caused, respectively, by the lentiviruses and the unclassified agents that cause the subacute spongiform encephalopathies.

Lentiviral Diseases

The lentiviruses are host species-specific, exogenous, nononcogenic retroviruses which are tropic for cells of the macrophage lineage *in vivo*,

TABLE 10-3

Slow Infections: Long Preclinical Phase, Slowly Progressive Fatal Disease

Group	Virus or agent	Host	Sites of infection	Antibodies	Disease
Lentivirus infections	Visna/maedi virus, ovine progressive pneumonia virus	Sheep	Macrophages, brain, lung	+ (Nonneutralizing)	Slowly progressive pneumonia or encephalitis
	Caprine arthritis–encephalitis virus	Goat	Macrophages, brain, joints	+ (Nonneutralizing)	Arthritis, encephalitis
	Human immunodeficiency viruses	Human	Helper T cells	+ (Nonneutralizing)	Acquired immunodeficiency syndrome (AIDS)
	Feline immunodeficiency virus	Cat	?Helper T cells	+(Nonneutralizing)	Feline acquired immunodeficiency syndrome
Subacute spongiform encephalopathies	Scrapie agent	Sheep	Central nervous system and lymphoid tissue	None	Slowly progressive encephalopathy
	Wasting disease agent	Deer, elk			
	Kuru agent	Human			
	Creutzfeldt-Jakob agent	Human			
	Bovine spongiform encephalopathy agent	Cattle			
	Mink encephalopathy agent	Mink			

virus expression being curtailed to a low level in precursor cells and increased when the cells become differentiated and/or immunologically activated. During replication, the DNA provirus is integrated into the host cell chromosomal DNA. The viruses replicate continuously *in vivo* and escape host defenses by a variety of mechanisms including the sequestration of neutralization epitopes by carbohydrate molecules, resistance to inactivation by proteolytic enzymes, antigenic variation, and infection of macrophages, which may be enhanced by nonneutralizing antibodies. In most cases the incubation period extends for several years. A feature of lentivirus infections is the occurrence of antigenic drift in the envelope glycoproteins during the progress of infection in a single animal.

The genus *Lentivirus* has been divided into a number of subgenera of which three contain only a single species: equine infectious anemia virus, bovine immunodeficiency virus, and feline immunodeficiency virus. Two subgenera contain more than one species: the ungulate lentiviruses (maedi/ovine progressive pneumonia of sheep and caprine arthritis–encephalitis) and the primate immunodeficiency viruses (human immunodeficiency viruses 1 and 2 and the simian immunodeficiency viruses) (see Chapter 33).

Subacute Spongiform Viral Encephalopathies

The term subacute spongiform viral encephalopathy is used as a generic name for seven diseases that have strikingly similar clinicopathological features and causative agents, namely, scrapie of sheep and goats, bovine spongiform encephalopathy, mink encephalopathy, wasting disease of deer and elk, and kuru, Creutzfeldt-Jakob disease, and Gerstmann-Sträussler syndrome in man. The basic lesion is a progressive vacuolation in neurons and, to a lesser extent, in astrocytes and oligodendrocytes, an extensive astroglial hypertrophy and proliferation, and finally a spongiform change in the gray matter.

The prototype of this group, scrapie, is an infection of sheep, usually transmitted from ewe to lamb. Infection was widely disseminated in Britain by the inoculation of sheep with louping-ill vaccine that was contaminated with the scrapie agent. The preclinical phase (incubation period) is very long, up to 3 years, and once signs have appeared the disease progresses slowly but inevitably to paralysis and death. Research was limited until it was discovered that mice and hamsters could be infected, with incubation periods of less than 1 year. Experimental studies in mice reveal that scrapie behaves as a typical infectious disease, and filtration shows that the causative agent is the size of a very small virus. Unusual features are the absence of an immune response and the lack of effect of either interferon or measures that augment or depress the immune system. Tests on the inactivation of infectivity by a variety of physical and chemical treatments show that the scrapie agent has a much higher degree of resistance to inactivation than conventional viruses. These unusual biological and physicochemical properties are shared by the agents of the other forms of subacute spongiform encephalopathy. The nature of the scrapie agent is still unclear; various hypotheses are discussed in Chapter 34.

PATHOGENESIS OF PERSISTENT INFECTIONS

The term "persistent infections" embraces such a wide variety of different conditions that it is not surprising to find that there are several mechanisms whereby the causative viruses bypass the host defenses that eliminate virus in acute infections. These include factors related primarily to the virus on the one hand and to the host defenses on the other, although the two kinds of factors interact in some instances.

Unique Properties of the Virus

Nonimmunogenic Agents. The uncharacterized agents that cause the subacute spongiform encephalopathies seem to be completely nonimmunogenic; they do not induce interferon, nor are they susceptible to its action. There seems to be no mechanism whereby the susceptible host can restrict the replication and pathologic effects of these agents.

Integrated Genomes. Retroviruses whose proviral DNA is integrated are maintained indefinitely, from one generation to the next, as part of the genome of the host; this proviral DNA may be implicated in oncogenesis (see Chapter 11). The lentiviruses of ungulates, on the other hand, have an integrated provirus only during their replication cycle, and after a long incubation period they cause systemic disease, with lesions in the lungs, brain, lymphoid tissues, and joints. Viruses of the acquired immunodeficiency disease subgroup of lentiviruses destroy Th lymphocytes, and this permits the unchecked proliferation of a variety of opportunistic infectious agents.

Growth in Protected Sites. During their latent phase, most alphaherpesviruses avoid immune elimination by remaining within cells of the nervous sytem, as episomal DNA in ganglion cells during the intervals between disease episodes and as viral DNA, subviral particles, or virions within axons prior to acute recurrent episodes of disease. Betaherpesviruses (e.g., cytomegalovirus) and gammaherpesviruses avoid immune elimination by maintaining serial infection by cell-to-cell contact.

Certain other viruses grow in epithelial cells on lumenal surfaces, for example, kidney tubules, salivary gland, or mammary gland, and are shed more or less continuously in the corresponding secretions. Most such viruses are not acutely cytopathic, and perhaps because they are released on the lumenal borders of cells they avoid cellular immune or inflammatory reactions. Secretory IgA, which is present in the secretions at such sites, does not activate complement, hence complement-mediated cytolysis or virolysis does not occur.

Antigenic Variation. Visna/maedi and equine infectious anemia viruses are lentiviruses which in part avoid the immune response of the host by antigenic drift. During the persistent infection, a series of antigenic variants develop within the infected animal, enabling each successive variant to evade the immune response. In equine infectious anemia clinical signs occur in cycles, each cycle being initiated by a new antigenic variant of the virus. The primate immunodeficiency viruses also undergo antigenic drift, but they utilize a number of other mechanisms to evade host defenses. In addition to providing a mechanism for escape from immune elimination, these variants may be more virulent and may directly affect the severity and progression of the disease.

Modification of Host Defense Mechanisms

Modification of the immune response is achieved in a variety of ways, some of which are also seen in nonpersistent viral infections (Table 10-4). They fall into several broad categories: ineffective antibodies, disturbance of function of cells of the immune system, avoidance of immune lysis of infected cells, and antigenic variation of the virus. Persistent infections often become reactivated when another disease, form of treatment, or physiologic condition interferes in some way with an immune response which was formerly operating effectively.

Defective Antibody Response. Viruses that replicate in lymphoid tissue and macrophages cause persistent plasma-associated viremia and also induce production of nonneutralizing antibodies. These antibodies combine with viral antigens and virions in the serum to form immune complexes which may produce "immune complex disease," usually by deposition in sites such as the renal glomeruli. It has been suggested that such antibodies may also block immune cytolysis of virus-infected target cells by T cells.

Many persistent infections are associated with a very weak antibody response, and such antibodies as are produced are nonneutralizing. The severe specific hyporeactivity found in conditions like congenital bovine

TABLE 10-4
Ineffective Immune Responses in Persistent Viral Infections[a]

Phenomenon	Mechanism	Examples[b]
No antibody	Nonimmunogenic agent	Scrapie
Nonneutralizing antibody	Small amounts, or low affinity, or reacting with irrelevant epitopes	Aleutian disease virus, African swine fever virus, lymphocytic choriomeningitis virus
Enhancing antibody	Antibody attached to virus enhances infection of macrophages	Cytomegaloviruses, lactate dehydrogenase virus, dengue viruses, feline infectious peritonitis virus
Disturbance/destruction of lymphocyte functions	Infection of lymphocytes	Infectious bursal disease virus, cytomegaloviruses, feline panleukopenia virus, human immunodeficiency virus, feline immunodeficiency virus
Disturbance of macrophage functions	Infection of macrophages	Lactate dehydrogenase virus, African swine fever virus
Antigen-specific suppression	Clonal deletion of T cells	Lymphocytic choriomeningitis virus, herpesviruses
Avoidance of immune lysis	Little or no antigen on cell membrane	Herpes simplex virus in ganglion cells; Marek's disease virus in T cells
	Loss of viral antigen by "stripping"/endocytosis	Canine distemper virus in neurons
	Antigen on inaccessible membrane	Cytomegaloviruses, rabies virus
	Fc receptor induced on infected cell; IgG binds nonspecifically	Alphaherpesviruses, cytomegaloviruses
Antigenic variation	Antigenic drift within host	Visna/maedi virus, equine infectious anemia virus

[a] Some of these mechanisms are also operative in nonpersistent infections.

[b] The examples are somewhat speculative. In several instances an association exists, but no cause-and-effect relationship has been demonstrated between the immunologic phenomenon and the persistent infection listed.

virus diarrhea virus infection, hog cholera, lymphocytic choriomeningitis, and some retrovirus infections is a form of immunological tolerance. Nonresponsiveness to other viral antigens is genetically determined, in the main by the MHC genes (see Chapter 8).

Defective Cell-Mediated Immunity. Persistent infections may be caused by partial suppression of the cell-mediated immune response of the host, as a result of any one or a combination of several factors: immunosuppression by the causative virus, immunological tolerance, the presence of "blocking" antibodies or virus–antibody complexes, failure of immune lymphocytes to reach target cells, decrease in the numbers of Th lymphocytes, inadequate expression of viral antigens on the surface of the target cell, or stripping/endocytosis of surface antigens. These factors are probably important in persistent infections caused by lentiviruses and herpesviruses.

Growth in Macrophages. In many chronic infections the virus appears to grow mainly in reticuloendothelial tissue, especially in macrophages. This may have two effects relevant to persistence: (1) impairment of the humoral and cell-mediated immune response and (2) impairment of the phagocytic and cytotoxic activities of the reticuloendothelial system. Furthermore, some persistent viruses replicate in lymphocytes; for example, helper T cells are virtually eliminated from the body in AIDS in humans.

FURTHER READING

Ahmed, R., and Stephen, J. G. (1990). Viral persistence. *In* "Fields Virology" (B. N. Fields, D. M. Knipe, R. M. Chanock, M. S. Hirsch, J. L. Melnick, T. P. Monath, and B. Roizman, eds.), 2nd Ed., p. 241. Raven, New York.

Chesebro, P. (1990). Spongiform encephalopathies: The transmissible agents. *In* "Fields Virology" (B. N. Fields, D. M. Knipe, R. M. Chanock, M. S. Hirsch, J. L. Melnick, T. P. Monath, and B. Roizman, eds.), 2nd Ed., p. 2325. Raven, New York.

Gibbs, E. P. J. (1981). Persistent viral infections of food animals: Their relevance to the international movement of livestock and germplasm. *Adv. Vet. Sci. Comp. Med.* **25,** 71.

Mahy, B. W. J. (1985). Strategies of virus persistence. *Br. Med. Bull.* **41,** 50.

Mims, C. A., and White, D. O. (1984). "Viral Pathogenesis and Immunology." Blackwell, Oxford.

Narayan, O., and Clements, J. E. (1989). Biology and pathogenesis of lentiviruses. *J. Gen. Virol.* **70,** 1617.

Notkins, A. L., and Oldstone, M. B. A., eds. (1984, 1986, 1989). "Concepts in Viral Pathogenesis," Vols. 1, 2, and 3. Springer-Verlag, New York.

Roizman, B., and Sears, A. E. (1990). Herpes simplex viruses and their replication. *In* "Fields Virology" (B. N. Fields, D. M. Knipe, R. M. Chanock, M. S. Hirsch, J. L. Melnick, T. P. Monath, and B. Roizman, eds.), 2nd Ed., p. 1824. Raven, New York.

Wittmann, G., Gaskell, R. M., and Rziha, H.-J., eds. (1984). Latent herpesvirus infections in veterinary medicine. *Curr. Top. Vet. Med. Anim. Sci.* **27,** 1.

CHAPTER 11

Mechanisms of Viral Oncogenesis

Tumors are initiated by alterations in one or more genes that regulate cell growth and/or differentiation. The genetic alterations may be caused by chemical or physical agents or by certain viruses, all of which appear to operate by common intracellular molecular pathways. Study of the infections caused by *oncogenic viruses,* which cause about 15% of human cancers and an unknown but substantial number of cancers of domestic animals, has provided major insights into the nature of these pathways, the elucidation of which is one of the most active fields in animal virology and is providing insights into the elaborate biochemical circuitry that regulates cell growth, division, and differentiation.

First we must define a few commonly used terms. Oncology is the study of tumors. A *benign tumor* is a growth produced by abnormal cell proliferation which remains localized and does not invade adjacent tissue; a *malignant tumor,* in contrast, is usually locally invasive and may also be *metastatic,* that is, may spread by lymphatic and blood vessels to other parts of the body. Such malignant tumors are often referred to as *cancers.* Malignant tumors of epithelial cell origin are known as *carcinomas,* those arising from cells of mesenchymal origin as *sarcomas,* and those from leukocytes as *lymphomas* (if solid tumors) or *leukemia* (if circulating cells are involved). The process of development of tumors is termed *oncogenesis*, synonyms for which are *tumorigenesis* and *carcinogenesis*. The capacity to study oncogenesis at a molecular level was greatly facilitated when it became possible to induce the essential genetic changes in cultured cells, a process called *cell transformation*.

The discoveries of the viral etiology of avian leukemia by Ellerman and Bang and of avian sarcoma by Rous in 1908 and 1911, respectively, were for many years regarded as curiosities unlikely to be significant in the understanding of cancer in general. However, these avian viruses have come to occupy a central place in oncology, and since the 1950s there has been a steady stream of discoveries clearly incriminating other viruses in a variety of benign and malignant tumors of numerous species of mammals, birds, amphibia, and reptiles (Table 11-1). Avian retroviruses are not merely good models for the study of oncogenesis, however; they are also major pathogens of poultry.

ONCOGENES AND TUMOR SUPPRESSOR GENES

An important element in our present understanding of oncogenesis has come from the discovery of *oncogenes*, which were originally found in retroviruses, where they are collectively referred to as v-*onc* genes. In a sense, the term oncogene is unfortunate in that for each of the more than 60 v-*onc* genes so far identified there is a corresponding normal cellular gene, which is referred to as a c-*onc* gene, or as a *protooncogene*, a term which suggests the origin of the v-*onc* genes of retroviruses. The term oncogene is now applied broadly to any genetic element associated with cancer induction, including some cellular genes not known to have a viral homolog and relevant genes of the oncogenic DNA viruses which do not have a cellular homolog. In the normal cell c-*onc* genes are involved in cellular growth control, in which four types of proteins participate: growth factors, growth factor receptors, intracellular signal transducers, and nuclear transcription factors.

Recently a second major class of cellular genes called *tumor suppressor genes* has been discovered which also play an essential regulatory role in normal cells. Their protein products are involved in negative regulation of growth. This regulatory role may be removed by mutation in the tumor suppressor gene, which may permit excess activity of a c-*onc* gene, leading to cancer. Although half of all cancers may be associated with altered tumor suppressor genes, they are only indirectly involved in cancers caused by viruses and thus will not be discussed further.

TABLE 11-1
Viruses That Can Induce Tumors in Domestic or Laboratory Animals

Family/genus	Virus	Kind of tumor
DNA viruses		
Papovaviridae		
Polyomavirus	*Polyomavirus muris* 1	Solid tumors in newborn rodents
	Polyomavirus macacae (SV40)	Solid tumors in newborn rodents
Papillomavirus	*Papillomavirus sylvilagi*	Papillomas, skin cancers in rabbits
	Bovine papillomavirus 4	Papillomas, carcinoma of intestine, bladder
	Bovine papillomavirus 7	Papillomas, carcinoma of eye
Adenoviridae	*Mastadenovirus*, many types	Solid tumors in newborn rodents, no tumors in natural hosts
Hepadnaviridae	Human, duck, woodchuck hepadnaviruses	Carcinoma of liver in natural hosts
Herpesviridae		
Alphaherpesvirinae	Marek's disease virus	Lymphoma
Rhadinovirus	Ateline herpesvirus 2	Lymphomas, leukemia in some primates
	Saimirine herpesvirus 1	Lymphomas, leukemia in some primates
Poxviridae[a]		
Leporipoxvirus	Rabbit fibroma virus	Benign fibromas in rabbits
	Squirrel fibroma virus	Benign fibromas in squirrels
Yatapoxvirus	Yaba monkey tumor virus	Histiocytoma in monkeys
RNA viruses		
Retroviridae		
HTLV-BLV group	Bovine leukemia virus	Leukemia
Mammalian type C retrovirus group	Feline leukemia virus	Leukemia
	Feline sarcoma virus	Sarcoma
	Avian reticuloendotheliosis virus	Reticuloendotheliosis
Avian type C retrovirus group	Avian leukosis virus	Leukosis, osteopetrosis, nephroblastoma
	Rous sarcoma virus	Sarcoma
	Avian erythroblastosis virus	Erythroblastosis
	Avian myeloblastosis virus	Myeloblastosis

[a] Poxviruses are not true oncogenic viruses; they differ from all other viruses listed in that they replicate in the cytoplasm and do not affect the cellular genome.

CELL TRANSFORMATION

Oncogenic viruses greatly change the growth characteristics of cultured cells, the process being called cell transformation, which is the *in vitro* equivalent of tumor formation. Transformation by DNA viruses is usually nonproductive (i.e., the transformed cells do not yield infectious progeny virus); transformation by retroviruses, on the other hand, is often productive. Viral (or proviral) DNA in transformed cells is integrated into the cell DNA, except in the case of papillomavirus and herpesvirus DNAs, which remain episomal.

Transformed cells differ in many ways from normal cells (Table 11-2, Fig. 11-1). One of the changes is a loss of control of cell growth; transformed cells acquire a capacity to divide unrestrictedly, which can be demonstrated in a variety of ways, including the capacity to produce tumors in athymic mice, which have defective T-cell immunity but do not support the growth of normal foreign cells.

Virus-Specific Antigens in Transformed Cells

Malignant tumors or transformed cells express distinctive antigens, called *tumor-associated antigens.* Cells transformed by nondefective retroviruses also express the full range of viral proteins, and new virions bud from their plasma membranes. In contrast, transformation by DNA viruses usually occurs in cells undergoing nonproductive infection; nev-

TABLE 11-2

Characteristics of Cells Transformed in Vitro *by Viruses*

1. Viral DNA sequences present, integrated into cellular DNA or as episomes
2. Greater growth potential *in vitro*
   (a) Formation of three-dimensional colonies of randomly oriented cells in monolayer culture, usually due to loss of contact inhibition
   (b) Capacity to divide indefinitely in serial culture
   (c) Higher efficiency of cloning
   (d) Capacity to grow in suspension or in semisolid agar (anchorage independence)
   (e) Reduced serum requirement for growth
3. Altered cell morphology
4. Altered cell metabolism and membrane changes
5. Chromosomal abnormalities
6. Virus-specified tumor-associated antigens present
   (a) Some at the cell surface behave as tumor-specific transplantation antigens
   (b) New intracellular antigens (e.g., T antigens) appear
7. Capacity to produce malignant neoplasms when inoculated into isologous or severely immunosuppressed animals

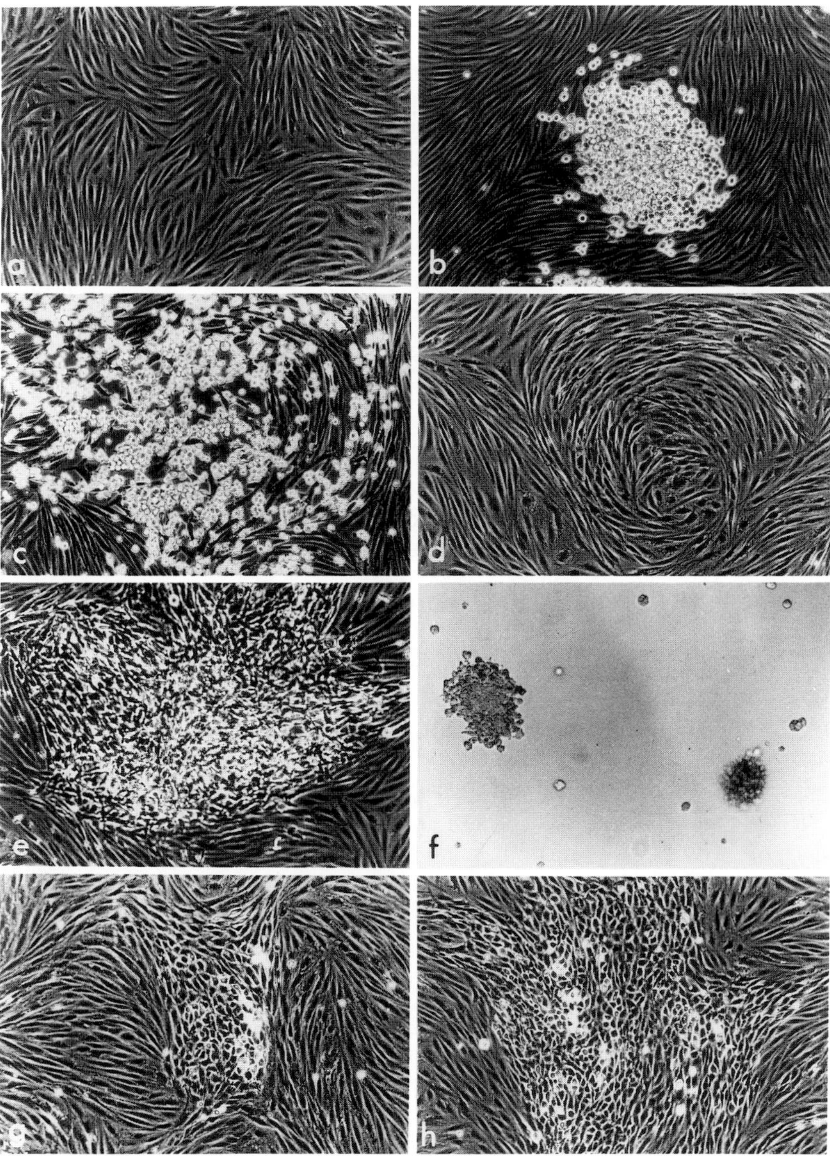

FIG. 11-1. *Transformation of a rat fibroblast cell line by different viral oncogenes. (a) Normal F111 cells. (b) Cells transformed by Rous sarcoma virus. (c) Cells transformed by Harvey murine sarcoma virus. (d) Cells transformed by Abelson leukemia virus. (e) Cells transformed by mouse polymavirus. (f) Polyomavirus-transformed cells in soft agar. (g) Cells transformed by SV40. (h) Cells transformed by simian adenovirus 7. [From T. Benjamin and P. K. Vogt,* In *"Fields Virology" (B. N. Fields, D. M. Knipe* et al., *eds.), 2nd ed., p. 322. Raven, New York, 1990; courtesy Dr. T. Benjamin.]*

ertheless, certain virus-specific antigens are regularly demonstrable. Some tumor-associated antigens are located in the plasma membrane, where they elicit transplantation rejection responses and are referred to as *tumor-specific transplantation antigens.*

TUMOR INDUCTION BY RETROVIRUSES

Retroviruses are the major cause of leukemias and lymphomas in many species of animals, including cattle, cats, apes, mice, and chickens, and cause a rare form of leukemia in humans.

Categories of Oncogenic Retroviruses

Retroviruses of five genera may produce tumors (see Chapter 33). Oncogenic retroviruses are subdivided according to whether they are *defective* or nondefective, endogenous or exogenous.

Defective and Nondefective Retroviruses. The genome of a typical nondefective retrovirus (Fig. 11-2A) consists of two identical copies of a ssRNA molecule, each of which has three genes: *gag,* encoding the four core proteins; *pol,* encoding the unique viral polymerase, reverse transcriptase; and *env,* encoding the two envelope glycoproteins. A second kind of rapidly oncogenic exogenous retrovirus carries a fourth gene, v-*onc,* which is responsible for the rapid malignant change in the infected cell. Because the oncogene has been incorporated into the viral RNA in place of part of one or more normal viral genes (Fig. 11-2C), the genome is defective; hence, such viruses are dependent on nondefective helper retroviruses for their replication. Rous sarcoma virus, on which many of the classic studies were made, is atypical in that its genome contains a viral oncogene (v-*src*) in addition to complete copies of the retrovirus genes *gag, pol,* and *env* (Fig. 11-2D).

Endogenous and Exogenous Retroviruses. A complete DNA copy of the genome (*provirus*) of one, or sometimes more than one, of many retroviruses may be transmitted in the germ-line DNA from parent to offspring and may thus be perpetuated in the DNA of every cell of every individual of certain vertebrate species. Proviral genomes are under the control of cellular regulatory genes and are normally totally silent in normal animals. Such retroviruses are said to be *endogenous* (Table 11-3). However, proviruses can be induced by various factors such as irradiation, exposure to mutagenic or carcinogenic chemicals, and hormonal or immunologic stimuli, so that virions are synthesized. In contrast, other retroviruses behave as more typical infectious agents, spreading horizon-

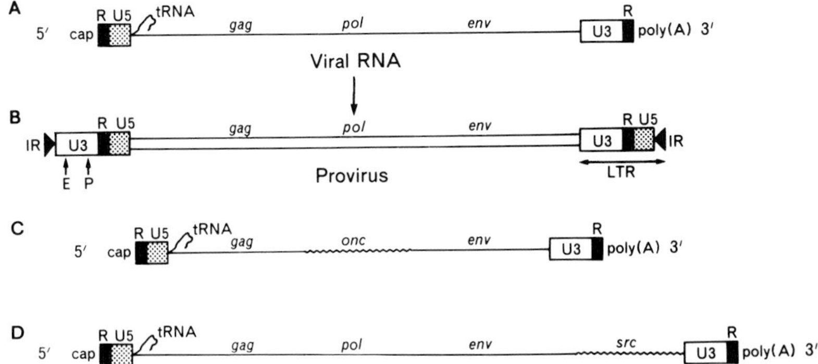

FIG. 11-2. *Simplified diagrams of the structure of retrovirus genomes and integrated provirus; in A, C, and D only one of the two identical RNA molecules is shown. (A) The genome of a replication-competent slowly transforming retrovirus. The major coding regions* gag, pol, *and* env *encode the viral proteins. The 5′ terminus is capped and the 3′ terminus is polyadenylated. A short sequence, R, is repeated at both ends of the molecule, while unique sequences, U5 and U3, are located near the 5′ and 3′ termini, immediately proximal to R. There is a 16- to 18-nucleotide sequence adjacent to U5, the primer binding site (PBS, Fig. 33-2), which is complementary to the 3′ terminus of a tRNA, which binds to it and acts as a primer for reverse transcriptase. (B) Provirus, a dsDNA, is integrated into cellular DNA. The genome is flanked at each terminus by additional sequences to form the long terminal repeat (LTR). Each LTR comprises U3, R, and U5 plus short inverted repeat sequences (IR) at the distal end. U3 contains the promoter (P) and enhancer (E) sequences, as well as several other sequences with important functions. (C) The genome of a replication-defective rapidly transforming retrovirus. A v-onc gene (wavy line) has replaced all of the* pol *and part of the* gag *and* env *genes. (D) The genome of a Rous sarcoma virus, a replication-competent rapidly transforming retrovirus. A v-*onc *gene (v-*src*) is present in addition to complete* gag, pol, *and* env *genes.*

tally to contacts, and are said to be *exogenous*. Exogenous retroviruses are also sometimes formed in animals exposed to environmental factors, as a result of mutation or recombination events within the host.

The host species from which a particular retrovirus is recovered is not necessarily is native host. Some endogenous retroviruses are *ecotropic*, that is, they replicate only in the host species from which they originate, while others are *amphotropic*, that is, they replicate in native and certain foreign hosts, and yet others are *xenotropic*, that is, they cannot replicate in the host species in whose genome they are carried as provirus, but can in certain other, not necessarily related, species.

Most endogenous retroviruses never produce disease, cannot transform cultured cells, and contain no oncogene in their genome. Most

TABLE 11-3
Comparison of Endogenous and Exogenous Retroviruses

Characteristic	Endogenous retroviruses	Exogenous retroviruses: Slowly transforming or *cis*-acting retrovirus	Exogenous retroviruses: Rapidly transforming or transducing retrovirus
Transmission	Vertical (germ line)	Horizontal	Horizontal
Expression	Usually not, but inducible	Yes	Yes
Genome	Complete	Complete	Defective[a]
Replication	Productive	Productive	Requires helper[a]
Oncogene	No	No	Yes
Tumorigenicity	Nil, or rarely leukemia	Leukemia after long incubation period	Sarcoma, leukemia, or carcinoma, after short incubation period
In vitro transformation	No	No	Yes

[a] Except for Rous sarcoma virus.

exogenous retroviruses, on the other hand, are oncogenic; some characteristically induce leukemia or lymphoma, others sarcoma, and yet others carcinoma, usually displaying a predilection for a particular type of target cell. Exogenous retroviruses can be further subdivided into rapidly oncogenic and slowly oncogenic variants (Table 11-3). The rapidly oncogenic sarcoma viruses, like Rous sarcoma virus, are the most rapidly acting carcinogens known, causing death in as short a time as 2 weeks after infection in certain host species, and rapidly transforming cultured cells *in vitro*. These properties are attributable to the v-*onc* gene which they carry as part of their genome. There are over 60 known v-*onc* genes, the characters of some of which are shown in Table 11-5; most exogenous retroviruses carry only one particular type of v-*onc* gene, for example, v-*src* in the case of Rous sarcoma virus. The genomes of weakly oncogenic ("slowly transforming") viruses contain no v-*onc* gene, but they can induce B-cell, T-cell, or myeloid leukemia with low efficiency and after a much longer incubation period. For example, the avian *leukosis* viruses, which are endemic in many chicken flocks, produce lifelong viremia in some chickens, which usually causes no disease but in a small percentage of birds leads later in life to a wide variety of diseases involving the hemopoietic system or rarely solid tumors, namely, sarcomas, carcinomas, and endotheliomas (see Chapter 33).

Replication of Retroviruses

The complete replication cycle of retroviruses is described in Chapter 33, but certain aspects associated with the integration of the DNA copy of the RNA genome into the cellular DNA need to be described here in order to explain viral oncogenesis. When released in the cytoplasm, the ssRNA genome is converted to dsDNA which is integrated into the chromosomal DNA as provirus (Fig. 11-2A,B). The expression of mRNA from the provirus is under the control of the viral transcriptional regulator sequences, which include promoter and enhancer elements, both of which are located in the *long terminal repeat (LTR).* In other ways the proviral DNA behaves as other chromosomal genes, segregating like other markers and being transmitted via the germ line. The strong promoter in the LTR influences the expression of genes in the vicinity of the insertion site, such that the provirus may acquire and transduce cellular genes, and it may increase the expression of downstream cellular genes or occasionally inactivate a cellular gene at the point of insertion.

Mechanisms of Tumor Production by Retroviruses

Retroviruses produce tumors by affecting the action of a c-*onc* gene in one of three ways (Table 11-4): (1) the *transducing retroviruses* introduce a v-*onc* gene, which is controlled by viral regulatory sequences present in the LTR of the viral genome, into the chromosome of a normal cell; (2) *cis-activating retroviruses,* which lack a v-*onc* gene, transform cells by integrating close to a c-*onc* gene and thus usurping normal cellular regulation of this gene; and (3) viral sequences that code for nonstructural regulatory proteins may either increase transcription from the viral LTR or interfere with the transcriptional control of specific cellular genes (*trans*-activating retroviruses). Transducing retroviruses transform cells rapidly both *in vitro* and *in vivo. cis*-Activating retroviruses are replication-competent, induce tumors more slowly, and do not transform cells in culture.

Modes of Action of Transduced Retroviral Oncogenes

A great variety of structural and regulatory changes, including mutation, translocation, retroviral insertion, and amplification, can activate the same oncogene in different naturally occurring tumors. The oncoprotein products of all retroviral oncogenes appear to act by interfering either with *signal transduction,* namely, the transfer of signals from the membrane to the cell interior, or directly with the regulation of cellular genes. Although the total pathway through which any oncoprotein stim-

TABLE 11-4

Mechanisms of Oncogenicity of Retroviruses[a]

Virus category	Tumor latency period	Efficiency of tumor formation	Oncogenic effector	State of viral genome	Ability to transform cultured cells
Transducing retroviruses	Short (days)	High (can reach 100% of animals)	Cell-derived oncogene carried in viral genome	Viral–cellular chimera, replication-defective	Yes
cis-Activating retroviruses	Intermediate (weeks, months)	High to intermediate	Cellular oncogene activated *in situ* by provirus	Intact, replication-competent genome	No
trans-Activating retroviruses	Long (months, years)	Very low (<1%)	Virus-coded regulatory protein controlling transcription	Intact, replication-competent genome	No

[a] From B. N. Fields, D. M. Knipe, R. M. Chanock, M. S. Hirsch, J. L. Melnick, T. P. Monath, and B. Roizman, eds., "Fields Virology," 2nd Ed., p. 328. Raven, New York, 1990.

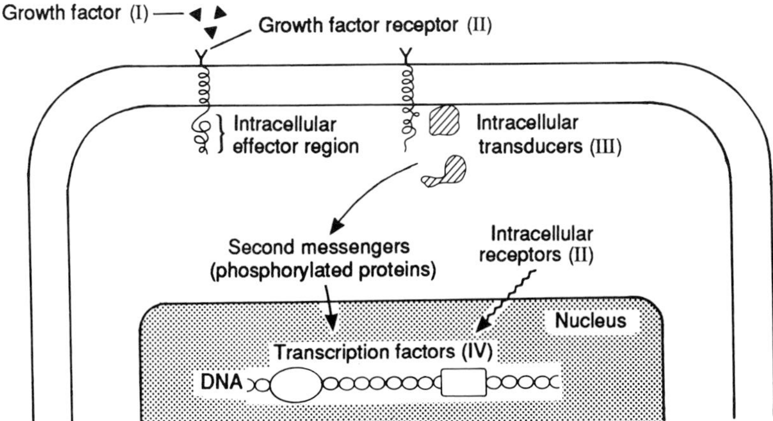

FIG. 11-3. *Cellular growth control involves four types of proteins, the genes for which can give rise to oncogenes. They are (I) growth factors, (II) receptors, (III) intracellular transducers, and (IV) intranuclear factors. See Table 11-5 for examples and text for explanation. (Modified from J. E. Darnell, H. Losish, and D. Baltimore, "Molecular Cell Biology," 2nd Ed., p. 985. Scientific American Books, New York, 1990.)*

ulates cell growth is not understood, there is information on where they fit into the overall picture of growth control (Fig. 11-3, Table 11-5).

Growth Factor (Class I). Only one example of oncogene acting as a growth factor is known, v-*sis*, the cellular counterpart of which codes for one of the two polypeptide chains of platelet-derived growth factor (PDGF), which is not normally expressed in fibroblasts. Activation of the gene by the retroviral v-*onc* gene, under the control of the powerful enhancer/promoter complex in the LTR, induces the fibroblast to manufacture its own growth factor, leading to immortalization of fibroblasts in culture and possibly the induction of malignant tumors.

Growth Factor Receptors (Class II). In the normal cell, growth factor receptors bind a specific factor and then the receptor sends a growth signal to the cell. The receptors can be turned into oncogenes by a variety of structural changes. For example, the v-*erbB* oncogene is a truncated epidermal growth factor (EGF) receptor gene, which lacks most of the extracellular ligand-binding domain. As a result there is deregulation of normal tyrosine kinase activity.

Hormone Receptors (Class II). The product of the v-*erbA* gene is derived from the intracellular receptor for thyroid hormone, which normally acts by transforming the intracellular receptor into a transcription

TABLE 11-5

Retroviral Oncogenes and Locations and Functions of Their Proteins[a]

Oncogene	Retrovirus	Subcellular location of protein	Nature of oncogene product
Class I: Growth factors			
sis	Simian sarcoma virus	Secreted	Platelet-derived growth factor β chain
Class II: Receptors			
A. Cell-surface receptors with protein-tyrosine kinase activity			
erbB	Avian erythroblastosis virus[b]	Plasma membrane	Truncated epidermal growth factor receptor
fms	Feline sarcoma virus	Plasma membrane	Mutated CSF-1 receptor
B. Intracellular receptors			
erbA	Avian erythroblastosis virus[b]	Nuclear	Thyroxine receptor; activated form prevents differentiation
Class III: Intracellular transducers			
A. *Ras* proteins			
H-*ras*	Harvey murine sarcoma virus	Plasma membrane	Guanine nucleotide-binding proteins with GTPase activity
Ki-*ras*	Kirsten murine sarcoma virus	Plasma membrane	Guanine nucleotide-binding proteins with GTPase activity
B. Protein-tyrosine kinase			
src	Rous sarcoma virus	Cytoplasm	Protein kinases that phosphorylate tyrosine residues
fps[c]	Fujinami avian sarcoma virus	Cytoplasm	Protein kinases that phosphorylate tyrosine residues
fes[c]	Feline sarcoma virus	Cytoplasm	Protein kinases that phosphorylate tyrosine residues
C. Protein serine/threonine kinases			
mos	Moloney murine sarcoma virus	Cytoplasm	Cytoplasmic serine kinase (cytostatic factor)
Class IV: Nuclear transcription factors			
myc	Avian myelocytoma virus	Nuclear matrix	Binds to DNA; regulates transcription
myb	Avian myeloblastosis virus	Nuclear matrix	Binds to DNA; regulates transcription
fos	Murine osteosarcoma virus	Nucleus	Transcription factor AP-1
jun	Avian sarcoma virus	Nucleus	Transcription factor AP-1

[a] Oncogenes are designated by three letters in lowercase italics, oncogene products (oncoproteins) by the same three letters in roman type, with an initial capital.

[b] Transducing retrovirus with two oncogenes.

[c] *fps* and *fes* are the same oncogene derived from avian and feline genomes, respectively.

factor. The modified receptor, ErbA, acts by competing with the endogenous thyroid hormone receptor, causing growth without control. In the avian erythroblastosis virus, v-*erbA* and v-*erbB* act synergistically to give full oncogenicity.

Intracellular Transducers (Class III). By far the largest class of oncogenes is derived from genes encoding proteins that act as intracellular transducers, that is, proteins that transmit signals from a receptor to a cellular target. The best understood are the Ha-*ras* ahd Ki-*ras* oncogenes; their cellular equivalents were the first nonviral oncogenes to be recognized. Most Ras molecules exist in an inactive state in the resting cell, where they bind guanosine diphosphate. When they receive a physiologic stimulus from a transmembrane receptor they are temporarily activated, leading to the synthesis of guanosine triphosphate. The *ras* genes acquire transforming properties by mutational changes, mostly point mutations at specific sites, which may stabilize Ras proteins in their active state. This may cause a continuous flow of signal transduction, leading to malignant transformation.

Many class III oncogenes encode a protein-tyrosine kinase, which differs from the products of the class II oncogenes in that they are cytoplasmic or nuclear proteins, lacking any transmembrane or extracellular domain. Oncogene kinases recognize and phosphorylate a broad range of target proteins, one or more of which may be crucial to the transformed state.

Nuclear Transcription Factors (Class IV). By one mechanism or another, all oncogenes must eventually cause changes in the cell nucleus. The class IV oncogenes directly affect transcription or bind to DNA. The v-*jun* oncogene is closely homologous to AP-1, a transcription factor gene, and it can bind tightly to another nuclear oncoprotein, Fos. The growth factors and oncoproteins that can induce *jun* are components of mitotic signal chains, and there is evidence that *jun* induces cancer through its role as a transcriptional regulator.

The phosphoprotein genes, of which *myc, myb,* and *fos* are the best known examples, can transactivate other genes and can stimulate DNA replication directly or indirectly. After having been activated by structural and/or regulatory changes, they may contribute to tumor development or progression.

Activation of Cellular Oncogenes

There is evidence that c-*onc* genes may be responsible for some transformations. It is not difficult to imagine a tumor arising from overexpression of a c-*onc* gene, or inappropriate expression, for example, in the wrong cell or at the wrong time. Such abnormal c-*onc* transcription may occur in a variety of ways, in several of which oncogenic viruses play a role.

Insertional Mutagenesis. The presence upstream from a c-*onc* gene of an integrated provirus, with its strong promoter and enhancer elements, may greatly amplify the expression of the c-*onc* gene. This is the likely mechanism whereby the weakly oncogenic avian leukosis viruses, which lack a v-*onc* gene but have an LTR in which the promoter and enhancer elements are located, produce tumors. When avian leukosis viruses cause malignancy, the viral genome is generally integrated at a particular location, immediately upstream from a c-*onc* gene. Integrated avian leukosis provirus increases the synthesis of the normal c-*myc* oncogene product 30- to 100-fold. Experimentally, only the LTR need be integrated, and furthermore by such a mechanism c-*myc* may be expressed in cells in which it is not normally expressed. In some instances a quantitative rather than a qualitative difference in the c-*onc* gene-product may be sufficient for oncogenicity.

Transposition. Transposition of c-*onc* genes may result in enhanced expression by bringing them under the control of strong promoter and enhancer elements. For instance, the 8 : 14 chromosomal translocation that characterizes Burkitt's lymphoma (a tumor associated with Epstein-Barr herpesvirus infection, occurring in African children) brings the c-*myc* gene into position just downstream of the strong immunoglobulin promoter. Perhaps v-*onc* genes may sometimes be transposed from their initial site of integration in a similar way.

Gene Amplification. Amplification of oncogenes is a feature of many tumors. For example, a 30-fold increase in the number of c-*ras* gene copies is found in one human cancer cell line, while the c-*myc* gene is amplified in several human tumors. The increase in gene copy number leads to a corresponding increase in the amount of oncogene product, thus producing cancer.

Mutation. Mutation in a c-*onc* gene, for example, c-*ras*, may alter the function of the corresponding oncoprotein. Such mutations can occur either *in situ*, as a result of chemical or physical mutagenesis, or in the course of recombination with retroviral DNA. Given the high error rate of reverse transcription, v-*onc* gene homologs of c-*onc* genes will always carry mutations, and the strongly promoted production of the viral oncoprotein will readily exceed that of the cellular oncoprotein.

TUMOR INDUCTION BY DNA VIRUSES

DNA tumor viruses interact with cells in one of two mutually exclusive ways: (1) productive infection in which the virus completes its replication cycle, resulting in cell lysis, or (2) nonproductive infection in which the virus transforms the cell without completing its replication cycle. During such nonproductive infection part or all of the viral DNA is integrated into the cellular DNA and continues to express its early gene functions. The molecular basis of oncogenesis by DNA viruses is best understood for polymaviruses, papillomaviruses, and adenoviruses, all of which contain genes that act as oncogenes (Table 11-6). These appear to act by mechanisms similar to those described for retrovirus oncogenes, primarily in the nucleus, where they alter patterns of gene expression and regulation of cell growth. In every case the relevant genes are "early" proteins having a dual role in viral replication and cell transformation. With a few possible exceptions, the oncogenes of DNA viruses have no homologs or direct ancestors (c-*onc* genes) among cellular genes of the host.

The protein products of DNA virus oncogenes are multifunctional, with particular functions related to particular domains of the folded

TABLE 11-6
Oncogenes of Adenoviruses and Papovaviruses, and Their Products

		Product	
Virus	Oncogene	Function	Location
Adenoviruses	E1A	Regulates transcription	Nucleus
	E1B	?	Nucleus, membranes
Papillomaviruses	E5	Signaling	Nuclear membrane
	E6	Transcription/replication	Nucleus, cytoplasm
	E7	Transcription/replication	Nucleus, cytoplasm
Polyomavirus	Py-t	Regulates phosphatase activity	Cytoplasm, nucleus
	Py-mT	Binds and regulates product of c-*src* and related kinases	Plasma membrane
	Py-T	Transcription/replication	Nucleus
SV40	SV-t	Regulates phosphatase activity	Cytoplasm, nucleus
	SV-T	Initiates DNA synthesis, regulates transcription	Plasma membrane, nucleus

protein, which mimic functions of normal cellular proteins. They interact with host cell proteins at the plasma membrane or within the cytoplasm or nucleus. Polyoma middle T protein, for example, interacts with c-*src*, resulting in increased levels of the protein kinase activity of the Src protein.

Polyomaviruses and Adenoviruses

During the 1960s and 1970s two members of the genus *Polyomavirus*, polyomavirus of mice and simian virus 40 (SV40), as well as certain human adenoviruses (types 12, 18, and 31), were found to induce malignant tumors following inoculation into baby hamsters and other rodents. Although they replicate productively in and destroy cultured cells of their native host species, they transform cultured cells of certain other species (see Fig. 11-1) and provide good experimental models for analysis of the biochemical events in cell transformation.

The polyomavirus- or adenovirus-transformed cell does not produce virus. Viral DNA is integrated at multiple sites on the chromosomes of the cell. Most of the integrated viral genomes are complete in the case of the polymaviruses, but defective in the case of the adenoviruses. Only certain early viral genes are transcribed, albeit at an unusually high rate. By analogy with retrovirus genes, they are called oncogenes (see Table 11-6). Their products, demonstrable by immunofluorescence, are known as *tumor (T) antigens*. A great deal is now known about the role of these proteins in transformation. For example, Py-mT of polyoma virus (like the product of the v-*ras* gene of retroviruses) seems to bring about the change in cell morphology and enables the cells to grow in suspension in semisolid agar medium as well as on solid substrates (*anchorage independence*), whereas Py-T, like the product of the v-*myc* gene of retroviruses, is responsible for the reduction in dependence of the cells on serum and enhances their life span in culture.

Virus can be rescued from polyomavirus-transformed cells (i.e., induced to replicate) by irradiation, treatment with certain mutagenic chemicals, or cocultivation with certain types of permissive cells. This cannot be achieved with adenovirus-transformed cells, as the integrated adenoviral DNA contains substantial deletions.

It should be stressed that integration of viral DNA does not necessarily lead to transformation. As discussed in Chapter 10, persistent infections with some herpesviruses are characterized by integration of the viral genome without any indication of cellular transformation. Many or most episodes of integration of papovavirus or adenovirus DNA have no recognized biological consequence. Transformation by these viruses in experimental systems is a rare event, requiring that the viral transforming genes be integrated in the location and orientation needed for their expression. Even then, many transformed cells revert (*abortive transformation*). Furthermore, cells displaying the characteristics of transformation (see Table 11-2) do not necessarily produce tumors. This needs to be demonstrated independently by transplantation of cells into athymic or syngeneic mice. Further, certain ostensibly normal cell lines commonly used for *in vitro* transformation assays, such as 3T3 cells, are in fact "premalignant"; moreover, transformation of normal cells to the fully malignant state may require the cooperation of more than a single oncogene, for example, either polyoma large T, adenovirus E1A, or retrovirus v-*myc*, together with at least one other.

Papillomaviruses

Papillomaviruses produce papillomas (warts) on the skin and mucous membranes. These benign tumors are hyperplastic outgrowths which generally regress spontaneously. Occasionally, however, they may progress to malignancy. There is evidence that a cofactor may be required.

One of the most instructive models is the bovine papillomavirus, of which seven types are recognized (see Chapter 17). Different bovine papillomavirus are associated with the development of tumors in different sites. In hot, sunny climates, such as in northern Australia and in Texas, viral papillomas around the eye and on hairless or nonpigmented patches of skin may become malignant; the cofactor is postulated to be ultraviolet irradiation. In the Scottish Highlands, multiple benign papillomas are common, but only cattle consuming bracken fern will sometimes develope carcinoma of the alimentary tract or bladder. Mature virions are readily demonstrable in the papillomas but are absent from the carcinomas. However, *in situ* hybridization with a labeled bovine papillomavirus 4 DNA probe reveals that the cells of carcinomas contain the viral genome, not integrated but free, in the form of a closed circular molecule of DNA. Viral DNA is also found in distant metastatic tumors, ruling out the possibility that it represents contamination from papillomas. The fact that it is all episomal indicates that integration of viral DNA is not required for the induction of malignancy. Bovine papillomaviruses, as well as those from man and other animals, will transform bovine or murine cells *in vitro* and induce fibromas in rodents. Examination of the transformed cells also reveals no virions but episomal viral DNA in essentially every cell. Moreover, the viral DNA, which is infectious, induces tumors in rodents and transforms cultured rodent cells. Indeed, transfection with a fragment of bovine papillomavirus 1 DNA representing 69% of the genome also transforms cultured cells. Only a small part of the corresponding papillomavirus genome is transcribed in bovine or rabbit carcinoma cells. Nevertheless, more of the viral DNA may be required for maintenance of the transformed state, as treatment with interferon has been reported to "cure" mouse cells transformed by bovine papillomavirus 1; revertants (abortively transformed cells) had lost their viral DNA.

Hepadnaviruses

All three mammalian hepadnaviruses are strongly associated with naturally occurring hepatocellular carcinomas in their native hosts. Chronically infected woodchucks almost inevitably develop carcinoma even in the absence of other carcinogenic factors. The duck hepatitis virus is probably not oncogenic by itself, but its integrated DNA has been found in mycotoxin-associated hepatocellular carcinomas in Pekin ducks. Oncogenesis by mammalian hepadnaviruses is a multifactorial process. These viruses contain a protein, HBx, which stimulates transcription of many growth-activating host cell genes (e.g., c-*myc* and c-*fos*) and possibly inhibits cellular growth suppressor proteins. HBx protein can complement E1A-defective adenoviruses. Deregulated overexpression of HBx and viral surface proteins is often found in the early stages of hepatocellular carcinoma. In carcinoma cells the viral genome is integrated at 5–7 sites scattered through the genome. Insertional activation of positive growth factors, such as N-Myc in woodchucks, has been described. Furthermore, host cell DNA seems to be destablized by hepadnavirus DNA, leading to gene rearrangements, deletions, and even chromosomal translocation, and the chronic regeneration accompanying cirrhosis of the liver also promotes the development of tumors. The likelihood of hepadnavirus-associated carcinoma is greatest in animals (and humans) infected perinatally.

Herpesviruses

Herpesviruses of the subfamily *Gammaherpesvirinae* are the etiological agents of lymphomas or carcinomas in hosts ranging from amphibia, through birds, to primates including man. Marek's disease virus, formerly considered a gammaherpesvirus but now classified as an alphaherpesvirus, transforms T lymphocytes, causing them to proliferate to produce a lethal generalized lymphomatosis. The disease is contagious, being transmitted via virus shedding in cells of the feather follicles, and is a major problem for the poultry industry.

The mechanism by which herpesviruses produce malignancy has been best studied in Burkitt's lymphoma, a malignant B-cell lymphoma found in children in East Africa, which is associated with Epstein-Barr (EB) virus infection. The EB virus genome DNA is present in multiple copies in each cell of most African Burkitt's lymphomas. Although sometimes integrated into host chromosomes, the EB virus genome generally occurs in the form of closed circles of the complete viral DNA molecule, found free as autonomously replicating episomes. The cells express EB virus nuclear antigen detectable by immunofluorescence, but they do not produce virus until induced to do so by cultivation *in vitro*. The malignant cells also contain a characteristic 8 : 14 chromosomal translocation. The human c-*myc* oncogene, located on the distal segment of chromosome 8, is transposed to one of three chromosomes that contain genes for immunoglobulin (usually chromosome 14, sometimes 2 or 22), leading to its enhanced expression.

Poxviruses

Although some poxviruses are regularly associated with the development of benign tumorlike lesions, there is no evidence that these ever become malignant, nor is there evidence that poxvirus DNA is ever integrated into cellular DNA. A very early viral protein produced in poxvirus-infected cells displays homology with epidermal growth factor, and it is probably responsible for the epithelial hyperplasia characteristic of many poxvirus infections. For some poxviruses, for example, fowlpox, orf, and rabbit fibroma viruses, epithelial hyperplasia is a dominant clinical manifestation and may be a consequence of a more potent form of the poxvirus epidermal growth factor.

COOPERATION BETWEEN ONCOGENES: MULTISTEP ONCOGENESIS

Tumors other than those induced by rapidly transforming retroviruses like Rous sarcoma virus generally do not arise as the result of a single event, but rather by a series of steps leading to progressively greater loss of regulation of cell division. Significantly, the genome of some retroviruses (e.g., avian erythroblastosis virus) carries two different oncogenes (and that of polyomavirus, three), while two or more distinct oncogenes are activated in certain human tumors (e.g., Burkitt's lymphoma). Cotransfection of normal rat embryo fibroblasts with the mutant c-*ras* gene plus the polyomavirus large T gene (Py-T), or with c-*ras* plus the E1A early gene of oncogenic adenoviruses, or with v-*ras* plus v-*myc*, converts them to tumor cells. It should be noted that, whereas v-*ras* and v-*myc* are typical v-*onc* genes, originally of c-*onc* origin, the other two had been assumed to be typical viral genes. Furthermore, a chemical carcinogen can substitute for one of the two v-*onc* genes; following immortalization of cells *in vitro* by treatment with the carcinogen, transfection of a cloned oncogene converts the cloned continuous cell line to tumor cell line.

Such experiments resurrect earlier unifying theories of cancer causation that viewed viruses as analogous to other mutagenic carcinogens, both being capable of initiating a chain of two or more events leading eventually to malignancy. If viruses or oncogenes are to be considered as cocarcinogens in a chain of genetic events culminating in a tumor, it will be necessary to determine whether their role is that of initiator or promoter, or both. The most plausible hypothesis may be that (1) a limited number of c-*onc* genes represent targets for carcinogens (chemicals, radiation, and tumor viruses) and (2) the full expression of malignancy may generally require the mutation or enhanced expression of more than one class of oncogene.

FURTHER READING

Aaronson, S. A. (1991). Growth factors and cancer. *Science* **254,** 1146.

Benjamin, T., and Vogt, P. K. (1990). Cell transformation by viruses. *In* "Fields Virology" (B. N. Fields, D. M. Knipe, R. M. Chanock, M. S. Hirsch, J. L. Melnick, T. P. Monath, and B. Roizman, eds.), 2nd Ed., p. 317. Raven, New York.

Bishop J. M. (1991). Molecular themes in oncogenesis. *Cell (Cambridge, Mass.)* **64,** 235.

Darnell, J. E., Lodish, H., and Baltimore, D. (1990). "Molecular Cell Biology," 2nd Ed., p. 955. Scientific American Books, New York.

Dulbecco, R. (1990). Oncogenic viruses I: DNA-containing viruses. *In* "Microbiology" (B. D. Davis, R. Dulbecco, H. N. Eisen, and H. S. Ginsberg, eds.), 4th Ed., p. 1103. Lippincott, Philadelphia, Pennsylvania.

Dulbecco, R. (1990). Oncogenic viruses II: RNA-containing viruses (retroviruses). *In* "Microbiology" (B. D. Davis, R. Dulbecco, H. N. Eisen, and H. S. Ginsberg, eds.), 4th Ed, p. 1123. Lippincott, Philadelphia, Pennsylvania.

Kung, H.-J., and Vogt, P. K., eds. (1991). Retroviral insertions and oncogene activation. *Curr. Top. Microbiol. Immunol.* **171,** 1.

Weinberg, R. A. (1991). Tumor suppressor genes. *Science* **254,** 1138.

zur Hausen, H. (1991). Viruses in human cancers. *Science* **254,** 1167.

CHAPTER 12

Laboratory Diagnosis of Viral Diseases

Tests for the specific diagnosis of a viral infection in an animal are of two general types: (1) those that demonstrate the presence of infectious virus, viral antigen(s), or viral gene sequences and (2) those that demonstrate the presence of specific viral antibody. The provision, by a single laboratory, of a comprehensive service for the diagnosis of viral infections of domestic animals is a formidable undertaking. Over 200 individual viruses, belonging to some 20 different viral families, cause infections of veterinary significance in the eight major domestic animal species (cattle, sheep, goat, swine, horse, dog, cat, and chicken). If antigenic types are considered, and if the number of animal species is broadened to include turkey, duck, laboratory animals, and wildlife, then the number of known viruses exceeds 1000. If is therefore not surprising that no single laboratory could have available the necessary specific reagents, nor the skills and experience, for the identification of such a large number of viruses. For this reason, veterinary diagnostic laboratories tend to specialize, for example, in diseases of food animals, companion animals, poultry, or "exotic" viruses. Within these specialized laboratories there is considerable scope for the development of rapid diagnostic methods that short-circuit the need for the isolation and identification of viruses, which is expensive, time-consuming, and rarely necessary.

Over the past few years there have been major advances in viral diagnosis based on nucleic acid hybridization techniques, whereby viral nucleic acid present in a sample is detected by use of an appropriate probe, either directly or following amplification by the polymerase chain reaction (PCR). It is theoretically possible for a single laboratory with access to a complete panel of oligonucleotide primers to use the PCR to provide a comprehensive diagnostic service within 24 hours from sample submission, and it is probable that such services will develop rapidly. There have also been great changes in techniques commonly used for the detection of antibodies in animals that have recovered from viral infections, namely, the replacement of a variety of methods such as virus neutralization, complement fixation, and immunofluorescence by enzyme-linked immunosorbent assays (ELISA), which can be done speedily by automated techniques. In response to the development and refinement of these techniques, manufacturers have produced efficient and reliable test kits for use by laboratories for large-scale testing or by practicing veterinarians on individual animals.

RATIONALE FOR SPECIFIC DIAGNOSIS

Many viral diseases can be diagnosed clinically and others with the assistance of the pathologist, but there are several circumstances under which laboratory confirmation of the specific virus involved is desirable or, indeed, essential.

Exotic Diseases. The industrialized countries of Europe, North America, Australasia, and Japan are free of many devastating diseases of livestock that are still endemic in other parts of the world, such as foot-and-mouth disease, African swine fever, rinderpest, and fowl plague. Clearly it is of the utmost importance that the clinical diagnosis of a suspected exotic virus should be confirmed quickly and accurately (see Chapter 15). All industrialized countries maintain or share the use of specialized biocontainment laboratories devoted to diagnosis and research on such "exotic" viruses.

Zoonoses. Several viral diseases such as rabies, Rift Valley fever, and Eastern, Western, and Venezulean equine encephalitis, are zoonotic and are of sufficient human public health significance as to require the maintenance of specialized diagnostic laboratories. For example, confirmation of the diagnosis of rabies in a skunk that has bitten a child provides the basis for postexposure treatment. Confirmation and early warning of an equine encephalitis virus epidemic allow implementation of mosquito control and other measures such as restriction of the movement of horses.

Certification of Freedom from Specific Infections. For diseases in which there is lifelong infection, such as bovine and feline leukemia, equine infectious anemia, and herpesvirus infections, a negative test certificate is often required as a condition of sale, particularly export sale, for exhibition at a state fair or show, or for competition, as at race meetings.

Artificial Insemination, Embryo Transfer, and Blood Transfusion. Males used for semen collection and females used in embryo transfer programs, especially in cattle, and blood donors of all species, are usually screened for a range of viral infections to minimize the risk of transmission to recipient animals.

Test and Removal Programs. For retrovirus infections, Marek's disease, pseudorabies, and certain other diseases, it is possible to reduce substantially the incidence of disease or eliminate the causative virus from the herd or flock by test and removal programs. The elimination of pseudorabies from Britain is a recent example. Laboratory diagnosis is essential for the effective implementation of such operations.

Veterinary Health Investigations. Provision of a sound veterinary service in any state or country depends on a knowledge of prevailing viral diseases; hence, epidemiologic studies to determine the prevalence and distribution of particular viral infections are frequently undertaken, usually based on the detection of specific antibody.

Clinical Management Dependent on Precise Diagnosis. Many relatively nonspecific disease syndromes, such as respiratory disease (e.g., kennel cough and shipping fever), diarrhea, and some skin diseases, may be caused by a variety of agents, viral and bacterial. Proper management of individual cases or infected herds or flocks may require specific viral diagnosis.

COLLECTION, PACKAGING, AND TRANSPORT OF SPECIMENS

It requires at least as much effort, and often more, to process a negative specimen as it does one from which virus is isolated or a positive diagnosis made. It is therefore important to maximize the possibility of success;

this depends critically on the knowledge, care, and attention of the veterinarian who collects the specimen (Fig. 12-1). Obviously such a specimen must be taken from the right place and at the right time. The right time is generally as soon as possible after the onset of clinical signs; virus is usually present in maximum amounts at about this time and diminishes, sometimes quite rapidly, in the ensuing days.

The site from which the specimen is collected will be influenced by the clinical signs and a knowledge of the pathogenesis of the suspected disease (Table 12-1). Having collected the appropriate specimen(s), it should be properly labeled and sent to the laboratory, with a history, including the provisional diagnosis. Where ambient temperatures are moderate and transit time to the laboratory is less than 1 day, ice or cold

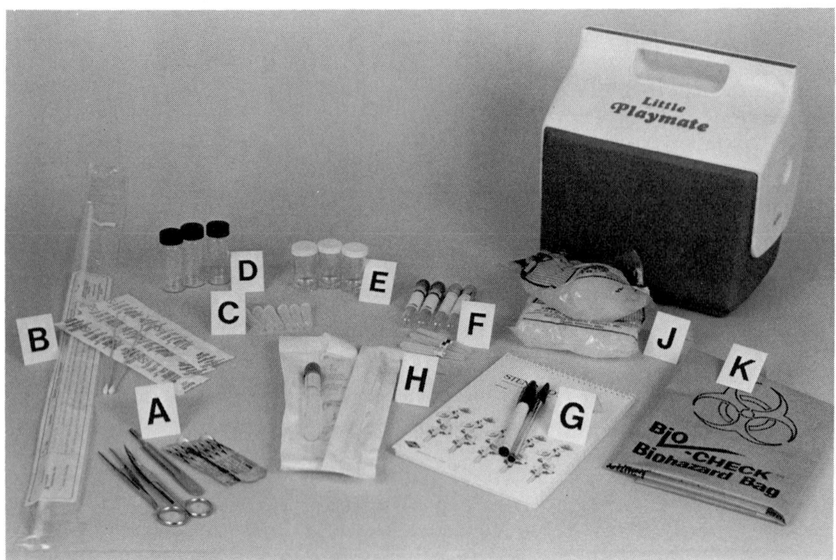

FIG. 12-1. *Equipment required for collection of virus samples. (A) Sterile forceps, scissors, and scalpels. (B) Selection of sterile swabs. (C) Vials containing virus transport medium (with antibiotics) for collection of samples for virus isolation or identification. (D) Bottles for collection of feces, blood, and other samples that do not require virus transport medium. (E) Bottles containing formol saline or Bouin's fixative for tissues to be examined by histology. (F) Blood collection equipment, without additive for serum and with anticoagulant for virus isolation. (G) Notebook and equipment for labeling specimens. (H) Swabs and transport medium for bacteriological investigation. (J) Cool-box. (K) Heavy-duty plastic bags for postmortem material.*

TABLE 12-1

Specimens Appropriate for Laboratory Diagnosis of Various Clinical Syndromes

Syndrome	Specimen
Respiratory	Nasal or throat swab; nasopharyngeal aspirate
Enteric	Feces
Genital	Genital swab
Eye	Conjunctival swab
Skin	Vesicle swab or scraping; biopsy of solid lesion
Central nervous system	Cerebrospinal fluid, feces, nasal swab
Generalized	Nasal swab,[a] Feces,[a] blood leukocytes[a]
Necropsy/biopsy	Relevant organ
Any	Blood for serology[b]

[a] Depending on known or presumed pathogenesis.
[b] Blood allowed to clot, then serum kept for assay of antibody.

packs (4°C) in a Styrofoam box are frequently used. If the environmental temperature is high and transit times longer than 1 day, dry ice (−70°C) may be used, although wet ice with provision to replenish it in transit is better. Styrofoam boxes must be enclosed within sturdy, double-walled containers, in some cases with absorbent padding, according to local regulations. Appropriate permits must be obtained for interstate and international transportation, and in such circumstances the collection and transport arrangements need to be discussed beforehand with the laboratory and/or the appropriate government regulatory agency.

METHODS OF VIRAL DIAGNOSIS

Virus isolation remains the benchmark against which other methods are measured, and it is essential when decisions of major economic importance depend on the diagnosis, for instance, with suspected introduction of exotic diseases such as foot-and-mouth disease or fowl plague. However, the direct demonstration of virions or viral constituents provides more rapid and less expensive diagnosis, particularly when large numbers of samples must be tested. Epidemiologic surveys, eradication programs, and the provision of certificates of freedom from specific infections are usually based on detection of antibodies. The advantages and disadvantages of various diagnostic techniques are outlined in Table 12-2.

TABLE 12-2
Advantages and Disadvantages/Problems of Various Diagnostic Methods

Diagnostic method	Advantages	Disadvantages/problems
Virus isolation	Permits further study of agent; usually highly sensitive; readily available	Slow, time-consuming, can be difficult; useless for nonviable virus; selection of cell type, etc., may be critical
Direct observation by electron microscopy, including immunoelectron microscopy	Rapid; detects viruses that cannot be isolated; detects nonviable virus	Equipment expensive, hence may not be available; relatively insensitive; limited to a few viral infections
Serologic identification of virus or antigen, e.g., ELISA	Rapid and sensitive; provides information on serotypes; readily available, often in diagnostic kits	Not applicable to all viruses; interpretation may be difficult
Nucleic acid probes (with or without gene amplification by PCR)	Rapid; very sensitive, especially after PCR; potentially applicable to all viruses	May not be readily available; risk of DNA contamination in PCR
Recognition of cellular pathology by light microscopy	Rapid; readily available	Limited to a few viral infections
Antibody conversion (acute and convalescent sera)	Useful in relating cases to a disease outbreak	Slow, late (retrospective); interpretation may be difficult

DIRECT IDENTIFICATION OF VIRUS, VIRAL ANTIGEN, OR VIRAL NUCLEIC ACID

A wide selection of techniques is available for the detection of virus, viral antigen, or viral nucleic acid. Several even fulfill the five criteria for acceptance in the small clinical laboratories of a veterinary practice (speed, simplicity, sensitivity, specificity, and cost) and, as mentioned earlier, are readily available in kits from several manufacturers. Most of these kits are based on an ELISA.

We use the term direct identification, in contrast to virus isolation, to encompass a variety of methods that can be used to detect and often identify the etiological agent by the direct demonstration of virions, viral antigens, or viral nucleic acids in the tissues, secretions, or excretions of infected animals. Although these methods do not provide the laboratory worker with a culture of the causative virus for further study, if the original samples are held at a low temperature they can be used later for virus isolation, if necessary.

Detection of Virions by Electron Microscopy

The introduction of negative staining procedures, together with a realization that in many clinical situations the concentration of virions frequently exceeds the critical lower limit of 10^6 per milliliter required for visualization in the electron microscope, has led to the use of this instrument for rapid viral diagnosis (Fig. 12-2). The procedure is particularly suited to enteric infections, in which a crude fecal suspension can be clarified by low-speed centrifugation, followed by high-speed centrifugation to yield a pellet for negative staining. In addition to its value in the recognition of known viruses, this technique has led to the discovery in diarrheal diseases of new viruses of etiological importance which were, and in some cases remain, uncultivatable (e.g., some adenoviruses, astroviruses, caliciviruses, coronaviruses, parvoviruses, and rotaviruses).

The procedure is also suited to viral infections of the skin and mucous membranes, the appropriate specimens being scabs, vesicular fluid, or scrapings made with a scalpel blade. Electron microscopy can be used for the rapid identification of viruses isolated in cell culture, allowing immediate and definitive diagnosis to the family or sometimes the genus or species level.

The sensitivity of electron microscopic methods can be enhanced by the use of immune serum, by a procedure known as immunoelectron microscopy. The sample, usually clarified by low-speed centrifugation, is mixed with antibody, and, after overnight interaction, the immune complexes are pelleted by low-speed centrifugation and the pellet negatively stained. The antibody used may be serum from an old animal hyperimmune to a large number of viruses, or it may be type-specific polyclonal or monoclonal antibody, or such antibodies may be used sequentially. To improve visualization, the antibody may be labeled with gold. Solid-phase immunoelectron microscopy procedures have also been developed, in which virus-specific antibody is first bound to the plastic supporting film on the copper grid. Sensitivity is enhanced by a double-layering procedure, in which staphylococcal protein A (which binds the Fc moiety of IgG) is bound to the film, then virus-specific antibody, then the sample.

Detection of Viral Antigen(s)

Detection of viral antigen is based on direct interaction between virions or viral antigens, *in situ* in tissues or in excretions or secretions, and

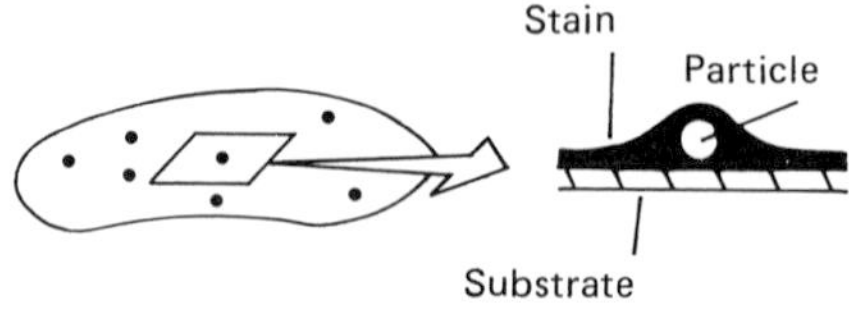

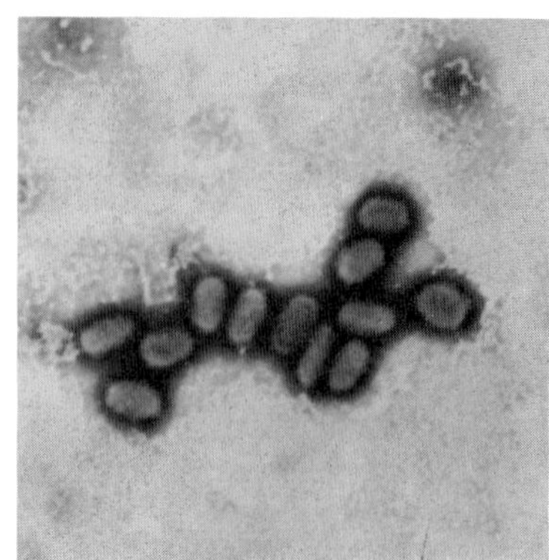

A

Antigen (virus) reacted with antibody (serum)

Virus particles

Negatively stained

Antibody

B

FIG. 12-2. *Negative staining for electron microscopy. (A) Direct staining of virions of bovine papular stomatitis virus. A suspension of the scraping was made in distilled water and a drop added to a plastic (Formvar)-coated copper grid. After 5 minutes the excess fluid was removed by touching filter paper to the edge of the grid. A drop of an electron-opaque stain (1% phosphotungstic acid) was added to the grid, and after 5 minutes the excess stain was removed. After drying the film was ready for examination. Magnification: ×13,000. (B) Immunoelectron microscopy. An isolate of foot-and-mouth disease virus type O was incubated with homotypic antiserum and stained with phosphotungstic acid. Magnification: ×100,000. [From E. P. J. Gibbs* et al., Vet. Rec. **106,** *451, (1980).]*

specific antibodies which are prelabeled in some way so as to permit the ready recognition of the interaction. The methods are specified by the type of labeling used: enzyme-linked immunosorbent assay (ELISA), radioimmunoassay, immunofluorescence, or immunoperoxidase staining. Viral antigens can also be detected by such time-honored serologic procedures as precipitation and complement fixation.

Enzyme-Linked Immunosorbent Assays. The ELISA [also known as enzyme immunoassay (EIA)] has revolutionized diagnostic virology. The ELISA is extremely sensitive and can be designed in different formats to detect antigen or antibody. A variety of direct, indirect, and reversed assays have been described; most involve a solid-phase ELISA, in which the "capture" antibody is attached (by simple adsorption or by covalent bonding) to a solid substrate, typically the wells of polystyrene or polyvinyl microtiter plates, thus facilitating washing steps. The simplest format is the direct ELISA (Fig. 12-3, left). Virus and soluble viral antigens from the specimen are allowed to absorb to the capture antibody. After unbound antigen has been washed away, an enzyme-labled antiviral antibody (the "detector" antibody) is added. Various enzymes can be linked to antibody; horseradish peroxidase and alkaline phosphatase are the most commonly used. After a final washing step, readout is based on the color change that follows addition of an appropriate organic substrate for the particular enzyme. The colored product of the action of the enzyme on the substrate should be clearly recognizable by eye. The test can be made quantitative by serially diluting the antigen to obtain an end point or by using spectrophotometry to measure the amount of enzyme-conjugated antibody bound to the captured antigen.

A further refinement takes advantage of the very high binding affinity of avidin for biotin. The antibody is conjugated to biotin, a reagent of

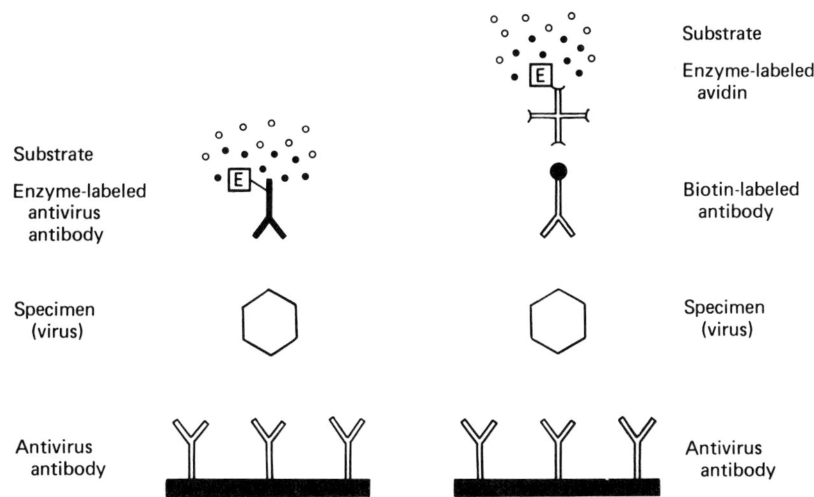

FIG. 12-3. *Enzyme-linked immunosorbent assay (ELISA) for detection of virus and/or viral antigen.* Left: *Direct;* right: *avidin–biotin.*

low M_r which gives reproducible binding and does not alter antigen-binding capacity. The antigen–antibody complex is recognized with high sensitivity simply by adding avidin-labeled enzyme, then substrate (Fig. 12-3, right). Subsequent modifications have been aimed at increasing sensitivity even further; for example, high-energy substrates can be used that release fluorescent, chemiluminescent, or radioactive products that can be identified in very small amounts.

Indirect immunoassays are widely used because of their somewhat greater sensitivity and avoidance of the need to label each antiviral antibody. Here, the detector antibody is unlabeled and a further layer of labeled (species-specific) anti-immunoglobulin is added as the "indicator" antibody; of course, the antiviral antibodies constituting the capture and detector antibodies must be raised in different animal species (Fig. 12-4, right). Alternatively, labeled staphylococcal protein A, which binds to the Fc moiety of IgG of most mammalian species, can be used as the indicator in indirect immunoassays.

Increasingly, monoclonal antiviral antibodies (MAbs) are being used as capture and/or detector antibodies in ELISA. It is important to select MAbs of high affinity but not of such high specificity that some strains of the virus sought might be missed in the assay. Indeed, the specificity of the assay can be predetermined by selecting MAb directed at an epitope that is either confined to a particular viral serotype or common to all serotypes within a species of genus.

ELISA procedures have been developed for a wide variety of applica-

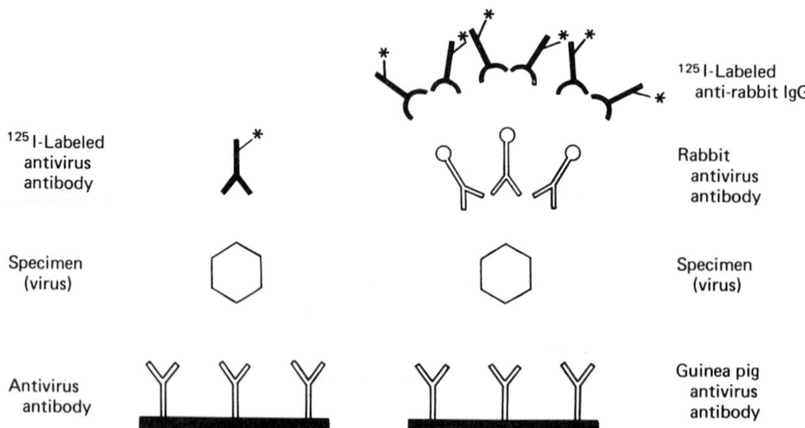

FIG. 12-4. *Radioimmunoassays for detection of virus and/or viral antigen.* Left: *Direct;* right: *indirect.*

tions in veterinary medicine. At one level, kits have been marketed for the rapid disgnosis of a number of important viral diseases for use by veterinary practitioners themselves. At another level, the assays have been automated by the introduction of automatic dispensing, washing, and spectrophotometric reading and recording instruments, which permit hundreds of samples to be processed in 1 day.

Radioimmunoassay. Radioimmunassay (RIA) predates ELISA but is being progressively superseded by it. The only significant difference is that the label is not an enzyme but a radioactive isotope such as ^{125}I, and the bound antibody is measured in a gamma counter (Fig. 12-4). Radioimmunoassay is a highly sensitive and reliable assay that lends itself well to automation, but the cost of equipment and the health hazard of working with radioisotopes are disadvantages.

Immunofluorescence. Its specificity, sensitivity, rapidity, and relative simplicity has made immunofluorescence a procedure of singular importance in the rapid diagnosis of viral infections. The prototypic example of immunofluorescence is the diagnosis of rabies (Fig. 12-5), for which it

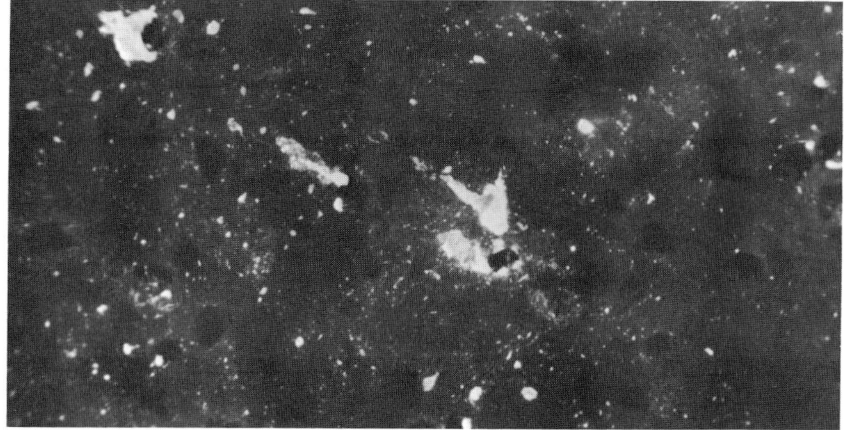

FIG. 12-5. *Immunofluorescence of cells infected with rabies virus. Tissue impressions are made from the medulla, cerebellum, and hippocampus of the suspect animal by lightly touching tissues to microscope slides. After staining, the slide is examined with a microscope that is set for observing the fluorescent emission of fluorescein isothiocyanate. Rabies antigen, identified by its specific apple-green fluorescence, may appear as dustlike particles or as large masses, equivalent to Negri bodies in histologic sections. The immunofluorescence technique has a 97–98% correlation with virus isolation techniques, which are very slow and cumbersome.*

has been the standard teste for more than 20 years. It is now being used for a wide range of viruses. Immunofluorescence can be applied to cultured cells, smears, or frozen sections of tissues or organs.

Two alternative staining procedures are used: (1) direct immunofluorescence, in which the antiviral antibody is conjugated to the fluorescent dye, fluorescein, and (2) indirect ("sandwich") immunofluorescence, in which an anti-immunoglobin specific for the animal species providing the antiviral antibody is conjugated to fluorescein (Fig. 12-6). For instance, an acetone-fixed smear or frozen tissue section is treated with virus-specific antibody (prepared, say, in rabbits), then rinsed before the second antibody, a fluorescein-conjugated anti-rabbit immunoglobulin made in goats, is added. Indirect procedures have two significant advantages over direct staining procedures: (1) if antibodies to different viruses are raised in a single animal species, for example, rabbits, then only a single conjugated antibody is required, and (2) the amount of bound labeled antibody is greatly augmented, hence the method is much more sensitive. Although simple in principle, the effective use of immunofluorescence demands careful attention to many technical details if false-positive results are to be avoided.

Immunoperoxidase Staining. An alternative method for locating and identifying viral antigen in infected cells employs an enzyme-labeled antibody. The procedure requires less expensive equipment than immunofluorescence (an ordinary light microscope is used) and produces a morphologically clearer, nonfading, permanent preparation. The procedures and principles are similar to those of immunofluorescence. The conjugated antibody, bound to antigen by a direct or indirect procedure, is detected by adding a substrate appropriate to the particular enzyme; in the case of peroxidase this is H_2O_2 mixed with a benzidine derivative which forms a colored, insoluble precipitate in the presence of enzyme. A disadvantage of the technique is that endogenous peroxidase present in the cells of many tissues, particularly leukocytes, produces false-positive results. This problem can be circumvented by adequate controls and experience.

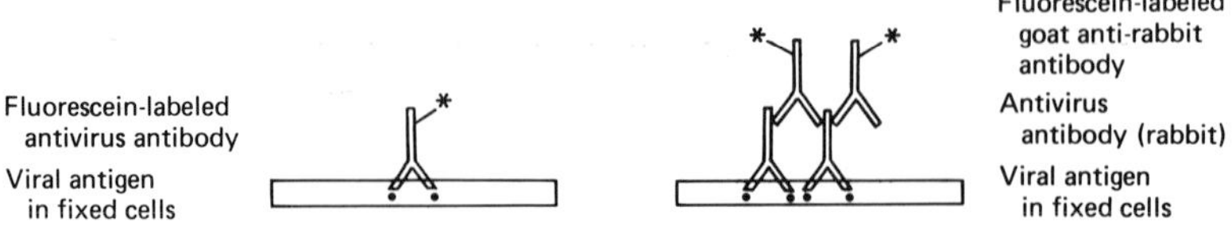

FIG. 12-6. *Immunofluorescence.* Left: *Direct;* right: *indirect.*

Detection of Viral Nucleic Acid

The detection of specific viral nucleic acid by hybridization to a labeled nucleic acid probe is being increasingly used as a preferred means of rapid diagnosis. If the specimen contains insufficient nucleic acid molecules for detection, the polymerase chain reaction may be used to amplify the copy number prior to probing by hybridization.

The principle of nucleic acid hybridization is that ssDNA will hybridize by hydrogen-bonded base pairing to another strand of DNA (or RNA) of complementary base sequence. The two strands of the target DNA molecule are first separated by boiling, then following cooling are allowed to hybridize with a ssDNA or ssRNA probe present in excess. The reaction can be accomplished in solution, and the percentage homology between the two sequences calculated from the kinetics of annealing. The conditions set for annealing, especially temperature and ionic strength, determine the degree of discrimination of the test. Under conditions of low stringency a number of mismatched base pairs are tolerated, whereas at high stringency such a heteroduplex is unstable.

The other major factor determining the specificity of the test is the nature of the probe itself, which may correspond in length with the whole viral genome, or a single gene, or a much shorter nucleotide sequence deliberately chosen to represent either a variable or a conserved sequence of the genome, depending on whether it is intended that the probe be type-specific or more versatile. The oligonucleotide sequence intended as a probe may be produced by chemical synthesis or by cloning in a bacterial plasmid or bacteriophage.

Traditionally, radioactive isotopes such as ^{32}P or ^{35}S have been used to label nucleic acids or oligonucleotides intended as probes for hybridization tests, the signal being read by counting or autoradiography. The trend is now toward nonradioactive labels. Some of these, such as fluorescein and peroxidase, produce a signal directly, whereas others, such as biotin and digoxigenin, act indirectly by binding to another labeled compound which then emits the signal. Biotinylated probes can be combined with various types of readout (e.g., an avidin-based ELISA).

Dot-Blot Hybridization. Most of the nucleic acid hybridization methods used today are two-phase systems, generically known as filter hybridization. In its simplest format, dot (blot) hybridization, DNA or RNA extracted from virus or infected cells is denatured, then spotted directly onto a charged nylon or nitrocellulose membrane filter to which it binds tightly on baking. The single-stranded DNA or RNA probe is then hybridized to the target nucleic acid *in situ* on the membrane, and unbound probe is washed away. The signal generated by the bound probe is measured by autoradiography if the probe is radioactive, or by the formation of a colored precipitate if an enzyme is used. Sensitivity can be improved by using RNA as a probe and the incidence of false positives reduced by treating the filters with RNase before counting.

***In Situ* Hybridization.** The probe may be used to detect the presence of viral nucleic acid in frozen sections of infected cells, the intracellular location of viral sequences being revealed by autoradiography or immunoperoxidase cytochemistry.

Southern Blot Hybridization. The introduction of *Southern blotting* introduced a higher level of sophistication. Restriction endonucleases are used to cleave the DNA into shorter oligonucleotides which are then separated by electrophoresis on agarose or acrylamide gels before alkali denaturation and transfer ("blotting") onto nylon or nitrocellulose membrane filters, where the individual bands are revealed by autoradiography or a color development process. *Northern blotting* of RNA follows similar principles but is generally not as sensitive.

Polymerase Chain Reaction

The polymerase chain reaction (PCR) (Fig. 12-7) probably constitutes the greatest advance in molecular biology since the advent of recombinant DNA technology. It enables a single copy of any gene sequence to be amplified 1 millionfold within a few hours. Thus viral DNA extracted from a small number of virions or infected cells may be amplified to the point where it can be readily identified using labeled probes in a hybridization assay. The method may be modified for the detection of viral RNA by incorporating a preliminary step in which reverse transcriptase converts the RNA to DNA. For diagnostic purposes it is not necessary or usual to amplify the whole genome, but it is necessary to know at least part of the nucleotide sequence in order to synthesize two oligonucleotide primers representing the extremities of the region to be amplified.

There are three steps in the process: (1) melting the target DNA, (2) binding of two oligonucleotide primers that have different sequences which lie on opposite strands of the template DNA and flank the segment of DNA that is to be amplified, and (3) extension from the oligonucleotide primers by DNA polymerase to form two DNA strands that are identical copies of the original target strands, namely, the DNA located between and including the two primers. The cycle of melting, primer binding, and primer extension is repeated many times, and the number of DNA copies increases exponentially. Thus after 30 cycles the number of DNA copies, beginning with a single copy of the target sequence, is about 1

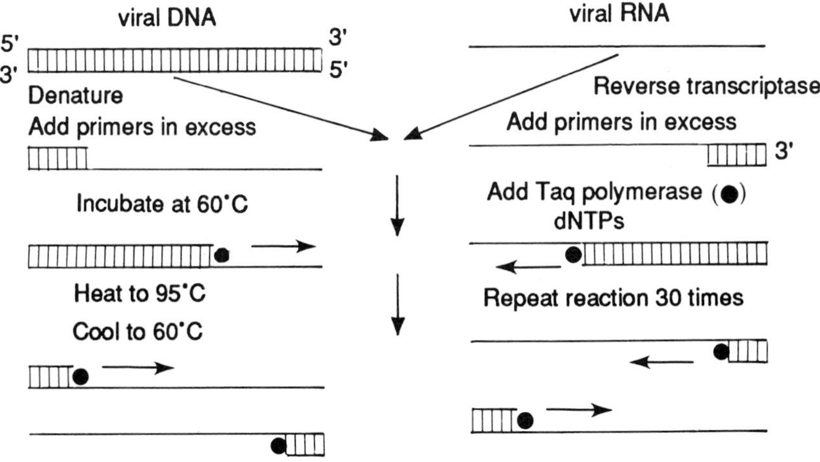

Result: one millionfold amplification

FIG. 12-7. *The polymerase chain reaction (PCR) for DNA amplification can be applied to viral DNA or viral RNA. Taq polymerase, a heat-resistant polymerase from* Thermus aquaticus, *is used to extend primers between two fixed points on a DNA molecule. All the components for chain elongation are heat-stable, so that multiple heating and cooling cycles result in alternate DNA synthesis and melting. DNA between the recognition sites of the two oligonucleotide primers accumulates exponentially.*

million. In the early cycles longer DNA strands are made, but these constitute less than 1% of the final product, which is predominantly the sequence between and including the two primers. The cycling process, which involves alternately heating the reaction mixture to 95°C followed by cooling to 50°–60°C (depending on the base composition of the primer), continues efficiently as the result of using the heat-stable DNA polymerase (Taq) of *Thermus aquaticus*, an organism naturally found in hot springs. Using a suitable automated thermal cycling device, 30 cycles can be completed within 4 hours. The amplified DNA may be detected by agarose gel electrophoresis either with or without restriction endonuclease digestion, or by probing.

Selection of the most suitable pair of primers is a matter of central importance. The primers may be chosen to be broadly reactive or to be highly specific for a particular virus strain. Reactions must be carried out under carefully controlled conditions of ionic strength, temperature, and primer and nucleotide concentration. Deviations can result in nonspecific amplification. Contamination of samples with extraneous DNA has been a serious problem in making the transition of PCR from a research tool to a routine diagnostic method, and great care is required to avoid such contamination. The most common cause of false positives is "carryover" of DNA sequences amplified in previous reactions, which may be present on laboratory equipment as well as in reagents. Methods have now been developed to overcome this problem, such as inclusion of a special wax plug in the top of the reaction tube to prevent cross-contamination after the reagents have been added.

A recently developed modification of the PCR, called isothermal amplification, eliminates the need for temperature cycling. Three enzymes involved in the replication of retroviruses are mixed with either a DNA or RNA template and DNA primers at a constant temperature, and 1 millionfold amplification is rapidly achieved.

The PCR has so enhanced the sensitivity and versatility of nucleic acid hybridization that probing for the vital genome may soon overtake probing for antigen as the method of choice in diagnostic laboratories. Even now, the procedure is invaluable when one is confronted with viruses that cannot be cultured readily, specimens that contain predominantly inactivated virus (as a result of prolonged storage or transport), or latent infections.

VIRUS ISOLATION

Despite the explosion of new techniques for rapid diagnosis of viral diseases that have just been described, virus isolation remains the "gold standard" against which newer methods must be compared. Further, it is the only method that can detect the unexpected, by identifying an unforeseen virus, or even discover a totally new agent. Accordingly, even laboratories well equipped for rapid diagnosis sometimes also inoculate cell cultures in an attempt to isolate the virus, even though isolation and identification of viruses from clinical specimens may require a week or more, and is expensive. In research and reference laboratories, in particular, viral isolation is essential to provide material for further study.

Preparation of Specimen for Inoculation. The sooner the specimen is processed and inoculated after arrival at the laboratory, the better. If delays of more than 1 day are anticipated, the specimen may be frozen to −70°C. Swabs are processed by twirling them in the transport medium and expressing the fluid by pushing the swab firmly against the side of the container. Feces are dispersed on a vortex mixer. Tissue specimens are finely minced with a pair of scissors and homogenized in a glass or mechanical homogenizer. Prior to inoculation, contaminating bacteria and molds are removed by filtering through membrane filters of average pore diameter 0.45 μm, although such filters allow the passage of mycoplasmas. Some of the original sample and some of the filtrate should be retained at 4°C or frozen until the isolation attempt is finalized. Virus can be grown from the suitably prepared specimen by inoculation into cell cultures, laboratory animals, or the species of host animal from which the specimen was obtained. By far the most widely used substrate is cultured cells.

Growth of Virus in Cultured Cells

Choice of Cultured Cells. The choice of the optimal cell culture for the primary isolation of a virus of unknown nature from clinical specimens is largely empirical. Primary or low-passage, homologous, monolayer cell cultures derived from fetal tissues usually provide the most sensitive substrate for isolation of the greatest variety of different viruses. Continuous cell lines derived from the homologous species are in most cases almost as good. Often the nature of the disease from which the material was obtained will suggest what virus may be found, and in such cases the optimum cell culture for that virus can be chosen, often in parallel with a second type of culture with a wide spectrum. Cell lines offer some advantages and are available for most domestic mammals.

Special types of cultures are utilized for particular viruses. For example, betaherpesviruses and gammaherpesviruses may be recovered from monolayer cultures propagated directly from tissues taken from the diseased animal, whereas inoculation of established monolayer cell cultures with cell-free material may be negative. For some coronaviruses and rhinoviruses that do not grow well in monolayer cultures, growth may occur in explant cultures (i.e., small cubes of tissue from the trachea or gut).

Recognition of Viral Growth. Cultures are usually incubated at 35°–37°C and are observed daily for cytopathic effects. The speed and nature of the cytopathic effect caused by different viruses vary considerably. Cytopathic effect must always be based on comparison with mock-inoculated cell cultures; this is particularly important for viruses requiring incubation periods longer than 1 week. Where none or a doubtful cytopathic effect is observed, it is usual to make a second or even a third ("blind") passage.

The speed and appearance of the cytopathic effect, coupled with the case history, may immediately suggest the diagnosis. Infected monolayers on glass coverslips or special slide/culture chambers may be fixed and appropriately stained, and the cells examined for inclusion bodies, syncytia, or other characteristic cell changes. Better, they may be stained with fluorescent antibody, which may provide an immediate, definitive diagnosis. Some viruses are relatively noncytopathogenic (see Chapter 5). In this case viruses such as orthomyxoviruses or paramyxoviruses in cell culture may sometimes be recognized by means of hemadsorption (see Fig. 5-2).

Growth of Virus in Laboratory Animals

Nowadays laboratory animals such as baby mice are little used for viral isolation. Intraamniotic inoculation of the developing chick embryo provides the most sensitive method for the isolation of influenza viruses and for several other avian viruses, and identification of orthopoxviruses can be done directly from the type of pock produced on the chick embryo chorioallantoic membrane. The natural host species, especially antibody-free susceptible young animals (e.g., calves, piglets, or chicks), can be used for the isolation of a virus not yet cultivatable *in vitro*, but this approach tends to be restricted to situations where there might be serious repercussions if the diagnosis were missed. Of course, the natural host is often used for research studies, for example, of pathogenesis, or for vaccine trials.

Identification of Viral Isolates

A newly isolated virus can usually be provisionally allocated to a particular family, and sometimes to a genus or species, on the basis of the clinical findings, the type of cell yielding the virus isolate, and the visible result of viral growth (cytopathic effect, hemadsorption, electron microscopy, etc.). Definitive identification, however, usually depends on antigen characterization with known antisera, using techniques similar to those for direct identification of virus in clinical material. Having allocated it to a particular family (e.g., *Adenoviridae*) with, say, an ELISA, one can then go on to determine the species or serotype (e.g., canine adenovirus) by a more discriminating procedure such as the virus neutralization test. This sequential approach is applicable only to families or genera with a common family/genus antigen.

The range of available immunologic techniques is now extremely wide (Table 12-3). Some are best suited to particular families of viruses. Each laboratory makes its own choice of favored procedures, based on considerations such as sensitivity, specificity, reproducibility, speed, convenience, and cost. Currently most immunologic procedures are carried out with "hyperimmune" sera comprising a polyclonal mixture of antibodies, sometimes after they have been absorbed to eliminate antibodies of certain specificities.

Monoclonal antibodies with defined specificity are now becoming

TABLE 12-3
Principal Serologic Procedures Used in Virology

Technique	Principle
Enzyme immunoassay (ELISA)	Antibody binds to antigen; enzyme-labeled anti-IgG binds to antibody; substrate changes color
Radioimmunoassay	Antibody binds to antigen; radiolabeled anti-IgG binds to antibody and can be counted
Western blot	Virus disrupted, proteins separated by polyacrylamide gel electrophoresis, transferred (blotted) onto nylon membrane; antiserum binds to viral proteins; labeled anti-IgG binds to particular bands; revealed by ELISA or autoradiography
Virus neutralization	Antibody neutralizes infectivity of virion; inhibits cytopathology, reduces plaques, or protects animals
Hemagglutination inhibition	Antibody inhibits viral hemagglutination
Immunofluorescence	Antibody binds to antigen in fixed cells; fluorescein-labeled anti-IgG binds; fluoresces by UV microscopy
Immunodiffusion	Antibodies and soluble antigens produce visible lines of precipitate in a gel

available. These reagents make it possible to proceed quickly to very specific diagnosis even to the level of subtypes, strains, or variants, for example, rabies viruses from different geographic areas. Family-, genus-, and type-specific monoclonal antibodies are also being developed. As the properties of MAbs are defined and they become commercially available, we can expect them to be widely used for most methods of immunologic identification.

Hemagglutination and Hemagglutination Inhibition. Virions of several viral families bind to red blood cells and cause hemagglutination. If specific antibody and virus are mixed prior to the addition of red blood cells, hemagglutination is inhibited (Fig. 12-8). The hemagglutination–inhibition test is sensitive and, except in the case of the togaviruses, highly specific, since it measures antibodies binding to the surface protein most subject to antigenic change. Moreover, it is simple, inexpensive, and rapid, and is therefore the serologic procedure of choice for identifying isolates of hemagglutinating viruses.

Virus Neutralization. After first "inactivating" the serum by heating at 56°C for 30 minutes, to inactivate complement and possibly nonspecific virus inhibitors, serum–virus mixtures are inoculated into appropriate cell cultures which are then incubated until the "virus only" controls develop cytopathology (Fig. 12-9). Antibody, by neutralizing the infec-

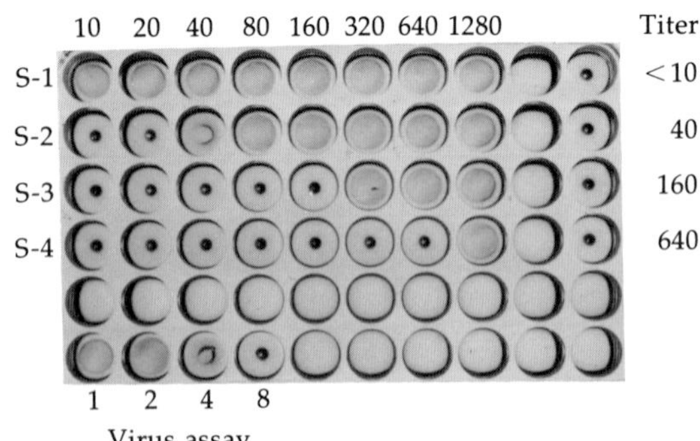

FIG. 12-8. *Hemagglutination–inhibition test, used for titrating antibodies to the influenza virus hemagglutinin. In the example illustrated, a horse was immunized against the prevalent strain of influenza virus. Serum samples S-1, S-2, S-3, and S-4 were taken, respectively, before immunization, 1 and 4 weeks after the first vaccine dose, and 4 weeks after the second. The sera were treated with periodate and heated at 56°C for 30 minutes to inactivate nonspecific inhibitors of hemagglutination, then diluted in wells of a multiwell plate in twofold steps from 1/10 to 1/1280. Each well then received 4 hemagglutinating (HA) units of the relevant strain of influenza virus. After incubation at room temperature for 30 minutes, 50 μl of a 0.5% suspension of red blood cells was added to each well. Where enough antibody is present to complex the virions, hemagglutination is inhibited, hence the erythrocytes settle to form a button on the bottom of the well. On the other hand, where insufficient antibody is present, erythrocytes are agglutinated by virus and form a mat. The virus titration (bottom row) indicates that the dilution of virus used gave partial agglutination (the end point) when diluted 1/4, in other words, that about 4 hemagglutinating units of virus was used in the assay.* ***Interpretation:*** *The horse originally had no hemagglutinin-inhibiting antibodies against the particular strain of influenza virus (top row). One dose of vaccine produced an antibody (titer 1/20); the second injection boosted the response to a titer of 1/640. (Courtesy I. Jack.)*

tivity of the virus, protects the cells against viral destruction. In keeping with the general trend toward miniaturization, neutralization tests are now usually conducted in disposable, nontoxic, sterile, plastic trays with 96 flat-bottomed wells in each of which a cell monolayer can be established.

Oligonucleotide Fingerprinting and Restriction Endonuclease Mapping

For most routine diagnostic purposes it is usually not necessary to "type" the isolate. Sometimes, however, important epidemiologic information can be obtained by going even further, to identify differences between subtypes within a given type. This may be accomplished using the PCR with appropriate primers, or by oligonucleotide fingerprinting of viral RNA or the determination of restriction endonuclease fragment

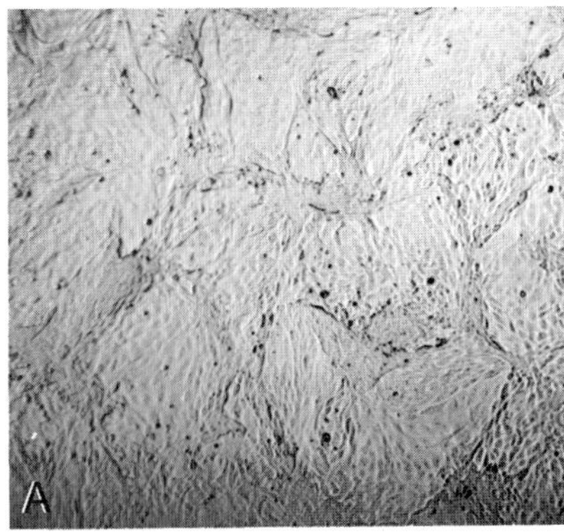

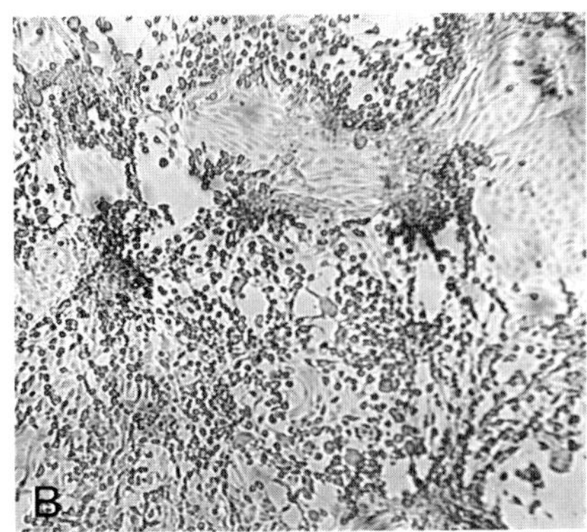

FIG. 12-9. *Virus neutralization test. A pig developed encephalitis during an epidemic of porcine enterovirus 1 infection. An enterovirus was isolated from the feces. One hundred tissue culture ID_{50} of this virus was incubated at 37°C for 60 minutes with a suitable dilution of "inactivated" (56°C, 30 minutes) porcine enterovirus 1 antiserum (a reference serum raised in a rabbit). The mixtures were inoculated onto a monolayer of swine kidney cells in the wells of a microculture tray (A). Virus similarly incubated with normal rabbit serum was inoculated into well B. The cultures were incubated at 37°C for several days and inspected daily for cytopathic effect. Unstained; magnification: ×23. (Courtesy I. Jack.)* ***Interpretation:*** *The infectivity of the virus isolate has been neutralized by the antiserum, thereby identifying the isolate as porcine enterovirus 1; the control culture (B) shows the typical cytopathic effect.*

patterns of viral DNA. An example of the use of oligonucleotide fingerprinting of viral RNA to trace the origin and spread of foot-and-mouth disease virus in Europe in 1981 is described in Chapter 22.

Viral DNA prepared from virions or infected cells can be cut with appropriately chosen restriction endonucleases and the fragments separated by agarose gel electrophoresis. When stained with ethidium bromide or silver, restriction endonuclease fragment patterns ("restriction maps") are obtained. The method has found application with all DNA virus families, particularly in epidemiologic studies. Depending on the viral family, the resolution of these methods is such that different isolates of the same virus are distinguishable. Minor degrees of genetic drift, often not reflected in serologic differences, can sometimes be detected in this way.

Interpretation

The isolation and identification of a particular virus from an animal with a given disease is not necessarily meaningful in itself. Concurrent subclinical infection with a virus unrelated to the illness in question is not uncommon. Koch's postulates are as applicable here as in any other microbiological context, but they are not always easy to fulfill. In attempting to interpret the significance of any virus isolation one must be guided by the following considerations. (1) The site from which the virus was isolated must be kept in mind. For example, one would be quite confident about the etiological significance of equine herpesvirus 1 isolated from the tissues of a 9-month-old aborted equine fetus with typical gross and microscopic lesions. On the other hand, recovery of an enterovirus from the feces or a herpesvirus from a nasal or throat swab may not necessarily be significant, because such viruses are often associated with inapparent infections at these sites. (2) Interpretation of the significance of the isolation in such instances will be facilitated by recovery of the same virus from several cases of the same illness during an epidemic. (3) Knowledge that the virus and the disease in question are often causally associated provides confidence that the isolate is significant.

MEASUREMENT OF SERUM ANTIBODIES

We discussed earlier the use of panels of antibodies of known specificity to identify viruses or their antigens. Serologic methods can be used the other way round, to identify antibody using panels of known antigens, either in individual animals or in populations. Such techniques are particularly useful in the latter context, since serum samples are readily obtained, in contrast to the special requirements, time, and effort needed for collecting samples for detection of virus, viral antigen, or viral nucleic acid. Furthermore, tests to detect and quantify antibody, such as the ELISA, lend themselves to automation, so that large numbers of samples can be tested; they form the basis of epidemiologic surveys and of control and eradication programs.

For diagnosis in the individual animal, paired sera are tested for specific viral antibody: the first sample is taken when the animal is initially examined (acute phase serum) and the second sample 2–4 weeks later (convalescent phase serum). A rise in antibody titer between first and second samples is a basis, albeit in retrospect, for a specific viral diagnosis; in some diseases, such as Eastern equine encephalitis, a significant rise can occur within 48 hours of the onset of clinical signs. Sometimes the demonstration of antibody in a single serum sample is diagnostic of current infection, for instance, with retroviruses and herpesviruses, since these viruses establish lifelong infections. However, in such circumstances there is no assurance that the persistent virus was responsible for the disease under consideration.

Detection of antiviral antibody in presuckle newborn cord or venous blood provides a basis for specific diagnosis of *in utero* infections. It was used, for example, in showing that Akabane virus was the cause of arthrogryposis–hydranencephaly in calves. Since transplacental transfer of immunoglobulins is rare in domestic animals (see Table 8-4), the presence of either IgG or IgM is indicative of exposure of the fetus to antigen.

Serologic methods based on the detection of IgM may also be used for the specific diagnosis of recent viral infection, since IgM appears first after primary infection and declines to relatively low levels, compared to IgG, by about 3 months after infection.

Immunoblotting (Western Blot). *Western blot* analysis (immunoblotting) can be used for the simultaneous detection of antibodies against several proteins of a particular virus. First, purified virus is solubilized with the anionic detergent sodium dodecyl sulfate (SDS) and the constituent proteins separated into discrete bands according to M_r by polyacrylamide gel electrophoresis (SDS-PAGE). Next, the separated proteins are electrophoretically transferred ("blotted") onto a nitrocellulose membrane. Finally, the test serum is allowed to bind to the viral proteins on the membrane, and their presence is demonstrated by using a radiolabeled or enzyme-labeled anti-species antibody. Thus immunoblotting permits demonstration of antibodies to some or all of the proteins of any given virus and can be used not only to discriminate between infection with closely related viruses sharing certain antigens, but also to monitor the presence of antibodies to different antigens at different stages of infection.

Applications of Serology

Technical advances such as miniaturization (multiwell plates), automation for large numbers of samples, and development of monoclonal antibodies have resulted in a revolution in the approach to diagnostic serology in human medicine, and their use is expanding in veterinary medicine. However, the major application is to test for immunity, especially in the context of epidemiologic surveys or for control or eradication programs (see Chapters 14 and 15).

LABORATORY SAFETY

It is appropriate to conclude this chapter with some remarks about safety precautions in virus diagnostic laboratories in general and regulations about exotic viruses in particular.

Safety of Laboratory Workers

Diagnostic virology is one of the less hazardous human occupations, but over the years many serious infections and a number of deaths have been caused by laboratory-associated infections. It is important to note that many of the procedures that may be dangerous for laboratory workers, particularly aerosolization, may also be sources of laboratory contam-

TABLE 12-4
Summary of Recommended Biosafety Levels for Infectious Agents[a]

Biosafety level	Practices and techniques	Safety equipment	Facilities
1	Standard microbiological practices	None: primary containment provided by adherence to standard laboratory practices during open-bench operations	Basic
2	Level 1 practices, plus laboratory coats, decontamination of all infectious wastes, limited access, protective gloves, and biohazard warning signs as indicated	Partial containment equipment (i.e., class I or II biological safety cabinets) used to conduct mechanical and manipulative procedures that have high aerosol potential which may increase the risk to personnel	Basic
3	Level 2 practices, plus special laboratory clothing, controlled access	Partial containment equipment used for all manipulations of infectious material	Containment
4	Level 3 practices, plus entrance through change room where street clothing is removed and laboratory clothing put on, shower on exit, all wastes are decontaminated on exit from the facility	Maximum containment equipment (i.e., class III biological safety cabinet or partial containment equipment in combination with full-body, air-supplied, positive-pressure personnel suit) used for all procedures and activities	Maximum containment

[a] From Centers for Disease Control/National Institutes of Health, "Biosafety in Microbiological and Biomedical Laboratories," 2nd Ed. U.S. Government Printing Office, Washington, D.C., 1988.

ination, which is something that may give rise to mistaken diagnoses and sometimes a great deal of misdirected administrative action.

Precautions to avoid these hazards consist essentially of good laboratory techniques, but special measures may be needed. Mouth-pipetting is banned. Special arrangements for disposal of "sharps" are essential. Laboratory coats must be worn at all times, and gloves used for handling potentially infectious materials. Various classes of biological safety cabinets providing increasing levels of containment are available for procedures of various degrees of biohazard; their use is summarized in Table

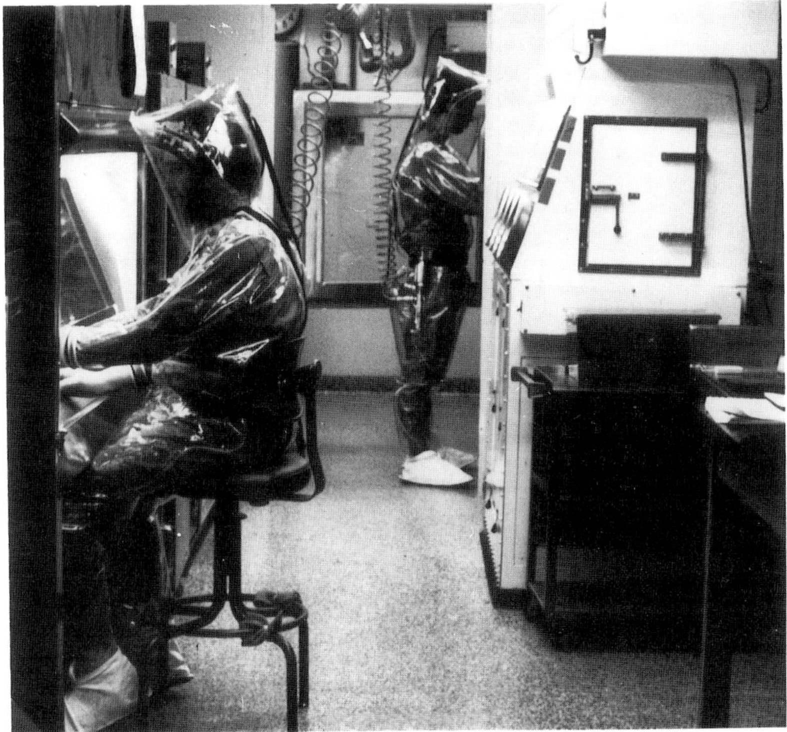

FIG. 12-10. *Maximum containment laboratory at the Centers for Disease Control, Atlanta, Georgia. Workers are protected by positive-pressure suits with an independent, remote source of breathing air. Primary containment of aerosols is achieved by the use of filtered vertical laminar-flow work stations. The ultracentrifuge is contained within an explosion-proof laminar-flow hood. A full range of sophisticated equipment is available, and animals as large as monkeys can be studied. (From J. S. Mackenzie, ed., "Viral Diseases in South-East Asia and the Western Pacific." Academic Press, Sydney, 1982. Courtesy Dr. K. M. Johnson.)*

TABLE 12-5

Animal Viruses the Importation of Which Is Restricted[a]

Virus	Family	Virus	Family
African horse sickness virus	*Reoviridae*	Nairobi sheep disease virus	*Bunyaviridae*
African swine fever virus	Unclassified	Newcastle disease virus (velogenic strains)	*Paramyxoviridae*
Borna disease virus	Unclassified	Porcine polioencephalomyelitis virus	*Picornaviridae*
Bovine ephemeral fever virus	*Rhabdoviridae*	Rift Valley fever virus	*Bunyaviridae*
Camelpox virus	*Poxviridae*	Rinderpest virus	*Paramyxoviridae*
Foot-and-mouth disease virus	*Picornaviridae*	Swine vesicular disease virus	*Picornaviridae*
Fowl plague virus	*Orthomyxoviridae*	Vesicular exanthema virus	*Caliciviridae*
Lumpyskin disease virus	*Poxviridae*	Wesselsbron disease virus	*Flaviviridae*

[a] For the United States. In other industrialized countries there are similar listings, some even longer; for example, the Australian list includes, in addition, bluetongue viruses, epidemic hemorrhagic disease of deer virus, hog cholera virus, malignant catarrhal fever virus, ovine progressive pneumonia virus, pseudorabies virus, rabies virus, the scrapie and bovine spongiform encephalopathy agents, and sheeppox virus, but it excludes bovine ephemeral fever virus, which is endemic in Australia.

12-4. Biosafety level 4 viruses, such as Ebola, Marburg, and Lassa viruses, can be handled only in maximum containment laboratories (Fig. 12-10).

Security for National Livestock Industries

Besides personal hazard, exotic animal viruses pose special community risks such that major industrialized countries with large livestock industries support special laboratories for their investigation. These are the so-called maximum containment laboratories, popularly designated by their location, for example, Plum Island in the United States, Pirbright in the United Kingdom, and Geelong in Australia. "Restricted" animal viruses are listed in Table 12-5, for the United States and Australia. The importation, possession, or use of these viruses is prohibited or restricted by law or regulation. The importation of some is totally prohibited (e.g., foot-and-mouth disease virus into Australia); more often their importation and study are restricted to the national maximum containment laboratories.

FURTHER READING

Balows, A., Hausler, W. J., Herrman, K. L., Isenberg, H. D., and Shadomy, H. J., eds. (1991). "Manual of Clinical Microbiology," 5th Ed. American Society of Microbiology, Washington, D.C.

Centers for Disease Control/National Institutes of Health. (1988). "Biosafety in Microbiological and Biomedical Laboratories," 2nd Ed. Publication NIH 88-8395. U.S. Government Printing Office, Washington, D.C.

Hierholzer, J. C. (1991). Rapid diagnosis of viral infection. *In* "Rapid Methods and Automation in Microbiology and Immunology" (A. Vaheri and A. Balows, eds.), pp. 556–573. Springer-Verlag, New York.

Innis, M. A., Gelfand, D. H., Sninsky, J. J., and White, T. J., eds. (1990). "PCR Protocols: A Guide to Methods and Applications." Academic Press, San Diego.

James, K. (1990). Immunoserology of infectious diseases. *Clin. Microbiol. Rev.* **3,** 132.

Johnson, F. B. (1990). Transport of viral specimens. *Clin. Microbiol. Rev.* **3,** 120.

Lennette, E. H., Halonen, P., and Murphy, F. A., eds. (1988). "Laboratory Diagnosis of Infectious Diseases. Principles and Practice. Volume II, Viral, Rickettsial and Chlamydial Diseases." Springer-Verlag, New York.

Palmer, E. L., and Martin, M. L. (1988). "Electron Microscopy in Viral Diagnosis." CRC Press, Boca Raton, Florida.

Rose, N. R., Friedman, H., and Fahey, J. L., eds. (1986). "Manual of Clinical Laboratory Immunology." American Society of Microbiology, Washington, D.C.

Sambrook, J., Fritsch, E. F., and Maniatis, T. (1989). "Molecular Cloning: A Laboratory Manual," 2nd Ed. Cold Spring Harbor Laboratory, Cold Spring Harbor, New York.

CHAPTER 13

Immunization against Viral Diseases

Immunization is the most generally applicable way of preventing viral diseases; in fact, the control of so many viral diseases of animals by immunization is probably the outstanding achievement of veterinary medicine in the twentieth century. Although vaccines of traditional types are still not fully utilized, the field of vaccinology is now being advanced by the application of recombinant DNA technologies.

There are some important differences between immunization practices in humans and animals. Except in developing countries, economic constraints are of little importance in human medicine, but very important in veterinary practice. There is greater agreement about the safest and most efficacious vaccines to be used in human medicine than there is with vaccines destined for use in animals. At the international level, the World Health Organization (WHO) exerts persuasive leadership for human vaccine usage and maintains a number of programs such as the Expanded Programme on Immunization, which is not matched for animal vaccine usage by its sister agency, the Food and Agriculture Organization. Further, within countries, more latitude is allowed in the manufacture and use of vaccines for animal diseases than is allowed by national regulatory authorities for human vaccines. As adduced from the tables in Chapter 35, at least 84 different viral vaccines are available for use in domestic animals whereas only 14 viral vaccines are available for use in humans. Finally, even a very small number of vaccine-associated illnesses or deaths constitute a major objection to the use of a vaccine in humans, whereas in animals mild disease (and even, in the past, occasional deaths) are tolerated if the vaccine is effective and the potential cost of failure to control the disease is sufficiently high.

There are two major strategies for the production of viral vaccines, one employing live virus and another employing inactivated virus or subunits of virions (Tables 13-1 and 13-2). These major strategies can be broken down into further categories, many of which represent progress based on modern recombinant DNA technologies.

Live-virus vaccines must replicate in the vaccine recipient in order to amplify the amount of antigen. There is an important benefit in this, since the replication of vaccine virus mimics infection to the extent that the host immune response is more similar to that occurring after natural infection than is ever the case with inactivated or subunit vaccine products. When inactivated virus vaccines are produced, the chemical or physical treatment used to eliminate infectivity is damaging enough to modify immunogenicity, especially cell-mediated immunogenicity, usually resulting in an immune response that is shorter in duration, narrower in antigenic specificity, weak in cell-mediated and mucosal immune response, and less effective in totally preventing viral entry.

LIVE-VIRUS VACCINES

If they can be developed and are safe, live-virus vaccines consisting of attenuated mutants are probably the best of all vaccines. Several have been dramatically successful in reducing the incidence of important diseases of animals and humans. Most live-virus vaccines are injected subcutaneously or intramuscularly, but some are delivered orally, and a few by aerosol or to poultry in their drinking water. The vaccine virus replicates in the recipient, eliciting a lasting immune response, but not causing disease. In effect, a live-virus vaccine produces a subclinical infection.

TABLE 13-1
Contemporary and Experimental Strategies for Production of Live-Virus Vaccines

Category	Strategy of production	Examples[a]
Wild-type virus	Unnatural route	Orf (C)
		Adenovirus (C) (human vaccine)
	Unnatural host	Marek's disease (C)
	Unnatural time of year	Equine arteritis (C)
Attenuated virus	Naturally occurring variant	Marek's disease (C)
		Bovine virus diarrhea (C)
		Vaccinia (C) (human vaccine)
	Adaptation to unnatural host	
	By animal passage	Rabies (C)
		Yellow fever (C) (human vaccine)
	By cell culture passage	Rabies (C)
		Rinderpest (C)
		Newcastle disease (C)
		Infectious bronchitis (C)
	Gene reassortment	Rift Valley fever (X)
		Rotavirus (X)
		Influenza (C) (human vaccine)
	Mutagenesis (temperature-sensitive, cold adapted)	Influenza (X) (human vaccine)
		Respiratory syncytial (X)
	Site-directed mutagenesis	Pseudorabies (C)
		Poliovirus (X) (human vaccine)
Virus vector	Heterologous gene expression (vectored vaccines/live vector)	Vaccinia:rabies (C, X)
		Vaccinia:rinderpest (C, X)
		Raccoonpox:rabies (X)
		Adenovirus:rabies (X) (vector is infectious canine hepatitis virus)
		Herpesvirus:bovine virus diarrhea virus (X) (vector is infectious bovine rhinotracheitis virus)
Bacterial vector	Heterologous gene expression (vectored vaccines/live vector)	Salmonella:rotavirus (X)
		Salmonella:rabies (X)

[a] (C), Contemporary vaccine, licensed and in use in some countries; (X), experimental vaccine, under development or in trials.

Naturally Occurring Viruses as Vaccines

The original vaccine (*vacca* = cow), introduced by Jenner in 1798 for the control of human smallpox, utilized cowpox virus, a natural pathogen of the cow. Cowpox virus produced only a mild lesion in man, but because it is antigenically related to smallpox virus, it conferred protec-

TABLE 13-2
Contemporary and Experimental Strategies for Production of Inactivated Virus and Subunit Vaccines

Category	Strategy of production	Examples
Whole virus	Cell culture	Rabies (C) Foot-and-mouth disease (C) Japanese encephalitis (C)
	Animal tissue (mouse brain)	Rabies (C) Japanese encephalitis (C)
Virus subunits	Naturally occurring subunits	Hepatitis B (C) (human vaccine; sole example)
	Detergent-split virus	Influenza (C) Fowl plague (X)
Virus proteins	Recombinant DNA expression	
	In bacteria	Foot-and-mouth disease (X)
	In yeast	Hepatitis B (C) (human vaccine; sole example)
	In mammalian cells	Hepatitis B (X) (human vaccine) Rabies (X) Human immunodeficiency virus (X)
	In insect cell culture or insect tissue	Avian influenza (X) Hepatitis B (X) (human vaccine)
	In heterologous virus (vectored vaccines/ inactivated)	Vaccinia:rabies (C, X) Vaccinia:avian influenza (X) Vaccinia:Venezuelan equine encephalitis (X) Vaccinia:Lassa (X) (human vaccine)
Virus peptides	*In vitro* chemical synthesis	Foot-and-mouth disease (X) Hepatitis B (X) (human vaccine)
Anti-idiotypic antibodies	Antigenic mimicry	Hepatitis B (X) (human vaccine) Reovirus (X)

[a] (C), Contemporary vaccine, licensed and in use in some countries; (X), experimental vaccine, under development or in trials.

tion against the severe human disease. The same principle has been applied to other diseases, for example, the protection of chickens against Marek's disease using a vaccine derived from a herpesvirus of turkeys and use of a bovine rotavirus to protect piglets against porcine rotavirus infection.

Virulent viruses given by an unnatural route have also been used as vaccines, for example, wild-type avian infectious laryngotracheitis virus via the cloaca, producing minimal disease but inducing good immunity.

Attenuated Live-Virus Vaccines

Most attenuated live-virus vaccines have been derived empirically, by serial passage of the wild-type virus through cell cultures, laboratory animals, or eggs. In the process, the accumulation of mutations generally leads not only to more vigorous growth in the particular type of cultured cell or animal tissue used, but also to progressive loss of virulence for the original host. On this serial passage series, it is important to "fix" the degree of attenuation, so that the vaccine virus retains the capacity to replicate sufficiently to produce the desired level of immunity but does not cause damaging morbidity.

An alternative approach in developing attenuated vaccine strains has been to select temperature-sensitive mutants; however, as with other point mutations, there have been problems with reversion to virulence. Temperature-sensitive mutant vaccines have been developed for infectious bovine rhinotracheitis, bovine respiratory syncytial disease, and bovine virus diarrhea. *Cold-adapted mutants* appear to be more stable, but they are often of low immunogenicity.

Genetic engineering can be used to construct deletion mutants by excising a sequence of nucleotides from a gene that is not essential for viral replication but contributes to virulence [e.g., the thymidine kinase (TK) gene in herpesviruses]. Since such mutants cannot revert, they are attractive candidates for attenuated live-virus vaccines. For example, pseudorabies virus vaccines have been constructed that are TK^- and also have a deletion in a glycoprotein gene(s) (gI, gII, or gX). The deleted glycoprotein may be used in an ELISA, so that vaccinated pigs can be distinguished from naturally infected pigs, enabling eradication programs to be conducted in parallel with continued vaccination.

Among viruses with segmented genomes, such as orthomyxoviruses and rotaviruses, attenuated reassortants can be constructed, with eggs or cultured cells being coinfected with a "master" strain of documented low virulence together with the virulent field strain bearing the particular antigens against which protection is sought. From the progeny of the coinfection, strains are selected that carry appropriate surface antigen genes (wild-type) and virulence genes (attenuated-type).

Virus-Vectored Vaccines

A new method of immunization, potentially of wide applicability in veterinary medicine, involves the use of viruses as vectors to carry the genes for the protective antigens of other viruses. For example, genes for many antigens from a variety of viruses have been incorporated into the genome of vaccinia virus, and immunization of animals with these vectored vaccines has produced good antibody responses (Fig. 13-1). Fowlpox virus is a logical choice for avian vaccines, and, surprisingly, as a vector fowlpox virus has been shown to evoke a good antibody response when inoculated in mammals, even though fowlpox virus does not replicate in mammalian hosts. Recent experimental work suggests that adenoviruses, herpesviruses, and hepatitis B virus can be used as vectors and may have advantages in terms of long-term antigen expression. Several RNA viruses, such as Sindbis virus and poliovirus, are also being developed as vectors.

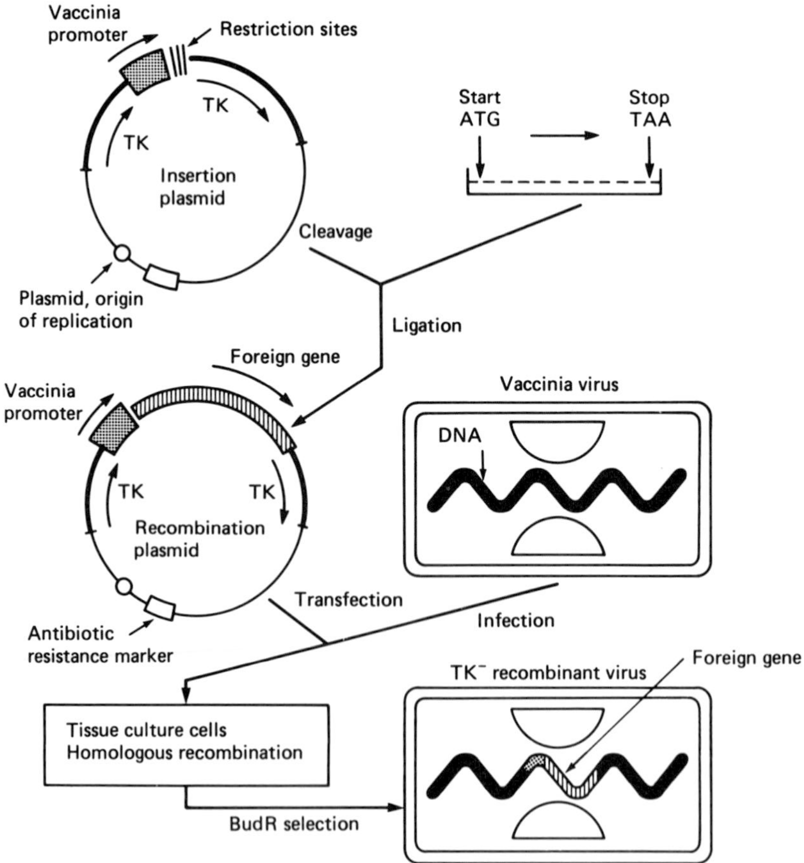

FIG. 13-1. *Method of constructing a vaccinia virus vector carrying a selected gene from another virus. TK, Thymidine kinase gene of vaccinia virus; BUdR, bromodeoxyuridine. (Courtesy Dr. B. Moss.)*

Although considerable research and development needs to be done, this approach opens the possibility of designing vaccines for the range of viral and bacterial and perhaps parasitic infections common in each species of domestic animal in any particular country. So far, however, the only vectored vaccines to be used in the field are vaccinia–rabies constructs used for vaccination of foxes in Europe and raccoons in the United States.

INACTIVATED VIRUS AND VIRUS SUBUNIT VACCINES

Inactivated vaccines are usually made from virulent virus; chemical or physical agents are used to destroy infectivity while maintaining immunogenicity. When properly prepared, such vaccines are safe, but they need to be injected in large amounts to elicit an antibody response commensurate with that attainable by a much smaller dose of attenuated live-virus vaccine. Normally the primary course comprises two or three injections, and further (*booster*) doses may be required at intervals over the succeeding years to maintain immunity.

The most commonly used inactivating agents are formaldehyde, β-propiolactone, and ethyleneimine. One of the advantages of β-propiolactone, used in the manufacture of human rabies vaccines, is that it is completely hydrolyzed within hours to nontoxic products. Because virions in the center of aggregates may be protected from inactivation, it is important that aggregates be removed. In the past, failure to do this occasionally resulted in vaccine-associated outbreaks of foot-and-mouth disease when formaldehyde was used to produce inactivated foot-and-mouth disease vaccine.

The logical extension from using whole inactivated virions as vaccines is to remove nonessential components of the virion and inoculate only the relevant *immunogen,* namely, the particular protein against which neutralizing antibodies are directed. Such "split" vaccines are in use against influenza, and they are feasible for a number of other viruses.

Viral Proteins from Cloned Genes

Recombinant DNA technology provides a means of producing large amounts of viral protein that can be readily purified. Selected viral genes are expressed in prokaryotic or eukaryotic cells, and the resultant proteins are harvested and purified. If the immunogenic protein is glycosylated, eukaryotic expression systems must be used, so that the expressed protein is glycosylated and produced in its proper conformation. Useful eukaryotic expression systems include insect cells, with the nuclear polyhedrosis baculovirus expression system; yeast cells, for which there is extensive experience with scaleup for industrial production; and mammalian cells. So far the only commercial vaccine produced in this way is the human hepatitis B vaccine, expressed in yeast cells.

SYNTHETIC VACCINES

Several techniques have been developed for locating and defining major epitopes on protective viral proteins, and it is possible to synthesize short peptides corresponding to these epitopes. Such synthetic peptides have been shown to elicit neutralizing antibodies against foot-and-mouth disease virus, rabies virus, and certain other animal pathogens. Further developments of this approach include linking a number of selected peptides corresponding to epitopes recognized by T and B lymphocytes. The preparation might contain certain additional sequences, such as a peptide facilitating fusion with a cell membrane, to enhance a desired response.

This new approach merits further research, although one limitation is that most epitopes which elicit humoral immunity are conformational, that is, they require the three-dimensional shape that they assume in the native protein molecule or virus particle. Since short synthetic peptides lack this tertiary or quaternary conformation, most antibodies raised against them are incapable of binding to virions; hence, the neutralizing titer may be orders of magnitude lower than that induced by inactivated whole virus vaccine or purified intact protein. However, peptides incapable of inducing protective levels of antibody may prime T cells so that on challenge with a small dose of inactivated virus an anamnestic response occurs.

ANTI-IDIOTYPIC ANTIBODIES

The antigen-binding site of the antibody produced by each B-cell clone contains a unique amino acid sequence known as its *idiotype* or idiotypic determinant (Id). Because anti-Id antibody is capable of binding to the same idiotype as binds the combining epitope on the original antigen, anti-Id antibody mimics the conformation of that epitope, so that anti-Id raised against a neutralizing monoclonal antibody to a particular virus could conceivably be used as a vaccine. Anti-Id antibodies raised against antibodies to hepatitis B surface antigen and reovirus S1 capsid antigen elicit an antiviral antibody response on injection into animals, and an anti-Id antibody generated against a T-cell receptor for Sendai virus has been shown to induce both humoral and cell-mediated immune responses in mice.

It is still uncertain whether this points the way to a novel vaccine strategy, but there are situations, probably in human rather than veterinary medicine, where such vaccines, if efficacious, would have advantages over orthodox vaccines, primarily because of their safety.

METHODS FOR ENHANCING IMMUNOGENICITY

The immunogenicity of inactivated vaccines, and to an even greater extent isolated viral proteins or synthetic peptides, usually needs to be enhanced. This may be achieved by mixing the antigen with an *adjuvant*, incorporation of the antigen in *liposomes*, or incorporation of the antigen in an immunostimulating complex (ISCOM).

Adjuvants

Adjuvants are materials that are mixed with vaccines to potentiate the immune response, both humoral and/or cellular, so that a lesser quantity of antigen is required and fewer doses need to be given. The mechanism of action of adjuvants includes (1) prolonged retention and slow release of antigen, (2) activation of macrophages, leading to secretion of lymphokines and attraction of lymphocytes, and (3) mitogenicity for lymphocytes. The adjuvants most widely used in animal vaccines are alum and mineral oils, and one of the most promising new adjuvants being developed is muramyl dipeptide, which can be coupled to synthetic antigens or incorporated into liposomes.

Liposomes

Liposomes consist of artificial lipid membrane spheres into which proteins can be incorporated. When purified viral envelope glycoproteins are used, the resulting "virosomes" (or "immunosomes") somewhat resemble the original envelope of the virion. This enables one not only to reconstitute viral envelope-like structures lacking viral nucleic acid and other viral components, but also to select nonpyrogenic lipids and to incorporate substances with adjuvant activity, thus regaining much of the immunogenicity lost when the viral glycoprotein was removed from its original milieu. Viral proteins can also be assembled into other types of membrane-bound micelles to restore immunogenicity. In practice, however, liposomes have not lived up to expectations as immunogens.

Immunostimulating Complexes

When virion proteins are solubilized by detergents and added to a sucrose gradient containing QUIL A, a glycoside extracted from the tree *Quillaga saponaria molina,* micelles are formed which are cagelike structures 35 nm in diameter in which viral glycoproteins are incorporated in a manner simulating their presence in the intact virion. These ISCOMs have been found to be effective immunogens in experimental animals but have not yet been used for commercial vaccines.

COMPARISON OF DIFFERENT CLASSES OF VACCINES

The relative advantages and disadvantages of live-virus vaccines compared with inactivated virus or subunit vasccines are summarized in Table 13-3.

TABLE 13-3
Advantages and Disadvantages of Live-Virus Vaccines and Inactivated Virus or Subunit Vaccines

Parameter	Live-virus vaccine	Inactivated virus or subunit vaccine
Route of administration	Natural[a] or injection	Injection
Antigen per dose	Low	High
Cost	Low	High
Number of doses needed	Single[b]	Multiple
Need for adjuvant	No	Yes
Duration of immunity	Many years	Months or years[c]
Antibody response	IgG; IgA[d]	IgG
Cell-mediated response	Good	Variable
Heat lability[e]	Yes[f]	No
Interference	Occasional[g]	No
Side effects	Occasional mild signs	Occasional local or general reactions
Dangerous in pregnant animals	Some	No
Reversion to virulence	Possible	No

[a] Oral or respiratory, in certain cases.
[b] For some a second dose may be required.
[c] Satisfactory with some.
[d] IgA if delivered via oral or respiratory route.
[e] Especially in hot climates.
[f] Stabilizers added to vaccine, plus maintenance of "cold chain" delay inactivation.
[g] If administered by oral or respiratory route.

Immunologic Considerations

The object of immunization is to protect against disease, and ideally to prevent infection and virus transmission within the population at risk. If, as immunity wanes over months or years following active immunization, or weeks following passive immunization, infection with wild-type virus does occur, the infection is likely to be subclinical, but will boost immunity. This is a frequent occurrence in farm animals and birds in crowded pens.

IgA is the most important class of immunoglobulin relevant to the prevention of infection of mucosal surfaces, such as those of the intestinal, respiratory, genitourinary, and ocular epithelia. One of the advantages of an attenuated live-virus oral vaccine, such as Newcastle disease vaccine, is that, by virtue of its replication in the intestinal tract, it leads to prolonged synthesis of local IgA antibody. By preventing infection, such a regime may make feasible the prospect of local eradication of the virus from the population.

Although neutralizing antibody is the key to prevention of infection, cell-mediated immunity plays a crucial role in recovery from many viral infections. Attenuated live-virus vaccines are more effective than other types of vaccine in eliciting cell-mediated immunity. Further, T-cell responses tend to display broader cross-recognition of related viral strains than do antibodies. Such cross-immunity is advantageous where several viral serotypes circulate simultaneously or sequentially, due to antigenic drift.

Vaccine Safety

Properly prepared and tested, all vaccines should be safe in immunocompetent animals. Licensing authorities insist on rigorous safety tests for residual live virus in "inactivated" vaccines. There are other safety problems that are unique to attenuated live-virus vaccines.

Contaminating Viruses. Because vaccines are grown in animals or cells derived from them, there is always a possibility that a vaccine will be contaminated with another virus from that animal or from the medium used for culturing its cells. An early example, which led to restrictions on international trade in vaccines and sera that are still in effect, was the introduction into the United States in 1908 of foot-and-mouth disease virus as a contaminant of smallpox vaccine produced in calves. The use of embryonated eggs to produce vaccines for use in chickens may pose problems, for instance, the contamination of Marek's disease vaccine with reticuloendotheliosis virus. Another important source of viral contaminants is bovine fetal calf serum, universally used in cell cultures; all batches must be screened for contamination with bovine virus diarrhea virus. Likewise, porcine parvovirus is a common contaminant of crude preparations of trypsin prepared from pig pancreases, which is commonly used in the preparation of animal cell cultures. The risk of contaminating viruses is greatest with live-virus vaccines but may also occur with inactivated whole virus vaccines, since some viruses are more resistant to inactivation than others.

The danger of contamination has triggered debate about which types of cultured cells should be licensed for use as substrates for vaccine production. If primary cell cultures are to remain legally acceptable for this purpose, the animals should be bred in a clean environment, preferably under specific-pathogen-free conditions, and the cultured cells must be rigorously tested for endogenous viruses. In general, however, for vaccine production primary cell cultures have been replaced by well-characterized diploid cells or continuous cell lines, which can be subjected to comprehensive screening, certified as safe, then stored frozen for many years as seed lots.

Heat Lability. Live-virus vaccines are vulnerable to inactivation by high ambient temperatures, a particular problem in the tropics. Since most tropical countries also have underdeveloped veterinary services, formidable problems are encountered in maintaining the "cold chain" from manufacturer to animals in remote, hot, rural areas. To some extent the problem has been alleviated by the addition of stabilizing agents to the vaccines and by packaging them in freeze-dried form, for reconstitution immediately before administration. In other cases simple portable refrigerators have been developed and placed in the field.

Unnecessary exposure to high temperatures should also be avoided with nonreplicating vaccines, since it may reduce the immunogenicity.

Adverse Effects in Pregnant Animals. Attenuated live-virus vaccines are not generally recommended for use in pregnant animals, since they may be abortifacient or teratogenic. For example, many infectious bovine rhinotracheitis vaccines are abortifacient, and feline panleukopenia, hog cholera, bovine virus diarrhea, and bluetongue vaccines are examples of teratogenic viruses. The adverse effects are usually due to primary immunization of a nonimmune pregnant animal. Proprietors of large dog and cat breeding establishments often wish to boost antibody titers in pregnant animals, especially to parvovirus, so as to provide high antibody levels for maternal transfer, but it is better to immunize the dam just before mating.

Underattenuation. Some inadequately attenuated live-virus vaccines have been associated with significant disease in some recipients. For example, some early canine parvovirus vaccines that had undergone few cell culture passages were used in an attempt to overcome residual maternal immunity, but they were found to produce an unacceptably high incidence of disease. Attempts to attenuate virulence further may be accompanied by a decline in the capacity of the virus to replicate in the host, with a corresponding loss of immunogenicity.

Such side effects as do occur with current animal virus vaccines are minimal and do not constitute a significant disincentive to immunization. However, it is important that attenuated live-virus vaccines should be used only in the species for which they were produced; for example, canine distemper vaccine may cause fatalities in some members of the Mustelidae, such as black footed ferrets (see Chapter 27).

Genetic Instability. Some vaccine strains may revert toward virulence during replication in the recipient, or in contact animals to which the vaccine virus has spread. Most vaccine viruses are incapable of such spread, but in those that do there may be an accumulation of back mutations that gradually leads to a restoration of virulence. The principal example of this phenomenon is the very rare reversion to virulence of poliovirus type 3 oral vaccine in man, but temperature-sensitive mutants of bovine virus diarrhea virus have also proved to be genetically unstable.

Adverse Effects from Nonreplicating Vaccines. Some inactivated whole virus vaccines have been found to potentiate disease. The earliest observations were made with inactivated vaccines for measles and human respiratory syncytial virus. In veterinary medicine attempts to produce a vectored vaccine for the coronavirus that causes feline infectious peritonitis illustrates the problem. A recombinant vaccinia virus that expressed the coronavirus E2 protein was used to immunize kittens. Despite the production of neutralizing antibodies, the kittens were not protected; instead when challenged they quickly died of feline infectious peritonitis, probably because of antibody-dependent enhancement of the disease.

FACTORS INTERFERING WITH VACCINE EFFICACY

Attenuated live-virus vaccines delivered by mouth or nose depend critically for their efficacy on replication in the intestinal or respiratory tract, respectively. Interference can occur between the vaccine virus and enteric or respiratory viruses with which the animal happens to be infected at the time, and in the past interference occurred between different attenuated live viruses contained in certain vaccine formulations (e.g., with bluetongue vaccines). More important currently is the fact that canine parvovirus infection may be immunosuppressive to such an extent that it interferes with the response of dogs to vaccination against canine distemper.

PASSIVE IMMUNIZATION

Instead of *actively immunizing* with viral vaccines it is possible to confer short-term protection by the intramuscular administration of antibody, as immune serum or immunoglobulin. Homologous immunoglobulin is preferred, because heterologous protein may provoke an anaphylactic response. Pooled normal immunoglobulin contains reasonably high concentrations of antibody against all the common viruses that cause systemic disease in the respective species. Higher titers occur in "convalescent" serum from donor animals that have recovered from infection or have been hyperimmunized by repeated vaccinations, and such hyperimmune globulin is the preferred product if commercially available (e.g., for canine distemper and canine parvovirus infection).

Vaccination of the dam is practiced in selected situations in order to provide the newborn with passive (maternal) immunity via antibodies present in the egg (in birds) or in colostrum and milk (in mammals). This is particularly important for diseases in which the major impact occurs during the first few weeks of life, when active immunization of the newborn cannot be accomplished early enough. With avian encephalomyelitis, this strategy is employed for the further reason that the attenuated live-virus vaccines themselves are pathogenic in young chicks.

VACCINATION POLICY

Economic Considerations

Cost–benefit factors are critical in determining the usage of veterinary vaccines. For example, good vaccines are available for the control of many diseases of swine and poultry, but the costs limit their use to large producers, and the diseases remain endemic elsewhere. Economic constraints are most evident in developing countries. For example, in the 1970s economic constraints led to the abandonment of vaccination against rinderpest in sub-Saharan Africa, in spite of the fact that a concerted vaccination program could well have led to regional elimination and eventually to global eradication of the virus (see Chapter 27).

Because of large markets (economy of scale of production), together with somewhat less stringent licensing requirements, veterinary vaccines are generally less expensive than those used in man. Some avian viral vaccines cost less than one cent per dose; many human (and some veterinary) viral vaccines cost dollars. The pattern of vaccine usage differs strikingly from country to country, with many of the principal diseases against which vaccines are employed in South Africa, for example, being exotic to the United States.

The decision to use a vaccine is governed by a complex equation, balancing expected extra profit against costs and risks. If the disease is lethal or causes major economic losses, the need for immunization is clear; both the owners and the vaccine-licensing authorities will accept a risk of occasional, quite serious side effects. If, on the other hand, the disease is perceived as trivial or economically unimportant, no vaccine would be used. Where equally satisfactory vaccines are available against a particular disease, considerations of cost and ease of administration tip the balance, for example, toward vaccines administered via drinking water in poultry.

Continuation of routine immunization after the risk of disease in an area has almost vanished, but the virus has not been totally eradicated, is difficult to sustain because of fading awareness of the risk. Yet it is essential, because reduction in circulation of wild-type virus leaves unimmunized animals highly susceptible, by removing the protective effect of repeated subclinical infections. Legislation for compulsory immunization against particular diseases is perhaps the most effective single measure for maintaining protection in the apparent absence of disease.

Vaccination Schedules

The available range of vaccines, often in multivalent formulations and with somewhat different recommendations from each manufacturer regarding immunization schedules, means that the practicing veterinarian needs expert guidance about vaccine choice and usage. Multivalent vaccine formulations, such as those available for canine distemper/hepatitis/parvovirus/coronavirus/parainfluenza virus/bordetella/leptospirosis for dogs, confer major practical advantages in minimizing the number of visits the owner must make to the veterinarian. Also, multivalent vaccines lead to the more extensive use of vaccines of secondary importance. However, unlike the situation in human medicine, where there is wide agreement on vaccine formulations and schedules for vaccination against all the common viral diseases of childhood, there is no such consensus in veterinary medicine. Furthermore, unlike the situation in human medicine where there are few vaccine manufacturers, there are many veterinary vaccine manufacturers, each promoting his own products. We outline below some of the principles underlying decisions on vaccination schedules, and we provide tables of schedules for the immunization of various domestic animals.

Optimal Age for Vaccination. The risk of most viral diseases is greatest in young animals. Most vaccines are therefore given during the first 6 months of life. Maternal antibody, whether transferred transplacentally or, as in domestic animals, in the colostrum, inhibits the immune response of the newborn to vaccines. Optimally, vaccination should be delayed until the titer of maternal antibody in the young animal has declined to near zero. However, waiting may leave the animal defenseless during the resulting "window of susceptibility." This is life-threatening in crowded, highly contaminated environments. There are a number of approaches to handling this problem in different animal species, but none is fully satisfactory.

Because the titer of passively acquired antibody in the circulation of newborn animal is proportional to that in the blood of the dam, and the rate of its subsequent clearance in different animal species is known, it is possible to estimate, for any given maternal antibody titer, the age at which no measurable antibody remains in the offspring. This can be plotted as a nomograph, from which the optimal age of vaccination against any particular disease can be read (Fig. 13-2). The method is not much used but could be considered for exceptionally valuable animals.

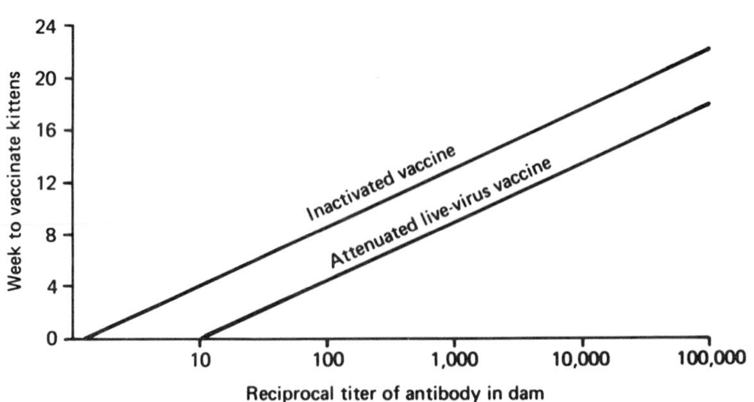

FIG. 13-2. *Nomograph indicating optimum times for vaccinating kittens with feline panleukopenia vaccines, based on the antibody titer of the dam and a half-life of IgG in the kitten of 9.5 days [Data from F. W. Scott, C. K. Csiza, and J. H. Gillespie,* J. Am. Vet. Med. Assoc. **156,** *439 (1970).]*

In practice, relatively few vaccine failures are encountered if one simply follows the instructions from the vaccine manufacturers, who have used averaged data on maternal antibody levels and rate of IgG decay in that animal species to estimate an optimal age for vaccination. Commonly it is recommended, even in the case of live-virus vaccines, that a number of doses of vaccine be administered, say, at monthly intervals, to cover the window of susceptibility in animals with particularly high maternal antibody titers. This precaution is even more relevant to multivalent vaccine formulations, because of the differences in maternal antibody titers against each virus.

Dam Vaccination. The aim of immunization is generally thought of as the protection of the vaccinee. This is usually so, but in the case of certain vaccines (e.g., those for equine abortion virus, rotavirus infection in cattle, parvovirus infection in swine, and infectious bursal disease of

TABLE 13-4

Schedule for Immunization against Viral Diseases of Cattle

Vaccine	Basic course	Revaccination
Attenuated live-virus vaccines		
Bovine virus diarrhea virus	4–9 months of age (single dose)[a, b]	Annual
Infectious bovine rhinotracheitis virus	3–4 months of age (single dose)	Annual
Rinderpest virus[c]	6–8 months of age (single dose)	None
Respiratory syncytial virus	4–6 months of age (2 doses with 4-week interval)	Annual
Parainfluenza virus type 3	4–6 months of age (2 doses with 4-week interval)	Annual
Inactivated virus vaccines		
Foot-and-mouth disease virus[d]	4 weeks of age (single dose)	4–12 months
Infectious bovine rhinotracheitis virus	3–4 months of age (2 doses at 4-week interval)	6–12 months
Parainfluenza virus type 3, reovirus, various adenovirus types	6 weeks, 3 months, 7 months of age	Annual
Rotavirus, coronavirus[e]	6–8 weeks and 2 weeks before end of gestation	Each pregnancy

[a] When vaccination is carried out at an early age, a second dose is recommended because of possible interference with maternal antibodies.

[b] Emergency vaccination: All animals older than 2 weeks except animals during the first trimester of pregnancy.

[c] Only in countries where the disease occurs

[d] Compulsory in some countries; multivalent vaccine.

[e] Dam vaccination.

chickens) the objective is to protect the vaccinee's offspring. This is achieved by vaccination of the female animal or laying hen, such that the level of maternal antibody transferred in the colostrum and milk or in the egg ensures that the offspring have a protective level of antibody during the critical early days of life. Since many attenuated live-virus vaccines are abortifacient or teratogenic, inactivated vaccines are recommended for dam vaccination.

Herd Effects of Vaccination. Under some circumstances an important auxiliary objective of a vaccination program may be to protect unvaccinated members of the population (e.g., against some avian virus diseases), either by natural spread of attenuated vaccine virus or by reducing the circulation of wild-type virus.

Available and Recommended Vaccines. The types of vaccines available for each viral disease (or the lack of any satisfactory vaccine) are discussed in each chapter of Part II of this book and in the tables in Chapter 35. There are obvious geographic variations in the requirements for particular vaccines, for example, between some countries in South America where vaccination against foot-and-mouth disease is practiced and the United States where it is not. There are also different requirements appropriate to various types of husbandry, for instance, for dairy cattle, beef cows, and their calves or cattle assembled in feedlots, and in poultry for breeders, commercial egg layers, and broilers (see Tables 13-4 through 13-10).

TABLE 13-5

Schedule for Immunization against Viral Diseases of Sheep and Goats

Vaccine	Basic course	Revaccination
Attenuated live-virus vaccines		
Bluetongue viruses[a] (polyvalent vaccines; up to 15 types)	3–6 months of age (2 doses with 3-week interval)	Annual
Sheeppox virus[a]	3 months of age (single dose)	2 years
Rinderpest virus[a] (peste des petits ruminants)	3 months of age (single dose)	None
Wild-type virus		
Orf virus[b]	2–3 months of age (single dose)	None
Inactivated virus vaccines		
Foot-and-mouth disease virus[a]	3–4 months of age (single dose)	Annual

[a] Only in countries where the disease occurs.

[b] In some countries; only on properties where scabby mouth is a problem.

TABLE 13-6
Schedule for Immunization against Viral Diseases of Swine

Vaccine	Basic course	Revaccination
Attentuated live-virus vaccines		
Hog cholera virus[a]	8 weeks of age (single dose)	None
Pseudorabies virus[a]	All ages (2 doses with 4-week interval)	4–6 months
Inactivated virus vaccines		
Pseudorabies virus[a]	4 weeks of age (2 doses with 4-week interval)	5–6 months
Porcine polioencephalitis virus[a]	8–12 weeks of age (2 doses with 4-week interval)	None
Parvovirus	Before mating (2 doses with 4-week interval)	Annual
Influenza virus	Any age (2 doses with 4-week interval)	Annual

[a] Depends on current policy in particular countries.

TABLE 13-7
Schedule for Immunization against Viral Diseases of Horses

Vaccine	Basic course	Revaccination
Attenuated live-virus vaccines		
Equine abortion virus (equine herpesvirus 1)	3 months of age (3 doses with 2- and 6-month intervals)	9–12 months
Equine arteritis virus[a]	3 months of age (2 doses with 4-week interval)	1–2 years
African horse sickness virus[a] (polyvalent vaccine)	6–8 months of age (single dose)	2–3 years
Inactivated virus vaccines		
Influenza virus (bivalent vaccine)	3–5 months of age (3 doses with 2- and 6-month intervals)	Every 3–6 months
Eastern, Western, and Venezuelan encephalitis viruses	3 months of age (2 doses with 3-week interval)	Annual
Equine abortion virus[b] (equine herpesvirus 1)	10 weeks of age (3 doses with 1- and 6-month intervals)	6–12 months

[a] Only recommended in areas where the disease occurs.
[b] Also in combination with influenza and reovirus types 1 and 3. Mares should be vaccinated additionally at 5, 7, and 9 months of pregnancy.

TABLE 13-8

Schedule for Immunization against Viral Diseases of Dogs

Vaccine	Basic course	Revaccination
Attenuated live-virus vaccines		
Canine distemper virus[a]	6–8 weeks of age (3 doses with 1- and 2-month intervals)	Every 2 years
Measles virus (for distemper)	8–10 weeks of age	Annual
Canine hepatitis virus	6–8 weeks of age (3 doses with 1- and 2-month intervals)	Every 2 years
Parvovirus[b, c]	6 weeks of age (3 doses with 1- and 2-month intervals)	Annual
Rabies virus	12 weeks of age	Annual
Inactivated virus vaccines		
Rabies virus	8–10 weeks of age (2 doses with 4- to 6-week interval)	Annual
Parvovirus[b]	6–8 weeks of age (3 doses with 1- and 2-month intervals)	Annual
Coronavirus	6–8 weeks of age (3 doses with 1- and 2-month intervals)	Annual
Parainfluenza virus	6–8 weeks of age (3 doses with 1- and 2-month intervals)	Annual

[a] Emergency vaccination with measles virus possible shortly after birth.

[b] Animals at risk should be revaccinated every 6–9 months. Bitches in heavily infected kennels can be vaccinated during pregnancy with inactivated vaccines in order to increase colostral antibody titers.

[c] A high-titer vaccine is available which obviates the need for the third dose (14–16 weeks).

TABLE 13-9

Schedule for Immunization against Viral Diseases of Cats

Vaccine	Basic course	Revaccination
Attenuated live-virus vaccines[a]		
Panleukopenia virus[b]	8–10 weeks of age (2 doses with 1-month interval)	Annual
Calicivirus	8–12 weeks of age (2 doses with 1-month interval)	Annual
Herpesvirus	8–12 weeks of age (2 doses with 1-month interval)	Annual
Rabies virus	12 weeks	Annual
Inactivated virus vaccines		
Panleukopenia virus	8–10 weeks of age (2 doses with 1-month interval	Annual
Rabies virus	8–10 weeks of age (2 doses with 1-month interval)	Annual
Calicivirus	8–10 weeks of age (2 doses with 1-month interval)	Annual
Herpesvirus	8–10 weeks of age (2 doses with 1-month interval)	Annual
Feline leukemia virus		
Subunit	9 weeks of age (2 doses with 3- to 15-week interval)	Annual
Whole virus	10 weeks of age (2 doses with 1-month interval)	Annual

[a] All vaccines are also available in combinations.

[b] Live panleukopenia virus vaccines should not be used in pregnant cats because of the risk of placental passage of the vaccine virus.

TABLE 13-10

Schedule for Immunization against Viral Diseases of Poultry[a, b]

Poultry and age	Vaccine	Route
Broilers		
1 day	Infectious bronchitis	Spray
	Newcastle disease	Spray (if required)
18 days	Infectious bronchitis	Drinking water or spray
	Newcastle disease	Drinking water or spray (if required)
Chickens: broiler or layer breeders		
1 day	Marek's disease	Intramuscular injection
3 weeks	Newcastle disease	Drinking water
	Infectious bronchitis	Drinking water
	Marek's disease	Intramuscular injection
8 weeks	Infectious bronchitis	Drinking water or spray
	Newcastle disease	Drinking water or spray
10 weeks	Infectious bursal disease	Drinking water
14 weeks	Avian encephalomyelitis	Drinking water
16 weeks	Newcastle disease	Intramuscular injection
	Infectious bronchitis	Intramuscular injection
	Infectious bursal disease	Intramuscular injection
Chickens: commercial egg layers		
1 day	Marek's disease	Intramuscular injection
3 weeks	Newcastle disease	Drinking water or spray
	Infectious bronchitis	Drinking water or spray
7 weeks	Infectious bronchitis	Drinking water or spray
	Newcastle disease	Drinking water or spray
10 weeks	Avian encephalomyelitis	Drinking water
14 weeks	Newcastle disease	Intramuscular injection
	Infectious bronchitis	Intramuscular injection
	Egg drop syndrome	Intramuscular injection
Turkey breeders		
3 weeks	Newcastle disease	Spray
6 weeks	Newcastle disease	Spray
12 weeks	Newcastle disease	Intramuscular injection
	Paramyxovirus 3	Intramuscular injection
24 weeks	Newcastle disease	Intramuscular injection
	Paramyxovirus 3	Intramuscular injection

[a] All are attenuated live-virus vaccines except those for egg drop syndrome and infectious bursal disease virus used at 16 weeks for broiler or layer breeders.

[b] Based on F. T. W. Jordan, "Poultry Diseases," 3rd Ed. Baillière Tindall, London, 1990.

FURTHER READING

Ada, G. L. (1989). Vaccines. *In* "Fundamental Immunology" (W. E. Paul, ed.), 2nd Ed., p. 985. Raven, New York.

American Veterinary Medical Association. (1989). Canine and feline immunization guidelines—1989. *J. Am. Vet. Med. Assoc.* **195,** 314.

American Veterinary Medical Association. (1985). Guidelines for vaccination of horses. *J. Am. Vet. Med. Assoc.* **185,** 32.

Binns, M. M., and Smith, G. L., eds. (1992). "Recombinant Poxviruses." CRC Press, Boca Raton, Florida.

Bittle, J. L., and Muir, S. (1989). Vaccines produced by conventional means to control major infectious diseases of man and animals. *Adv. Vet. Sci. Comp. Med.* **33,** 1.

Brown, F., ed. (1990). Modern approaches to vaccines. *Semin. Virol.* **1,** 1.

Burbonboy, S., Charlier, P., Hertogs, J., Lobman, M., Wiseman, A., and Woods, S. (1991). Performance of high titre attenuated canine parvovirus vaccine in pups with maternally derived antibody. *Vet. Rec.* **128,** 377.

Chanock, R. M., Ginsberg, H. S., Brown, F., and Lerner, R. A., eds. (1992). "Vaccines 91." Cold Spring Harbor Laboratory, Cold Spring Harbor, New York, and preceding volumes.

Murphy, B. R., and Chanock, R. M. (1990). Immunization against viruses. *In* "Fields Virology" (B. N. Fields, D. M. Knipe, R. M. Chanock, M. S. Hirsch, J. L. Melnick, T. P. Monath, and B. Roizman, eds.), 2nd Ed., p. 469. Raven, New York.

CHAPTER 14

Epidemiology of Viral Infections

Epidemiology is the study of the determinants, dynamics, and distribution of diseases in populations. The risk of infection and/or disease in an animal or animal population is determined by characteristics of the virus (e.g., antigenic variation), the host and host population (e.g., innate and acquired resistance), and behavioral, environmental, and ecologic factors that affect virus transmission from one host to another. Epidemiology, which may be viewed as a part of the science of population biology, attempts to meld these factors into a unified whole.

Although originally derived from the root term *demos,* meaning people, the word epidemiology is widely used for the discipline whatever host is concerned, and the words endemic, epidemic, and pandemic are used to characterize disease states in communities, whether of humans or other animals. By introducing quantitative measurements of disease trends, epidemiology has come to have a major role in improving our understanding of the nature of diseases and in alerting and directing disease control activities. Epidemiologic study is also effective in clarifying the role of viruses in the etiology of diseases, understanding the interaction of viruses with environmental determinants of disease, determining factors affecting host susceptibility, unraveling modes of transmission, and large-scale testing of vaccines and drugs.

COMPUTATIONS AND DATA USED BY EPIDEMIOLOGISTS

Calculations of Rates

The comparison of disease experience in different populations is expressed in the form of rates, as set out below, the purpose of the multiplier (10^n = 1000, 100,000, 1,000,000, etc.) being to produce a rate that is a manageable whole number. Two rates are widely used; the *incidence rate* and the *prevalence rate.* In both cases the denominator (total number of animals at risk) may be as general as the total population in a country or as specific as the population known to be susceptible or at risk (e.g., the number of animals in a specified population that lack antibodies to the virus of interest).

$$\text{Incidence rate} = \frac{\text{number of cases} \times 10^n}{\text{population at risk}} \quad \text{in a specified period of time}$$

Incidence. *Incidence* is a measure of frequency over time, for example, monthly or annual incidence rate, and is especially useful for acute diseases of short duration. For acute infections three parameters determine the incidence rate of infection (disease): the proportion of animals that are susceptible, the proportion of the susceptible animals that are infected, and the percentage of infected animals with disease. The proportion of animals in the population that are susceptible to a specific virus reflects their past history of exposure to that virus and the duration of immunity. The proportion of susceptible animals infected during a year or a season may vary considerably, depending on factors such as number and density, season, and, for arbovirus infections, the vector population. Of those animals infected, only some develop overt disease; the ratio of inapparent infections to overt disease varies greatly with different viruses.

$$\text{Prevalence rate} = \frac{\text{number of cases} \times 10^n}{\text{population at risk}} \quad \text{at a particular time}$$

Prevalence. It is difficult to measure the incidence of chronic diseases, especially where the onset is insidious, and for such diseases it is customary to determine the prevalence rate, namely, the ratio of the number of cases occurring in a population to the size of the population at a particular point in time. *Prevalence* is thus a snapshot of the frequency that prevails at a given time, and it is a function of both incidence and the duration of the disease. *Seroprevalence* relates to the proportion of animals in a population that have antibody to a particular virus, and, because neutralizing antibodies often last for many years, seroprevalence rates usually represent cumulative experience with the virus.

Death Rates. Deaths from a disease can be categorized in two ways: the cause-specific mortality rate (the number of deaths from the disease in a given year, divided by the total population at midyear), usually expressed per 100,000, or the case–fatality rate (the percentage of animals with a particular disease that die from the disease).

Sources of Data. All these rates may be affected by various attributes that distinguish one individual from another: age, sex, genetic constitution, immune status, nutrition, and various behavioral parameters. The most widely applicable attribute is age, which may encompass, and can therefore be confounded by, immune status as well as various physiologic variables. The collection of accurate data about the occurrence of disease is more difficult than the computation of the rates just described. Even data for the denominator, namely, the total population, are often not available, let alone accurate information on the number of cases. Where such information is regarded as essential, government legislation proscribes the disease to be "notifiable," and in theory all cases should be reported to the relevant veterinary public health authorities.

Terms Used in Epidemiology

An infectious disease is characterized as *endemic* (the word *enzootic* is often used for diseases of animals) when there are multiple or continuous chains of transmission resulting in continuous occurrence of disease in a population of a limited region over a period of time. *Epidemics* (the word *epizootics* is often used for diseases of animals) are peaks in disease incidence that exceed the endemic baseline or expected rate of disease. The size of the peak required to constitute an epidemic is arbitrary and is related to the background endemic rate, the morbidity rate (frequency of illness), and the anxiety that the disease arouses because of its severity; thus, a few cases of velogenic Newcastle disease in poultry might be regarded as an epidemic, whereas a few cases of infectious bronchitis would not be. A *pandemic* (the word *panzootic* is often used for diseases of animals) is a worldwide epidemic, such as the canine parvovirus pandemic that swept around the world in the early 1980s.

The *incubation period* is the interval between infection and the onset of clinical signs of disease. In many diseases, such as avian influenza, there is a period of a day or so during which birds are infectious before they become clinically sick. Infected animals shed virus and remain infectious for a variable period, the period of infectivity, depending on the disease concerned. These variables are usually short in duration in acute infections, but both may be very long in chronic infections. For example, in lentivirus infections such as feline immunodeficiency virus infection, the incubation period is measured in years, but infected animals are infectious long before they develop clinical signs of disease. In such infections the level of infectivity may be very low, but since the period of infectivity is so long the virus is readily maintained in the population.

TYPES OF EPIDEMIOLOGIC INVESTIGATIONS

Investigation of Causation

Epidemiologic methods used to determine the incidence and prevalence of infectious diseases, the relationships between cause and effect, and the evaluation of the risk factors of disease include the *cross-sectional study*, the *case–control study*, and the *cohort study*. A cross-sectional study can be carried out relatively quickly and provides data on the prevalence of particular diseases in the population. In a case–control study, investigation starts after the disease has occurred, and attempts to identify the cause; it is thus a *retrospective study*. In human medicine this is the most common type of study. Although it does not require the creation of new data or records, it does require careful selection of the control group, matched to the test group so as to avoid bias. Because records are generally poorly maintained for most animal disease outbreaks, this can be difficult in veterinary medicine. The advantages of the retrospective study are that it makes use of existing data and is relatively inexpensive to carry out.

In cohort studies, also called *prospective studies*, investigation starts with a presumed cause, and a population exposed to the presumed causative virus is monitored for evidence of the disease. This type of study requires the creation of new data and the careful selection of a control group to be as similar as possible to the exposed group, except for the absence of contact with the presumed causative virus. Cohort studies do not lend themselves to quick analysis, as groups must be followed until disease is observed, often for long periods of time, which makes such studies expensive. However, when cohort studies are successful, proof of a cause–effect relationship is often incontrovertible.

Another kind of epidemiologic investigation that can provide etiologic information, and also data on the value of vaccines or therapeutic agents (see below), is the long-term herd study. Because of the present advanced state of diagnostic virology and computerized data files, such studies now yield a much greater amount of readily analyzed data than was possible a few years ago, but they are very expensive and require long-term dedication of both personnel and money. When used principally for the detection of virus in an area, such investigations are referred to as *sentinel studies,* and are widely used for studying the prevalence of arbovirus infections. For example, sentinel chickens are used for the early detection of Eastern equine and St. Louis encephalitis viruses in southern United States. When used for evaluating vaccines or therapeutic agents, long-term herd studies have the advantage that they include all of the variables attributable to the entire husbandry system.

The production of congenital defects in cattle by Akabane virus provides examples of both the case–control and cohort types of epidemiologic study. Case–control studies of epidemics of congenital defects in calves, characterized by deformed limbs and abnormal brain development and referred to as congenital arthrogryposis–hydranencephaly (see Chapter 30), were carried out in Australia in the 1950s and 1960s, but the cause was not identified. During the summer and early winter months from 1972 to 1975, approximately 42,000 calves were born with these congenital defects in central and western Japan, causing significant economic loss. Japanese scientists postulated that the disease was infectious but were unable to isolate a virus from affected calves. However, when precolostral sera from such calves were tested for antibody to a number of viruses, antibody to Akabane virus, a bunyavirus which was first isolated from mosquitoes in Akabane Prefecture in Japan in 1959, was found in almost all sera tested. A retrospective serologic survey indicated a very high correlation between the geographic distribution of the disease and the presence of antibody to the virus, suggesting that Akabane virus was the etiologic agent of congenital arthrogryposis–hydranencephaly in cattle. Cohort (prospective) studies were then organized. Sentinel herds were established in Japan and Australia, and it was soon found that the virus could be isolated from fetuses obtained by slaughter or cesarian section for only a short period after infection, thus explaining the earlier failures in attempts to isolate virus after calves were born. Experimental inoculation of pregnant cows with Akabane virus during the first two trimesters induced congenital abnormalities in calves similar to those seen in natural cases of the disease; clinical disease was not seen in the cows.

Vaccine Trials

The immunogenicity, potency, safety, and efficacy of vaccines are first studied in laboratory animals, followed by small-scale closed trials in the target animal species, and finally by large-scale open-field trials. The last-mentioned employ epidemiologic methods, rather like those of the cohort study just described. There is no alternative way to evaluate new vaccines, and the design of field trials has now been developed so that they yield maximum information with minimum risk and cost. Even with this system, however, a serious problem may be recognized only after a vaccine has been licensed for commercial use. This occurred after the introduction of attenuated live-virus vaccines for infectious bovine rhinotracheitis (caused by bovine herpesvirus 1) in the United States in the 1950s. Surprisingly, the vaccines had been in use for 5 years before it was recognized that abortion was a common sequel to vaccination.

Molecular Epidemiology

The term molecular epidemiology has been applied to the use of molecular biological methods for epidemiologic investigation of viral diseases. Many of the diagnostic techniques described in Chapter 12 can be used. With DNA viruses (e.g., equine herpesvirus 1 and pseudorabies virus), restriction endonuclease fingerprinting and comparative mapping can be used for the identification of field isolates with a precision that surpasses serologic methods. With viruses that have segmented genomes, such as orbiviruses and rotaviruses, polyacrylamide gel electrophoresis of genomic RNA provides valuable supplementation to serologic typing. Other techniques, such as nucleic acid hybridization and oligonucleotide fingerprinting, can also distinguish strains of virus within the same serotype. For example, the 1981 outbreak of foot-and-mouth disease in the United Kingdom was traced by oligonucleotide fingerprinting to the presence of noninactivated virus in a vaccine being used in France (see Fig. 22-4). With many viruses (e.g., foot-and-mouth disease virus, retroviruses, influenza A virus, and parvoviruses), epidemiologic information is now obtainable by determining complete or partial nucleotide sequences of representative viruses isolated from the field. The polymerase chain reaction (PCR) can be used to detect very low copy numbers of a particular viral DNA in diagnostic samples.

Seroepidemiology

Seroepidemiology is extremely useful in veterinary public health operations and in research. Because of the expense of collecting and properly storing sera, advantage is taken of a wide range of sources, such as abattoirs, culling operations (especially useful for assessment of wildlife populations), and vaccination programs. Such sera can be used to determine the prevalence or incidence of particular infections, to evaluate eradication and immunization programs, and to assess the impact, dynamics, and geographic distribution of new, emerging, and reemerging viruses. For example, bluetongue 20 virus was isolated from collections of *Culicoides* in Australia in 1977 and bluetongue 2 virus from similar collections in Florida in 1983 before any clinical disease was recognized. Serologic surveys were used to determine their geographic distribution and, using stored sera, to estimate how long they had been present. Monoclonal antibodies provide a powerful means of distinguishing viruses that cannot be readily differentiated by conventional serology employing polyclonal antibodies. This approach has been particularly useful in elucidating the relationships between rabies virus and rabieslike rhabdoviruses and in distinguishing geographic variants of rabies virus.

Traditional surveillance is based on the reporting of clinical disease. However, examination of appropriate numbers of sera for antibodies gives a more accurate index of the prevalence of a particular virus. By detecting antibodies to selected viruses in various age groups of the population, it is possible to determine how effectively viruses have spread or how long it has been since the last appearance of epidemic viruses. Correlation of serologic data with clinical observations makes it possible to determine the ratio of clinical to subclinical infections.

Serologic surveys may detect virus-infected herds and flocks. For example, serologic surveys have been used to detect infected breeding herds in hog cholera eradication campaigns; when they are found, the entire herd is sent for slaughter. Serologic surveys are also valuable in determining the success of immunization programs; for example, the gradual decrease in the percentage of animals with antibodies to rinderpest virus associated with reduced vaccination heralded the reemergence of epidemic rinderpest in Africa in the late 1970s.

Examination of sera from individual animals may also yield useful epidemiologic information. For example, when paired serum samples are obtained from an animal several weeks apart, the absence of antibody in the first serum sample and its presence in the second sample, or a rise in antibody titer (usually a fourfold or greater rise is considered significant), indicates recent infection. Likewise, the presence of specific IgM antibody in a single serum sample may indicate recent infection.

Mathematical Modeling

From the time of William Farr, who studied both medical and veterinary problems in the 1840s, mathematicians have been interested in "epidemic curves" and secular trends in the incidence of infectious diseases. With the development of mathematical modeling using the computer there has been a resurgence of interest in the dynamics of infectious diseases within populations. Since modeling involves predictions about future occurrences of diseases, models carry a degree of uncertainty; it is sometimes said that "for every model there is an equal and opposite model."

Although our present knowledge of the epidemiology of infectious diseases has been derived from the analysis of field data, mathematical models are now being developed to predict various epidemiologic parameters. These include the critical population sizes required to support the continuous transmission of animal viruses with short and long incubation periods, the dynamics of endemicity of viruses that establish persistent infection, and the important variables in age-dependent viral pathogenicity.

Computer modeling also provides insights into the effectiveness of disease control programs. In this regard, most attention has been given to the potential national and international spread of exotic virus diseases. Figure 14-1 illustrates the modeling of an outbreak of foot-and-mouth disease in the United States, commencing with the introduction of the virus, and progressing through discovery of its presence to the stage where the disease becomes well established and the traditional control measures (quarantine, slaughter, and disinfection) become ineffective. The model suggests that in the so-called worst-case scenario, 60% of the cattle herds in the United States could become infected within a 30-week period. In this model, if it were decided not to vaccinate or if sufficient vaccine of the correct antigenic type were not available, the disease would increase again in incidence after 60 weeks and begin a series of endemic cycles. Such models bring a number of issues into focus. The results are often unexpected, pointing to the need for better data and different strategies for disease control.

VIRUS TRANSMISSION

Viruses survive in nature only if they are able to be transmitted from one host to another, whether of the same or another species. Transmission cycles require virus entry into the body, replication, and shedding with subsequent spread to another host. These aspects of viral activity

---

FIG. 14-1. *(A) A state-transition model of a major epizootic of foot-and-mouth disease in the United States from the point of virus introduction, through the time of discovery of its presence, to the stage where the disease is well established and traditional control measures (quarantine, slaughter, and disinfection) are no longer effective. The model is based on data from a 1967–1968 epizootic in the United Kingdom, during which outbreaks*

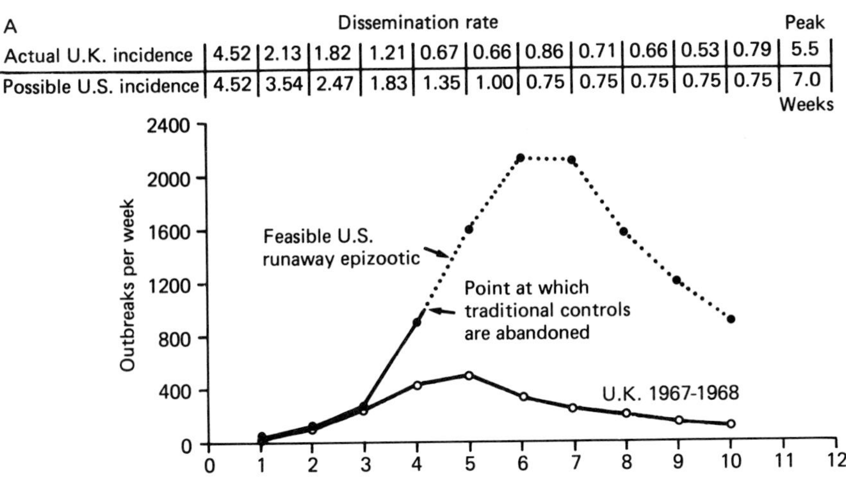

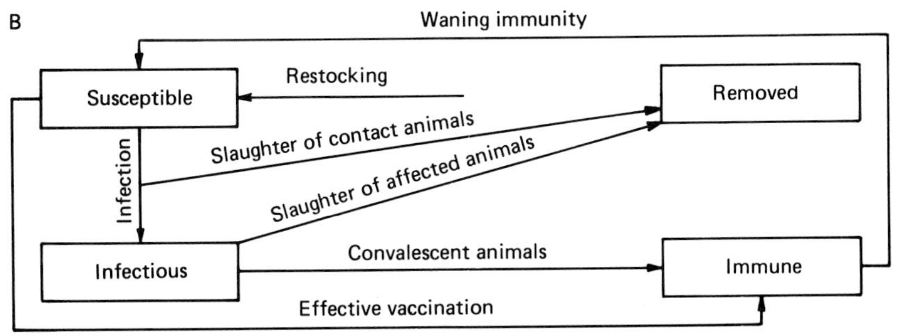

were recorded on 2364 farms. The model permits a variety of disease-control strategies to be examined. It illustrates several key characteristics of a useful model: its pathways are intuitively acceptable; it behaves in a biologically and mathematically logical way (i.e., it is sensitive to appropriate variables); it mimics real-life situations; and it is simple enough to be rigorously tested, but is not naively simplistic. (From M. W. Miller, 1979.) (B) In the model the basic unit is the herd. Each herd is considered to be in one of four mutually exclusive categories: "susceptible," "infectious," "immune," or "removed/dead." For each week the probability of transition from one category to another and the number of herds expected to be in each category during the next week are calculated. A key factor in determining the probability of a susceptible herd becoming infected in a particular week is the dissemination rate, which is the average number of herds to which the virus spreads from each infected herd. This depends on a number of factors such as topography, weather, husbandry, animal movement, and quarantine effectiveness. The dissemination rate used in the model is based on that calculated for the 1967–1968 epidemic in the United Kingdom. With this dissemination rate, a situation wherein traditional control methods fail is reached 4 to 5 weeks after introduction of the virus.

are described in relation to individual animals in Chapters 3 and 6; here we mention only those aspects that are relevant to epidemiology.

Virus transmission may be *horizontal* or *vertical*. Transmission is usually horizontal, that is, between individuals within the population at risk, and can occur via direct contact, indirect contact, or a common vehicle; or the virus may be airborne, vector-borne, or iatrogenic. Vertical transmission describes transmission from parent, usually the mother, to its offspring. Some viruses are transmitted in nature via several modes, others exclusively via one mode (Table 14-1).

TABLE 14-1
Common Modes of Transmission of Viruses of Animals

Virus family	Mode of transmission
Parvoviridae	Fecal–oral, respiratory, contact, transplacental (e.g., feline parvovirus)
Papovaviridae	Direct contact, skin abrasions (e.g., papillomaviruses)
Adenoviridae	Respiratory, fecal–oral
Herpesviridae	Sexual (e.g., equine coital exanthema virus)
	Respiratory (e.g., infectious bovine rhinotracheitis virus)
	Transplacental (e.g., pseudorabies)
Poxviridae	Contact (e.g., orf, cowpox)
	Arthropod (mechanical, e.g., myxoma virus)
African swine fever virus	Fecal–oral, respiratory, arthropod
Picornaviridae	Fecal–oral (e.g., swine enteroviruses)
	Respiratory (e.g., equine rhinoviruses)
	Ingestion of garbage (e.g., foot-and-mouth disease viruses to pigs)
Caliciviridae	Respiratory, fecal–oral, contact
Togaviridae	Arthropod (e.g., Venezuelan equine encephalitis virus)
Flaviviridae	Arthropod (e.g., Japanese encephalitis virus)
	Respiratory, fecal–oral, transplacental (e.g., bovine virus diarrhea virus)
Paramyxoviridae	Respiratory, contact
Coronaviridae	Fecal–oral, respiratory, contact
Rhabdoviridae	Arthropod and contact (e.g., vesicular stomatitis)
	Animal bite (e.g., rabies virus)
Orthomyxoviridae	Respiratory
Bunyaviridae	Arthropod (e.g., Rift Valley fever virus)
Arenaviridae	Contact with contaminated urine, respiratory
Reoviridae	Fecal–oral (e.g., calf rotavirus)
	Arthropod (e.g., bluetongue viruses)
Birnaviridae	Fecal–oral, water
Retroviridae	Contact, *in ovo* (germ line)
	Ingestion, mechanically by arthropods

Virus Entry

Portals of entry of viruses into the body include the skin, conjunctiva, respiratory tract, oropharynx, intestinal tract, and urogenital tract. In some cases, viruses make use of a particular portal of entry because of environmental or host behavioral factors and in other cases because of specific viral attachment or penetration factors. In many cases, failure of normal host defense mechanisms leads to entry that might not otherwise occur; for example, papillomaviruses may enter the deep layers of the skin via abrasions, acid-labile coronaviruses may enter the intestine protected by the buffering capacity of milk, and opportunistic bacteria may enter the lower respiratory tract because an ongoing respiratory viral infection has dampened the action of cilia on respiratory epithelium.

Horizontal Transmission

Direct Contact Transmission. Direct contact transmission involves actual physical contact between an infected animal and a susceptible animal [e.g., licking, rubbing, biting (rabies), and coitus (sexually or venereally transmitted diseases)].

Indirect Contact Transmission. Indirect contact transmission occurs via *fomites,* such as shared eating containers, bedding, dander, restraint devices, vehicles, clothing, improperly sterilized surgical equipment, or improperly sterilized syringes or needles.

Common Vehicle Transmission. Common vehicle transmission includes fecal contamination of food and water supplies (fecal–oral transmission, e.g., rotaviruses) and virus-contaminated meat or bone products (e.g., for the transmission of vesicular exanthema of swine, hog cholera, pseudorabies, and bovine spongiform encephalopathy).

Airborne Transmission. *Airborne transmission,* resulting in infection of the respiratory tract, occurs via droplets and droplet nuclei (aerosols) emitted from infected animals during coughing or sneezing (e.g., influenza) or from environmental sources such as dander or dust from bedding (e.g., Marek's disease). Large droplets settle quickly, but microdroplets evaporate to form droplet nuclei (less than 5 μm in diameter) which remain suspended in the air for extended periods. Droplets may travel only 1 meter or so, but droplet nuclei may travel long distances, even many kilometers if wind and other weather conditions are favorable (e.g., with foot-and-mouth disease virus).

Arthropod-Borne Transmission. Arthropod-borne transmission involves the bites of arthropod vectors; for example, mosquitoes transmit equine encephalitis viruses, ticks transmit African swine fever, and culicoid midges transmit bluetongue (see Table 14-4).

Vertical Transmission

The term vertical transmission is usually used to describe infection that is transferred from mother to embryo/fetus/newborn prior to, during, or shortly after parturition, although some writers prefer to restrict the term to situations where infection occurs before birth. Certain retroviruses are vertically transmitted via the integration of viral DNA into the germ-line DNA (see Fig. 33-5). Other viruses are transmitted to the fetus via the placenta; yet others are transmitted when the newborn passes through the birth canal. Another mode of vertical transmission is via colostrum and milk (e.g., caprine arthritis–encephalitis virus). Vertical transmission of a virus may cause early embryonic death or abortion (e.g., with several lentiviruses), or it may be associated with congenital disease (e.g., bovine virus diarrhea virus), or the infection may be the cause of congenital defects (e.g., Akabane virus). Herpesviruses of many species and parvoviruses of several species are important causes of congenital diseases.

Other Categories of Transmission

Other terms used to describe transmission may embrace more than one of the above routes.

Iatrogenic Transmission. *Iatrogenic* transmission (caused by the hand of the doctor) may involve the veterinarian (or other person) in the course of caring for animals. Iatrogenic transmission has been important in the spread of equine infectious anemia virus via multiple-use syringes and needles. Similarly, chickens have been infected with reticuloendotheliosis virus via contaminated Marek's disease vaccine.

Nosocomial Transmission. *Nosocomial* transmission occurs while an animal is in a hospital or clinic. During the peak of the canine parvovirus epidemic in the 1980s, many pups became infected in veterinary hospitals. Feline respiratory virus infections are also often acquired nosocomially.

Zoonotic Transmission. Because most viruses are host-restricted, most viral infections are maintained in nature within populations of the same or related species. However, there are a number of viruses that may have multiple hosts and spread naturally between several different species of animals (e.g., rabies and Eastern equine encephalitis viruses). The term *zoonosis* is used to describe infections that are transmissible from animals to man (Tables 14-2 and 14-5). The zoonoses, whether involving domestic or wild animals, usually represent important problems only under conditions where humans are engaged in activities involving close contact with animals.

TABLE 14-2
Nonarthropod-Borne Viral Zooneses

Virus family	Virus	Reservoir host	Mode of transmission to humans
Herpesviridae	B virus	Monkey	Animal bite
Poxviridae	Cowpox virus	Rodents, cattle, cats	Contact, through skin abrasions
	Monkeypox virus	Squirrels, monkeys	Contact, through oral and skin abrasions
	Pseudocowpox virus	Cattle	Contact, through skin abrasions
	Orf virus	Sheep, goats	Contact, through skin abrasions
Rhabdoviridae	Rabies virus	Terrestrial mammals and bats	Animal bite, scratch
	Vesicular stomatitis virus[a]	Cattle	Contact with oral secretions or vesicular fluids
Filoviridae	Ebola, Marburg viruses	?Monkeys	Contact, iatrogenic (injection) human-to-human spread
Orthomyxoviridae	Influenza A virus	Swine, birds	Respiratory
Bunyaviridae	Hantaan virus	Rodents	Contact with rodent urine
Arenaviridae	Lymphocytic choriomeningitis virus Junin virus Guanarito virus Machupo virus Lassa virus	Rodents	Contact with rodent urine

[a] May be arthropod-borne.

MECHANISMS FOR SURVIVAL OF VIRUSES IN NATURE

Survival of a virus in nature depends on the maintenance of serial infections; the occurrence of disease is neither required nor necessarily advantageous. As knowledge of the different features of the pathogenesis, species susceptibility, routes of transmission, and environmental stability has increased, epidemiologists have been able to recognize four different mechanisms by which viruses maintain serial transmission in their hosts: acute self-limiting infections, persistent infections, vertical transmission, and arthropod transmission. An appreciation of these mechanisms for viral perpetuation is valuable in designing and implementing control programs.

The resistance of a virus to destruction when exposed to the environment affects the efficiency of survival; in general it is found that viruses that are transmitted by the respiratory route have low environmental stability and those transmitted by the fecal–oral route have a higher stability. Sometimes this factor plays a major role in perpetuation. Thus stability of the virus, either in water, on fomites, or on the mouthparts of mechanical arthropod vectors, favors transmission, a mechanism that is particularly important in small or dispersed animal communities. For example, the parapoxvirus that causes orf in sheep survives for months on pastures, and during the winter myxoma virus can survive for many weeks on the mouthparts of mosquitoes.

Most viruses have a principal mechanism for survival in nature, but if this mechanism is interrupted, for example, by a sudden decline in population of the host species, a second, or even a third, mechanism may exist as a "backup." For example, in bovine virus diarrhea there is an acute fecal–oral primary transmission cycle, backed up by the persistent shedding of virus by congenitally infected calves. This feature should be remembered when relating the epidemiology of a specific disease to particular mechanisms of perpetuation, as proposed in Table 14-3.

Population size and density play a role in virus survival that depends in the main on whether the virus produces acute self-limiting or persistent infections. In general, local survival of viruses that produce acute nonpersistent infections requires that the susceptible host population should be large and relatively dense. Such viruses may disappear from a particular population because they exhaust the supply of susceptible hosts as they become immune. Whether or not the initial infection is acute, persistent viruses may survive in very small populations, sometimes by infecting progeny. Depending on the breeding characteristics of the animal (population turnover rate), duration of immunity, and the pattern of virus shedding, the *critical population size* varies considerably with different viruses and different host species.

TABLE 14-3
Modes of Survival of Viruses in Nature

Virus family	Example	Mode of survival
Papovaviridae	Papillomaviruses	Persistent in lesions; virus stable
Adenoviridae	Canine adenovirus 1	Persistent infection; virus stable
Herpesviridae	Bovine herpesvirus 1	Persistent infection
Poxviridae	Orf virus	Virus stable
African swine fever virus		Acute self-limiting infection; persistent infection in ticks
Picornaviridae	Foot-and-mouth disease virus	Acute self-limiting infection; sometimes persistent
Caliciviridae	Feline calicivirus	Acute self-limiting infection; virus stable
Togaviridae	Equine encephalitis viruses	Arthropod-borne
	Bovine virus diarrhea virus	Acute self-limiting infection; persistent after congenital infection
Flaviridae	Japanese encephalitis virus	Arthropod-borne
Coronaviridae	Feline infectious peritonitis	Acute self-limiting infection
Paramyxoviridae	Newcastle disease virus	Acute self-limiting infection; vertical with velogenic strains
Rhabdoviridae	Vesicular stomatitis virus	Acute self-limiting infection; virus stable, arthropod-borne
Orthomyxoviridae	Influenza A virus	Acute self-limiting infection
Bunyaviridae	Rift Valley fever virus	Arthropod-borne
Arenaviridae	Lassa virus	Persistent infection; vertical transmission
Reoviridae	Calf rotavirus	Acute self-limiting infection
	Bluetongue virus	Arthropod-borne
Birnaviridae	Infectious bursal disease virus	Acute self-limiting infection
Retroviridae	Avian leukosis virus	Persistent infection; vertical transmission

Acute Self-Limiting Infections

The most precise data on the importance of population size in acute, self-limiting infections come from studies of measles, which is a cosmopolitan human disease. Measles has long been a favorite disease for modeling epidemics, because it is one of the few common human diseases in which subclinical infections are rare, clinical diagnosis is easy, and postinfection immunity is lifelong. Measles virus is closely related to rinderpest and canine distemper viruses, and many aspects of the model apply well to these two viruses. Survival of measles virus in a population requires a continuous supply of susceptible hosts. Analyses of the incidence of measles in large cities and in island communities have shown that a population of about half a million persons is needed to ensure a large enough annual input of new susceptible hosts, by birth or immigration, to maintain measles virus in the population. Because infection depends on respiratory transmission, the duration of epidemics of measles is correlated inversely with population density. If a population is dispersed over a large area, the rate of spread is reduced and the epidemic will last longer, so that the number of susceptible persons needed to maintain transmission chains is reduced. On the other hand, in such a situation a break in the transmission chain is much more likely. When a large proportion of the population is initially susceptible, the intensity of the epidemic builds up quickly, and attack rates are almost 100% (*virgin-soil epidemic*). There are many examples of similar transmission patterns among viruses of domestic animals, but the quantitative data are not as complete as those for measles. *Exotic viruses*, that is, those which are not present in a particular country or region, represent the most important group of viruses with a potential for causing virgin-soil epidemics.

Persistent Infections

Persistent viral infections, whether or not they are associated with acute initial disease or with recurrent episodes of clinical disease, play an important role in the perpetuation of many viruses. For example, recurrent virus shedding by a persistently infected animal can reintroduce virus into a population of susceptible animals all of which have been born since the last clinically apparent episode of infection. This transmission pattern is important for the survival of bovine virus diarrhea virus, hog cholera virus, equine arteritis virus, and the herpesviruses, and such viruses have a much smaller critical population size than occur in acute self-limited infections, as small as a single farm, kennel, cattery, or breeding unit.

Sometimes the persistence of infection, the production of disease, and the transmission of virus are dissociated; for example, togavirus and arenavirus infections have little adverse effect on their reservoir hosts (arthropods, birds, and rodents) but transmission is very efficient. On the other hand, the persistence of infection in the central nervous system, as with canine distemper virus, is of no epidemiologic significance, since no infectious virus is shed from this site; infection of the central nervous system may have a severe effect on the dog, but it is of no consequence for survival of the virus. Infection with members of some viral families is characteristically associated with continuous or intermittent shedding;

certain other viruses cause acute infections which are associated with brief but high levels of virus shedding.

Vertical Transmission

Transmission of virus from the dam to the embryo, fetus, or newborn, as described above, can be important in virus survival in nature: all arenaviruses, several herpesviruses, parvoviruses, and retroviruses, some orbiviruses and togaviruses, and a few bunyaviruses and coronaviruses may be transmitted in this way (see Table 6-4). Indeed, if the consequence of vertical transmission is lifelong persistent infection, as in the case of arenaviruses and retroviruses, the long-term survival of the virus is assured. Virus transmission in the immediate perinatal period, by contact or via colostrum and milk, is also an important mode of transmission for some viruses. Vertical transmission in arthropod vectors is an important method of survival in nature of some arthropod-borne viruses.

Arthropod Transmission

Several arthropod-borne diseases are discussed in appropriate chapters of Part II; here we consider some common features that will be useful in understanding their epidemiology and control. Over 500 arboviruses are known, of which 16 cause disease in domestic animals (Table 14-4), and many viral zoonoses are caused by arboviruses (Table 14-5).

Rarely, arthropod transmission may be mechanical, as in myxomatosis and fowlpox, in which mosquitoes act as "flying pins." More commonly it involves replication of the virus in the arthropod vector, which may be a tick, a mosquito, a sandfly (*Phlebotomus*), or a midge (*Culicoides*). This is called *biological transmission.* The arthropod vector acquires virus by feeding on the blood of a viremic animal. Replication of the ingested virus, initially in the insect gut, and its spread to the salivary gland take several days (the *extrinsic incubation period*); the interval varies with different viruses and is influenced by ambient temperature. Virions in the salivary secretions of the vector are injected into new animal hosts during blood meals. Arthropod transmission provides a way for a virus to cross species barriers, since the same arthropod may bite birds, reptiles, and mammals that rarely or never come into close contact in nature.

Most arboviruses have localized natural habitats in which specific receptive arthropod and vertebrate hosts are involved in the viral life cycle. Vertebrate reservoir hosts are usually wild mammals or birds; domestic animals and humans are rarely involved in primary transmission cycles, although the exceptions to this generalization are important (e.g., Vene-

TABLE 14-4

Arthropod-Transmitted Viral Diseases of Domestic Animals

Virus family	Virus genus	Disease	Vertebrate hosts	Vector (replication[a])
Poxviridae	*Avipoxvirus*	Fowlpox, pigeonpox	Poultry, pigeons	Mosquito (−)
	Leporipoxvirus	Myxomatosis	Rabbit	Mosquito, flea, other arthropods (−)
African swine fever virus		African swine fever	Swine	Tick (+)
Togaviridae	*Alphavirus*	Equine encephalitides	Horse, human	Mosquito (+)
		Getah virus infection	Horse	Mosquito (+)
Flaviviridae	*Flavivirus*	Louping ill	Sheep	Tick (+)
		Wesselsbron disease	Sheep	Tick (+)
		Japanese encephalitis	Swine, human	Mosquito (+)
Bunyaviridae	*Phlebovirus*	Rift Valley fever	Sheep, cattle, human	Mosquito (+)
	Nairovirus	Nairobi sheep disease	Sheep	Tick (+)
	Bunyavirus (Akabane virus)	Arthrogyposis–hydranencephaly	Sheep, cattle	Mosquito (+)
Reoviridae	*Orbivirus*	Bluetongue	Sheep, cattle	*Culicoides* (+)
		Ibaraki virus infection	Cattle	?Species (+)
		Epizootic hemorrhagic disease of deer	Deer	*Culicoides* (+)
		African horse sickness	Horse	*Culicoides*, mosquitoes (+)
		Equine encephalosis	Horse	?Species (+)
Retroviridae	*Lentivirus*	Equine infectious anemia	Horse	Tabanids, other biting flies (−)

[a] (+), Biological transmission (viruses that replicate in their vector); (−), mechanical transmission.

TABLE 14-5

Arthropod-Borne Viral Zoonoses

Virus family	Virus genus	Disease	Reservoir hosts	Arthopod vector
Togaviridae	*Alphavirus*	Chikungunya virus infection	Mammals	
		Eastern equine encephalitis	Birds	
		Western equine encephalitis	Birds	Mosquitoes
		Venezuelan equine encephalitis	Mammals	
		Ross River virus infection	Mammals	
Flaviviridae	*Flavivirus*	Japanese encephalitis	Birds, swine	
		Murray Valley encephalitis	Birds	Mosquitoes
		Yellow fever	Monkeys	
		Kyasanur Forest disease	Monkeys	
		Louping ill	Mammals	
		Omsk hemorrhagic fever	Mammals	Ticks
		Powassan virus infection	Mammals	
		Tick-borne encephalitis	Mammals, birds	
Bunyaviridae	*Phlebovirus*	Rift Valley fever	Mammals	Mosquitoes
		Sandfly fever	Gerbils	*Phlebotomus*
	Nairovirus	Crimean–Congo hemorrhagic fever	Mammals	Ticks
	Bunyavirus	California encephalitis	Mammals	
		La Crosse encephalitis	Mammals	Mosquitoes
		Tahyna virus infection	Mammals	
Reoviridae	*Coltivirus*	Colorado tick fever	Mammals	Ticks

zuelan equine encephalitis virus in horses, yellow fever and dengue viruses in humans). Domestic animal species are in most cases infected incidentally, for example, by the geographic extension of a reservoir vertebrate host and/or a vector arthropod.

Most arboviruses that cause periodic epidemics have ecologically complex endemic cycles, which often involve different arthropod as well as different vertebrate hosts from those involved in epidemic cycles. Endemic cycles, which are generally poorly understood and inaccessible to effective control measures, provide for the amplification of virus and therefore are critical in dictating the magnitude of epidemics.

When arthropods are active, arboviruses replicate alternately in vertebrate and invertebrate hosts. A puzzle that has concerned many investigators has been to understand what happens to these viruses during the winter months in temperate climates, when the arthropod vectors are inactive. One important mechanism for "overwintering" is *transovarial* and *trans-stadial transmission.* Transovarial transmission occurs with the tick-borne flaviviruses and has been shown to occur with some mosquito-borne bunyaviruses and flaviviruses. Some bunyaviruses are found in high northern latitudes where the mosquito breeding season is too short to allow virus survival by horizontal transmission cycles alone; many of the first mosquitoes to emerge each summer carry virus as a result of transovarial and trans-stadial transmission, and the pool of virus is rapidly amplified by horizontal transmission in mosquito–mammal–mosquito cycles.

Vertical transmission in arthropods may not explain overwintering of all arboviruses, but other possibilities are still unproven or speculative. For example, hibernating vertebrates have been thought to play a role in overwintering. In cold climates, bats and some small rodents, as well as snakes and frogs, hibernate during the winter months. Their low body temperature has been thought to favor persistent infection, with recrudescent viremia occurring when the temperature rises in the spring. Although demonstrated in the laboratory, this mechanism has never been proven to occur in nature.

Many human activities disturb the natural ecology and hence natural arbovirus life cycles and have been incriminated in the geographic spread or increased prevalence of the diseases caused by these viruses: (1) population movements and the intrusion of man and domestic animals into new arthropod habitats, notably tropical forests; (2) deforestation, with development of new forest–farmland margins and exposure of domestic animals to new arthropods; (3) irrigation, especially primitive irrigation systems, which pay no attention to arthropod control; (4) uncontrolled urbanization, with vector populations breeding in accumulations of water and sewage; (5) increased long-distance air travel, with potential for carriage of arthropod vectors; (6) increased long-distance livestock transportation, with potential for carriage of viruses and arthropods (especially ticks); and (7) new routing of long-distance bird migrations brought about by new manmade water impoundments.

The history of the European colonization of Africa is replete with examples of "new" arbovirus diseases resulting from the introduction of susceptible European livestock into that continent, for example, African swine fever, African horse sickness, Rift valley fever, Nairobi sheep disease, and bluetongue. The viruses that cause these diseases are now feared in the industrialized countries as exotic viruses that may devastate their livestock. Another example of the importance of ecologic factors is the infection of horses in the eastern part of North America with Eastern equine encephalitis virus when their pasturage is made to overlap the natural swamp-based mosquito–bird–mosquito cycle of this virus. Similarly, in Japan and southeastern Asian countries, swine may become infected with Japanese encephalitis virus and become important amplifying hosts when they are bitten by mosquitoes that breed in rice fields.

Examples of the complexity of the life cycles of arboviruses are given in Chapters 21, 24, 25, 28, 30, 31, and 34. Mosquito-borne togaviruses and bunyaviruses cause several encephalitides in domestic animals (see Table 14-4). Most of these viruses cycle through wild birds or small mammals, with domestic animals being only incidental or dead-end hosts. However, in its epidemic cycle Venezuelan equine encephalitis virus can be maintained in a horse–mosquito–horse cycle, from which humans are easily infected by the same species of mosquitoes.

Tick-borne flaviviruses illustrate two features of epidemiologic importance. First, transovarial infection in ticks is often sufficient to ensure survival of the virus independently of a cycle in vertebrates; vertebrate infection amplifies the population of infected ticks. Second, for some of these viruses transmission from one vertebrate host to another, once initiated by the bite of an infected tick, can also occur by mechanisms not involving an arthropod. Thus, in central Europe and the eastern part of the Soviet Union, a variety of small rodents may be infected with tick-borne encephalitis virus. Goats, cows, and sheep are incidental hosts and sustain inapparent infections, but they excrete virus in their milk. Adult and juvenile ungulates may acquire the virus during grazing on tick-infected pastures, and newborn animals may be infected by drinking infected milk. Humans may be infected by being bitten by a tick or by drinking milk from an infected goat.

VARIATIONS IN DISEASE INCIDENCE ASSOCIATED WITH SEASONS AND ANIMAL MANAGEMENT PRACTICES

Many viral infections show pronounced seasonal variations in incidence. In temperate climates, arbovirus infections transmitted by mosquitoes or sandflies occur mainly during the summer months, when vectors are most numerous and active. Infections transmitted by ticks occur most commonly during the spring and early summer months. Other biological reasons for seasonal disease include both virus and host factors. Influenza viruses and poxviruses survive better in air at low rather than at high humidity, and in aerosols all viruses survive better at lower temperatures. It has also been suggested, without much supporting evidence, that there may be seasonal changes in the susceptibility of the host, perhaps associated with changes in the physiological status of nasal and oropharyngeal mucous membranes.

More important in veterinary medicine than any natural seasonal effects are the changes in housing and management practices that occur in different seasons. Housing animals such as cattle and sheep for the winter often increases the incidence of respiratory and enteric diseases. These diseases often have obscure primary etiologies, usually viral, followed by secondary infections caused by opportunistic pathogens (see Chapter 9). In such cases, infectious disease diagnosis, prevention, and treatment must be integrated into an overall system for the management of facilities as well as husbandry practices. In areas where animals are moved, for example, to feedlots or seasonally to distant pasturage, there are two major problems: animals are subjected to the stress of transportation, and they are brought into contact with new populations carrying and shedding different infectious agents. Often summer pasturage is at high altitude, adding the stress of pulmonary vascular dysfunction and pulmonary edema to the insult of respiratory virus infections. Secondary *Pasteurella* pneumonia, shipping fever, is not limited to animals subjected to the stress of transportation to feedlots.

In areas of the world where cattle are moved hundreds of miles each year, such as in the Sahelian zone of western Africa, viral diseases such as rinderpest are associated with the contact between previously separate populations brought about by this traditional husbandry practice. In southern Africa, the communal use of waterholes during the dry season promotes the exchange of viruses such as foot-and-mouth disease virus between different species of wildlife, and in certain circumstances between wildlife and domestic animals.

EPIDEMIOLOGIC ASPECTS OF IMMUNITY

Immunity acquired from prior infection or from vaccination plays a vital role in the epidemiology of viral diseases; in fact vaccination (see Chapter 13) is the single most effective method of controlling viral diseases. Canine distemper, caused by a single, antigenically stable virus, is associated with a very effective immune response. In industrialized countries widespread vaccination of puppies with attenuated live-virus canine distemper vaccine has sharply decreased the incidence of both canine distemper and its complications, old dog encephalitis and hard pad disease.

For some viruses immunity is relatively ineffective, because of the absence of antibodies at the site of infection (e.g., the respiratory or intestinal tract). Respiratory syncytial viruses cause mild to severe respiratory tract disease in cattle and sheep. Infections usually occur during the winter months when the animals are housed in confined conditions. The virus spreads rapidly by aerosol infection, and reinfection of the respiratory tract is not uncommon. Preexisting antibody, whether derived passively by maternal transfer or actively by prior infection, does not prevent viral replication and excretion, although clinical signs are usually mild where the antibody titer is high. Not surprisingly, vaccination is not very effective.

FURTHER READING

Anderson, R. M., and May, R. M. (1985). Herd immunity. *Nature* (*London*) **318,** 323.

Berg, E. (1987). "Methods of Recovering Viruses from the Environment." CRC Press, Boca Raton, Florida.

Black, F. L., and Singer, B. (1987). Elaboration versus simplification in refining mathematical models of infectious disease. *Annu. Rev. Microbiol.* **41,** 677.

Coyne, M. J., Smith, G., and McAllister, F. E. (1989). Mathematic model for the population biology of rabies in raccoons in the mid-Atlantic states. *Am. J. Vet. Res.* **50,** 2148.

Gibbs, E. P. J., ed. (1981). "Virus Diseases of Food Animals. A World Geography of Epidemiology and Control. Volume I, International Perspectives; Volume II, Disease Monographs." Academic Press, London.

Gloster, J. (1983). Forecasting the airborne spread of foot-and-mouth disease and Newcastle disease. *Philos. Trans. R. Soc. London Ser. B* **302,** 535.

James, A. D., and Rossiter, P. B. (1989). An epidemiological model of rinderpest. I. Description of the model. *Trop. Anim. Health Prod.* **21,** 59.

Kramer, M. S. (1988). "Clinical Epidemiology and Biostatistics." Springer-Verlag, New York.

Miller, W. M. (1979). A state-transition model of epidemic foot-and-mouth disease. *In* "A Study of the Potential Economic Impact of Foot-and-Mouth Disease in the United States"

(E. H. McCauley, N. A. Aulaqi, J. C. New, W. Sundquist, and W. M. Miller, eds.). U.S. Government Printing Office, Washington, D.C.

Mims, C. A. (1981). Vertical transmission of viruses. *Microbiol. Rev.* **41,** 267.

Pech, R. E., and Hone, J. (1988). A model of the dynamics and control of an outbreak of foot-and-mouth disease in feral pigs in Australia. *J. Appl. Biol.* **25,** 63.

Rossiter, P. B., and James, A. D. (1989). An epidemiological model of rinderpest. II. Simulations of the behavior of rinderpest in populations. *Trop. Anim. Health Prod.* **21,** 69.

Smith, G., and Grenfell, B. T. (1990). Population biology of pseudorabies in swine. *Am. J. Vet. Res.* **51,** 148.

CHAPTER 15

Disease Surveillance, Prevention, Control, and Treatment

Nowhere in veterinary medicine is the adage "an ounce of prevention is better than a pound of cure" more appropriate than in viral diseases. Apart from therapeutic regimes for ameliorating symptoms, for example, the administration of fluid in viral diarrheas, or using antibiotics to prevent secondary bacterial infections after viral respiratory diseases, there are no effective and practical treatments for viral diseases of domestic animals. However, there are many well proven approaches to their prevention, control, and eradication. The most generally useful control measure is the use of vaccines (see Chapter 13). On-farm hygiene and sanitation are important methods of controlling fecal–oral infections, and vector control on a regional basis may be useful for arbovirus diseases. Exotic diseases may be excluded by national quarantine programs. Finally, either local, regional, national, continental, or global eradication may be considered. Countrywide elimination is widely practiced in industrialized countries if serious exotic diseases gain entry.

CHANGING PATTERNS OF ANIMAL PRODUCTION

Since the 1950s there has been a revolution in systems of food animal management and production, and these changes have had profound effects on disease patterns and control. Throughout much of the industrialized and nearly all of the developing world, systems of animal production for food and fiber are traditional or extensive, typified by the grazing of sheep and cattle across vast areas in the Americas and Australia, or the movement of small herds of cattle or goats across the Sahel or in Somalia by nomadic tribes. Chickens and swine were penned and housed centuries ago, but intensive animal production systems, particularly for chickens and swine, were developed from the middle of this century. In the industrialized world, they are now almost the only method of production for these species, and similar intensive systems are used for some classes of cattle. Infectious diseases, particularly viral diseases, have often been the rate- and profit-limiting step in the development of such systems.

Significant aspects of intensive animal production include the following: (1) the bringing together of large numbers of animals, often from diverse backgrounds, and confining them to limited spaces, at high density; (2) asynchronous turnoff of animals for sale and the introduction of new animals; (3) the care of large numbers of animals by few, sometimes inadequately trained, personnel; (4) elaborate housing systems, with complex mechanical services for ventilation, feeding, waste disposal, and cleaning; (5) limitation of the husbandry system to one species; (6) manipulation of natural biological rhythms (artificial daylight, estrus synchronization, etc.); (7) use of very large batches of premixed, easily digestible foodstuffs; (8) improved hygienic conditions; and (9) isolation of animal populations.

Some figures from the United States illustrate the scale of operations of intensive animal production units. A large cattle feedlot operation in Colorado has at any one time 100,000 cattle held in 1-acre pens of 400 each, and 2.5 batches are processed each year. A single farrowing house in Iowa may hold 5000 sows; on a fully integrated "farrow-to-finish" farm there may at any one time be 50,000 swine, of which 45,000 are sold and replaced 2.2 times a year. A dairy farm in California may milk 5000 cows. A single broiler house in Georgia may house 50,000 birds, and the farm may comprise six such houses; several farms are often located in close proximity. The growing time for a broiler chicken is 9 weeks, so that 1.7 million chickens may be produced on a single farm each year. There are also intensive systems for producing veal calves and lambs. Three consequences follow from these situations. (1) The conditions favor the emergence and spread of endemic infectious diseases, as well as opportunistic infections. (2) The introduction of nonendemic viruses poses a great risk to such populations, although many farms are designed to provide reliable barriers against such introductions. (3) These conditions favor multiple infections working synergistically, further complicating diagnosis, prevention, and therapy.

None of the basic characteristics of intensive livestock production systems are going to change because of disease constraints; the economics of these systems is such that losses due to diseases are generally small relative to gains, due mainly to feed and labor efficiency. Nevertheless, there is great merit in improving these production systems by minimizing disease losses, and thereby increasing yields and lowering costs. The chief constraint is management, the solution requiring the introduction of modern epidemiologic methods into the training and experience of veterinarians and other animal scientists concerned with livestock production.

While intensive livestock production units are common in most industrialized countries, the production of sheep, goats, and in some cases cattle in these countries still follows traditional extensive farming methods, which resemble production systems that pertain to all species in most developing countries. In the latter, husbandry is often primitive, but requirements for animal products have greatly increased because of the continually expanding human populations. For example, in the Sahel installation of watering points has led to buildup of herds in good seasons, with disastrous results when droughts occur or when epidemic diseases enter the region. More frequent and extensive movement of stock and people exacerbates the spread of infectious diseases, especially in Africa where the large populations of wildlife harbor many viral diseases that affect introduced livestock. These are matters of national and international concern, not only for humanitarian reasons, but because of the risk of the international transfer of exotic viruses of livestock and the disastrous consequences such importations could have on animal production industries in the industrialized countries.

The situation with companion animals is very different. However, the risk of infectious diseases varies greatly between the single, mature-age household dog, cat, or pony and the large breeding establishments for these species, in which several hundred animals, of all ages, are kept and bred.

DISEASE SURVEILLANCE

The implementation of disease control programs is critically dependent on accurate information about the existence and extent of occurrence of particular viral diseases. *Surveillance* of infectious diseases provides this basic information; it is the systematic and regular collection, collation, and analysis of data on disease occurrence. Its main purpose is to detect changes in trends and distribution of diseases.

The need for data on the occurrence of infectious diseases has led to the concept of "reportable" (notifiable) diseases, whereby veterinary practitioners are required to report to a central authority such as the local or state veterinary authority. Clearly the list of such diseases must not be too large, or notification will be ignored. However, data provided by a system of notification influence decisions on resource allocation for the control of diseases and the intensity of follow-up. Such data can also provide useful information on strategies of prevention, especially by allowing calculations of cost/benefit ratios and indices of vaccine efficacy.

Sources of Surveillance Data

The methods of surveillance commonly used for animal diseases are (1) notifiable disease reporting, (2) laboratory-based surveillance, and (3) population-based surveillance. The key to surveillance is the veterinary practitioner. Although any one practitioner may see only a few cases of a particular disease, data from many practitioners can be accumulated and analyzed to reveal trends in the occurrence of diseases. An important component of effective surveillance, especially for exotic or unusual diseases, is the presence of a heightened awareness among veterinary practitioners. Once information is collected from the practitioners, it is collated by the regional veterinary public health office.

There are seven sources of information on disease incidence, not all of which are required for any one disease:

1. Morbidity and mortality data assessed through material submitted to national, state, and local diagnostic laboratories.
2. Case and outbreak investigations linked to diagnostic laboratories.
3. Analyses of vaccine manufacture and use.
4. Reviews of local media reports of disease.
5. Monitoring of virus activity by clinical, serologic, and virologic examination of animals presented for slaughter at abattoirs, tested for legal movement, or exposed as sentinels to detect arbovirus activity.
6. Monitoring of arthropod populations and virus infection rates to detect arbovirus activity.
7. Specific serologic and virologic surveys.

Having collected the data, it is important that they should be analyzed quickly enough to influence the institution of control measures. Dissemination of information, namely, the provision of feedback from the state veterinary authority to the local veterinary practitioner, is a vital component of an effective surveillance system.

Investigation and Action in Disease Outbreaks

When there is a disease outbreak, it must first be recognized, hopefully at the level of primary veterinary care. This is not always easy when a disease emerges in a new setting. The only way that shortcomings in recognition can be avoided is by an elevation in the "index of suspicion," which is instilled as part of professional training. The strategy for investigation and action is dictated by the diagnosis itself. For diseases that are identified as endogenous or sporadically present in the given animal population, outbreaks are usually handled by veterinary practitioners working directly with livestock producers. For diseases that are identified as exotic or as having epidemic potential, most further investigation and action depends on available organization and expertise. Early in an outbreak investigation is focused on (1) identification of the etiologic agent, (2) measurement of population susceptibility and acquired immunity, (3) quantitation of the magnitude of the outbreak and the rate of spread, and (4) a search for reservoirs and modes of transmission.

In the usual endemic circumstances, disease control may be based on routine activities such as immunizations or control of arthropods. However, in epidemic circumstances, control programs more commonly require delivery of a whole package of resources, including technically trained personnel, special equipment, supplies, transportation, and funds. Resource needs might be of such magnitude as to support large-scale tasks such as the limitation of movement of animals or even the implementation of quarantine under national or international regulations.

HYGIENE AND SANITATION

Intensive animal husbandry leads to a buildup in the local environment of feces, urine, hair, feathers, etc., which may be contaminated with viruses. For viruses that are thermostable, the buildup of such contamination provides a ready source of virus for infecting newly introduced livestock. To avoid this, many pork, veal, and poultry farmers operate an "all in, all out" management system, by which the animal houses are emptied, cleaned, and disinfected between groups of animals.

Hygiene and disinfection are most effective in the control of fecal–oral infections; they have much less effect on the incidence of respiratory infections. In general, attempts to achieve "air sanitation" have failed, and respiratory viral infections constitute the single most important group of diseases in intensive animal production systems.

Nosocomial Infections

Nosocomial infections are less common in large animal veterinary practice, since such animals are usually treated on the farm, than in companion animal medicine. The use of appointment systems in veterinary practices reduces the risk of disease transmission in the waiting room; further, the preference of many clients to wait in their cars so that their animals become less excited also cuts down the risk of disease transmission. Veterinary clinics should require that all inpatients have current immunization records or receive booster immunization. Clinics should be designed for easy disinfection, with wash-down walls and flooring, and as few permanent fixtures as possible. They should also have efficient ventilation or air conditioning, not only to minimize odors, but also to reduce the aerosol transmission of viruses. Frequent hand washing and decontamination of contaminated equipment are essential.

Disinfection and Disinfectants

Disinfectants are chemical germicides formulated for use on inanimate surfaces, in contrast to *antiseptics,* which are chemical germicides designed for use on the skin or mucous membranes. Disinfection of contaminated premises plays an important role in the control of diseases of livestock.

Viruses of different families vary greatly in their resistance to disinfectants, enveloped viruses usually being much more sensitive than nonenveloped viruses. However, most modern disinfectants rapidly inactivate all viruses. Their effective action is influenced by access, and virus trapped in heavy layers of mucus or fecal material will not always be inactivated. Standard requirements by the U.S. Environmental Protection Agency specify that test viruses must be suspended in 5% serum and dried on a hard surface before testing the efficacy of a disinfectant. There are special problems when surfaces cannot be cleaned thoroughly or where cracks and crevices are relatively inaccessible, as in old timber buildings or the fence posts and railings of cattle and sheep yards.

Table 15-1 sets out some common disinfectants and their potential uses. The first five classes of compounds listed can be used in animal quarters, although some are too expensive for large-scale use. The second five are of use primarily in the consulting room, hospital, or laboratory. Lye (2% NaOH) is inexpensive and has been the traditional agent for large-scale disinfection of farm premises following outbreaks of foot-and-

TABLE 15-1
Commercially Available Disinfectants Used to Inactivate Viruses[a]

Disinfectant	Uses	Remarks
Sodium hypochlorite (Clorox, Chlorize)	Drinking water, food and utensils, dairies, spot disinfection	Highly effective, but high protein concentrations interfere; inexpensive, nontoxic, rapid action
Detergent iodophores (Betadine, Wescadine, Redene)	Same as sodium hypochlorite	Action based on slow release of iodine and detergent action; less affected by high protein concentrations than sodium hypochlorite; expensive
Formaldehyde (formalin)	Laundry, bedding surfaces, and as vapor for surface sterilization	Low power of penetration, but useful for terminal disinfection; irritating, hypersensitivity develops
Phenol derivatives (Lysol, Dettol, Staphene, Sudol)	2.5% Aqueous solution for hands, examination tables, cages, hospital surfaces	Efficacy depends on concentration and temperature; high protein concentrations interfere
Chlorhexidine (Hibitane, Nolvasan)	Wide range, examination tables, cages, hospital surfaces	Little affected by body fluids, soap, organic compounds; expensive
Ethylene dioxide	For heat-sensitive medical supplies, plastic isolators	Toxic and explosive except as mixture, 10% with 90% CO_2, which is available commercially as compressed gas
Glutaraldehyde (Cidex)	Cold sterilization of instruments with lenses	2% Solution buffered with sodium bicarbonate is virucidal in 10 minutes at pH 7.5–8.5; expensive
Alcohol (ethyl, isopropyl)	Hands, thermometers	Moderately virucidal only in high concentrations (70–80%); ethanol preferable to methanol or isopropanol; nontoxic
Quaternary ammonium compounds (Zephiran, Roccal, Savlon)	Zephiran (benzalkonium chloride) used for cleansing wounds	Not very effective against many viruses; high protein concentrations interfere

[a] Based on data supplied by Professor J. Storz.

mouth disease and other exotic viral diseases. Hot water containing detergent and steam sterilization are also useful for the decontamination of livestock premises.

CONTROL OF ARTHROPOD VECTORS

Control of arbovirus infections relies, where possible, on the use of vaccines, because of the large areas and extended periods over which vectors may be active. However, vector control is an important adjunct control strategy. For example, aerial spraying with ultra-low-volume insecticides is used to prevent the establishment of mosquito populations carrying Western equine encephalitis and St. Louis encephalitis viruses in some parts of North America.

Elimination of cracks and crevices in pigpens (in which soft ticks can hide) has been important in the control of African swine fever in Spain (see Chapter 21). A similar approach has been found to be successful in South Africa, where swine are double-fenced to avoid contact with warthogs. In the case of many other arbovirus infections, vector arthropods breed over too wide an area to make vector control feasible. In Australia and New Zealand, spraying of the luggage bays of overseas aircraft with insecticides reduces the chances of intercontinental transfer of exotic arthropods, whether infected or not.

VACCINATION

As outlined in Chapter 13 and discussed at length in the chapters of Part II, there are now effective vaccines for many viral diseases of animals. These vaccines are especially effective against diseases with a viremic phase caused by monotypic viruses, such as canine distemper virus. It has proved much more difficult to immunize effectively against infections of the digestive or respiratory tracts, or the skin. The effect of vaccination programs in reducing the incidence of canine distemper in urban communities and foot-and-mouth disease in European livestock has been dramatic (Fig. 15-1).

The introduction of recombinant DNA vaccines containing deletion mutants, linked to the ability to differentiate by serologic tests animals that have been exposed to natural infection from those that have been vaccinated, has opened up a new arena whereby vaccination and elimination programs are conducted concurrently (see Chapter 13). Several such vaccines for pseudorabies, with corresponding ELISA test kits for differentiating vaccinated and naturally infected swine, are commercially avail-

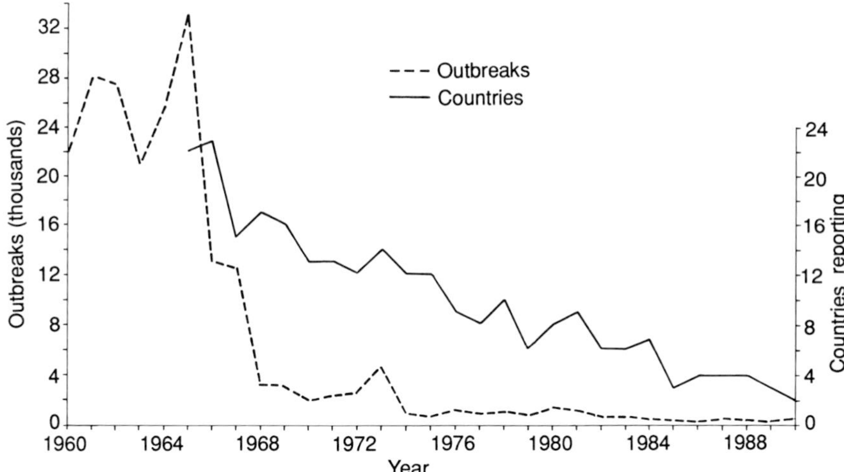

FIG. 15-1. *Foot-and-mouth disease in Europe, 1960–1990, showing numbers of outbreaks and numbers of countries reporting cases each year. The reduction since the mid-1960s is due to the effective use of trivalent inactivated vaccines (types A, O, and C). Since 1977 (with the exception of an epidemic in Italy in 1986–1987) over two-thirds of the outbreaks each year have occurred in the Anatolian (Asian) region of Turkey. In 1990, only Turkey and the U.S.S.R. reported foot-and-mouth disease; of the 547 outbreaks, 542 were in Anatolian Turkey; the location (Europe or Asia) of the five outbreaks in the U.S.S.R. was not available. (Data from the European Commission for the Control of Foot-and-Mouth Disease,* in *"Animal Health Yearbook." FAO, Rome, 1990.)*

able and in use in Europe, New Zealand, and the United States to eradicate the disease. Recombinant vaccinia-vectored rabies vaccines are currently being used in Europe, the United States, Canada, and some countries in Africa to control infection in wildlife species.

QUARANTINE

Movement of domestic animals across international and even state borders can be regulated, at least in the industrialized countries, where there are appropriate veterinary services and regulatory infrastructure, and quarantine remains a cornerstone in many animal disease control programs. A period of quarantine, with or without specific etiologic or serologic testing, is usually a requirement for the importation of animals from another country, and similar requirements may be enforced within a country or local area to assist in the control or eradication of specific infectious agents.

As international movement of live animals for breeding purposes and exhibition has increased, so also has the risk of introducing disease. Before the advent of air transport, the duration of shipment usually exceeded the incubation period of most diseases, but this is no longer the case. With the ever-increasing value of livestock, national veterinary authorities have tended to adopt stricter quarantine regulations to protect their livestock industries. Complete embargoes on importation are imposed for some animals by some countries. The original concept of quarantine, where animals were simply isolated and observed for disease for a given period of time, is now augmented by extensive laboratory testing designed to detect previous exposure to selected viruses or a carrier state. Laboratory testing requirements are set down in detailed protocols and supported by national legislation.

While dog and cat quarantine has been a successful method for preventing the introduction of many diseases, such as rabies into Australia, New Zealand, and Great Britain, other diseases may be introduced in animal products (e.g., foot-and-mouth disease in meat products) or by virus-infected arthropods (e.g., bluetongue). It must also be recognized that most countries have land boundaries with their neighbors and cannot easily control human and wildlife movement (e.g., the movement of rabies via foxes in Europe). For countries with long land borders, quarantine is difficult to enforce. To help overcome this problem, most countries have agreed to notify each other through the Office International des Epizooties (OIE) in Paris, France, of the disease status of their livestock. Although the recognition of internationally acceptable criteria for reporting the presence of specific diseases remains a problem, the system usually provides countries with an opportunity to take appropriate action (e.g., increased vigilance along a national boundary, maintenance of vaccine stocks). However, there is still a long way to go in developing standards for testing animals and controlling animal movement. The problems are often social, economic, and political rather than scientific; for example, smuggling of exotic birds may play a significant role in the introduction of Newcastle disease and fowl plague viruses.

ELIMINATION/ERADICATION OF VIRAL DISEASES

Control, whether by vaccination alone or by vaccination plus the various methods of hygiene and sanitation aimed at lessening the chance of infection, is an ongoing process which must be maintained as long as the disease is of economic importance. If a disease can be eradicated, so that the virus is no longer present anywhere except in microbiologically secure laboratories, control measures are no longer required. The term *eradication* is best restricted to elimination on a global or at least a continental scale; the lesser but still valuable goal of countrywide eradication is usually termed *elimination.* Both elimination and eradication of a disease that is endemic demand major financial commitments for a long period, often decades, if success is to be achieved. Close cooperation between veterinary services and the farming industry is essential. To achieve such cooperation the veterinary services of a country must justify their proposals by cost–benefit analyses and consult with all interested organizations. As the control program proceeds they must ensure feedback of information on progress (or problems) directly to those involved, or via the media.

Foot-and-mouth disease has now been eliminated from a number of countries in which it was once established: Japan, the United Kingdom, the United States, Mexico, and the countries of Central America. Rinderpest, once a devastating disease of cattle in Europe, was finally eliminated from that continent in 1949, and rabies was eliminated from the United Kingdom in 1901 and again in 1922, after reintroduction of the disease during World War I.

So far, global eradication has been achieved for only one disease, and that a disease of man. The last endemic case of smallpox occurred in Somalia in October 1977. Global eradication was achieved by an intensified effort that involved a high level of international cooperation and made use of a potent and very stable vaccine that was easy to administer. However, mass vaccination alone could not have achieved eradication of the disease from the densely populated tropical countries where it remained endemic in the 1970s, because it was impossible to achieve the necessary high level of vaccination. The effective strategy was to combine vaccination with *surveillance and containment,* by which cases were actively sought out, isolated, and their contacts vaccinated, first in the household and then at increasing distances from the index case.

The achievement of global eradication of smallpox led to discussions as to whether any other diseases could be eradicated worldwide. Smallpox was unusual in that, given an effective vaccine, all of its biological characteristics enhanced the possibility of global eradication (Table 15-2). Yet this was achieved only after an immense and sustained international effort.

The biological characteristics that would render more likely the elimination or global eradication of viral diseases of livestock are as follows: (1) no wildlife reservoir host, (2) no reservoir or carrier host, (3) lack of recurrent disease and virus shedding, (4) only one or few stable serotypes, and (5) an effective vaccine. No less important is the level of public

TABLE 15-2

Biological Characteristics Enhancing Chances of Eradication

Characteristic	Human smallpox	Canine distemper	Newcastle disease	Bovine rinderpest	Foot-and-mouth disease
Reservoir host in wildlife	No	No	Yes	Yes	Yes, in Africa
Persistent infection occurs	No	No	No	No	Yes, especially in buffalo
Subclinical cases occur	No	No	Yes	Unusual	Yes
Number of serotypes	1	1	1	1	7
Infectivity during prodromal stage	No	Yes	Yes	Yes	Yes, very infectious
Vaccine					
Effective	Yes	Yes	Yes	Yes	Usually but type-specific polyvalent formulation used
Heat-stable	Yes	Moderately	Moderately	No[a]	Yes
Number of doses	1	1	2	1	2, then annually or semiannually
Early containment of outbreak possible	Yes	No	Sometimes	Yes	Difficult
High level of public concern	Yes	No	Yes	Yes	Yes

[a] A vaccinia virus–rinderpest glycoprotein recombinant vaccine is available that overcomes this problem, but it has not yet (1991) been licensed.

concern, for any eradication program requires a sustained commitment of human and financial resources. Applying these criteria, it becomes obvious that rinderpest could be eradicated. In fact, several industrialized nations of the world eliminated the disease by a test and slaughter ("stamping out") policy before vaccines were available, in some cases even before the viral etiology of the disease was recognized. In the 1960s, when an effective pan-African vaccination program was in force, the prospect of global eradication for rinderpest was seriously discussed. Unfortunately, as the incidence of disease fell so did the momentum of the control program, and by 1984 Africa was again experiencing a large-scale epidemic of rinderpest. To combat this epidemic and to revitalize many of the veterinary services in Africa, the Organization of African Unity, with financial and technical assistance from the European Community and the Food and Agricultural Organization of the United Nations, launched a pan-African vaccination campaign in 1986. The success of this program has led to the establishment of similar campaigns in western Asia and the Indian subcontinent.

The possibility of global eradication of the other diseases listed in Table 15-2 is more remote. A low level of public concern and infectivity in the prodromal stage make the eradication of canine distemper difficult, and the existence of a widely dispersed wildlife reservoir makes the global eradication of Newcastle disease impossible. Foot-and-mouth disease has the largest constellation of unfavorable features, balanced in the industrialized countries by the very high level of concern about its presence or importation. However, by using test and slaughter policies, in conjunction with quarantine, licensed movement of animals, and in some diseases vaccination, several important viral diseases, such as sheeppox, hog cholera, and velogenic Newcastle disease, have been eliminated from most of the industrialized and some of the developing nations. Whether any widespread disease of domestic animals eventually proves to be globally eradicable depends biologically on whether there is a major wildlife reservoir, and politically on the setting of priorities for the use of human and financial resources, on an international scale.

ANTIVIRAL CHEMOTHERAPY

If this had been a book about bacterial diseases of domestic animals there would have been at least one chapter on antibacterial chemotherapy. However, the antibiotics that have been so effective against bacteria do not have the slightest effect on any virus. The reason is that viruses are intimately dependent on the metabolic pathways of the host cell for their replication; hence most agents that interfere with viral replication are toxic to the cell. In recent years, however, increased knowledge of the biochemistry of viral replication has led to a more rational approach to the search for antiviral chemotherapeutic agents, and a small number of such compounds have become a standard part of the armamentarium against particular human viruses. As yet there are no specifically antiviral chemotherapeutic agents in common use in veterinary practice, but that day is sure to come. Accordingly it is appropriate to outline briefly some potential developments in the field.

Strategy for Development of Antiviral Agents

Several steps in the viral replication cycle (see Chapter 3) represent potential targets for selective attack. Theoretically, all virus-coded enzymes are vulnerable, as are all processes (enzymatic or nonenzymatic) that are more essential to the replication of the virus than to the survival of the cell. Table 15-3 sets out the most vulnerable steps and provides examples of antiviral drugs that display activity, indicating also which have already been licensed for use in humans.

A logical approach to the discovery of new antiviral chemotherapeutic agents is to isolate or synthesize substances that might be predicted to serve as inhibitors of a known virus-coded enzyme such as a transcriptase, replicase, or protease. Analogs of this prototype drug are then synthesized with a view to enhancing activity and/or selectivity. A further refinement of this approach is well illustrated by the nucleoside analog acycloguanosine (acyclovir), an inhibitor of herpesvirus DNA

TABLE 15-3
Possible Targets for Antiviral Chemotherapy

Target	Prototype drug
Attachment of virion to cell receptor	Receptor analogs
Uncoating	Rimantadine[a]
Primary transcription from viral genome	Transcriptase inhibitors
Reverse transcription	AZT (Zidovudine[a])
Regulation of transcription	HIV *tat* inhibitors
Processing of RNA transcripts	Ribavirin[a]
Translation of viral mRNA into protein	Interferons[a]
Posttranslational cleavage of proteins	Protease inhibitors
Replication of viral DNA genome	Acycloguanosine (acyclovir[a])
Replication of viral RNA genome	Replicase inhibitors

[a] Licensed for human use.

polymerase. Acyclovir is in fact an inactive *prodrug* that requires another herpesvirus-coded enzyme, thymidine kinase, to phosphorylate it to its active form. Because this viral enzyme occurs only in infected cells, acyclovir is nontoxic for uninfected cells but very effective in herpesvirus-infected cells. Such drugs find limited use in veterinary medicine, for example, for treatment of feline herpesvirus 1 corneal ulcers.

The renaissance in X-ray crystallography has opened a major new approach to the search for antiviral agents. Now that the three-dimensional structure of icosahedral virions such as those of picornaviruses is known (see frontispiece), it has been possible to characterize the receptor-binding site on the critical capsid protein in atomic detail. Complexes of viral proteins with purified cell receptors can be crystallized and examined directly. The receptor-binding site on the virion has generally turned out to be a "canyon," cleft, or depression on the external surface of the protein. The next step is to analyze the structure of complexes of virions and compounds known to neutralize their infectivity by blocking adsorption or uncoating, thereby confirming the identity of the receptor-binding site and supplying information on the nature of the interaction between the two. Further information is provided by mapping the position of the particular amino acid residues found to be substituted in drug-resistant mutants, or by using site-specific mutagenesis to optimize the fit and the binding energy of the drug–virus interaction. Clearly, this approach lends itself best to the development of drugs that act by binding directly to the capsid or envelope of the virion itself, thereby blocking attachment, penetration, or uncoating.

A third approach has recently emerged from the discovery of several regulatory genes in the genome of the human immunodeficiency virus (HIV) and related viruses (see Chapter 3). Potentially, the replication of such viruses could be blocked by agents that bind either to the protein product of such a regulatory gene or to the recognition site in the regulatory region of the viral genome with which that protein normally interacts, such as the TAR region to which the product of the HIV *tat* gene binds.

FURTHER READING

FAO–WHO–OIE. (1991). "Animal Health Yearbook." FAO, Rome (produced annually).

Fenner, F., Henderson, D. A., Arita, I., Jezek, Z., and Ladnyi, I. D. (1988). "Smallpox and Its Eradication." World Health Organization, Geneva.

Hanson, R. P., and Hanson, M. G. (1983). "Animal Disease Control. Regional Programs." Iowa State Univ. Press, Ames.

Morris, R. S., ed. (1991). "Epidemiological Information Systems." *Rev. Sci. Tech. Off. Int. Epizoot., Paris* **10**, 7.

Quinn, P. J. (1991). Disinfection and disease prevention in veterinary medicine. *In* "Disinfection, Sterilization and Preservation" (S. S. Block, ed.), 4th Ed., p. 846. Lea & Febiger, Philadelphia, Pennsylvania.

Radostits, O. M., and Blood, D. C. (1985). "Herd Health. A Textbook of Health and Production Management of Agricultural Animals." Saunders, Philadelphia, Pennsylvania.

Schnurrenberger, P. R., Sharman, R. S., and Wise, G. H. (1987). "Attacking Animal Diseases: Concepts and Strategies for Control and Eradication." Iowa State Univ. Press, Ames.

Watson, W. A., and Brown, A. C. L. (1981). Legislation and control of virus diseases. *In* "Virus Diseases of Food Animals. Volume I, International Perspectives" (E. P. J. Gibbs, ed.). Academic Press, London.

White, D. O., and Fenner, F. (1993). Chemotherapy of viral diseases. *In* "Medical Virology," 4th Ed. (in press). Academic Press, San Diego.

PART II

Viruses of Domestic Animals

CHAPTER 16

Parvoviridae

Members of the family *Parvoviridae* (*parvus* = small) have a small icosahedral virion and a genome of ssDNA. There are three genera: *Parvovirus*, members of which infect vertebrates and replicate autonomously, *Dependovirus*, which are defective and depend on a helper virus, usually an adenovirus, for their replication, and *Densovirus*, all members of which infect insects. Only the genus *Parvovirus* will be further discussed; these viruses replicate selectively in cycling cells and cause important diseases in swine, cats, dogs, and geese (Table 16-1).

The parvoviruses responsible for infections in cats, dogs, and mink are closely related. Porcine parvovirus infection is usually subclinical but may affect the fetus; goose parvovirus causes a lethal disease in goslings. Rodent parvoviruses are used as models in studies of the pathogenesis of certain fetal abnormalities, and they are common contaminants of cultured rodent cells and tumors. A human parvovirus has been incriminated as the cause of a common exanthematous disease, erythema infectiosum. Parvoviruses have been isolated from chickens, rabbits, and an equine fetus, but their role in causing disease in these species has not been established.

TABLE 16-1
Diseases of Domestic Animals Caused by Parvoviruses[a]

Virus	Disease
Porcine parvovirus	Stillbirth, abortion, fetal death, mummification, and infertility
Feline panleukopenia virus[b]	Cerebellar hypoplasia, panleukopenia, enteritis
Canine parvovirus 1	Mild diarrhea
Canine parvovirus 2[b]	Generalized neonatal disease, enteritis, myocarditis, panleukopenia
Mink enteritis virus[b]	Panleukopenia, enteritis
Aleutian mink disease virus	Chronic immune complex disease, encephalopathy
Goose parvovirus	Hepatitis

[a]Parvoviruses have also been recovered from cattle and from laboratory rodents, but under natural conditions they are not known to cause disease in these species.
[b]Closely related viruses; mink enteritis virus and canine parvovirus 2 were probably derived from feline panleukopenia virus in the 1940s and 1970s, respectively.

PROPERTIES OF PARVOVIRUSES

As determined by X-ray crystallography, the icosahedral virions of canine parvovirus 2 are 25.5 nm in diameter, although estimates from electron micrographs had suggested a diameter of 22 nm (Table 16-2). The capsid is composed of 60 protein subunits that are predominantly VP2 (~65 K), but including some copies of VP1 (~84 K). VP1 and VP4 are formed by alternative splicing of the same mRNA, and the entire sequence of VP2 is contained within VP1. A third structural protein, VP3, is formed only in "full" (DNA-containing) capsids by cleavage of 15–20 amino acids from the amino terminus of VP2.

As determined by X-ray crystallography, the central structural motif of VP2 of canine parvovirus 2 has the same eight-stranded antiparallel β

TABLE 16-2
Properties of Parvoviruses

Icosahedral virion, 18–26 nm diameter, composed of 60 protein subunits
Minus sense ssDNA genome, 5.2 kb
Replicate in nucleus of cycling cells, producing large intranuclear inclusion bodies
Very stable, resisting 60°C for 60 minutes and pH 3–9
Three genera: *Parvovirus*, replication-competent; *Dependovirus*, defective, requires helper adenovirus; *Densovirus*, infects insects
Most species hemagglutinate

barrel as has been found in several other icosahedral viruses (see Fig. 1-4); however, it represents only about one-third of the capsid protein. There is a 22 Å long protrusion at the threefold axes, a 15 Å deep canyon about each of the five cylindrical structures at the fivefold axes, and a 15 Å deep depression at the twofold axes. The canyon is probably the site of receptor binding. Within the capsid there is a minus sense ssDNA genome, 5.2 kb in size. There are eleven nucleotides in each of the 60 symmetry-related pockets on the inner surface of the capsid. These 660 nucleotides (13% of the total) form loops nestled into the pockets on the internal protein surface.

Parvoviruses of all genera may package either a plus sense or a minus sense strand, in proportions ranging from 1% to 50%, but members of the genus *Parvovirus* preferentially package minus sense DNA. The complete nucleotide sequences of several parvoviruses are now available.

Parvoviruses are remarkably stable to environmental condtions (extremes of heat and pH); hence disinfection of contaminated premises is difficult.

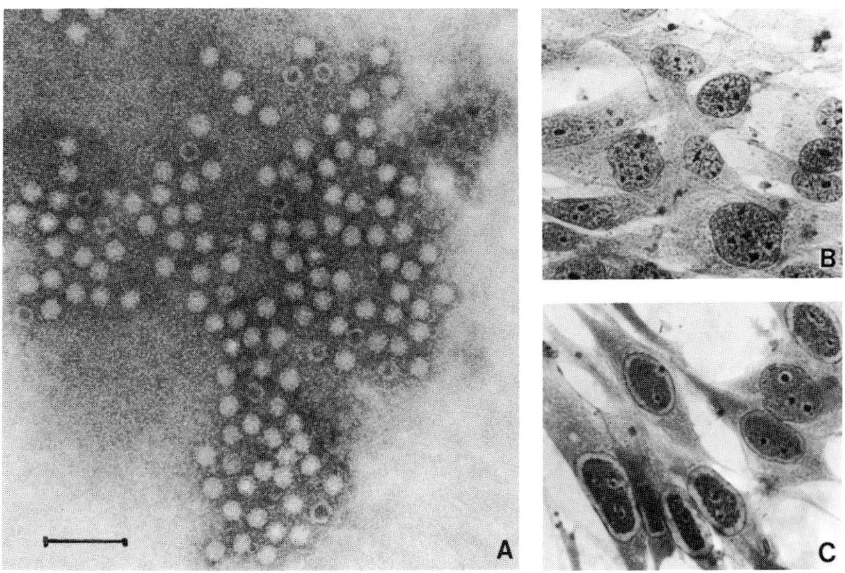

FIG. 16-1. Parvoviridae. *(A) Negatively stained virions of canine parvovirus (bar; 100 nm). (B) Normal feline embryo cells. (C) Feline embryo cells infected with feline panleukopenia virus. All nuclei show inclusion bodies in various stages of development. Hemotoxylin and eosin; magnification: ×550. [B and C from M. J. Studdert* et al., Vet. Rec. **93,** *156 (1973).]*

VIRAL REPLICATION

Members of the genus *Parvovirus* replicate in the nucleus of cycling cells. They require cell functions which are only provided during the late S or early G_2 phases of the cell cycle (Fig. 16-2A). Because of their small size, parvoviruses have been intensively studied as a model for understanding DNA replication and gene expression. Two main overlapping transcription units have been identified, from which three major mRNA species are transcribed. The mRNAs have a common 3′ terminus, and they are polyadenylated and spliced. The most abundant mRNA codes for structural proteins late in infection, the relevant information mapping in the right-hand half of the genome (Fig. 16-2B), whereas the information for a nonstructural protein involved in DNA replication resides in the left-hand half of the DNA.

DNA replication occurs via a double-stranded replicative form, initiated by a self-priming mechanism via the 3′ terminal palindromic sequence (Fig. 16-2B). Following DNA replication, viral capsids assemble, into which progeny ssDNA is packaged.

PATHOGENESIS AND IMMUNITY

The pathogenesis of parvoviruses is determined by the requirement for cycling cells for viral replication. Following infection of the fetus (pig or cat) or newborn (dog or cat), the virus may infect a wide range of cells

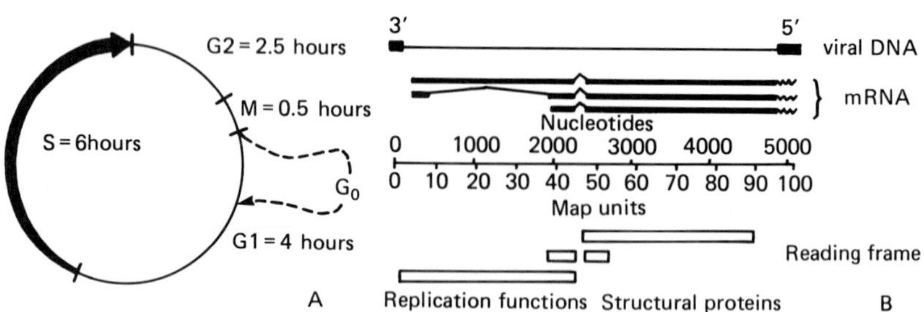

FIG. 16-2. *(A) Phases of the cell cycle of feline embryo cells. The total cell cycle time is 13 hours. Autonomous parvovirus replication depends on events that occur in the S phase. (B) Diagram illustrating the organization of the genome of a* Parvovirus. *The palindromic termini (thick lines) occupy approximately 2 map units at the left-hand end and 4 map units at the right-hand end of the viral DNA. The three major cytoplasmic transcripts are represented by thick black lines; the thin lines indicate the introns spliced out of the mature mRNA. The open reading frames are shown as open blocks. [From S. F. Cotmore* et al., Virology **129,** *333 (1983).]*

in various tissues and organs. In older animals a narrower range of cells is affected; the degree of cell cycling in a particular organ or tissue and the presence of appropriate virus receptors on the cells are the important factors determining susceptibility. Both factors are influenced by the age of the animal. Thus, the cerebellum is selectively destroyed in feline fetuses or kittens infected in the perinatal period, and the myocardium is highly susceptible in pups 3–8 weeks of age and goslings 0–2 weeks of age. At all ages, the continuous cycling of cells of the lymphoid tissue and intestinal epithelium renders them highly susceptible, hence the common occurrence of enteritis and panleukopenia with concomitant immunosuppression.

Following natural infection there is a rapid immune response. Different antigenic determinants appear to be involved in neutralization and hemagglutination–inhibition. Neutralizing antibody can be detected within 3–5 days of infection and may rise to very high titers before there is clinical recovery. The presence of high-titer antibody is correlated with protection, and immunity after natural infection appears to be lifelong. In cats and dogs, some maternal antibody may be transferred transplacentally, but most is transferred with colostrum. The titer of natural passive antibody in kittens or pups parallels the maternal antibody titer and is therefore quite variable, providing protection for only a few weeks or for as long as 22 weeks. Cytotoxic T cells are generated after both infection and vaccination.

PORCINE PARVOVIRUS INFECTIONS

Porcine parvovirus was originally identified as a contaminant in cell cultures prepared from apparently healthy piglets. It was also recognized as a contaminant of cell cultures of nonporcine origin; the source of such contamination was traced to trypsin prepared from swine pancreases (widely used in the preparation of cell cultures), in which it survived because of the great stability of parvoviruses. There is only a single serotype of porcine parvovirus.

Disease in Swine

Porcine parvovirus infection is an important disease of swine, and the virus has been isolated in association with reproductive failure in swine, which includes stillbirth, mummification, embryonic death, infertility (Fig. 16-3) (in respect of which the acronym SMEDI has been applied), abortion, neonatal death, and low fertility of boars. Virus has been recovered from semen, vaginal mucus, and diseased piglets as well as from

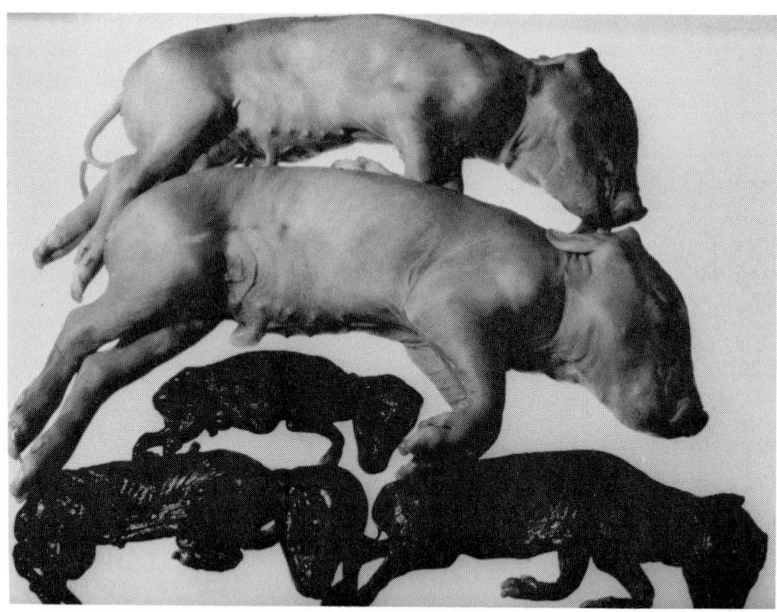

FIG. 16-3. *Porcine parvovirus infection. Infected fetuses in various stages of mummification, compared with normal fetuses. (Courtesy Dr. R. H. Johnston and Dr. H. S. Joo.)*

the tissues of healthy piglets. In young pigs, parvoviruses have been associated with a vesicular disease of the feet and mouth.

Serologic surveys show that the incidence of infection is far higher than the incidence of reported disease. SMEDI syndromes are most noticeable when the virus is first introduced into a herd, and are then an important component of fetal loss. For the many herds in which the virus remains endemic, losses are less serious or less obvious. Inactivated vaccines are used in selected herds to control reproductive losses.

FELINE, CANINE, AND MINK PARVOVIRUS INFECTIONS

Feline panleukopenia has been recognized for about 100 years, mink enteritis was first described in 1947, and canine parvovirus 2 was recognized as a new pathogen in 1978. The three parvoviruses that cause these diseases are closely related, and the mink and canine viruses appear to have arisen as host range mutants of feline parvovirus.

Feline and mink parvoviruses are indistinguishable antigenically by hemagglutination–inhibition and serum neutralization tests and by DNA analysis with restriction endonucleases; although closely related, canine parvovirus can be distinguished from the other two viruses by these criteria. Most strains of feline and mink parvovirus hemagglutinate pig and rhesus monkey red blood cells to low titer at 4°C at pH 6.5, the hemagglutination patterns being unstable at room temperature. On the other hand, under the same conditions canine parvovirus agglutinates these cells to high titer, and the hemagglutination patterns are stable at room temperature.

The diseases in cats, mink, and dogs are remarkably similar, particularly with respect to panleukopenia and enteritis. In animals infected in the perinatal period, the feline virus produces cerebellar hypoplasia while the canine virus produces myocarditis.

Feline Panleukopenia

It is thought that all Felidae are susceptible to infection with feline panleukopenia virus, which is probably the most important of all feline viral infections and occurs worldwide.

Clinical Signs. Feline panleukopenia is most common in kittens about the time of weaning, but cats of all ages are susceptible (see Table 16-3). Infection usually occurs via the oral route but may also be acquired by inhalation. The incubation period averages 5 days (range 2–10 days). Beginning 2–5 days after infection, leukopenia develops and is most marked at 5–6 days after infection, when there may be fewer than 100 circulating white blood cells per cubic millimeter. The severity of clinical disease and the mortality rate parallel the severity of the leukopenia. Clinical signs include fever (>40°C) which persists for about 24 hours and during which, in the peracute form of the disease, death occurs. The temperature returns to normal and rises again on the third or fourth day, at which time clinical illness is apparent, with lassitude, inappetence, a rough coat, and repeated vomiting. A profuse, persistent, frequently bloody diarrhea develops 2–4 days after the initial fever. Dehydration due to the severe enteritis is a major contributing factor to death. The prognosis is grave if total white blood cell counts fall below 1000 cells per cubic millimeter. For reasons that are not well understood, the severe disease often observed after natural infection is not seen following experimental infection.

Kittens that have been infected from 2 weeks before to about 2 weeks after birth develop cerebellar hypoplasia (Fig. 16-4). Affected kittens are noticeably ataxic when they become ambulatory at about 3 weeks of age; they have a wide-based stance and move with exaggerated steps, tending to overshoot the mark and to pause and oscillate about an intended goal.

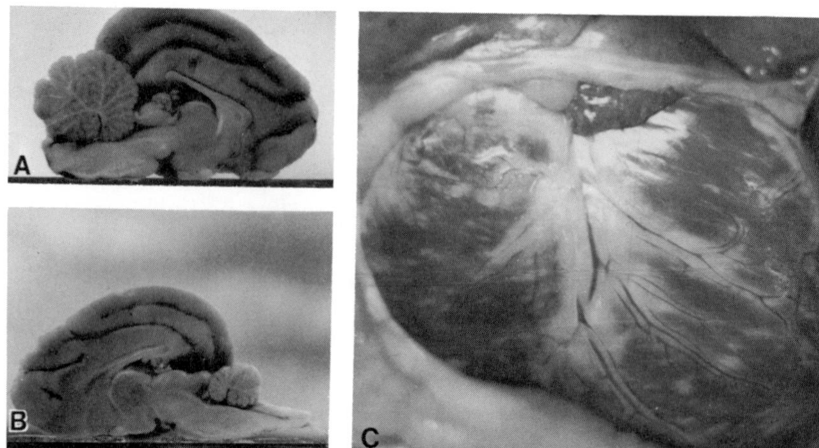

FIG. 16-4. *Cerebellar hypoplasia caused by feline parvovirus infection in a 3-month-old kitten (A) and matched control (B). (C) Canine parvovirus myocarditis, showing scar tissue throughout the myocardium. [From C. Lenghaus and M. J. Studdert,* Am. J. Pathol. **115,** *316 (1984).]*

Pathogenesis. Following initial proliferation in pharyngeal lymphoid tissue, virus is distributed to all organs and tissues via the bloodstream, with infection and lysis of cells which have appropriate receptors and are cycling, since virus replicates in cells in the S phase of the cell cycle. Following viral replication, these cells are blocked from entering mitosis. There may be profound panleukopenia in which all white blood cell elements—lymphocytes, granulocytes, monocytes, and platelets—are destroyed, both those present in the circulation and those in the lymphoid organs, including thymus, bone marrow, lymph nodes, spleen, and Peyer's patches. Resting peripheral leukocytes may be stimulated to proliferate, and these dividing cells can become permissive for viral replication. Alternatively, the presence of virus bound to the surface of cells may render these cells a target for cytotoxic lysis. Polymorphonuclear leukocytes may be lost across the gut wall.

The rapidly dividing intestinal epithelial cells in the crypts of Lieberkuhn are also very susceptible. Epithelial cells at the tips of the intestinal villi are continuously lost into the lumen of the gut and are normally replaced by division of the cells in the crypts, the cell cycle time for which is 8–12 hours. After feline parvovirus infection, the normal loss of cells from the villus tips and the failure of replacement with cells from the crypts lead to greatly shortened, nonabsorptive villi, and hence to the rapid accumulation of fluid and ingesta in the gut lumen and diarrhea. Where the clinical course is more prolonged, dehydration is a major factor contributing to death; most cats given adequate fluid therapy will recover.

At necropsy, lesions in the small intestine are usually patchy in their distribution; the entire small intestine needs to be carefully examined for evidence of slight congestion and thickening, which is visible from the serosal as well as the lumenal surface. Where enteritis has been present for several days before death the intestinal lesions are usually obvious and consist of segments in which the gut wall is greatly thickened into a rigid, hoselike structure. The lymph nodes may be enlarged and edematous. The bone marrow, for example, at the proximal end of the femur, normally a jelly-firm, red cylinder, may be pale and fluid, so that it can be poured from the marrow cavity.

Histologically, the villi are greatly shortened and blunted; necrotic but still adherent cells may be present at the tips of the villi. The crypts are dilated and distended with mucus and cell debris. Rarely intranuclear inclusions may be found in cells near the base of the crypts. There is evidence of widespread destruction of lymphoid cells and massive infiltration with polymorphonuclear cells.

In fetuses infected during the last 2 weeks of pregnancy and the first 2 weeks of life, lesions are found only in cells of the external granular layer of the cerebellum. During this period of development, these cells undergo rapid cell division and migrate to form the internal granular and Purkinje cell layers of the cerebellum, which control motor functions. Like the young of most animal species, the newborn kitten is somewhat ataxic for at least 1 week after birth. Motor neurons that are destroyed by feline parvovirus are not replaced; hence affected kittens remain permanently ataxic. If the cells of the cerebellum are affected during a generalized infection, this organ remains permanently damaged while other cells in the body are rapidly replaced. The high immunogenicity of the virus leads to a rapid immune response, which may be significant in limiting the extent of cell damage associated with these generalized infections.

Diagnosis. The clinical disease and postmortem findings are characteristic and usually suggests the diagnosis. Confirmatory procedures include hematologic examination to demonstrate leukopenia, the direct hemagglutination of pig or rhesus monkey red blood cells by suitably prepared fecal samples, or isolation of the virus in cell culture. Fluorescent antibody staining may be used for detection of antigen, and ELISA for detection of either antigen or antibody.

Epidemiology. Feline panleukopenia is highly contagious. The virus may be acquired by direct contact with other cats or via fomites (bedding, food dishes); fleas and humans may act as mechanical vectors. Virus is shed in the feces, vomit, urine, and saliva. The incidence of specific antibody in the cat population is much higher than the combined reported incidence of clinical disease and vaccination, indicating that subclinical infection is common. Recovered cats may excrete small amounts of virus for many months. Neither the exact duration of such excretion nor the underlying basis for persistent infection has been determined.

The stability of the virus and the very high rates of viral excretion (up to 10^9 virus particles per gram of feces) result in persistent high levels of environmental contamination; hence it may be extremely difficult to disinfect contaminated premises. Because of this, close contact between cats is not essential for transmission. The virus may be acquired from premises following the introduction of susceptible cats months, even up to 1 year, after previously affected cats have been removed, and the virus may be carried a considerable distance on wind-blown fomites.

Control. Vaccination is universally practiced, both attenuated live-virus and inactivated vaccines being used. In large catteries strict hygiene and quarantine of incoming animals are essential. Sick cats should be isolated, and cats introduced into the colony should be held in isolation for several weeks before introduction to the main cattery. For disinfection 1% sodium hypochlorite applied to clean areas will destroy residual contaminating virus, but treatment is ineffective if the area is dirty or if the viral concentration is high. Organic iodine and phenolic disinfectants are also used.

Canine Parvovirus Disease

Two parvoviruses affect dogs. Canine parvovirus 1 was identified in the feces of dogs in 1967, but it has not been confirmed as a major cause of disease, although mild diarrhea may occur. It is antigenically and genetically quite distinct from canine parvovirus 2, which emerged as a major new pathogen of dogs in 1978 and caused a worldwide pandemic. Since then canine parvovirus 2 has become endemic in dogs throughout the world and is firmly entrenched in wild canine species in many countries. Two subtypes are recognized which are distinguishable antigenically and by restriction enzyme analysis.

Clinical Signs. Three distinct age-related syndromes have been recognized in dogs (Table 16-3). Generalized neonatal disease is rare. The panleukopenia/enteritis syndromes precisely parallel the same syn-

TABLE 16-3

Relations between Age of Host and Occurrence of Various Disease Syndromes after Feline Panleukopenia Virus or Canine Parvovirus Infection

Syndrome	Animal species	Age
Generalized neonatal disease	Cat and dog	2–12 days
Panleukopenia/enteritis	Cat and dog	2–4 months
Enteritis	Cat and dog	4–12 months
Cerebellar hypoplasia	Cat	2 weeks before birth to 2 weeks
Myocarditis		
Acute	Dog	3–8 weeks
Chronic	Dog	8 weeks

dromes in cats, but the cerebellar hypoplasia found in cats has not been recognized in dogs. Myocarditis due to canine parvovirus infection is usually recognized as an acute disease in pups characterized by sudden death, usually without any clinical signs. However, even though the lesions are extensive, the pup may survive with a scarred myocardium (Fig. 16-4C).

Pathogenesis. The pathogenesis of canine parvovirus infections in the dog is similar to that of feline parvovirus infections of the cat, but the absence of cerebellar hypoplasia and the occurrence of myocarditis are somewhat surprising, since myocardial cells are not normally considered as rapidly cycling.

Diagnosis. The simplest procedure for the laboratory diagnosis of canine parvovirus infection is hemagglutination of pig or rhesus monkey red blood cells (pH 6.5, 4°C) by fecal extracts, titrated in parallel in the presence of normal and immune dog serum. Fecal samples from dogs with acute enteritis may contain up to 20,000 HA units of virus per milliliter, which is the equivalent of about 10^9 virions per gram of feces. Electron microscopy, virus isolation, and ELISA procedures can also be used for laboratory confirmation of the clinical diagnosis.

Epidemiology. When canine parvovirus disease was first recognized in 1978, the canine population all over the world was completely susceptible. Generalized neonatal disease was then rarely recognized, but myocarditis and panleukopenia/enteritis were common. Like cerebellar hypoplasia in cats caused by feline parvovirus, myocarditis is now rare, since passively derived maternal antibody usually protects pups beyond the 2-week and 8-week periods which appear to be the age limits for the development of generalized neonatal disease and myocarditis, respectively. Canine parvovirus disease, occurring predominantly as panluekopenia/enteritis, is now an endemic worldwide disease of dogs, its epidemiology being similar to that of feline panleukopenia.

Control. Major control problems are encountered in large, crowded breeding colonies where hygiene is difficult to implement and maintain. Subclinical infections are common, particularly in single, well-cared-for pups, emphasizing the importance of hygiene and general good health in limiting the occurrence of clinical disease. While vaccination with either attenuated live-virus or inactivated vaccines is effective, considerable problems are encountered in devising effective vaccination schedules because of the variable levels of maternal antibodies transferred to pups.

Mink Enteritis

Mink enteritis and Aleutian disease of mink (see below) are caused by two antigenically different parvoviruses. The virus causing mink enteritis is closely related to the feline panleukopenia virus and produces in mink syndromes similar to panleukemia in cats, except that cerebellar hypoplasia has not been recognized.

Origins of Mink Enteritis Parvovirus and Canine Parvovirus

The restriction endonuclease maps of mink enteritis virus and feline panleukopenia virus are virtually identical, and the disease in minks appears to have been due to the introduction of feline panleukopenia virus into commercial mink farms in Ontario, Canada, about 1946. Canine parvovirus was recognized simultaneously in five continents in 1978, although serologic surveys show that it was present in dogs in Greece in 1974 and in some other countries in Europe in 1977. Genetic mapping studies showed that three or four sequence differences within the VP1/VP2 gene determine all the properties that distinguish canine parvovirus from feline parvovirus, including the host range for canine cells and dogs. The two antigenic subtypes of canine parvovirus appear to have been derived from a common ancestor (probably a feline parvovirus) before 1978.

Aleutian Disease of Mink

Aleutian disease of mink is a chronic disease caused by a parvovirus and characterized by plasmacytosis, hypergammaglobulinemia, splenomegaly, lymphadenopathy, glomerulonephritis, arteritis, focal hepatitis, anemia, and death. The lesions are the result of the continued production of virus and a failure to eliminate virus–antibody complexes; the persistence of virus induces a virus-specific plasmacytosis, antibody-specific hypergammaglobulinemia, and immune complex-mediated disease. It occurs primarily in mink that are homozygous for the recessive pale ("Aleutian") coat color. This commercially desirable light pelt color gene is linked to a gene associated with a lysosomal abnormality of the Chediak–Higashi type, whereby, following phagocytosis, immune complexes are not destroyed. The level of the hypergammaglobulinemia is cyclical, death occurring during a peak response between 2 and 5 months after infection.

Despite the extremely high levels of virus-specific antibody, this does not "neutralize" infectivity, and infectious virus can be recovered from immune complexes. Immunization of mink carrying the Aleutian gene with killed virus vaccine increases the severity of the disease. Conversely, immunosuppression diminishes the severity of the response.

GOOSE PARVOVIRUS INFECTIONS

Goose parvovirus causes a highly lethal disease of goslings 8–30 days old, which is characterized by focal or diffuse hepatitis and widespread acute degeneration of striated and smooth muscle including myocardium. Inclusion bodies are found mainly in the liver, but also in the spleen, myocardium, thymus, thyroid, and intestines. Control is achieved by the vaccination of laying geese with attenuated live-virus vaccine, after which antibody persists in goslings for at least 4 weeks.

FURTHER READING

Mengeling, W. L. (1986). Porcine parvovirus infection. *In* "Diseases of Swine" (A. D. Leman, B. Straw, R. D. Glock, W. L. Mengeling, R. H. C. Penny, and E. Scholl, eds.), 6th Ed., p. 411. Iowa State Univ. Press, Ames.

Parrish, C. R. (1990). Emergence, natural history and variation of canine, mink and feline parvoviruses. *Adv. Virus Res.* **38,** 404.

Siegl, G., Bates, R. C., Berns, K. I., Carter, B. J., Kelly, D. C., Kurstak, E., and Tattersall, P. (1985). Characteristics and taxonomy of *Parvoviridae. Intervirology* **23,** 61.

Tijssen, P., ed. (1990). "CRC Handbook of Parvoviruses," Vols. 1 and 2. CRC Press, Boca Raton, Florida.

Tsao, J., Chapman, M. S., Agbandje, M., Keller, W., Smith, K., Wu, M. L., Smith, T. J., Rossman, M. G., Compans, R. W., and Parrish, C. R. (1991). The three-dimensional structure of canine parvovirus and its functional implications. *Science* **251,** 1456.

CHAPTER 17

Papovaviridae

The family *Papovaviridae* includes two genera, *Papillomavirus* and *Polyomavirus*. Viruses in both genera have a nonenveloped icosahedral capsid enclosing a circular dsDNA genome (Table 17-1). Papillomaviruses produce papillomas (warts) in many different species. Only those affecting cattle, horses, and dogs are likely to require veterinary attention. They are commonly seen in young animals as areas of simple hyperplasia or as benign neoplasms and usually regress spontaneously. However, in association with certain cofactors, bovine, human, and rabbit papillomaviruses may produce carcinomas (Table 17-2).

Papillomaviruses have not yet been grown in cell culture, which until recently restricted study to the pathology of the lesions, the ultrastructure of the virion, and experiments on transmission. With the introduction of recombinant DNA or PCR technology, it is now possible to clone papillomavirus DNA obtained from virions purified from papillomas, and the genomes of several papillomaviruses have now been completely sequenced. These advances have greatly increased our knowledge of the genomic structure/function of papillomaviruses and, in conjunction with the development of *in vitro* transformation assays in the 1980s, have stimulated renewed interest in their mechanism of oncogenesis.

Polyomaviruses are highly species-specific. Except for a rare disease in humans and a disease in budgerigars, infections are not generally associated with clinical disease in their natural hosts, but mammalian

TABLE 17-1

Properties of Papovaviruses

Nonenveloped icosahedral virion, 72 capsomers, 45[a] or 55[b] nm in diameter
Circular, supercoiled dsDNA genome, 5[a] or 7–8[b] kbp
Members of both genera replicate in nucleus; members of genus *Polyomavirus* grow in cultured cells; members of genus *Papillomavirus* have not been grown in culture but will transform cultured cells; infectious virions produced only in terminally differentiated epithelial cells
During replication, polyomavirus DNA is transcribed from both strands, papillomavirus DNA from one strand
Integrated[a] or episomal[b] DNA may be oncogenic

[a]*Polyomavirus.*
[b]*Papillomavirus.*

TABLE 17-2

Diseases Caused by Papillomaviruses

Virus[a]	Principal species affected	Disease
Bovine papillomavirus		
Type 1	Cattle	Cutaneous fibropapilloma
	Horse	Sarcoid
Type 2	Cattle	Cutaneous fibropapilloma
	Horse	Sarcoid
Type 3	Cattle	Cutaneous papilloma
Type 4	Cattle	Alimentary tract papilloma (may become malignant)
Type 5	Cattle	Teat fibropapilloma ("rice grain")
Type 6	Cattle	Teat papilloma ("frond")
Ovine papillomavirus	Sheep	Cutaneous fibropapilloma
Equine papillomavirus	Horse	Cutaneous papilloma
Porcine genital papillomavirus	Swine	Cutaneous papilloma
Canine oral papillomavirus	Dog	Oral papilloma
Cottontail rabbit papillomavirus[b] (*Sylvilagus floridanus*)	Rabbit	Cutaneous papilloma (may become malignant)
Human papillomavirus (>60 types)	Human	Cutaneous and mucosal papillomas (some become malignant)

[a]In addition, papillomaviruses have been recovered from several species of deer, from birds, and from hamsters, in all of which they cause small cutaneous papillomas or fibropapillomas.

[b]Also called Shope papillomavirus, the virus was much used in early studies of oncogenic viruses.

polyomaviruses are oncogenic when inoculated into newborn rodents. In contrast to papillomaviruses, they grow readily in cell cultures. During the 1960s and 1970s mouse polyomavirus and simian virus 40 (SV40) were intensively studied by tumor virologists, and a great deal is known about their replication cycles (see Fig. 3-6). However, apart from noting that, in contrast to the papillomaviruses, transcripts are made from both strands of DNA, polyomavirus replication will not be described since viruses of this genus are of minor veterinary importance.

PAPILLOMAVIRUSES

Properties

The virion of papillomaviruses is a nonenveloped icosahedral capsid, approximately 55 nm in diameter, with 72 capsomers (Table 17-1). Both "empty" and "full" virus particles are seen by electron microscopy (Fig. 17-1). Tubular and other aberrant morphological forms are common. The genome of papillomavirus is a double-stranded, covalently closed, circular, supercoiled DNA molecule, varying in size from 6.7 kbp for bovine papillomavirus 3 to 8.2 kbp for canine oral papillomavirus. Ten polypeptides have been identified by polyacrylamide gel electrophoresis, with two capsid proteins of 50K–63K. Papillomaviruses are ether-resistant, acid-stable, and thermostable.

Although antisera to intact virions of different papillomaviruses show

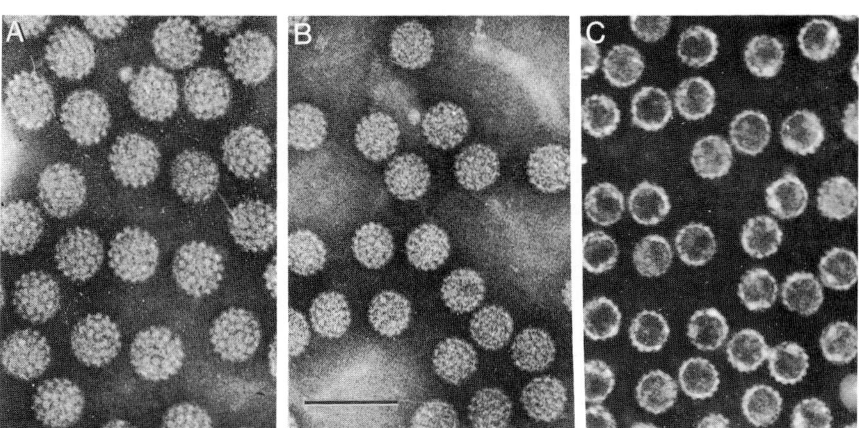

FIG. 17-1. Papovaviridae. *(A)* Papillomavirus. *(B)* Polyomavirus. *(C)* Polymavirus, *empty virions. Bar: 100 nm. (Courtesy Dr. E. A. Follett.)*

no cross-reactivity, wide serologic cross-reactivity can be demonstrated with antisera to detergent-disrupted virions, indicating that there are conserved epitopes on internal proteins. There is only a limited sequence homology between the DNAs of papillomaviruses of different species, but substantial sequence homologies exist between those derived from any given species (human or bovine, for example). Sequence homology has been used to distinguish different "types" among the papillomaviruses infecting a given species. The convention has been adopted that to be classified as a new type, there should be less than 50% homology between the DNAs and significant serologic differences in reciprocal assays. Six types of bovine papillomaviruses and at least 60 types of human papillomaviruses have been identified so far.

The bovine papillomaviruses can be divided into two groups. Bovine papillomavirus 1, 2, and 5 are more closely related immunologically, have the same genome size, and share DNA sequences. Viruses of the other group, bovine papillomavirus 3, 4, and 6, have a smaller genome and also have DNA sequences in common. The two groups are only distantly related.

Replication

Transcription takes place from only one strand of the papillomavirus DNA; in productive infections the whole genome is transcribed, in nonproductive infections only the early region. The late viral genes that encode the two viral capsid proteins are expressed only in the terminally differentiated epithelial cells; hence mature virions are seen only in these cells. However, although they do not replicate in cultured cells, bovine papillomavirus 1 and 2 and their DNAs can transform cells *in vitro.* In contrast to other oncogenic or transforming DNA viruses, papillomavirus DNA is rarely integrated into the cellular genome, but remains episomal. Several mRNAs are expressed in such cells; these encode viral factors concerned with viral episome replication, regulation of viral transcription, and cellular transformation. Fragments of the bovine papillomavirus 1 genome have been cloned and expressed in *E. coli,* and antisera to some of the proteins expressed inhibit transformation of cells by bovine papillomavirus 1. Bovine papillomavirus 1 DNA and a subgenomic fragment of it (the 5.4-kb transforming fragment) have been used as eukaryotic vectors for foreign DNA.

Pathogenesis and Immunity

Based on host response, papillomaviruses can be subdivided according to tissue tropism and histology of the lesion. There is a good correlation between histopathologic appearance and viral type as determined by

DNA sequence (Table 17-3). The cells of the dermal layer of a papilloma proliferate excessively, but neither virions nor viral antigen can be detected in the proliferating cells, although many copies of the viral DNA are present. Viral antigen and virions can be detected only in the keratinized cells at the surface of the papilloma.

Papillomas develop after the introduction of virus through abrasions of the skin. Infection of the epithelial cells results in hyperplasia of cells of the stratum spinosum with subsequent degeneration and hyperkeratinization. Clinically, the epithelium overlying the area of hyperplasia begins to proliferate 4–6 weeks after infection. In general, fibropapillomas persist for 4–6 months before spontaneous regression; multiple warts regress simultaneously. The level of antibody does not appear to be correlated with either growth or regression of papillomas, and the mechanisms inducing regression are unknown.

Bovine Papillomatosis

Warts are more commonly seen in cattle than any other domestic animal. All ages are affected, but the incidence is highest in calves and yearlings.

Clinical Features. Warts caused by bovine papillomavirus 1 and 2 have a fibrous core covered to a variable depth with stratified squamous epithelium, the outer layers of which are hyperkeratinized. The lesions vary from small firm nodules to large cauliflower-like growths; they are grayish to black in color, and rough and spiny to the touch. Large fibropapillomas are subject to abrasion and may bleed. Fibropapillomas

TABLE 17-3
Host Responses to Papillomaviruses

Host response	Virus
Group 1	
Neoplasia of cutaneous stratified epithelium (cutaneous papilloma)	Bovine 3 and 6, equine, and cottontail rabbit papillomaviruses[a]
Group 2	
Hyperplasia of normal nonstratified squamous epithelium or metaplastic squamous epithelium	Bovine 4[b] and canine oral papillomaviruses
Group 3	
Cutaneous papilloma with underlying fibroma of connective tissue	Bovine papillomavirus 1, 2, and 5

[a]May progress to squamous carcinoma.
[b]With cofactors, alimentary tract and bladder papillomas may progress to carcinomas.

can occur on the udder and teats and around the genitalia (Fig. 17-2A), but they are most common on the head, neck, and shoulders.

Cutaneous papillomas, lacking a fibrous core, are also seen in cattle. They are caused by bovine papillomavirus 3 and have a tendency to persist. This type of wart is usually flat with a broad base, in contrast to fibropapillomas which protrude and are often pedunculated. In upland areas of Scotland and northern England, papillomas due to bovine papillomavirus 4 occur commonly in the alimentary tract and in the urinary bladder (Fig. 17-2B) of cattle, and may progress to squamous cells carcinomas (see Chapter 11). Ingestion of bracken fern (*Pteridium aquilinum*) appears to be a major contributing factor (cocarcinogen) in the transition from benign papilloma to invasive carcinoma of the alimentary tract or bladder, the latter leading to so-called chronic endemic hematuria.

Papillomas on the teats are common in dairy cattle throughout the world. Generally they are of little concern, but large lesions may interfere with milking. Pedunculated fibropapillomas ("frond papillomas"), caused by bovine papillomavirus 6, and "rice grain" papillomas, caused

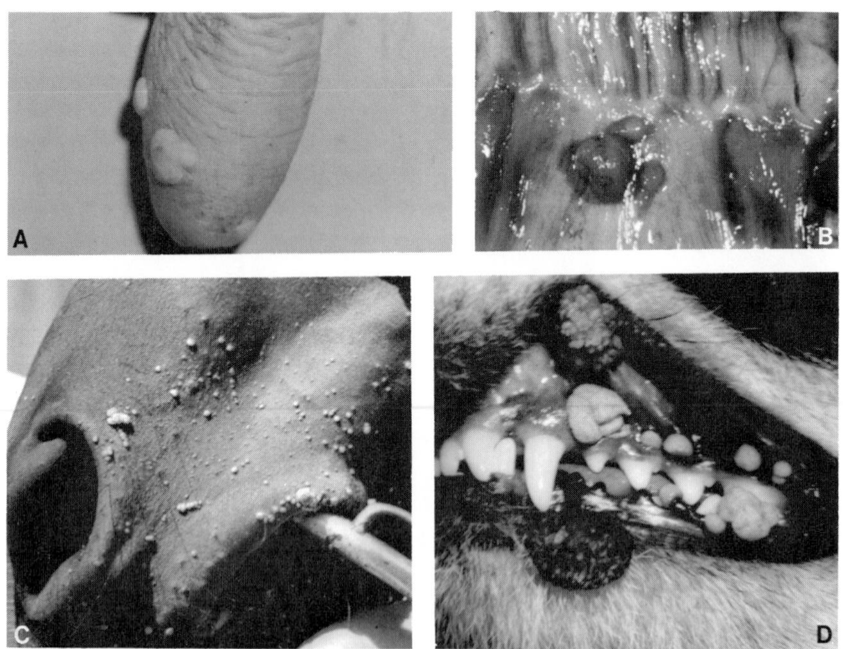

FIG. 17-2. *Warts affecting different species. (A) Bovine teat warts, fibropapilloma (bovine papillomavirus 5). (B) Bovine bladder papilloma (bovine papillomavirus 4). (C) Equine papillomatosis. (D) Canine oral papillomatosis.*

by bovine papillomavirus 5, may also occur on the teats of cattle (Fig. 17-2A).

Laboratory Diagnosis. The clinical appearance of papillomas is characteristic, and laboratory diagnosis is seldom necessary. Virus particles can be found by electron microscopic examination of lesion biopsies. Hybridization assays and the PCR can be used to detect papillomavirus DNA, but they are seldom used for routine diagnosis in veterinary medicine.

Epidemiology. Virus is transmitted between animals by contaminated halters, nose leads, grooming and earmarking equipment, rubbing posts, and other articles contaminated by contact with diseased cattle. Cattle that have been groomed for show may have extensive lesions. The disease is more common in housed cattle than in cattle at pasture.

Prevention and Control. Despite their wide use, there is little evidence that autologous vaccines are effective. The disease is self-limiting, and apart from surgical removal of fibropapillomas on the teats of milking cattle, veterinary intervention is rarely justified. Carcinomas associated with alimentary and urinary tract papillomatosis can be prevented by restricting or eliminating the ingestion of bracken fern.

Equine Papillomatosis and Sarcoids

Warts due to equine papillomavirus occasionally appear as small, elevated, keratinized papillomas around the lips and noses of horses (Fig. 17-2C). They generally regress after a few months. Warts that interfere with the bit or bridle can be surgically removed.

Sarcoids are naturally occurring skin tumors of horses that have the histological appearance of a fibrosarcoma. Although they do not metastasize, they persist for life and are locally invasive, often recurring after surgical or radiation implant removal. The horse is susceptible to experimental infection with bovine papillomavirus 1 and 2, and the tumors produced are similar to sarcoids. Bovine papillomavirus DNA sequences have been detected in high copy number of molecular hybridization in both experimental and natural lesions. These data, together with the observation that sarcoids can occur in epidemic form, suggest that bovine papillomavirus 1 and 2 may be the cause of equine sarcoids.

Canine Papillomatosis

Warts in dogs usually begin on the lips and can spread to the buccal mucosa, tongue, palate, and pharynx before regressing spontaneously (Fig. 17-2D). The lesions occasionally become extensive, requiring veterinary attention and sometimes euthanasia.

Papillomatosis in Other Species

Classic studies on viral oncogenesis were carried out 40–50 years ago with the Shope rabbit papilloma virus. These papillomas often progress to carcinoma in both naturally infected cottontail rabbits and experimentally infected laboratory rabbits. Papillomaviruses of other species are of little importance in veterinary medicine, but one isolated from the multimammate mouse (*Mastomys natalensis*) causes keratinizing squamous epithelial cell carcinomas, which resemble spontaneous human keratoacanthomas.

POLYOMAVIRUSES

Two polyomaviruses are of some interest to veterinarians: a bovine and an avian polyomavirus.

Bovine Polyomavirus. About 60% of calf sera, including fetal and neonatal calf sera, contain a bovine polyomavirus, which grows well in monkey kidney cells. A construct containing its early genes transforms rodent cells, and these cells induce tumors in immunocompromised rats. In a survey in the Netherlands, sera from about 60% of veterinarians tested were found to contain antibodies to this virus.

Budgerigar Fledgling Disease. An avian polyomavirus that has been called budgerigar fledgling disease virus causes an acute generalized disease, with a high mortality, in fledgling budgerigars. The same virus may also be responsible for French molt, which is a milder disease of budgerigars that results in chronic disorders of feather formation, and it is also widespread among chickens as a subclinical infection. The virus is similar to the polyomaviruses of mammals but has a smaller large T antigen and differs in the organization of its origin of replication.

FURTHER READING

Dalgleish, A. G. (1991). Viruses and cancer. *Br. Med. Bull.* **47,** 21.

Dimaio, D. (1991). Transforming activity of bovine and human papillomaviruses in cultured cells. *Adv. Cancer Res.* **56,** 133.

Gaskin, J. M. (1989). Psittacine viral diseases: A perspective. *J. Zoo Wildl. Med.* **20,** 249.

Lambert, P. F. (1991). Papillomavirus DNA replication. *J. Virol.* **65,** 3417.

Olson, C. (1987). Animal papillomas: Historical perspectives. *In* "The *Papovaviridae,* Volume 2: The Papillomaviruses" (N. P. Salzman and P. M. Howley, eds.), p. 39. Plenum, New York.

Onions, D. (1991). Integration of viruses into chromosomal DNA. *J. Pathol.* **163,** 191.

Sundberg, J. P. (1987). Papillomavirus infections in animals. *In* "Papillomaviruses and Human Disease" (K. Syrjanen, L. Gissman, and L. G. Koss, eds.), p. 40. Springer-Verlag, Berlin.

CHAPTER 18

Adenoviridae

In 1953 Rowe and colleagues, having observed that explant cultures of human adenoids degenerated spontaneously, isolated a new virus which they named "adenovirus." The next year Cabasso and colleagues demonstrated that the etiological agent of infectious canine hepatitis was an adenovirus. Subsequently many serotypes of adenoviruses, each of which appeared to be highly host-specific, were isolated from humans and many other species of animals and birds, usually from the upper respiratory tract but sometimes from feces. Most of the viruses produce subclinical infections, with occasional evidence of upper respiratory disease, but the avian adenoviruses are associated with a variety of syndromes (Table 18-1).

PROPERTIES OF ADENOVIRUSES

The morphology of the virion is shown in Fig. 18-1 (see also Fig. 1-1A). The capsid is an icosahedron 70–90 nm in diameter, composed of 252 capsomers (see Table 18-2): 240 hexamers which occupy the faces and

TABLE 18-1
Diseases of Domestic Animals Associated with Adenoviruses

Animal species	Number of serotypes	Disease
Horse	2	Usually asymptomatic or mild upper respiratory disease; generalized disease in foals with congenital immunodeficiency
Cattle	9	Usually asymptomatic, or mild upper respiratory disease
Swine	4	
Sheep	6	
Goat	2	
Dog	2	Infectious canine hepatitis (type 1); infectious canine tracheobronchitis (type 2)
Chicken	12	Rarely, inclusion body hepatitis and egg drop syndrome
Turkey	3	Bronchitis, marble spleen disease, enteritis, egg drop syndrome
Duck	2	Rarely, duck hepatitis
Quail	?	Bronchitis
Goose	3	Isolated from liver, intestine

edges of the 20 equilateral triangles of an icosahedron and 12 pentamers which occupy the vertices. From each pentamer projects a fiber 20 to 50 nm in length, with a terminal knob; avian adenovirus fibers are bifurcated. There are several other minor structural proteins, some of which are associated with the capsid and some with the core, which also contains the viral genome. This is linear dsDNA, 30–37 kbp in size, with inverted terminal repeats. This molecule, in association with a 55K protein covalently linked to each 5′ terminus, is infectious.

Many adenoviruses agglutinate red blood cells, hemagglutination occurring when the tips of the fiber bind to an appropriate receptor on the surface of the erythrocyte. The species of erythrocytes agglutinated and the optimal conditions of assay have been empirically established for each viral species or serotype. Once established, hemagglutination and hemagglutination–inhibition assays provide the simplest and most convenient assays for virus and antibody.

Classification

Classification is based primarily on antigenic relationships. Restriction endonuclease fragment patterns of the viral DNA are useful for detailed comparisons of strains. Shared antigenic determinants associated with the inner part of the hexamers define two genera: *Mastadenovirus*, the mammalian adenoviruses, and *Aviadenovirus*, the avian adenoviruses.

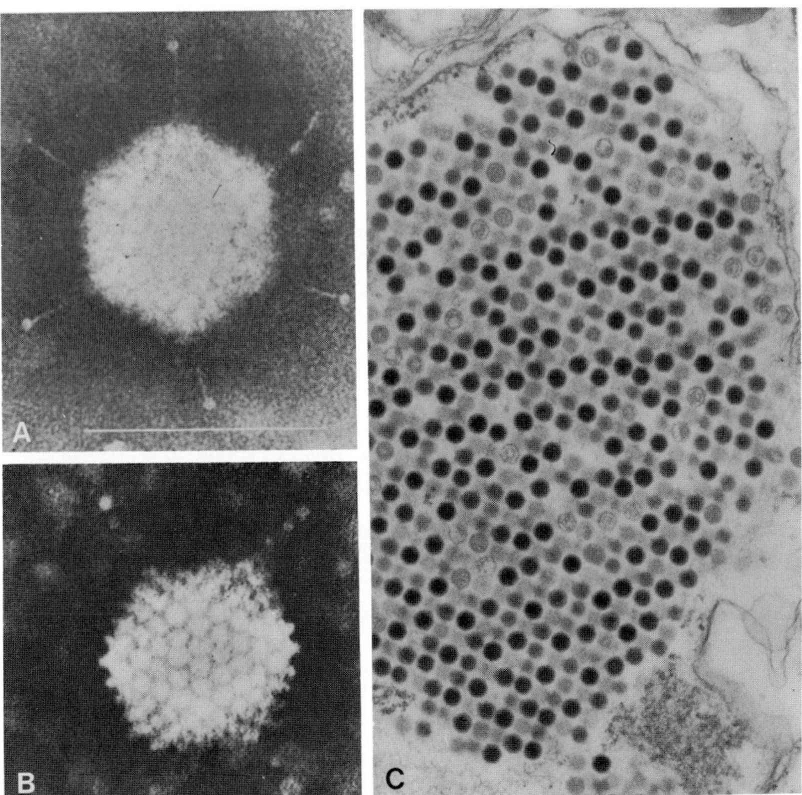

FIG. 18-1. Adenoviridae. *(A and B) Negatively stained preparations of* Mastadenovirus. *(A) Virion showing the fibers projecting from the vertices. (B) Virion showing the icosahedral array of capsomers. Capsomers at the vertices (pentons) are surrounded by five nearest neighbors, all the others (hexons) by six. (C) Section showing crystalline array of mature virions of a human adenovirus in the nucleus of a human fibroblast cell. bar: 100 nm. [A and B, from R. C. Valentine and H. G. Periera,* J. Mol. Biol. **13,** *13 (1965); C, courtesy of Dr. A. K. Harrison.]*

There are also genus-specific antigenic determinants on the pentamer. Type-specific antigenic determinants, which are defined by neutralization and hemagglutination–inhibition assays, are located on the outward-facing surface of the hexamers. The fiber contains type-specific determinants, which can also be detected by neutralization assays. Although the fiber binds to specific cell receptors during absorption, antibody to the fiber or fiber–pentamer complex is only weakly neutralizing.

The number of adenovirus serotypes within each animal species is

TABLE 18-2
Properties of Adenoviruses

Two genera: *Aviadenovirus* and *Mastadenovirus*
Icoahedral virion, 70–90 nm in diameter, composed of 252 capsomers, with one (*Mastadenovirus*) or two (*Aviadenovirus*) fibers (glycoprotein) projecting from each vertex
Linear dsDNA genome, 30–37 kbp, associated with a 55K protein that plays role in DNA replication
Replicate in nucleus of cell, by a complex program of early and late transcription (before and after DNA replication), virions released by cell lysis
Produce intranuclear inclusion bodies containing virions in paracrystalline array
Virus agglutinates red blood cells
Some are oncogenic in rodents

shown in Table 18-1. Some 41 different types are recognized in man, and certain serotypes, which can be grouped together, tend to be associated with particular clinical syndromes. The number of serotypes defined for each domestic animal species is usually small.

VIRAL REPLICATION

Adenovirus fibers attach to cell receptors, and virions enter the cell via clathrin-coated pits. The pentons are removed in the cytoplasm, and the core migrates to the nucleus. In the nucleus the genome is transcribed according to a complex program. RNA transcribed from five separate regions, situated on both strands of the DNA, is spliced, then translated into about a dozen, mainly nonstructural, early proteins. Viral DNA replication, using the 5′-linked 55K protein as primer, proceeds from both ends by a strand displacement mechanism. Following DNA replication, late mRNAs are transcribed; these are translated into structural proteins, which are made in considerable excess. Virions are assembled in the nucleus, where they form crystalline aggregates (Fig. 18-1C) which can be seen by light microscopy as intranuclear inclusion bodies. Shutdown of host macromolecular synthesis occurs progressively during the second half of the replication cycle. Virions are released by cell lysis.

PATHOGENESIS AND IMMUNITY

Most of the adenoviruses listed in Table 18-1 cause acute, mild, or subclinical respiratory disease, which is usually confined to the upper respiratory tract, but may include conjunctivitis and bronchopneumonia.

Some adenoviruses cause mild or subclinical gastroenteric disease. All infections with adenoviruses are associated with long periods of latency, and adenoviruses can often be recovered from the lymphoid organs of apparently healthy animals.

In contrast to the usual mild effects of most adenoviruses, canine adenovirus 1 causes a severe generalized disease of dogs, and several other adenoviruses are pathogenic in immunodeficient animals. These include generalized infections in certain Arabian foals with primary severe combined immunodeficiency and in avian species whose immune systems are compromised by other infections, such as avian leukosis, infectious bursal disease, or chicken anemia.

LABORATORY DIAGNOSIS

Virus can be isolated from swabs, fecal samples, or tissue homogenates by inoculation of cell cultures derived from the homologous species. Cytopathic changes are usually evident on first passage, although for some more slowly growing viruses a second passage is required. Some enteric adenoviruses are difficult to grow in cell cultures. Hemagglutination–inhibition and neutralization assays are universally used for typing viral isolates.

EPIDEMIOLOGY AND CONTROL

Adenoviruses are highly species-specific, and persistent, subclinical, productive infection permits the survival of the virus and provides a source of infection for each new generation of animals. For most adenoviruses the pharyngeal region, particularly the associated lymphoid tissues, is the site of persistent infection, which is concomitant with the presence of antibody. Enteric adenoviruses presumably persist by similar mechanisms, probably in gut-associated lymphoid tissues. Transmission occurs by droplet or a fecal–oral route. Following localization of the virus in the kidney, urine is an important mode of excretion of canine adenovirus 1.

Only the canine adenoviruses cause sufficiently troublesome diseases to warrant vaccination, and attenuated live or inactivated canine adenovirus 1 or 2 vaccines are widely used for the control of canine hepatitis and canine respiratory disease. Avian adenoviruses may be important contaminants of live vaccines produced in eggs or avian cell cultures.

EQUINE ADENOVIRUS INFECTIONS

Most adenovirus infections in horses produce an asymptomatic or mild upper respiratory tract disease. However, certain Arabian foals that suffer from primary severe combined immunodeficiency disease, in which there is an almost total absence of both T and B cells, are particularly susceptible to adenoviruses. As maternal antibody wanes, these foals are increasingly susceptible to a wide range of pathogens before they die, which invariably occurs within 3 months. Among diverse pathogens, the dominant role of equine adenovirus 1 in the total pathology is intriguing. In addition to the extensive adenovirus bronchiolitis and pneumonia, the virus destroys cells in a wide range of other tissues, particularly the pancreas and salivary glands, but also renal, bladder, and gastrointestinal epithelium.

CANINE ADENOVIRUS INFECTIONS

The two diseases caused by canine adenoviruses are much the most important adenovirus infections. Infectious canine hepatitis, caused by canine adenovirus 1, was first recognized as fox encephalitis. As well as causing hepatitis in dogs, canine adenovirus 1 may cause respiratory or ocular disease, encephalopathy, chronic hepatitis, and interstitial nephritis. Canine adenovirus 2 causes respiratory disease: tonsillitis, pharyngitis, tracheitis, bronchitis, and bronchopneumonia.

Infectious Canine Hepatitis

Most infections with canine adenovirus 1 are asymptomatic, a situation probably enhanced by the introduction of vaccination. The virus is acquired as a nasooral or conjunctival infection, and it is a recognized cause of pharyngitis and tonsillitis. It is one of the several causes of "kennel cough," although in this context it is probably less important than canine adenovirus 2. Most canine adenovirus 1 infections are subclinical, but occasionally generalization via the bloodstream occurs, with destruction of vascular endothelium and mesothelium, leading to petechial hemorrhages in many tissues and sometimes massive destruction of hepatocytes, resulting in a peracute fatal disease. In addition to the initial respiratory disease, the pattern of systemic canine adenovirus 1 is divisible into three overlapping syndromes, which are usually seen in pups less than 6 months old: (1) peracute disease in which the pup is found dead either without apparent preceding illness or after an illness lasting only 3 or 4 hours; (2) an acute illness, which may be fatal, with fever, depression, loss of appetite, vomiting, bloody diarrhea, petechial hemorrhages of the gums, pale mucous membranes, and jaundice; and (3) mild cases.

Postmortem findings may include edematous lymph nodes, excess (and sometimes bloody) fluid in the abdominal cavity, hemorrhages in many tissues, and jaundice. The liver may show slight enlargement, congestion, and yellowish mottling, and histologic examination invariably reveals characteristic inclusion bodies in hepatocytes (Fig. 18-2A).

In the convalescent stages of natural infection, or 8–12 days after vaccination with attenuated live canine adenovirus 1, corneal edema ("blue eye") is occasionally observed (Fig. 18-2B). Though clinically dramatic and alarming, especially after vaccination, the edema usually resolves after a few days without consequence. The edema is due to virus–antibody complexes, deposited in the small blood vessels of the ciliary body, interfering with normal fluid exchange within the cornea. A similar pathogenesis underlies glomerulonephritis due to canine adenovirus 1. Infection of the kidney is associated with viruria, which is a significant mode for transmission.

Both killed and attenuated live canine adenovirus 1 vaccines are in general use. Attenuated live canine adenovirus 2 vaccines are also used. The antigenic relationship between canine adenoviruses 1 and 2 is sufficiently close for the canine adenovirus 2 vaccine to be cross-protective; it has the advantage that it does not cause corneal edema.

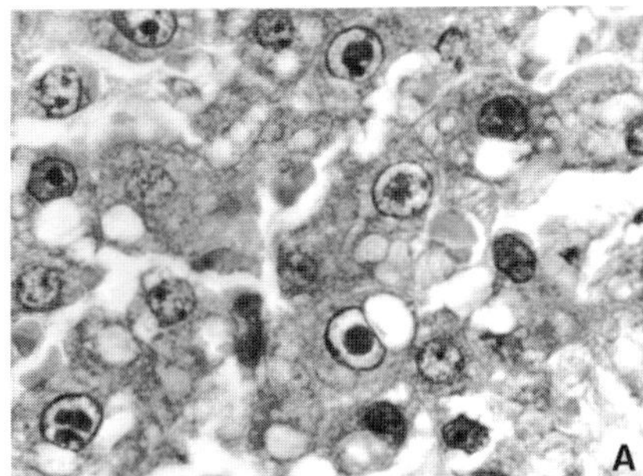

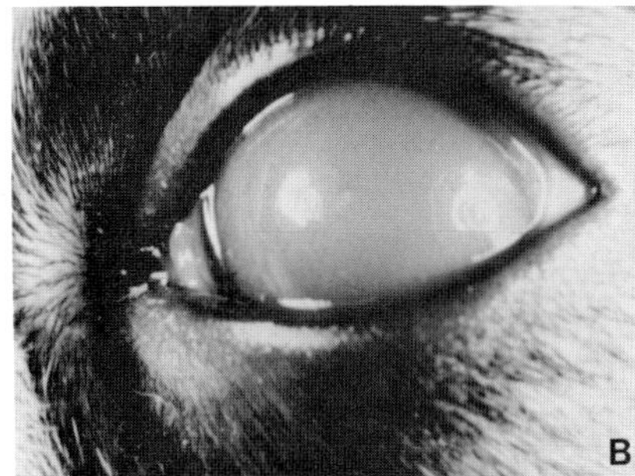

FIG. 18-2. *Canine adenovirus 1 infections. (A) Inclusion bodies within hepatocytes in peracute infectious canine hepatitis. (B) "Blue eye" in a pup 9 days after vaccination with canine adenovirus 1 vaccine. (Courtesy Dr. L. E. Carmichael.)*

AVIAN ADENOVIRUS INFECTIONS

Adenoviruses commonly infect chickens and other avian species including quail, turkey, duck, geese, and pheasants. Initially, avian adenoviruses were considered to be nonpathogenic for domestic poultry, although they were lethal following inoculation of chick embryos. Avian adenoviruses have been assigned to three groups. Group I viruses share a common group antigen and have been isolated from chickens, turkeys, geese, and other species. Group II viruses share a different group antigen and include viruses from turkey hemorrhagic enteritis, marble spleen disease, and some chicken isolates associated with splenomegaly. Group III avian adenoviruses are partially related antigenically to Group I viruses and are associated with egg drop syndrome in chickens and ducks.

Although the recovery of the virus and the accompanying pathology, as seen in inclusion body hepatitis of chickens, suggest that adenoviruses play a specific role in the production of disease, these varied syndromes are difficult or impossible to reproduce experimentally with adenoviruses alone. There is a strong suspicion that the pathogenicity of adenoviruses is enhanced by immunodeficiency, particularly that caused by intercurrent infections with agents such as avian leukosis, infectious bursal disease, or chicken anemia viruses.

Adenoviruses persist as subclinical infections in breeding flocks and contaminate eggs and cell cultures used as substrate for the production of vaccines; hence they have caused concern as contaminants of avian live-virus vaccines.

FURTHER READING

Horwitz, M. S. (1990). Adenoviridae and their replication. *In* "Fields Virology" (B. N. Fields, D. M. Knipe, R. M. Chanock, M. S. Hirsch, J. L. Melnick, T. P. Monath, and B. Roizman, eds.), 2nd Ed., p. 1679. Raven, New York.

Ishibashi, M., and Yasne, H. (1984). Adenoviruses of animals. *In* "The Adenoviruses" (H. S. Ginsberg, ed.), p. 497. Plenum, New York.

Kopotopoulos, G., and Cornwell, H. J. C. (1981). Canine adenoviruses: A review. *Vet. Bull.* **51,** 135.

McFerran, J. B. (1991). Adenovirus infections. *In* "Diseases of Poultry" (B. W. Calnek, ed.), 9th Ed., p. 552. Iowa State Univ. Press, Ames.

McGuire, T. C., and Perryman, L. E. (1981). Combined immunodeficiency of Arabian foals. *In* "Immunologic Defects in Laboratory Animals" (M. E. Gershwin and B. Merchant, eds.), Vol. 2, p. 185. Plenum, New York.

Wigand, R., Bartha, A., Dreizin, R. S., Esche, H., Ginsberg, H. S., Green, M., Hierholzer, J. C., Kalter, S. S., McFerran, J. B., Pettersson, U., Russell, W. C., and Wadell, G. (1982). *Adenoviridae:* Second report. *Intervirology* **18,** 169.

CHAPTER 19

Herpesviridae

About one hundred herpesviruses have been at least partially characterized. They have been found in insects, reptiles, and amphibia as well as in virtually every species of bird and mammal that has been investigated. At least one major disease of each domestic animal species except sheep is caused by a herpesvirus, including such important diseases as infectious bovine rhinotracheitis, pseudorabies, and Marek's disease.

Herpesvirus particles are fragile and do not survive well outside the body. In general transmission requires close contact, particularly the kinds of physical contact that brings mucosae into apposition, for example, coitus, or licking and nuzzling as between mother and offspring or between foals or kittens. In large, closely confined populations, such as are found in a cattle feedlot, multiple farrowing unit, cattery, or broiler chicken run, sneezing and short distance droplet spread are major modes of transmission.

Herpesviruses can survive from one generation to the next by establishing latent infections, from which virus is periodically reactivated and shed, and in some infections shedding may be continuous.

PROPERTIES OF HERPESVIRUSES

The herpesvirus virion is enveloped and about 150 nm in diameter (Table 19-1). The DNA genome is wrapped around a fibrous spoollike core which has the shape of a torus and appears to be suspended by fibrils which are anchored to the inner side of the surrounding capsid and pass through the hole of the torus. The capsid is an icosahedron, 100 nm in diameter, composed of 162 hollow capsomers: 150 hexamers and 12 pentamers (see Fig. 19-1B). Surrounding the capsid is a layer of globular material, known as the "tegument," which is enclosed by a typical lipoprotein envelope with numerous small glycoprotein peplomers (Fig. 19-1A). Because of the envelope, the virion is somewhat pleomorphic and can range in diameter from 120 to 200 nm.

The virion contains over 30 proteins, of which 6 are present in the nucleocapsid, 2 being DNA-associated. The glycoproteins, of which there are about 10, are located in the envelope, from which some project as peplomers. One of the peplomer glycoproteins possesses Fc receptor activity and binds normal IgG. Other structural proteins are tegument-associated. Antigenic relationships are complex. There are some shared antigens within the family, but different species have distinct envelope glycoproteins.

The herpesvirus genome (Fig. 19-2) consists of a linear dsDNA molecule which is infectious under appropriate experimental conditions. There is a remarkable degree of variation in the composition, size, and structure of herpesvirus DNAs; for example, the percentage of guanine

TABLE 19-1
Properties of Herpesviruses

Enveloped virions, 120–200 nm (usually about 150 nm) in diameter, with several different peplomers up to 8 nm long in envelope
Icosahedral capsid with 162 capsomers
Linear dsDNA genome, 120–240 kbp; G + C ratio varies from 32% to 74%
Replicates in nucleus, with sequential transcription and translation of immediate early (α), early (β), and late (γ) genes producing α, β, and γ proteins, respectively, the earlier of which regulate transcription from later genes
Produce eosinophilic intranuclear inclusion bodies
DNA replication and encapsidation occur in nucleus; envelope is acquired by budding through nuclear membrane
Establish latent infections, with recurrent or continuous shedding of infectious virus

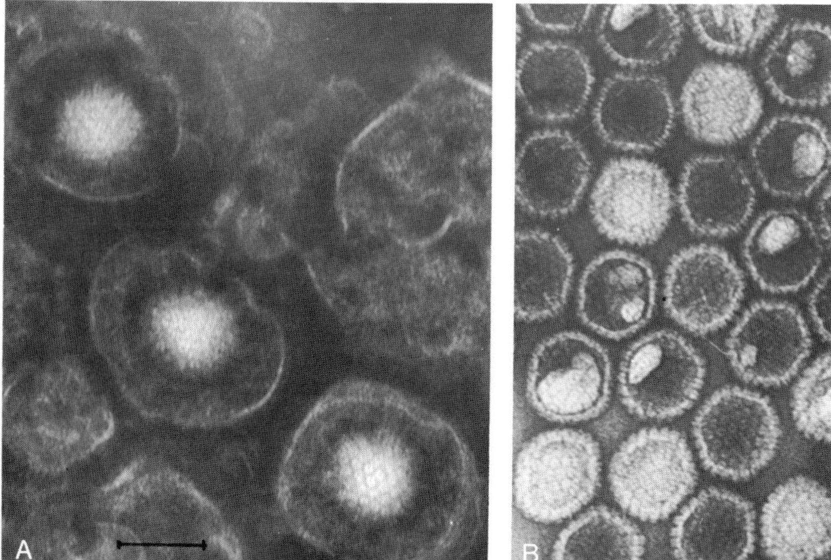

FIG. 19-1. Herpesviridae. *Negatively stained preparations of the prototype herpesvirus, herpes simplex virus type 1. (A) Enveloped particles. (B) Icosahedral capsids with 162 capsomers. Bar: 100 nm. (Courtesy Dr. E. L. Palmer.)*

plus cystosine varies between 32% and 74%, a range far exceeding that found in the DNAs of all eukaryotes, and the genome size varies between 121 and 227 kbp. Physical maps based on ordering of restriction endonuclease fragments are available for many herpesviruses, and DNA fragment patterns (fingerprints) are useful for epidemiologic analysis.

The genomes of several herpesviruses have been sequenced, including at least one member of each subfamily. The genomes of the alphaherpesviruses appear to be colinear, that is, the presence and order of the individual genes are similar. While it is clear that the genome is complex, 24 of the total 72 genes of herpes simplex virus are not required for replication in cell culture. The role of these "nonessential" genes in intact animals remains to be defined.

Classification

Subdivision of the family into subfamilies is based on biological properties, which in general coincide with genome structure, as shown in Fig. 19-2. Many herpesviruses, however, have not yet been allocated to a subfamily.

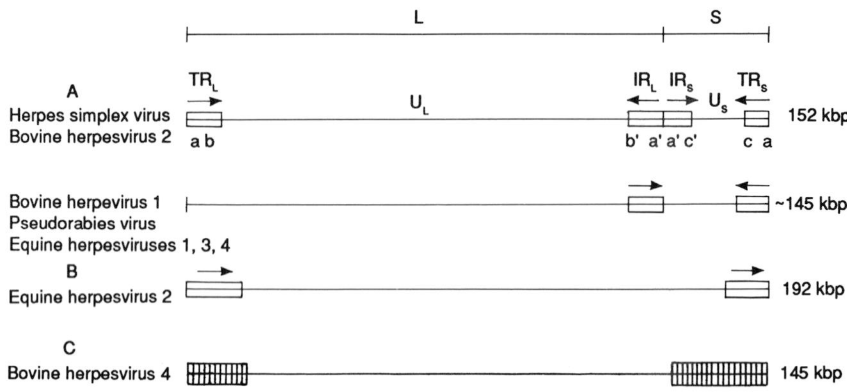

FIG. 19-2. *The genome structure of herpesviruses. (A) Alphaherpesvirus genomes comprise two regions designated long (L) and short (S). Terminal repeat (TR) and internal repeat (IR) sequences may bracket unique sequences (U_L, U_S) of both L and S, or only S. Repeat sequences are shown as boxes and are indirect as indicated by the direction of the arrows. The repeat sequences allow the DNA they bracket to invert relative to the rest of the genome such that where both U_L and U_S are bracketed by repeat sequences four isomers are made and packaged in equimolar amounts into virions. Where only S is bracketed by repeat sequences two equimolar isomers are made. (B) The genome of equine herpesvirus 2, a betaherpesvirus, contains terminal direct repeat structures. (C) The genome of bovine herpesvirus 4, a gammaherpesvirus, contains multiple direct terminal repeat sequences (small boxes) in a nonequal, variable number of copies.*

***Alphaherpesvirinae*.** The prototype viruses of this subfamily are herpes simplex type 1 and varicella viruses (Fig. 19-2A). They grow rapidly and lyse infected cells, and they establish latent infections primarily in sensory nerve ganglia. Some alphaviruses have a broad host range.

***Betaherpesvirinae*.** Individual cytomegaloviruses (genome, Fig. 19-2B) have a restricted host range. Their replicative cycle is slow, and cell lysis does not occur until several days after infection. The virus may remain latent in secretory glands, lymphoreticular tissue, kidneys, and other tissues.

***Gammaherpesvirinae*.** The subfamily *Gammaherpesvirinae* (Fig. 19-2C) was defined in terms of Epstein-Barr virus. Members have a narrow host range, and they replicate in lymphoid cells; some also cause cytocidal infections in epithelial and fibroblastic cells. Latent virus is frequently demonstrable in lymphoid tissue.

VIRAL REPLICATION

Herpesvirus replication has been most extensively studied with herpes simplex virus. Betaherpesviruses and gammaherpesviruses probably follow a similar pattern, but replicate more slowly. Following adsorption via the glycoprotein peplomers of the envelope to host cell receptors, one of which is heparin sulfate proteoglycan, the nucleocapsid penetrates to the cytoplasm either by fusion of the virion envelope to the cell membrane or via a phagocytic vacuole. A DNA–protein complex is then freed from the nucleocapsid and enters the nucleus, shutting off host cell macromolecular synthesis.

Three classes of mRNA, α, β, γ, are transcribed in sequence by the cellular RNA polymerase II (Fig. 19-3). Thus α (immediate early) RNAs, when appropriately processed to mRNAs, are translated to α proteins, which initiate transcription of β (early) mRNAs, whose translated product(s), β (proteins, suppress transcription of further α mRNAs. Viral DNA replication then commences, utilizing some of the α and β proteins as well as host cell proteins. The program of transcription then switches again, and the resulting γ (late) mRNAs, which are transcribed from sequences situated throughout the genome, are translated into the γ proteins. Over 70 virus-coded proteins are made during the cycle,

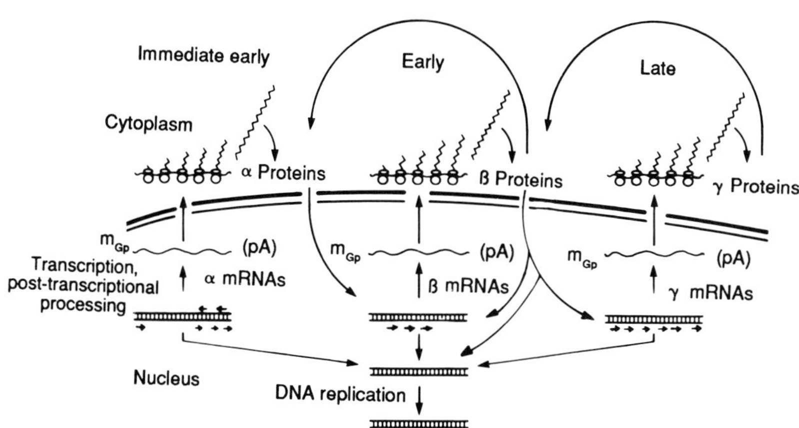

FIG. 19-3. *Diagram representing transcription, translation, and DNA replication of herpes simplex virus (see text). Transcription and posttranscriptional processing occur in the nucleus, translation takes place in the cytoplasm, and some of the α and β proteins are involved in further transcription and some β proteins in DNA replication. (Courtesy Dr. B. Roizman.)*

many of the α and β proteins being enzymes and DNA-binding proteins, whereas most of the γ proteins are structural. Intricate controls must regulate expression at the level of both transcription and translation. Viral DNA is replicated in the nucleus, and newly synthesized DNA is spooled into preformed immature capsids.

Maturation involves the encapsidation of DNA into nucleocapsids and the association of nucleocapsids with altered areas of the inner layer of the nuclear membrane, followed by envelopment by budding. Mature virions accumulate within vacuoles in the cytoplasm, and they may be released by exocytosis or cytolysis. Virus-specific proteins are also found in the plasma membrane, where they are involved in cell fusion, may act as Fc receptors, and are presumed to be targets for immune cytolysis.

Intranuclear inclusion bodies are characteristic of herpesvirus infections and can usually be found both in tissues from herpesvirus-infected animals and in appropriately fixed and stained cell cultures (Fig. 19-4).

PATHOGENESIS AND IMMUNITY

Collectively and individually herpesviruses are versatile pathogens. Transmission is generally associated with close contact of mucosae, but droplet infection is also common. Many alphaherpesviruses produce localized lesions, particularly in the skin or on the mucosal surfaces of the respiratory and genital tracts. These are characterized by the sequential production of vesicles, pustules, and shallow ulcers which become covered by a pseudomembrane and heal after 10–14 days, usually without scar formation.

Generalized alphaherpesvirus infection, characterized by foci of necrosis in almost any organ or tissue, is seen when animals less than 3 months of age are infected without the protection provided by maternal antibody. In pregnant animals a mononuclear cell-associated viremia may result in transfer of virus across the placenta, leading to abortion, focal necrotic lesions being found throughout the fetus. Betaherpesviruses are associated with respiratory and generalized disease, while gammaherpesviruses may produce systemic disease and tumors.

Persistent infection with periodic or continuous shedding occurs in all herpesvirus infections. In alphaherpesvirus infections, multiple copies of viral DNA are demonstrable either as episomes or more rarely integrated into the chromosomal DNA of latently infected neurons, having arrived there via axonal spread from lesions located in the skin and mucous membranes. Only a small percentage of neurons carry the viral genome, although in any one neuron there are multiple copies suggesting that the genome replicates within the neuron. The latent genome

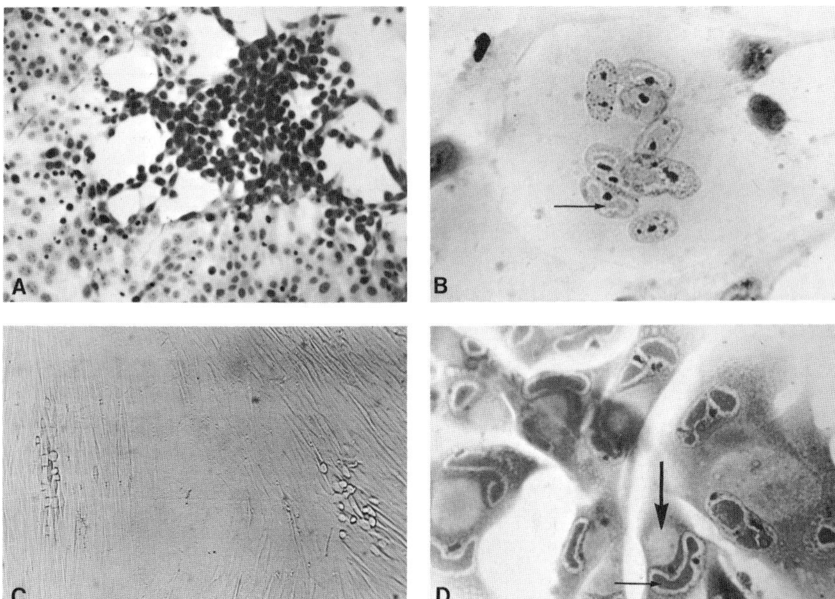

FIG. 19-4. *Cytopathic effects induced by herpesvirus. (A) Alphaherpesvirus in HEp-2 cells showing early focal cytopathology (top right) and (B) virus in kidney cells (hematoxylin and eosin stain; magnification: ×228), showing multinucleated giant cell containing acidophilic intranuclear inclusions (arrow). Cytomegalovirus in embryo fibroblasts, (C) showing two foci of slowly developing cytopathology, (unstained; magnification: ×35) and (D) showing giant cells with acidophilic inclusions in the nuclei (small arrow) and cytoplasm (large arrow), the latter being characteristically large and round (hematoxylin and eosin stain; magnification: ×228). (Courtesy I. Jack.)*

is essentially silent except for the production of a latency-associated transcript that is overlapping with the immediate early gene $\alpha 0$ but is read from the opposite DNA strand. This antisense RNA transcript is not known to code for any protein; its significance in the establishment, maintenance, or reactivation of latent virus has not yet been established.

Reactivation is usually intermittent and may be associated with stress, such as is occasioned by intercurrent disease, shipping, cold, or crowding. Shedding of virus in nasal, oral, or genital secretions provides the source of infection for other animals, including transfer from mother to offspring. In domestic animals reactivation is frequently subclinical, partly because the sites involved, on nasal or genital mucosae, are not readily observed. Some betaherpesviruses and gammaherpesviruses cause a persistent, cell-associated viremia and appear to be shed continuously via epithelial surfaces.

Neutralizing antibody is primarily directed at envelope glycoproteins and reaches a maximum titer about 14 days after infection. Early neutralizing antibody can only be demonstrated in the presence of complement; later complement is not required, but its presence enhances the titer four- to eightfold. Following primary infection, antibody titers may drop to nondetectable levels, but with advancing age titers are generally high, presumably as a consequence of recurrent production of virus. In adult animals antibody titers tend not to rise in association with syndromes such as abortion or encephalitis.

Viral antigens expressed on the surface of infected cells are targets for cell-mediated immune lysis. It is generally assumed that late glycoproteins are important targets for cytotoxic T cells, although for both alphaherpesviruses and betaherpesviruses immediate early antigens have been identified as target antigens for cytotoxic T cells. Although both antibody and cell-mediated immune responses develop following primary infection, they are without effect on virus in latently infected neurons, or in preventing its egress via sensory nerve pathways to sites of epithelial infection. However, in recurrent episodes viral spread at epithelial sites is restricted by the immune response to contiguous cells, so that recurrent lesions are usually milder than primary lesions.

Herpesvirus infections are much more severe following primary infection of young animals that have lost or lack maternally derived antibodies.

LABORATORY DIAGNOSIS

Rapid diagnostic methods include electron microscopy of vesicular fluid or scrapings and immunofluorescent staining of smears or tissue sections. Viral isolation and characterization provide a definitive diagnosis. Herpesviruses are most readily grown in cell cultures derived from their natural host. With adaptation, the host range of a particular herpesvirus in cell culture can be extended, though for some herpesviruses only cells from the natural host are permissive. Alphaherpesviruses produce a rapid cytopathic effect, some species producing syncytia, and characteristic eosinophilic intranuclear inclusion bodies are readily demonstrated in infected cells. Betaherpesviruses and gammaherpesviruses are slowly cytopathic in cell culture but produce similar intranuclear inclusion bodies.

TREATMENT

Chemotherapy is possible in some herpesvirus diseases; because of the expense, however, it is feasible only for individual valuable animals. Antiherpetic drugs such as 5-iodo-2′-deoxyuridine (iodouridine), cytosine arabinoside (cytarabine), and acycloguanosine (acyclovir) represent a progression in the development of increasingly effective drugs for the treatment of human alphaherpesvirus diseases. Such drugs are not used nor seriously contemplated for use in veterinary medicine, with the possible exception of the treatment of feline herpesvirus 1 corneal ulcers.

DISEASES CAUSED BY ALPHAHERPESVIRUSES

Viruses of the subfamily *Alphaherpesvirinae* cause infections of veterinary importance in a wide range of animals (Table 19-2).

Infectious Bovine Rhinotracheitis (Bovine Herpesvirus 1)

Bovine herpesvirus 1 (infectious bovine rhinotracheitis virus) causes a variety of diseases in cattle, which include rhinotracheitis, pustular vaginitis, conjunctivitis, abortion, enteritis, a generalized disease of newborn calves, and possibly encephalitis.

The rapid expansion of feedlots in the United States during the 1950s led to the recognition of new disease syndromes including "infectious bovine rhinotracheitis," from which a herpesvirus was isolated. Comparison of the herpesviruses isolated from infectious bovine rhinotracheitis and from infectious pustular vulvovaginitis in dairy cattle in the eastern United States showed that the viruses were indistinguishable. Bovine herpesvirus 1 and the diseases it causes are now known to occur worldwide.

Clinical Features of Genital Disease. Infectious pustular vulvovaginitis is most commonly recognized in dairy cows. Affected cows develop fever, depression, anorexia, and stand apart, often with the tail held away from contact with the vulva; micturition is frequent and painful. The vulval labia are swollen, there is a slight vulval discharge, and the vestibular mucosa is reddened with many small pustules (Fig. 19-5A). Adjacent pustules usually coalesce to form a fibrinous pseudomembrane which covers an ulcerated mucosa. The acute stage of the disease lasts 4–5 days, and uncomplicated lesions usually heal by 10–14 days. Many cases are subclinical or go unnoticed.

TABLE 19-2
Herpesviruses That Cause Diseases in Domestic Animals

Virus	Disease
Subfamily *Alphaherpesvirinae*	
Bovine herpesvirus 1	Infectious bovine rhinotracheitis, infectious pustular vulvovaginitis, infectious balanoposthitis, abortion
Bovine herpesvirus 2	Bovine mammillitis, pseudo-lumpyskin disease
Bovine herpesvirus 5	Encephalitis
Caprine herpesvirus 1	Conjunctivitis, respiratory disease
Porcine herpesvirus 1	Pseudorabies
Equine herpesvirus 1	Abortion
Equine herpesvirus 3	Coital exanthema
Equine herpesvirus 4	Rhinopneumonitis
Canine herpesvirus 1	Hemorrhagic disease of pups
Feline herpesvirus 1	Feline viral rhinotracheitis
Avian herpesvirus 1	Infectious laryngotracheitis
Avian herpesvirus 2	Marek's disease
Duck herpesvirus 1	Duck plague
Cercopithecine herpesvirus 1	Herpes simplex-like disease in macaques, paralysis in man (also called B virus)
Subfamily *Betaherpesvirinae*	
Equine herpesvirus 2	Equine cytomegalovirus infection
Equine herpesvirus 5	Unknown
Porcine herpesvirus 2	Inclusion body rhinitis, generalized cytomegalovirus infection
Subfamily *Gammaherpesvirinae*	
Alcelaphine herpesvirus 1	Bovine malignant catarrhal fever
Bovine herpesvirus 4	Unknown

The lesions of infectious balanoposthitis in bulls and the clinical course of disease are similar (Fig. 19-5B). Where lesions are extensive and acute there is reluctance or complete refusal to serve. Semen from recovered bulls may be contaminated with virus as a result of periodic shedding. However, cows may conceive to the service or artificial insemination from which they acquire infectious pustular vulvovaginitis, and pregnant cows that develop the infection rarely abort. Bovine herpesvirus 1 has occasionally been isolated from cases of vaginitis and balanitis in swine and from stillborn piglets.

Clinical Features of Respiratory Infection. Infectious bovine rhinotracheitis occurs as a subclinical, mild, or severe disease. Morbidity approaches 100% and mortality may reach 10%, particularly if complications occur. Initial signs include fever, depression, inappetence, and a profuse nasal discharge, initially serous and later mucopurulent. The nasal mu-

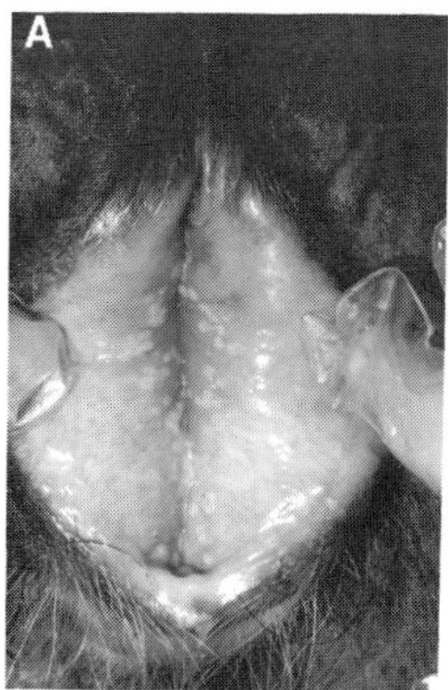

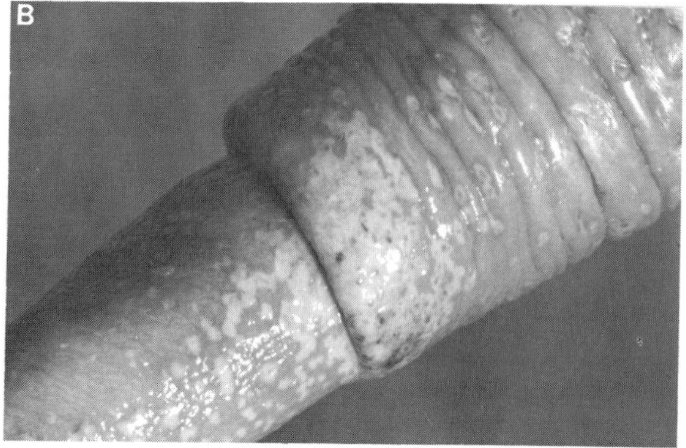

FIG. 19-5. *Genital disease caused by bovine herpesvirus 1. (A) Infectious pustular vulvovaginitis. (B) Infectious pustular balanoposthitis. [A from D. F. Collings* et al., Vet Rec. **91,** *214 (1972); B from M. J. Studdert* et al., Am. J. Vet. Res. **105,** *303 (1964).]*

cosa is hyperemic, and lesions within the nasal cavity, which may be difficult to see, progress from focal pustular necrosis to large areas of shallow, hemorrhagic, ulcerated mucosa which is covered by a cream-colored diphtheritic membrane. The breath may be fetid. Dyspnea, mouth breathing, salivation, and a deep bronchial cough are common. Acute, uncomplicated cases last 5–10 days.

Unilateral or bilateral conjunctivitis, often with profuse lacrimation, is a common clinical sign in cattle with infectious bovine rhinotracheitis but may occur in a herd as an almost exclusive clinical sign. Gastroenteritis may occur in adult cattle and is a prominent finding in the generalized disease of neonatal calves, which is often fatal. Abortion may occur at 4–7 months gestation, and the virus has also been reported to cause mastitis.

Pathogenesis and Pathology. Genital disease may result from coitus or artificial insemination, although some outbreaks, particularly in dairy cows, may occur in the absence of coitus. Respiratory disease and conjunctivitis result from droplet transmission. Within the animal, dissemination of the virus from the initial focus of infection probably occurs via a cell-associated viremia.

Lifelong latent infection with periodic virus shedding occurs after bovine herpesvirus 1 infection, the sciatic and trigeminal ganglia being the sites of latency following genital and respiratory disease, respectively. The administration of corticosteroids results in reactivation of the virus, and this approach has been used as a means of detecting and eliminating carrier bulls in artificial insemination centers.

In both the genital and respiratory forms of the disease the lesions are focal areas of epithelial cell necrosis in which there is ballooning of epithelial cells; typical herpesvirus inclusions may be present in nuclei at the periphery of necrotic foci. There is an intense inflammatory response. Gross lesions are not observed in aborted fetuses, but microscopic necrotic foci are present in most tissues and the liver is consistently affected.

Epidemiology and Control. Genital and respiratory disease are rarely diagnosed in the same herd at the same time. Infectious bovine rhinotracheitis is an uncommon disease in range cattle but is of major significance in feedlots. In cattle not in feedlots, the incidence of antibody varies between 10% and 35%. Primary infection often coincides with transport and introduction to a feedlot of young, fully susceptible cattle from diverse sources. Adaptation from range to feedlot conditions and dietary changes including the high-protein diet contribute to a stressful environment which may potentiate disease, although in well managed operations these factors are minimized, with a corresponding reduced incidence of severe disease. The damaged necrotic mucosa provides a substrate for bacterial infection in stressed cattle and contributes to the complex syndrome called "shipping fever" (see Chapter 9).

Iatrogenic transmission has occurred among bulls in artificial insemination centers when a common sponge was used for washing the prepuce prior to semen collection. Virus may also be spread by artificial insemination.

Bovine herpesvirus 1 vaccines (mostly attenuated live-virus vaccines) are used extensively, alone or in formulations containing other viral vaccines. Recombinant DNA vaccines have been constructed in which the thymidine kinase and other genes have been deleted. Although they do not prevent infection, vaccines significantly reduce the incidence of disease.

Because of the low incidence of bovine herpesvirus 1 infections in cattle in Switzerland and Denmark, successful eradication programs based on test and slaughter, combined with control of cattle movements, were initiated there in the early 1980s. Vaccines were not used, so as to avoid problems of masking latently infected animals. With the probable commercial introduction of better vaccines in the near future, other countries in Europe are now considering eradicating the virus by an integrated program involving vaccination, movement control, and slaughter of all cattle with serologic evidence of exposure to wild virus.

Bovine Mammillitis/Pseudo-Lumpyskin Disease (Bovine Herpesvirus 2)

Two clinical forms of bovine herpesvirus 2 infections are known: lesions localized to the teats, occasionally spreading to the udder (bovine mammillitis), and a generalized skin disease (pseudo-lumpyskin disease). Bovine herpesvirus 2 was first isolated in 1957 from cattle in South Africa with a generalized lumpyskin disease. The disease was mild, however, and its major significance lay in the need to differentiate it from a more serious lumpyskin disease found in South Africa and caused by a poxvirus (see Chapter 20). A similar herpesvirus was isolated from cattle with extensive erosions of the teats elsewhere in Africa, and subsequently from similar lesions in cattle in many countries of the world.

Bovine herpesvirus 2 is antigenically related to human herpes simplex virus, and the DNAs of these viruses show 15% sequence homology, compared with less than 6% homology between bovine herpesvirus 2 and bovine herpesvirus 1.

Clinical Features. Pseudo-lumpyskin disease has as incubation period of 5–9 days and is characterized by a mild fever, followed by the sudden appearance of skin nodules: a few, or many, on the face, neck, back, and perineum. The nodules have a flat surface with a slightly depressed center and involve only the superficial layers of the epidermis, which undergo necrosis. Within 7–8 days, the local swelling subsides, and healing, without scar formation, is complete within a few weeks.

In many countries, the generalized skin disease is not seen and bovine herpesvirus 2 is recognized only as a cause of mammillitis, but experimentally, virus isolated from cases of mammillitis can cause generalized skin disease. Lesions usually occur only on the teats, but in severe cases most of the skin of the udder may be affected. Occasionally heifers may develop fever, coinciding with the appearance of lesions. Milk yield may be reduced by as much as 10% as a result of difficulty in milking the affected cows and intercurrent mastitis.

Pathogenesis. The distribution of lesions in mammillitis suggests local spread. The generalized distribution of lesions in pseudo-lumpyskin disease suggests viremic spread, but viremia is difficult to demonstrate.

Diagnosis. The benign nature of of pseudo-lumpyskin disease, the characteristic central depression on the surface of the nodules, the superficial necrosis of the epidermis, and the shorter course of the disease are helpful in differentiating the condition from true lumpyskin disease, in countries where both occur.

The clinical differentiation of the various conditions that affect the teats of cattle (see Fig. 20-3A,B) can be difficult; other virus diseases causing teat lesions are warts, cowpox, pseudocowpox, vesicular stomatitis, and foot-and-mouth disease. For this reason it is advisable to examine the whole herd, as a comparison of the early developmental stages helps considerably in the diagnosis. Advanced lesions are often similar, irrespective of the cause. Demonstration of virus in scrapings or vesicular fluid by electron microscopy, coupled with virus isolation, is used for confirming a diagnosis.

Epidemiology. Pseudo-lumpyskin disease occurs most commonly in southern Africa, in moist low-lying areas, especially along rivers, and it has its highest incidence in the summer months and early fall. Susceptible cattle cannot be infected by placing them in contact with diseased cattle if housed in insect-proof accommodation. It is therefore assumed that mechanical transmission of the virus by arthropods occurs, but attempts to identify the vectors have failed. Buffalo, giraffe, and other African wildlife may be naturally infected with bovine herpesvirus 2.

Although milking machines were initially thought to be responsible for transmission of mammillitis in dairy herds, there is evidence of arthropod transmission. The infection may spread rapidly through a herd, but in some outbreaks disease is confined to newly calved heifers or heavily pregnant cattle. Serologic surveys suggest that many infections are subclinical.

Bovine Herpesvirus Encephalitis (Bovine Alphaherpesvirus 5)

Encephalitis due to bovine herpesvirus 5 has been recognized in several countries. It is believed to result from direct neural spread from the nasal cavity, pharynx, and tonsils via the maxillary and mandibular branches of the trigeminal nerve. Lesions initially occur in the midbrain and later involve the entire brain. The natural history of the causative virus is obscure. Although frequently stated to cause encephalitis, bovine herpesvirus 1 has not been confirmed as a cause of this disease.

Infections with Caprine Herpesvirus 1

Herpesviruses have been isolated from goats in several parts of the world, in association with a variety of clinical signs, including conjunctivitis, disease of the respiratory, digestive, and genital tracts, and abortion. Caprine herpesvirus 1 is antigenically related to bovine herpesvirus 1 in a one-way cross-reaction; however, it is not infectious for cattle or lambs, and its restriction endonuclease map is quite different from that of bovine herpesvirus 1.

Pseudorabies (Porcine Herpesvirus 1)

Pseudorabies (synonym Aujeszky's disease) is primarily a disease of swine, which serve as a reservoir and the principal source of natural infection for a diverse range of secondary hosts, which include horse, cattle, sheep, goats, dogs, and cats, and many feral species. The diverse host range is also demonstrated *in vitro;* cell cultures derived from almost any animal species support the replication of pseudorabies virus.

Pseudorabies is endemic in swine in most parts of the world. The eradication of hog cholera from the United States and the United Kingdom (see Chapter 24) has brought pseudorabies to greater prominence, and it is now economically the most important viral disease of swine, causing multimillion dollar losses each year in countries where it is found.

Clinical Features in Swine. In herds in which the disease is endemic, reactivation of virus occurs without obvious clinical signs, but the spread of the virus within a nonimmune herd may be rapid, the consequences of primary infection being markedly influenced by age and, in sows, by pregnancy. Pruritus, which is such a dominant feature of the disease in secondary hosts such as cattle, is rare in swine.

Pregnant Sows. In nonimmune herds, up to 50% of pregnant sows may abort over a short period of time, due to rapid spread of infection from an index case or carrier. Infection of a sow before the thirtieth day of gestation results in death and resorption of embryos, after that time in abortion. Infection in late pregnancy may terminate with the delivery of a mixture of mummified, macerated, stillborn, weak, and normal swine, and some of these pregnancies may be prolonged for 2–3 weeks beyond the normal gestation period. Up to 20% of aborting sows are infertile on the first subsequent breeding but do eventually conceive.

Piglets. Mortality rates among piglets born to nonimmune dams depend somewhat on their age, but approach 100%. Maternal antibody is protective, and disease in piglets born to recovered or vaccinated sows is greatly diminished in severity, with recovery the usual outcome.

Weaned, Growing, and Mature Swine. The incubation period is about 30 hours. In younger animals the course is typically about 8 days but may be as short as 4 days. Initial signs include sneezing, coughing, and moderate fever (40°C) which increases up to 42°C in the ensuing 48 hours. There is constipation during the fever, the feces are hard and dry, and vomiting may occur. Pigs are listless, depressed, and tend to remain recumbent. By the fifth day there is incoordination and pronounced muscle spasm, circling, and intermittent convulsions accompanied by excess salivation. By the sixth day swine become moribund and die within 12 hours. In mature swine the mortality rate is low, usually less than 2%, but there may be significant weight loss and poor growth rates after recovery.

Clinical Features in Secondary Hosts. Important secondary hosts include cattle ("mad itch"), dogs ("pseudorabies"), and cats. Disease in secondary hosts is sporadic and occurs where there is direct or indirect contact with swine. Infection is usually by ingestion, less commonly inhalation, and possibly via minor wounds. In cattle the dominant clinical sign is intense pruritus. Particular sites, often on the flanks or hind limbs, are licked incessantly; there is gnawing and rubbing such that the area becomes abraded. Cattle may become frenzied. There is progressive involvement of the central nervous system; following the first signs, the course leading to death may be as short as a few hours but is never longer than 6 days.

In dogs, the frenzy associated with intense pruritus, paralysis of the jaws and pharynx accompanied by drooling of saliva, and plaintive howling simulates true rabies; however, there is no tendency for the dogs to attack other animals. In cats, the disease may progress so rapidly that pruritus is not observed.

Pathogenesis and Pathology. Following primary oral or intranasal infection of swine, virus replicates in the oropharynx. There is no viremia during the first 24 hours, and it is difficult to demonstrate at any time. However, within 24 hours virus can be isolated from various cranial nerve ganglia and the medulla and pons, to which virions have traveled via the axoplasm of the cranial nerves. Virus continues to spread within the central nervous systems; there is ganglioneuritis at many sites including those controlling vital functions.

The relative lack of gross lesions even in young swine is notable. Tonsillitis, pharyngitis, tracheitis, rhinitis, and esophagitis may be evident. Occasionally small necrotic foci may be found in the liver and spleen. Microscopically the principal findings in both swine and secondary hosts are in the central nervous system. There is a diffuse nonsuppurative meningoencephalitis and ganglioneuritis, marked perivascular cuffing, and focal gliosis associated with extensive necrosis of neuronal and glial cells. There is a correlation between the site and severity of clinical signs and the histologic findings. Typical intranuclear herpesvirus inclusions are rarely found in the lesions in swine.

Some swine that have recovered from pseudorabies may shed virus continuously in their nasal secretions. Others from which virus cannot be isolated by conventional means may yield virus when explant cultures of tonsillar tissue are made. Pseudorabies virus DNA can be demonstrated in the trigeminal ganglia of recovered swine by DNA hybridization and PCR, but there is debate about the relative significance of lymphoreticular cells and nerve cells as a site for latency.

Diagnosis. The history and clinical signs often suggest the diagnosis. ELISA has been approved as a standard test in several countries, and it is used in association with vaccination and eradication programs. Fluorescent antibody staining of frozen tissue sections, virus isolation, and serum neutralization tests are used for confirmation.

Epidemiology and Control. Swine are the primary host and reservoir for pseudorabies virus, and the virus causes a uniformly fatal disease when transmitted to a wide variety of secondary hosts. Virus is shed in the saliva and nasal discharges of swine, so that licking, biting, and aerosols could result in transmission. Virus is not shed in the urine or feces. The contamination of livestock feed or the ingestion of infected carcasses by swine is common, and ingestion of virus-contaminated material including pork is probably the most common source of infection for secondary hosts. Rats may contribute to farm-to-farm transfer, and sick or dead rats and other feral animals are probably the source of infection for dogs and cats. In the United States raccoons, because of their scavenging habits, have received particular attention, but they probably play a minor role in the natural spread of pseudorabies virus.

Management practices influence epidemiologic patterns of infection and disease in swine. Losses from severe overt disease occur when nonimmune pregnant sows or swine less than 3 months old, born to nonimmune sows, are infected. Such a pattern is likely to be seen when the virus is newly introduced into a herd or unit within a farm. When breeding sows are immune with adequate antibody levels, overt disease in their progeny is not observed or is greatly reduced. Where breeding and growing/finishing operations are conducted separately, significant losses from pdeudorabies occur when weaned swine from several sources are brought together in the growing/finishing unit, but the disease in these older swine is less severe than that in piglets. If care is taken to prevent the entry of pseudorabies, the move toward complete integration of swine husbandry, so-called farrow to finish operations, provide an ideal situation by which to produce and maintain pseudorabies-free herds and thus avoid the costs of disease losses and the problems associated with vaccination.

Vaccination of swine in areas where the virus is endemic and spreading can reduce losses. Both recombinant DNA and inactivated vaccines are used, but they do not prevent infection or the establishment of latent infection by the wild-type virus. A pseudorabies vaccine from which both the thymidine kinase and a glycoprotein gene have been deleted, and the E1 gene of hog cholera virus inserted, provides protection against both pseudorabies and hog cholera. Vaccination of secondary hosts is rarely undertaken because of the sporadic incidence of the disease.

Eradication programs have been established in several countries including the United Kingdom and United States, and in 1991 the national herd in the United Kingdom was considered free of pseudorabies.

Equine Alphaherpesvirus Infections

Three alphaherpesviruses, designated 4, 1, and 3, have been identified as causes of disease in horses. Equine herpesvirus 4 causes acute upper respiratory disease in foals during the first year or two of life, and it has been recovered from sporadic cases of abortion. Equine herpesvirus 1 is the major cause of epidemics of equine abortion ("abortion storms") and occasionally causes respiratory disease. Equine herpesvirus 3 causes equine coital exanthema.

Equine Rhinopneumonitis (Equine Herpesvirus 4)

Equine herpesvirus 4 is the most important of the several viruses that cause acute respiratory disease of foals.

Clinical Features. Acute respiratory disease due to equine herpesvirus 4 occurs commonly in foals over 2 months old, weanlings, and yearlings. There is fever, anorexia, and a profuse serous nasal discharge which later becomes mucopurulent. Most affected foals recover completely, and mild or subclinical infections are common. More severe disease including bronchopneumonia and death may occur when there is crowding, stress, poor hygiene, and secondary infection.

Epidemiology and Control. The source of virus is thought to be older horses in which inapparent virus shedding occurs, following reactivation of the latent virus. Both inactivated and attenuated live equine herpesvirus 1 vaccines are used to control both respiratory disease and abortion. Inactivated vaccines incorporating both equine herpesvirus type 1 and type 4 viruses are licensed for use in the United States.

Equine Abortion Caused by Equine Herpesvirus 1

Abortion may occur as early as the fourth month of gestation, although most cases occur during the last four months. It occurs without premonitory signs, and there are usually no complications. The fetus is usually born dead.

Perinatal infection may result in a fatal generalized disease in which respiratory distress due to interstitial pneumonia is the dominant clinical feature. Encephalitis occurs sporadically or as epidemics, usually in association with respiratory disease and abortion. Clinical signs vary from mild ataxia to complete recumbency with forelimb and hindlimb paralysis, leading to death.

Pathology. In fetuses aborted before 6 months there is diffusely scattered cell necrosis with inclusion bodies and a lack of an inflammatory cell response. Gross lesions are sometimes present in fetuses aborted after 6 months and may include small necrotic foci in the liver. Characteristic microscopic lesions include bronchiolitis, pneumonitis, severe necrosis of splenic white pulp, and focal hepatic necrosis, accompanied by a marked inflammatory cell response. Typical herpetic intranuclear inclusion bodies are readily demonstrated in these lesions.

Only certain strains of equine herpesvirus 1 cause encephalitis, which is characterized by vasculitis leading to thrombosis and hypoxic degeneration of adjacent neural tissue. In contrast to alphaherpesvirus encephalitis in other species, it is usually difficult or impossible to isolate virus from neural tissues; it is thought that the vasculitis is caused by virus–antibody complexes.

Epidemiology. Abortion, perinatal mortality, and less commonly encephalitis affecting up to 70% of horses in a herd may follow the occurrence of abortion in the index case, usually a recently introduced mare.

Equine Coital Exanthema (Equine Herpesvirus 3)

A disease that was probably equine coital exanthema has long been known, but its causative agent was not shown to be an alphaherpesvirus (equine herpesvirus 3) until 1968. Equine herpesvirus 3 shows no serologic cross-reactivity with other equine herpesviruses by neutralization tests, but it shares antigens with equine herpesvirus 1, demonstrable by complement fixation and immunofluorescence. Equine herpesvirus 3 grows only in cells of equine origin and produces large plaques. Although rapidly cytopathic, the virus tends to remain cell-associated.

Equine coital exanthema is an acute, usually mild disease characterized by the formation of pustular and ulcerative lesions on the vaginal and vestibular mucosa, on the skin of the penis, prepuce, and the perineal region, especially of the mare, and occasionally on the teats, lips, and the respiratory mucosa. The incidence of antibody in sexually active horses is much higher (about 50%) than the reported incidence of clinical disease. The incubation period may be as short as 2 days, and in uncomplicated cases healing is usually complete by 14 days. Where the skin of the vulva, penis, and prepuce is black, white depigmented spots mark for life the site of earlier lesions and identify potential carriers.

Although genital lesions may be extensive, there are no systemic signs, and unless the affected areas are carefully examined cases are readily missed. Abortion or infertility are not associated with equine herpesvirus 3 infection; indeed, mares usually conceive to the service in which they acquire the disease, although abortion occurs following experimental *in utero* inoculation.

Affected stallions show decreased libido, and the presence of the disease may seriously disrupt breeding schedules. Recurrent disease is more likely to occur when stallions are in frequent use. Management of the disease consists of the removal of stallions from service until all lesions have healed, along with symptomatic treatment.

Equine herpesvirus 3 can cause subclinical respiratory infection in yearling horses and has been isolated from vesicular lesions on the muzzles of foals in contact with infected mares.

Infections with Canine Herpesvirus 1

Canine herpesvirus 1 was first recognized in the United States in 1965 as the cause of a highly fatal, generalized hemorrhagic disease of pups under 4 weeks of age. The syndrome is rare, and the prevalence of the virus, based on antibody surveys, is low (<20%). It probably occurs worldwide. In sexually mature dogs canine herpesvirus 1 causes genital disease, although this is rarely diagnosed clinically.

Clinical Features. The incubation period varies from 3 to 8 days, and in fatal disease the course is brief, 1–2 days. Signs include painful crying, abdominal pain, anorexia, and dyspnea. In older dogs there may be vaginal or prepucial discharge, and on careful examination a focal nodular lesion of the vaginal, penile, and prepucial epithelium may be seen. The virus may also cause respiratory disease and may be part of the "kennel cough" syndrome.

Pathogenesis and Pathology. Pups born to presumably seronegative bitches are infected oronasally either from the vagina of their dam or from other infected dogs. Pups less than 4 weeks old which become hypothermic develop the generalized, often fatal disease. There is a cell-associated viremia followed by viral replication in blood vessel walls. The optimal temperature for viral replication is about 33°C, namely, the temperature of the genital and upper respiratory tracts. The hypothalmic thermoregulatory centers of the pup are not fully operative until about 4 weeks of age. Accordingly, in the context of canine herpesvirus 1 infection, the pup is critically dependent on ambient temperature and maternal contact for the maintenance of its normal body temperature. The more severe the hypothermia, the more severe and rapid is the course of the disease.

The gross findings in pups are frequently dramatic. Large ecchymotic hemorrhages are particularly obvious in the kidney, adrenal, and gastrointestinal tract. Microscopically they are seen as necrotic foci, however not all such necrotic foci are marked by gross hemorrhage.

Diagnosis. This sporadic disease is rarely diagnosed during life. The gross postmortem findings, particularly the ecchymotic hemorrhages of the kidney and gastrointestinal tract, are characteristic. Inclusion bodies may be present in liver cells, and the causative virus can be readily isolated in canine cell cultures.

Control. The low incidence of severe disease in pups and the mild nature of infections in older dogs have not warranted the development of vaccines. Losses may be prevented or arrested if the ambient temperature minimizes the risk of hypothermia. Raising the body temperature early in the course of infection may have therapeutic value.

Feline Herpesvirus Disease (Feline Herpesvirus 1)

About half of the cats presenting with respiratory disease have feline herpesvirus 1 infection, about half calicivirus infection, and a few *Chlamydia psittaci* infection. The incidence of feline herpesvirus antibody in colony cats is over 70%, whereas for household cats the figure is less than 50%. All species of the family Felidae are believed to be susceptible.

Feline herpesvirus 1 causes acute disease of the upper respiratory tract in the first year or so of life. After an incubation period of 24–48 hours there is a sudden onset of bouts of sneezing, coughing, profuse serous nasal and ocular discharges, frothy salivation, dyspnea, anorexia, weight loss, and fever. Occasionally there may be ulcers on the tongue. Keratitis associated with punctate corneal ulcers are common. In fully susceptible kittens up to 4 weeks old the extensive rhinotracheitis and an associated bronchopneumonia may be fatal. Clinically, the acute disease is very similar to that cause by caliciviruses. Profuse frothy salivation and corneal ulcers suggest feline herpesvirus infection, while ulcers of the tongue, palate, and pharynx are more frequently encountered in calicivirus infections. Infection of cats over 6 months of age is likely to result in mild or subclinical disease. Pregnant queens may abort, although there is no evidence that the virus crosses the placenta and fatally infects fetuses, and virus has not been isolated from aborted placenta or fetuses; abortion is thought to be secondary to fever and toxemia.

There is necrosis of epithelia of the nasal cavity, pharynx, epiglottis, tonsils, larynx, and trachea and in extreme cases, in young kittens, a bronchopneumonia. Typical intranuclear inclusion bodies may be detected if death occurs within 7–9 days after infection.

Inactivated and attenuated live-virus vaccines are used for the control of infections due to feline herpesvirus 1; they reduce disease but do not prevent infection.

Avian Infectious Laryngotracheitis (Avian Herpesvirus 1)

Identified as a specific viral disease of chickens in the United States in 1926, infectious laryngotracheitis, caused by avian herpesvirus 1, occurs among chickens worldwide. Rarely this virus causes disease in other avian species. Strains of the virus vary considerably in virulence.

Clinical Features. Chickens of all ages are susceptible, but disease is most common in those aged 4–18 months. After an incubation period of 2–8 days, mild coughing and sneezing are followed by nasal and ocular discharge, dyspnea, loud gasping and coughing, and depression. In severe cases the neck is raised and the head extended during inspiration, which is known as "pump handle respiration." Head shaking with coughing is characteristic and may be associated with expectoration of bloody mucus and frank blood which appear on the beak, face, and feathers. Morbidity approaches 100%, and for virulent strains the mortality may be 50–70%, and for strains of low virulence, about 20%. Strains of low virulence are associated with conjunctivitis, ocular discharge, swollen infraorbital and nasal sinuses, and lowered egg production.

Pathology and Pathogenesis. There is severe laryngotracheitis characterized by necrosis, hemorrhage, ulceration, and the formation of diphtheritic membranes. The latter may form a second tube for the length of the trachea, greatly restricting, and in some cases totally occluding, air flow. The extensive diphtheritic membrane formation and death from asphyxia prompted the designation "fowl diphtheria." The virus probably persists as a latent infection, and virus has been recovered from tracheal explant cultures over 3 months after infection.

Diagnosis. Clinical and postmortem findings are characteristic. Fluorescent antibody staining of smears and tissues and isolation of the virus by inoculation on the chorioallantoic membrane of embryonated eggs or inoculation of cell cultures are also used. Neutralizing antibody may be detected by pock or plaque reduction assays, and ELISAs have been developed.

Epidemiology and Control. Infectious laryngotracheitis virus is usually introduced into a flock via carrier birds and is transmitted by droplet and inhalation, less commonly by ingestion. Although virus spreads rapidly through a flock, new clinical cases may occur over a period of 2 to 8 weeks; thus, it spreads somewhat more slowly than Newcastle disease, influenza, and infectious bronchitis.

It is feasible to establish and maintain flocks free of infectious laryngotracheitis, and, where management systems allow, this practice is increasingly adopted, particularly in the broiler industry where birds are harvested at 9 weeks of age and where "all-in, all-out" management is possible. However, for breeding and egg production flocks vaccination is still widely practiced, using attenuated live-virus vaccine. This protects birds against clinical disease, but not against infection with virulent virus or the development of a latent carrier status for either the virulent or the vaccine viruses.

Marek's Disease (Avian Herpesvirus 2)

The specific herpesvirus etiology of Marek's disease, which occurs worldwide, was established in 1967. Prior to the introduction of vaccination in 1970, Marek's disease was the most common lymphoproliferative disease of chickens, causing annual losses in the United States of $150 million and in the United Kingdom of $40 million. Vaccination has dramatically reduced the incidence of disease, but not of infection. Because of continuing losses from disease and the costs of vaccination, it remains an important disease of chickens. The virus is slowly cytopathic and remains highly cell-associated, so that cell-free infectious virus is virtually impossible to obtain except as dander from feather follicles. Although it used to be classified as a gammaherpesvirus on the basis of its pathologic features, its genome closely resembles that of other alphaherpesviruses.

Clinical Features. Marek's disease is a progressive disease with variable signs; four overlapping syndromes are described.

Neurolymphomatosis, or so-called classical Marek's disease, is associated with an asymmetric paralysis of one or both legs or wings (Fig. 19-6). Incoordination is a common early sign; one leg is held forward and the other backward when stationary because of unilateral paresis or paralysis. Wing dropping and lowering of the head and neck are common. If the vagus nerve is involved there may be dilation of the crop and gasping.

Acute Marek's disease occurs in explosive outbreaks in which a large proportion of birds in a flock show depression followed after a few days by ataxia and paralysis of some birds. Significant mortality occurs without localizing neurologic signs.

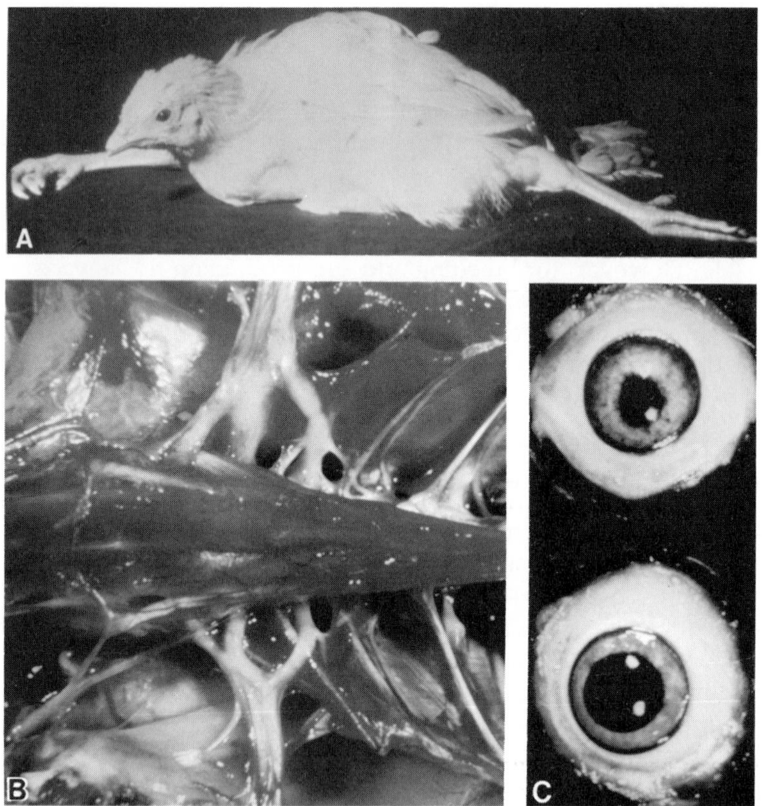

FIG. 19-6. *Marek's disease of chickens. (A) Paralysis. (B) Enlargement of sciatic nerves. (C) Ocular lesions. The lower eye is normal, with dilated pupil; the pupil of the upper eye failed to dilate and has an irregular outline owing to infiltration of transformed lymphocytes.*

Ocular lymphomatosis leads to greying of the iris of one or both eyes because of lymphoblastoid cell infiltration; the pupil is irregular and eccentric, and there is partial or total blindness.

Cutaneous Marek's disease is readily recognized after plucking, when round, nodular lesions up to 1 cm in diameter are seen, particularly at feather follicles.

Pathology. Enlargement of one or more peripheral nerve trunks is the most constant gross finding. In the vast majority of cases a diagnosis can be made if the celiac, cranial, intercostal, mesenteric, brachial, sciatic, and greater splanchnic nerves are examined. In a diseased bird, the nerves are up to three times their normal diameter, show loss of striations, and are edematous, gray, or yellowish and somewhat translucent in appearance. Because enlargement is frequently unilateral it is especially helpful to compare contralateral nerves.

Lymphomatous lesions, indistinguishable from those of avian leukosis, are usually small, diffuse, grayish, and translucent. They are most common in acute Marek's disease and occur in the gonads, particularly the ovary, and other tissues.

Pathogenesis. The outcome of infection of chickens by Marek's disease virus is influenced by the virus strain, dose, and route of infection, and by the age, sex, immune status, and genetic susceptibility of the chickens. Subclinical infection with virus shedding is common. Infection is acquired by inhalation of dander. Epithelial cells of the respiratory tract are productively infected and contribute to a cell-associated viremia involving macrophages. By the sixth day there is productive infection of lymphoid cells in a variety of organs, including the thymus, bursa of Fabricius, bone marrow, and spleen, resulting in immune suppression. During the second week after infection there is a persistent cell-associated viremia followed by a proliferation of T lymphoblastoid cells, and 1 week later deaths begin to occur, although regression may also occur from this time.

T lymphocytes are transformed by the virus, and up to 90 genome equivalents of Marek's disease virus DNA can be demonstrated in transformed cells in both plasmid and integrated forms.

The lesions of Marek's disease result from the infiltration and *in situ* proliferation of T lymphocytes, which may result in leukemia, but in addition there is often a significant inflammatory cell response to the lysis of nonlymphoid cells by the virus. Lesions of the feather follicle are invariably a mixture of lymphoblastoid and inflammatory cells. Epithelial cells at the base of feather follicles are exceptional in that productive infection of these cells is also associated with the release of cell-free infectious virus.

The basis for genetic resistance is not fully defined, but resistance has been correlated with birds that carry the B21 alloantigen of the B red blood cell group. Maternal antibody may persist in newly hatched chicks for up to 3 weeks, and infection of such chicks with virulent Marek's disease virus may not produce disease, but may lead to an active immune response. Chickens that are bursectomized and then actively immunized also survive challenge infection.

Many apparently healthy birds are lifelong carriers and shedders of virus, but the virus is not transmitted *in ovo*. When fully susceptible 1-day-old chicks are infected with virulent virus, the minimum time for detection of microscopic lesions is 1–2 weeks, and gross lesions are present by 3–4 weeks. Maximal virus shedding occurs at 5–6 weeks after infection.

Diagnosis. Where sufficient numbers of birds are examined, history, age, clinical signs, and gross postmortem findings are adequate for the diagnosis, which can be confirmed by histopathology. Detection of viral antigen by immunoflourescence is the simplest reliable laboratory diagnostic procedure. Gel diffusion, indirect immunofluorescence, or virus neutralization are used for detection of viral antibody.

A variety of methods can be used for viral isolation: inoculation of cell cultures, the chorioallantoic membrane, or the yolk sac of 4-day-old embryonated eggs with suspensions of buffy coat or spleen cells. The presence of virus can be demonstrated by immunofluorescence or electron microscopy.

Marek's disease and avian leukosis are usually present in the same flock, and both diseases may occur in the same bird. The two diseases were long confused, but they can be differentiated by clinical and pathologic features, or by specific tests for virus, viral antigens, or viral antibody.

Epidemiology and Control. Most birds have antibody to Marek's disease virus by the time they are mature; infection persists and virus is released in dander from the feather follicles. Congenital infection does not occur, and chicks are protected by maternal antibody for the first few weeks of life. They then become infected by the inhalation of virus in the dust. Epidemics of Marek's disease usually involve sexually immature birds 2–5 months old; there is a high mortality (about 80%) which soon peaks and then declines sharply.

Isolates of Marek's disease virus vary considerably in virulence and in the types of lesions different strains produce. Avirulent strains are recognized and used for vaccine, although the antigenically related turkey herpesvirus is preferred as a vaccine strain, primarily because it infects cells productively. Marek's disease virus and turkey herpesvirus are about 95% homologous by DNA : DNA hybridization.

Vaccination if the principal method of control. One-day-old chicks are vaccinated parenterally, the vaccine being available as either a lyophilized cell-free preparation or a cell-associated preparation. The cell-free vaccine does not take in chicks with maternal antibody, whereas the cell-associated vaccines do. Protective immunity develops within about 2 weeks. Vaccination decreases the incidence of disease, particularly of lymphomatous lesions in visceral organs, and it has been most successful in the control of acute Marek's disease. Neurologic disease continues to occur in vaccinated flocks, but at reduced incidence.

A further level of control can be achieved if flocks are built up with birds carrying the B21 alloantigen. It is possible to establish flocks free of Marek's disease, but commercially it is extremely difficult to maintain the disease-free status. The production of chickens on the "all-in, all-out" principle, whereby they are hatched, started, raised, and dispersed as a unit, would improve the efficacy of vaccination as a control measure.

Duck Plague (Anatid Herpesvirus 1)

Duck plague occurs worldwide among domestic and wild ducks, geese, swans, and other waterfowl, migratory waterfowl contributing to the spread within and between continents. Major epidemics have occurred in duck farms in the United States.

Strains of virus vary in virulence, although only a single antigenic type has been recognized. The virus grows readily on the chorioallantoic membrane of embryonated duck eggs and in duck embryo fibroblast cell cultures, but only poorly or not at all in similar substrates of chicken origin, although it may be adapted to grow in chicken cells.

Clinical Features. Attention is drawn to the disease by the occurrence of a sudden and persistent increased mortality within flocks of ducks. The incubation period is 3–7 days. There is anorexia, depression, nasal discharge, ruffled, dull feathers, adherent eyelids, photophobia, extreme thirst, ataxia leading to recumbency with outstretched wings with head extended forward, tremors, watery diarrhea, and soiled vents. Egg production drops 25% to 40%. Morbidity and mortality vary from 5% to 100%. Most ducks that develop clinical signs die. Sick wild ducks conceal themselves and die in vegetation at the water's edge.

Pathology. Ingested virus causes enteritis, and viremic spread leads to vasculitis and widespread focal necrosis. Blood is present in the body cavities including gizzard and intestinal lumens, and petechial hemorrhages are present in many tissues. There may be elevated crusty plaques of diphtheritic membrane in the esophagus, cecum, rectum, cloaca, and bursa. Herpesvirus inclusions are most readily demonstrated in hepatocytes, intestinal epithelium, and lymphoid tissues.

Diagnosis. Clinical and gross postmortem findings may be confirmed by the finding of herpesvirus inclusion bodies or positive immunofluorescence. Duck plague needs to be differentiated from duck hepatitis (due to a picornavirus) and from Newcastle disease and influenza.

Epidemiology and Control. Ingestion of contaminated water is thought to be the major mode of transmission, although the virus may also be transmitted by contact. Virus has been isolated from wild ducks up to 1 year after infection. A chick embryo-adapted attenuated live-virus vaccine has been used in the United States. However, despite the continued threat of reintroduction from wild birds, the disease has been eliminated from the duck farms of Long Island, New York, and vaccination is not now routinely practiced.

Infections with B Virus of Macaques (Cercopithecid Herpesvirus 1)

Macaques suffer from a herpesvirus infection caused by B virus, the natural history of which in these animals is very like that of herpes simplex type 1 infection in man. A number of fatal cases of ascending paralysis and encephalitis in animal handlers have occurred, infection being transmitted by monkey bite, and the virus poses a continuing risk to personnel working with primates.

Alphaherpesviruses of Other Species

A few species of alphaherpesviruses of other animals warrant brief mention. They have been associated with fatal diseases in hedgehogs, kangaroos, wallabies, wombats, and harbor seals. Major epidemics of fatal illness due to alphaherpesviruses have occurred in a variety of tortoise species in captivity, and the viruses are recognized as significant causes of mortality in channel catfish and salmonid species. Alphaherpesviruses antigenically related to bovine herpesvirus 1 have been isolated from several ruminant species including red deer, reindeer, and buffalo.

DISEASES CAUSED BY BETAHERPESVIRUSES

The betaherpesviruses replicate more slowly than alphaherpesviruses and often produce greatly enlarged cells, hence the designation "cytomegalovirus." Their host range is narrow, and in latent infections viral DNA is believed to be sequestered in cells of secretory glands, lymphoreticular organs, and kidneys. Rather than being subject to periodic reactivation, betaherpesviruses are often associated with continuous viral excretion. They have been associated with diseases of economic importance in horses and swine (see Table 19-2).

Porcine Cytomegalovirus Infections (Porcine Herpesvirus 2)

First recognized in 1955, porcine herpesvirus 2 is endemic in many swine herds worldwide. In the United Kingdom some 50% of herds are infected, while a survey in Iowa indicated infection in 12% of herds.

Within a herd up to 90% of swine may carry the virus. Often disease is not seen in herds in which the virus is endemic; it is more likely to be associated with recent introduction of the virus or with environmental factors such as poor nutrition and intercurrent disease. Virus-free herds have been established.

Clinical Features. Rhinitis occurs in swine up to 10 weeks of age, after which infection is subclinical, and it is most severe in swine less than two weeks old. There is sneezing, coughing, serous nasal and ocular discharge, and depression. The discharge becomes mucopurulent and may block the nasal passages, which interferes with suckling; such piglets lose weight rapidly and die within a few days. Survivors are stunted. A generalized disease following viremic spread is also recognized in young swine. Porcine herpesvirus 2 crosses the placenta and may cause fetal death or result in generalized disease in the first 2 weeks after birth, or there may be runting and poor weight gains.

Pathology. Large basophilic intranuclear inclusions are found in enlarged cells of the mucous glands of the turbinate mucosa (hence the synonym "inclusion body rhinitis").

Epidemiology and Control. When newly introduced into a susceptible herd, virus is transmitted both transplacentally and horizontally. In herds in which the virus is endemic, transmission is predominantly horizontal, but since young swine are infected when maternal antibody is present the infection is subclinical. Disease occurs when the virus is introduced into susceptible herds or if susceptible swine are mixed with carrier swine. Virus-free swine can be produced by hysterotomy, although because the virus crosses the placenta swine produced in this way must be monitored carefully for antibody for at least 70 days after delivery.

Equine Cytomegalovirus Infections (Equine Herpesvirus 2)

Equine cytomegalovirus (equine herpesvirus 2) may be isolated from nasal swab filtrates or from buffy coat cells of some 70% of all horses. Horses are infected in the first weeks of life even in the presence of maternal antibody. Neutralization tests suggest that several antigenic types exist; more than one antigenic type may be recovered at different times from the same horse.

Equine cytomegalovirus has been recovered from horses with respiratory disease sometimes characterized by coughing, swollen submaxillary and parotid lymph nodes, and pharyngeal ulceration, from conjunctivitis, and from the genital tract. The role of the virus is these and other diseases is uncertain. A second, distinctly different, slowly growing herpesvirus (equine herpesvirus 5) has been isolated from nasal swabs and from buffy coat cells; its pathologic significance is unknown.

DISEASES CAUSED BY GAMMAHERPESVIRUSES

Gammaherpesviruses are characterized by replication in lymphoblastoid cells, different members of the subfamily being specific for either B or T lymphocytes. In lymphocytes, infection is frequently arrested at a prelytic stage, with persistence and minimum expression of the viral genome. Infection may enter a lytic stage, causing cell death without production of virions. Latent infection can be demonstrated in lymphoid tissue.

Apart from Epstein-Barr virus, which causes human disease and is the prototype of the subfamily, and some related viruses of primates, assignments of viruses to this family are still debated. Bovine malignant catarrhal fever virus caused by alcelaphine herpesvirus 1 and bovine herpesvirus 4 have been tentatively classified as gammaherpesviruses.

Marek's disease virus has been removed from the family, even though it produces lymphoblastoid tumors, because the genome structure of the virus resembles that of alphaherpesviruses.

Bovine Malignant Catarrhal Fever (Alcelaphine Herpesvirus I)

Malignant catarrhal fever is an invariably fatal, generalized disease of cattle and some wild ruminants (deer, buffalo, antelope), primarily affecting lymphoid tissues and epithelial cells of the respiratory and gastrointestinal tracts. Three distinct epidemiologic patterns are recognized from only one of which has a herpesvirus been isolated. In Africa (and zoos) epidemics of the disease occur in cattle (and captive, susceptible wild ruminants) following transmission of the virus from wildebeest (*Connochaetes gnou* and *C. taurinus*), and to a lesser extent from hartebeest (*Alcelaphus buselaphus*) and topi (*Damaliscis korrigum*), particularly at calving time. A herpesvirus (alcelaphine herpesvirus 1) has been isolated from this African form of malignant catarrhal fever and shown experimentally to reproduce the disease; it has been tentatively classified as a gammaherpesvirus.

Outside Africa and zoos, a disease described as malignant catarrhal fever in cattle and deer occurs when these species are kept in close contact with sheep, especially during lambing time. This sheep-associated form can be transmitted by inoculation of cattle or deer with blood from known carrier sheep. It has been shown that sheep have antibody that is cross-reactive with alcelaphine herpesvirus 1. Although the virus responsible for the ovine form of the disease has not been isolated, a DNA clone corresponding to it has been characterized.

A third epidemiologic form of the syndrome described as malignant catarrhal fever is recognized in feedlot cattle in North America, in the absence of contact with sheep. It occurs as minor epidemics; the identity and source of virus in this third form are unknown. Both alcelaphine herpesvirus 1 and the putative sheep-associated herpesvirus produce a disease resembling malignant catarrhal fever in rabbits. The description which follows refers to the African form of the disease.

Clinical Features. After an incubation period of about 3 weeks malignant catarrhal fever is characterized by fever, depression, leukopenia, profuse nasal and ocular discharges, bilateral ophthalmia, generalized lymphadenopathy, extensive mucosal erosions, and central nervous system signs. The ophthalmia is associated with corneal opacity which begins peripherally and progresses centripetally, often leading to blindness. Erosions of the gastrointestinal mucosa lead to diarrhea. Death occurs about 1 week after the onset of clinical signs.

Pathology and Pathogenesis. Postmortem findings vary according to the duration of the disease. There are usually extensive erosions, edema, and hemorrhage throughout the gastrointestinal tract. There is a generalized lymphadenopathy; all lymph nodes are enlarged, edematous, sometimes hemorrhagic. Frequently there are multiple raised necrotic lesions accompanied by ecchymotic hemorrhages in the kidney, as well as erosions of the mucosa of the turbinates, larynx, and trachea. Histologically there is widespread lymphoid cell proliferation and multifocal areas of necrosis, centered on small blood vessels.

Diagnosis. The history and clinical signs, particularly the presence of bilateral ophthalmia, suggest the diagnosis of malignant catarrhal fever. The virus can be isolated when washed, peripheral blood leukocytes are inoculated in calf thyroid cells. Cell-free inocula do not yield virus. The cytopathic changes require at least 3 days to appear, and often several passages in cell culture are necessary. They are characterized by synctia and the presence of typical herpesvirus intranuclear inclusion bodies.

Epidemiology and Control. The virus does not appear to be pathogenic for wildebeest, and in this species it appears to be transmitted from mother to offspring in the immediate postcalving period, via nasal secretions. Cattle are believed to be infected via the relatively large amounts of virus present in the nasal secretions of wildebeest calves. The virus is not transmitted between cattle, which appear to be dead-end hosts. Attempts to develop a vaccine have been unsuccessful.

Bovine Herpesvirus 4 Infections

Bovine herpesvirus 4, which has a genome organization similar to that of Epstein-Barr virus, has been isolated throughout the world from cattle suffering from a variety of diseases including conjunctivitis, respiratory disease, vaginitis, metritis, skin nodules, and lymphosarcoma. However, there is no proven etiologic association between the disease and the virus occasionally isolated from cases. When experimentally inoculated into susceptible cattle these viruses produce no disease. Strains of bovine herpesvirus 4 have been isolated when cell cultures are prepared from tissues of apparently normal cattle; they have also been isolated from semen of normal bulls.

FURTHER READING

Bridgen, A., and Reid, H. W. (1991). Derivation of a DNA clone corresponding to the viral agent of sheep associated malignant catarrhal fever. *Res. Vet. Sci.* **50,** 38.

Calnek, B. W., and Witter, R. L. (1991). Marek's disease. *In* "Diseases of Poultry" (B. W. Calnek, ed.), 9th Ed., p. 342. Iowa State Univ. Press, Ames..

Campbell, T. M., and Studdert, M. J. (1983). Equine herpesvirus type 1 (EHV1). *Vet. Bull.* **53,** 135.

Carmichael, L. E., and Greene, C. E. (1990). Canine herpesvirus infection. *In* "Infectious Diseases of the Dog and Cat" (C. E. Greene, ed.), p. 252. Saunders, Philadelphia, Pennsylvania.

Edington, N. (1986). Porcine cytomegalovirus. *In* "Diseases of Swine" (A. D. Leman, B. Straw, R. D. Glock, W. L. Mengeling, R. H. C. Penny, and E. Scholl, eds.), 6th Ed., p. 330. Iowa State Univ. Press, Ames.

Hanson, L. E., and Bagust, T. J. (1991). Laryngotracheitis. *In* "Diseases of Poultry" (B. W. Calnek, ed.), 9th Ed., p. 485. Iowa State Univ. Press, Ames.

Kit, S. (1989). Recombinant-derived modified-live herpesvirus vaccines. *Adv. Exp. Med. Biol.* **251,** 219.

Povey, R. C. (1990). Feline viral rhinotracheitis (FVR). *In* "Infectious Diseases of the Dog and Cat" (C. E. Greene, ed.), p. 346. Saunders, Philadelphia, Pennsylvania.

Roizman, B. (1990). Herpesviridae: A brief introduction. *In* "Fields Virology" (B. N. Fields, D. M. Knipe, R. M. Chanock, M. S. Hirsch, J. L. Melnick, T. P. Monath, and B. Roizman, eds.), 2nd Ed., p. 1787. Raven, New York.

Roizman, B., Desrosiers, D. C., Fleckenstein, B., Lopez, C., Minson, A. C., and Studdert, M. J. (1992). The family *Herpesviridae:* An update. *Arch. Virol.* **123,** 432.

Straub, O. C. (1990). Infectious bovine rhinotracheitis virus. *In* "Virus Diseases of Ruminants" (Z. Dinter and B. Morein, eds.), p. 71. Elsevier, Amsterdam.

Van Oirschot, J. T., ed. (1989). "Vaccination and Control of Aujeszky's Disease." Kluwer Academic Publ., Dordrecht, The Netherlands.

Wagner, E. K. (1990). "Herpesvirus Transcription and Its Regulation." CRC Press, Boca Raton, Florida.

CHAPTER 20

Poxviridae

The family *Poxviridae* includes several viruses of veterinary and medical importance. Poxvirus diseases occur in most animal species, and they are of considerable economic importance in some regions of the world. Diseases such as sheeppox are now eradicated in the industrialized countries but are still a cause of major losses in some developing countries.

The history of the poxviruses has been dominated by smallpox. This disease, once a cosmopolitan and greatly feared infectious disease of man, has now been eradicated by use of a simple live-virus vaccine that traces its ancestry to the cowsheds of Gloucestershire in England (see Chapter 15). With the eradication of smallpox, use of smallpox vaccine was discontinued throughout the world, but it is possible that it may be widely used again, since recombinant DNA vaccines using vaccinia virus as a vector for delivering a wide range of viral antigens are the subject of intensive research (see Chapter 13). The use of other poxviruses as vaccine vectors is also being vigorously investigated.

PROPERTIES OF POXVIRUSES

The family *Poxviridae* is subdivided into two subfamilies: *Chordopoxvirinae* (poxviruses of vertebrates) and *Entomopoxvirinae* (poxviruses of insects). The subfamily *Chordopoxvirinae* is subdivided into eight named genera (Table 20-1), and there are several other chordopoxviruses that have not yet been classified; indeed new poxviruses are constantly being discovered, in lizards, deer, and kangaroos among other wild animals. Each of the named genera except *Molluscipoxvirus* include species that cause diseases in domestic or laboratory animals.

The poxviruses are the largest and most complex of all viruses. Figure 20-1A,C,D illustrates the structure of the virion of vaccinia virus. Virions of all other genera of the chordopoxviruses are similar, except those belonging to the genus *Parapoxvirus* (Fig. 20-1B) and some ungrouped viruses from reptiles, which are shaped like orthopoxviruses but have a surface detail similar to the parapoxviruses (Fig. 20-1B). There is no nucleocapsid conforming to either of the two types of symmetry found in most other viruses (see Chapter 1); hence it is called a "complex" virion. An outer membrane encloses a dumbbell-shaped core and two "lateral bodies" of unknown nature. The core contains the viral DNA together with several proteins. In particles released naturally from cells, rather than by cellular disruption, there is an envelope which contains cellular lipids and several virus-specified polypeptides.

TABLE 20-1
Classification of Poxviruses of Vertebrates[a]

Genus	Prototype virus
Orthopoxvirus	Vaccinia virus
Parapoxvirus	Pseudocowpox virus
Capripoxvirus	Sheeppox virus
Suipoxvirus	Swinepox virus
Leporipoxvirus	Myxoma virus
Avipoxvirus	Fowlpox virus
Molluscipoxvirus	Molluscum contagiosum virus[b]
Yatapoxvirus	Yaba monkey tumor poxvirus

[a] Family *Poxviridae*, subfamily *Chordopoxvirinae*.
[b] Specific for humans.

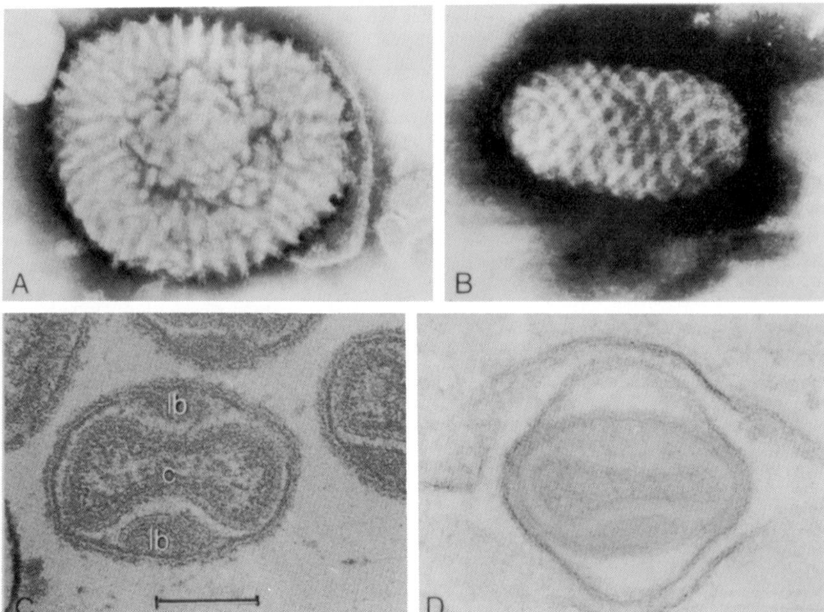

FIG. 20-1. Poxviridae. *(A) Negatively stained vaccinia virion, showing the surface structure of tubules characteristic of the outer membrane of all genera except* Parapoxvirus. *(B) Negatively stained orf virion, showing characteristic surface structure of the outer membrane of* Parapoxvirus. *(C) Thin section of a vaccinia virion in its narrow aspect, showing the biconcave core (c) and the two lateral bodies (1b). (D) Thin section of mature enveloped extracellular virion lying between two cells. Bar: 100 nm. [A and D, from S. Dales,* J. Cell Biol. **18,** *51 (1963); B from J. Nagington* et al, Virology **23,** *461 (1964); C from B. G. T. Pogo and S. Dales,* Proc. Natl. Acad. Sci. U.S.A. **63,** *820 (1969).]*

The nucleic acid is dsDNA, varying in size from 130 kbp (parapoxviruses) to 280 kbp (fowlpox virus) (Table 20-2). The genome of vaccinia virus (191,636 bp) has been completely sequenced. Within the genus *Orthopoxvirus,* restriction endonuclease maps provide the definitive criteria for the allocation of strains of virus recovered from various sources to a particular species (e.g., cowpox virus, see Table 20-3). Species of other genera that have been tested (e.g., *Parapoxvirus*) cannot be as readily grouped in this way.

There are over 100 polypeptides in the virion: the core proteins including a transcriptase and several other enzymes. The virion contains numerous antigens recognizable by immunodiffusion, most of which are common to all members of a genus, although each species is character-

TABLE 20-2
Properties of Poxviruses of Vertebrates

Eight genera (see Table 20–1)
Most genera: brick-shaped virion, 300 × 240 × 100 nm, irregular arrangement of tubules on outer membrane; *Parapoxvirus*: ovoid, 260 × 160 nm, with regular spiral arrangement of "tubules" on outer membrane
Complex structure with core, lateral bodies, outer membrane, and sometimes envelope
Linear dsDNA genome, 130 kbp (*Parapoxvirus*), 165–210 kbp (*Orthopoxvirus*), 280 kbp (*Avipoxvirus*)
Transcriptase, poly(A) polymerase, capping enzyme, methylating enzymes in virion
Cytoplasmic replication, enveloped particles released by exocytosis, nonenveloped particles released by cell lysis

ized by certain specific polypeptides. A few other antigens appear to be shared by all poxviruses of vertebrates. There is extensive cross-neutralization and cross-protection between viruses belonging to the same genus, but none between viruses of different genera. Genetic recombination occurs readily between viruses of the same genus, but very rarely between those of different genera.

Poxviruses are resistant to ambient temperatures and may survive many years in dried scabs. Orthopoxviruses and most avipoxviruses are ether-resistant, but parapoxviruses, capripoxviruses, and leporipoxviruses are ether-sensitive.

VIRAL REPLICATION

Replication of poxviruses occurs in the cytoplasm and can be demonstrated in enucleated cells. After fusion of the virion with the plasma membrane or via endocytosis, the viral core is released into the cytoplasm (Fig. 20-2). Transciption is initiated by the viral transcriptase, and functional capped and polyadenylated mRNAs are produced within minutes after infection. The polypeptides produced by translation of these mRNAs complete the uncoating of the core, and transcription of about 100 genes, distributed throughout the genome, occurs before viral DNA synthesis begins. Early proteins include thymidine kinase, DNA polymerase, and several other enzymes.

With the onset of DNA replication 2–5 hours after infection, there is a dramatic shift in gene expression; almost the entire genome is transcribed, but transcripts from the early genes (i.e., those transcribed before DNA replication begins) are not translated. Virion formation occurs

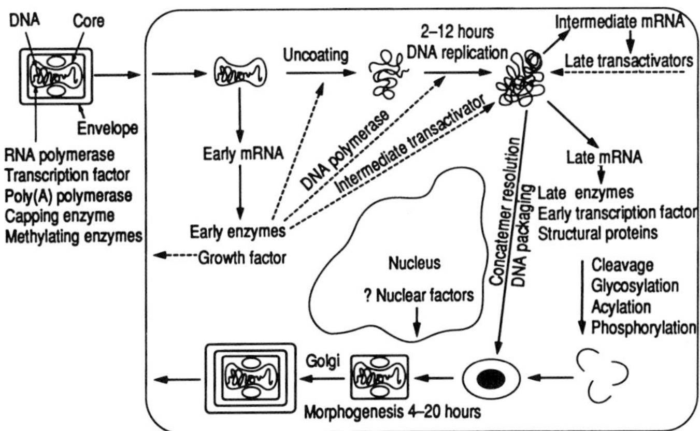

FIG. 20-2. *Replication cycle of vaccinia virus. [From B. Moss,* Science **252,** *1662 (1991).]*

in circumscribed areas of the cytoplasm ("viral factories"). Spherical immature particles can be visualized by electron microscopy; their outer bilayer becomes the outer membrane of the virion, and the core and lateral bodies differentiate within it. Some of the mature particles move to the vicinity of the Golgi complex, acquire an envelope, and are released from the cell by exocytosis. However, most particles are not enveloped and are released by cell disruption. Both enveloped and nonenveloped particles are infectious.

Several poxvirus genes code for proteins that are secreted from infected cells and affect the response of the host to infection. Among these are homologs of epidermal growth factor and complement regulatory proteins; other proteins appear to confer resistance to interferon and suppress the immune response (see Table 7-2). Now that the complete sequence of vaccinia virus is known, we can anticipate the discovery of many additional genes affecting the host response to infection.

PATHOGENESIS AND IMMUNITY

All poxvirus infections are associated with lesions of the skin. These may affect only one part of the animal, for example, the teats of milking cows with cowpox, or the disease may be generalized, for example, lumpyskin disease in cattle. The lesions associated with these two diseases and many other pox diseases are essentially pustular; with other poxviruses the lesions may be more proliferative, such as the nodules of pseudocowpox, or they may be tumor-like, as in myxomatosis. Several poxviruses, for example, sheeppox, cause generalized disease with lesions throughout the viscera and are associated with a significant mortality.

Generalized poxvirus infections have a stage of cell-associated viremia, which leads to localization in the skin and to a lesser extent in internal organs. Immunity to such infections is prolonged. However, in some localized poxvirus infections, notably those produced by parapoxviruses, immunity is short-lived and reinfection is common.

LABORATORY DIAGNOSIS

Because of the large size and distinctive structure of the virions, electron microscopic examination of lesion material usually allows ready identification of the virions of poxviruses and is the preferred method of laboratory diagnosis. Parapoxviruses have a distinctive structure (Fig. 20-1B); other poxviruses are morphologically similar to each other, but their source (species of animal, type of lesion) should make specific diagnosis easy.

Most poxviruses, except for parapoxviruses and molluscum contagiosum virus, grow readily in cell culture. They also produce pocks on the chorioallantoic membrane of embryonated hen's eggs, the morphology of which is used to differentiate orthopoxviruses from each other.

EPIDEMIOLOGY AND CONTROL

Poxviruses can be transmitted between animals by several routes: by introduction of virus into small skin abrasions from other infected animals or from a contaminated environment (e.g., orf), by droplet infection of the respiratory tract (e.g., sheeppox), or through mechanical transmission by biting arthropods (e.g., swinepox, fowlpox, and myxomatosis).

DISEASES CAUSED BY ORTHOPOXVIRUSES

Six of the ten recognized species of *Orthopoxvirus* cause infections in domestic or laboratory animals (Table 20-3).

Vaccinia

Vaccinia virus has long been the "model" poxvirus for laboratory studies. In its biological properties and restriction endonuclease map it

TABLE 20-3

Orthopoxviruses That Affect Domestic, Laboratory, and Wild Animals: Host Ranges and Geographic Distribution

Virus	Animals found naturally infected	Host range in laboratory animals	Geographic range; natural infections
Vaccinia virus	Numerous: man, cow,[a] buffalo,[a] pig,[a] rabbit[a]	Broad	Worldwide
Cowpox virus	Numerous: cow, man, rats, cats, gerbils, large felines, elephant, rhinoceros, okapi	Broad	Europe, Turkmenia
Camelpox virus	Camel	Narrow	Asia and Africa
Ectromelia virus	Mice, ?voles	Narrow	Europe
Monkeypox virus	Numerous: squirrels, monkeys, great apes, man	Broad	Western and central Africa
Uasin Gishu disease virus	Horse	Broad	Eastern Africa
Tatera poxvirus	Gerbil (*Tatera kempi*)	?	Western Africa
Raccoon poxvirus	Raccoon	Broad	North America
Vole poxvirus	Vole (*Microtus californicus*)	?	California
Seal poxvirus	Gray seal (*Halichoerus grypus*)	?	North Sea

[a] Infected from man.

is clearly different from cowpox virus, as originally used by Jenner. Because of its widespread use and its wide host range, vaccinia virus sometimes caused naturally spreading diseases in domestic animals. (e.g., teat infections of cattle) and also in laboratory rabbits ("rabbitpox"). In Holland in 1963, 8 of 36 outbreaks of cowpox were found to be caused by vaccinia virus and the rest by authentic cowpox virus (see below).

Buffalopox. Buffalopox occurs in water buffaloes (*Bubalus bubalis*) in Egypt, the Indian subcontinent, and Indonesia. By restriction mapping, the causative virus appears to be vaccinia virus, although differing from laboratory strains in some properties. The disease is characterized by pustular lesions on the teats and udders of milking buffaloes; occasionally, especially in calves, a generalized disease is seen. Outbreaks still occur in Egypt and India, sometimes producing lesions on the hands and face of milkers, who are no longer protected by vaccination against smallpox.

Cowpox

Cowpox virus can be differentiated from vaccinia virus by its biological properties in laboratory animals, and it also has a larger genome (220 kbp compared with 192 kbp for vaccinia virus) and a different restriction endonuclease map. Usually seen as a lesion on the teats or udders of cows, the virus occasionally infects milkers and may be transferred by them from one animal to another.

Since the early 1960s outbreaks of severe generalized poxvirus infection, in a variety of zoo and circus animals including elephants and large felines, have been shown to be caused by cowpox virus. Cowpox virus appears to be maintained in nature as an infection of rodents, and infection of domestic cats is not uncommon in the United Kingdom. Since the virus has a wide host range, sporadic cases occur in many other species, presumably due to contact with infected rodents. Infections in large felines may be severe and often fatal.

The incubation period of cowpox in cattle and in humans is about 5 days. Local erythema and edema are followed by the development of a multiloculate vesicle, then a pustule, which ruptures and suppurates. A scab can then form, but in milking cows ulceration is common. The lesions, which are often found on all four teats as well as the skin of the udder, may take several weeks to heal. The diagnosis of cowpox cannot be made without laboratory assistance, since a parapoxvirus (see Fig. 20-3A,B) and a herpesvirus (bovine mammillitis virus, see Chapter 19) cause similar lesions on the teats of cows.

Camelpox

Camelpox causes a severe generalized disease in camels, with extensive skin lesions. It is an important disease, especially in countries of Africa and southwestern Asia where the camel is used as a beast of burden and milch animal. The more severe cases usually occur in young animals, and in epidemics the case–fatality rate may be as high as 25%.

The causative virus is a distinctive species, and its restriction endonuclease map differentiates it from other orthopoxviruses. It has a narrow host range; in spite of the frequent exposure of unvaccinated humans to florid cases of camelpox, human infection has not been seen.

Ectromelia

Ectromelia virus causes mousepox, a disease known only in laboratory mice. Its veterinary importance derives from the fact that it is endemic in many mouse colonies in Europe, China, and Japan and has periodically been imported to the United States, where devastating outbreaks have occurred in mouse colonies. Depending mainly on the genotype of the mouse, the infection may cause inapparent disease or acute death with extensive necrosis of the liver and spleen. Mice that survive the acute infection often develop widespread skin lesions.

Demonstration of poxvirus particles in lesion material is diagnostic, since no other poxvirus causes a naturally spreading disease in mice. If a positive result is found in a country normally free of the disease, like the United States, it should be checked by other tests, since infected laboratory colonies may have to be destroyed.

Vaccination with vaccinia virus provides some protection and can be used for particularly valuable mouse stocks, but spread of mousepox can occur in vaccinated mice. Hence the usual recommendation is that infected mouse stocks should be destroyed and the mouse breeding quarters thoroughly disinfected before reestablishing the colony.

Monkeypox

First observed in captive Asian monkeys in a laboratory in Copenhagen in 1958, the generalized poxvirus infection known as monkeypox was subsequently diagnosed in eight similar outbreaks in Europe and the United States between 1958 and 1968. Affected monkeys developed a generalized rash, the disease being especially severe in great apes. At that time no infections occurred among animal attendants. The virus has a distinctive restriction endonuclease map, and its biological properties also distinguish it clearly from other orthopoxviruses. It has a wide host range.

In 1970 it was discovered that in western and central Africa monkeypox virus caused a disease in humans, with a generalized pustular rash indistinguishable from that of smallpox. The human disease is a rare zoonosis, occurring only among Africans living in small villages in tropical rainforests. Monkeys and squirrels are the sources of most human infections, but occasionally person-to-person transmission occurs. Originally important to veterinarians as a sporadic generalized pox disease of captive monkeys, in laboratories or zoos, monkeypox now derives its significance as being the only smallpoxlike disease of man.

Other Species of Orthopoxvirus

Uasin Gishu disease is a rare disease that produces papular skin lesions in horses in Kenya and Zambia, and is caused by an orthopoxvirus. It is presumably contracted from a wildlife source. Other species of orthopoxviruses have been isolated from a gray seal (*Halichoerus grypus*) in the North Sea affected with skin lesions, from raccoons (*Procyon lotor*) in North America, from a skunk in Iowa, and from a vole in California. Raccoon poxvirus has been used to produce a recombinant rabies vaccine for the oral vaccination of raccoons.

DISEASES CAUSED BY PARAPOXVIRUSES

Parapoxviruses infect a range of species but are most important in cattle, sheep, goats, camels, and seals (Table 20-4). The viruses are zoonotic; farmers, shearers, veterinarians, butchers, and others who handle infected livestock can develop a localized lesion, usually on the hands (Fig. 20-3E). The lesion, which is identical irrespective of the source of the virus, begins as an inflammatory papule, then enlarges to form a granulomatous lesion before regressing. It may persist for several weeks. If the infection is acquired from milking cattle, the lesion is known as "milker's nodule"; if from sheep, as "orf."

Pseudocowpox

Pseudocowpox occurs as a common endemic infection in cattle in most countries of the world. It is an chronic infection in many milking herds and occasionally occurs in beef herds.

The first clinical sign of pseudocowpox is a small papule on the teat; this soon develops into a small, dark red scab, the edges of which extend while the center becomes umbilicated and then scabbed. The central part of the scab desquamates, leaving a "ring" or "horseshoe" scab that is pathognomonic for the disease (Fig. 20-3B). Several such lesions may

TABLE 20-4

Other Poxviruses of Veterinary Importance: Host Ranges and Geographic Distribution

Genus	Virus	Animals found naturally infected	Host range in laboratory animals	Geographic range
Parapoxvirus	Pseudocowpox virus	Cattle, man	Narrow	Worldwide
	Bovine papular stomatitis virus	Cattle, man	Narrow	Worldwide
	Orf virus	Sheep, goat, man	Narrow	Worldwide
	Ausdyk virus	Camel	Narrow	Africa, Asia
	Seal parapoxvirus	Seal, man	Narrow	Worldwide
Capripoxvirus	Sheeppox virus	Sheep, goat	Narrow	Africa, Asia
	Goatpox virus	Goat, sheep	Narrow	Africa, Asia
	Lumpyskin disease virus	Cattle, buffalo	Narrow	Africa, Israel
Suipoxvirus	Swinepox virus	Swine	Narrow	Worldwide
Leporipoxvirus	Myxoma virus	Rabbits (*Oryctolagus* and *Sylvilagus*)	Narrow	Americas, Europe, Australia
Avipoxvirus	Fowlpox virus	Chickens, turkey, other birds	Narrow	Worldwide
Yatapoxvirus	Yaba monkey tumor poxvirus	Monkeys	Narrow[a]	West Africa

[a] Animal handlers have been infected.

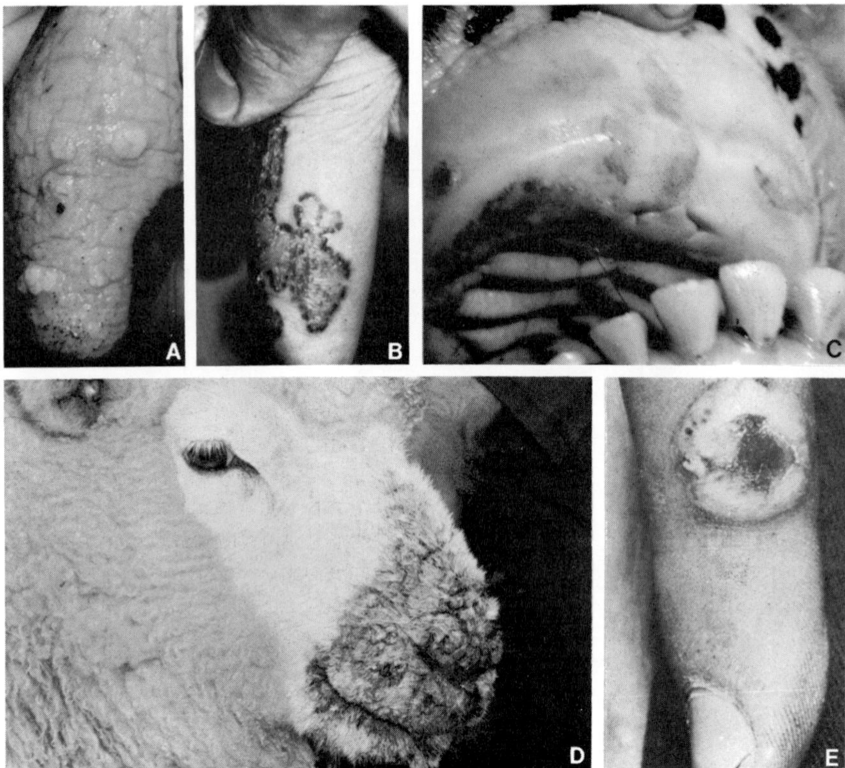

FIG. 20-3. *Parapoxvirus infections: pseudocowpox, bovine papular stomatitis, and orf in animals and man. (A and B) Pseudocowpox lesions on the teats of a cow, at the pustular and scab stages. (C) Bovine papular stomatitis. (D) Scabby mouth caused by orf virus, in a lamb. (E) Orf lesion on the hand of a man. (A and B, courtesy Dr. D. C. Blood; D, courtesy of Dr. A. Robinson; E, courtesy of Dr. J. Nagington.)*

coalesce to form linear scabs. Ulceration is unusual, and the lesions usually heal within 6 weeks without scarring, although occasionally cattle develop chronic infection. Similar lesions can develop on the muzzles and within the mouths of nursing calves.

Infection is transmitted by cross-suckling of calves, improperly disinfected teat clusters of milking machines, and probably by the mechanical transfer of virus by flies. Attention to hygiene in the milking shed and the use of teat dips reduces the risk of transmission.

Bovine Papular Stomatitis

Bovine papular stomatitis is usually of little clinical importance, but it occurs worldwide, affecting cattle of both sexes and all ages, although the incidence is higher in animals less than 2 years old. The development of lesions on the muzzle, margins of the lips, and the buccal mucosa is similar to that of pseudocowpox in calves (Fig. 20-3C). Immunity is of short duration, and cattle can become reinfected. Demonstration by electron microscopy of the characteristic virions in lesion scrapings can be used to confirm the clinical diagnosis.

Orf

Orf (contagious pustular dermatitis, scabby mouth) is a more important disease in sheep and goats than either pseudocowpox or bovine papular stomatitis in cattle, and it is common throughout the world. Orf, which is the Old English for "rough," commonly involves only the muzzle and lips (Fig. 20-3D), although lesions within the mouth affecting the gums and tongue can occur, especially in young lambs. The lesions can also affect the eyelids, feet, and the teats of ewes. Human infection can occur among persons occupationally exposed (Fig. 20-3E).

Lesions of orf progress from papules to pustules, and then to thick crusts. The scabs are often friable and mild trauma causes the lesions to bleed. Orf may prevent lambs from suckling. Severely affected animals may lose weight and be predisposed to secondary infections. Morbidity is high in young sheep, but mortality is usually low. Clinical differentiation of orf from other diseases seldom presents a problem, but if necessary electron microscopy can be used to confirm the diagnosis.

Sheep are susceptible to reinfection, and chronic infections can occur. These features, and the resistance of the virus to desiccation, explain how the virus, once introduced to a flock, can be difficult to eradicate. Spread of infection can be by direct contact or through exposure to contaminated feeding troughs and similar fomites, including wheat stubble and thorny plants.

Ewes can be vaccinated several weeks before lambing, using commercial live-virus vaccines derived from infected scabs collected from sheep. These are applied to scarified skin, preferably in the axilla, where a localized lesion develops. A short-lived immunity is generated; ewes are thus less likely to develop orf at lambing time, thereby minimizing the risk of an epidemic of orf in the lambs.

DISEASES CAUSED BY CAPRIPOXVIRUSES

The genus *Capripoxvirus* comprises sheeppox virus, goatpox virus, and lumpyskin disease virus, which affects cattle. Although the geographic distributions are different, indicating that the viruses are distinct, the viruses are indistinguishable by conventional serology; sheeppox vaccine has been used to protect cattle from lumpyskin disease. Restriction endonuclease analyses of the DNA of several isolates of sheeppox, goatpox, and lumpyskin disease confirm that the viruses are closely related. The African strains of sheeppox and lumpyskin disease are more closely related to each other than sheeppox is to goatpox. However, while sheeppox and goatpox are often considered to be host-specific, in parts of Africa where sheep and goats are herded together both species may show clinical disease during an outbreak, indicating that some strains may affect both sheep and goats.

For presumptive diagnosis, negative-staining electron microscopy can be used to demonstrate virus particles in clinical material, the virions being indistinguishable from those of vaccina virus. Capripoxviruses can be isolated in various cell cultures derived from sheep, cattle, or goats, in which cytoplasmic inclusions are formed.

Sheeppox and Goatpox

Sheeppox and goatpox are the most important of all pox diseases of domestic animals, causing high mortality in young animals and significant economic loss. They occur as endemic infections in southwestern Asia, the Indian subcontinent, and most parts of Africa except southern Africa.

Sheeppox has a documented history almost as old as that of smallpox. The disease was apparently present in Europe as early as the second century A.D., and its infectious nature was recognized in the mid-eighteenth century. Eradication was achieved in Britain in 1866, but in other areas of Europe eradication was more difficult, probably because of the extensive live animal trade between countries.

The clinical signs vary in different hosts and in different geographical areas. Sheep and goats of all ages may be affected, but the disease is generally more severe in young animals. An epidemic in a susceptible flock of sheep can affect over 75% of the animals, with a mortality as high as 50%; case–fatality rates in young sheep may approach 100%.

After an incubation period of 4–8 days, there is a rise in temperature, an increase in respiratory rate, edema of the eyelids, and a mucous discharge from the nose. Affected sheep may lose their appetite and stand with an arched back. One to two days later, cutaneous nodules 0.5–1.5 cm in diameter develop, which may be widely distributed over the body. The nodules are most obvious in the areas of skin where the wool/hair is shortest, such as the head, neck, ears, axillae, and under the tail (Fig. 20-4A). The nodules usually scab and persist for 3–4 weeks, healing to leave a permanent depressed scar. Lesions within the mouth affect the tongue and gums and ulcerate. Such lesions constitute an important source of virus for infection of other animals. In some sheep,

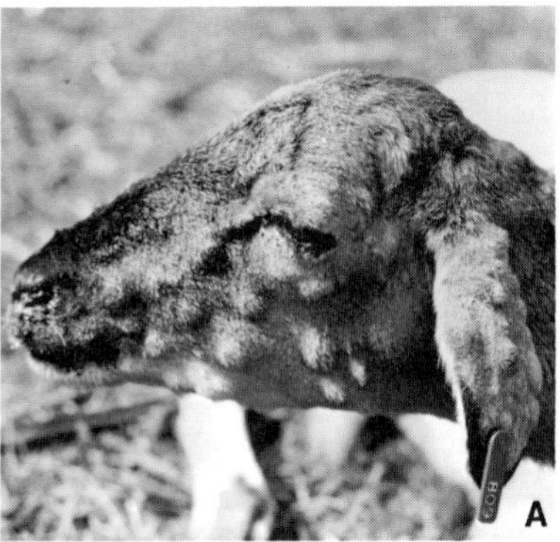

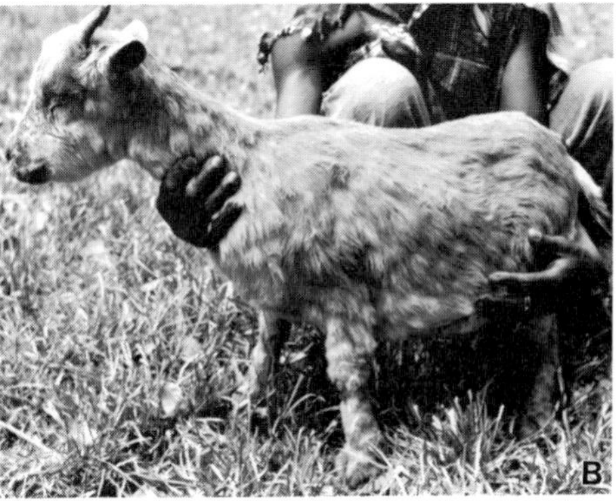

FIG. 20-4. *(A) Sheeppox and (B) goat pox in native breeds in Ghana. (Courtesy Dr. M. Bonniwell.)*

lesions develop in the lungs, as multiple consolidated areas 0.5–2.0 cm in diameter. Goatpox is clinically similar to sheeppox (Fig. 20-4B).

Sheeppox and goatpox are notifiable diseases in most countries of the world, and any clinical suspicion of disease should be reported to the appropriate authorities. Apart from occasional outbreaks in partly immune flocks, where the disease may be mild, or when the presence of orf complicates the diagnosis, sheeppox and goatpox present little difficulty in clinical diagnosis. When confirmation is required, the most rapid diagnosis is by electron microscopy.

As with most poxviruses, environmental contamination with sheeppox or goatpox virus can lead to introduction of virus into small skin wounds. Scabs that have been shed by infected sheep remain infective for several months. The common practice of herding sheep and goats into enclosures at night in the countries where the disease occurs provides adequate exposure to maintain endemic infection. During an outbreak, the virus is probably transmitted between sheep by aerosol, and there is evidence that mechanical transmission of virus by biting arthropods such as stable flies may also occur.

In countries where the diseases are endemic, attenuated live-virus and inactivated vaccines are available. Recombinant vaccines based on the use of capripoxviruses as vectors are in development.

Lumpyskin Disease

Lumpyskin disease affects cattle breeds derived from both *Bos taurus* and *Bos indicus*, and it was first recognized in an extensive epidemic in Zambia in 1929. An epidemic in 1943–1944, which involved other countries including South Africa, emphasized the importance of the disease, which remained restricted to southern Africa until 1956, when it spread to central and eastern Africa. Since the 1950s, it has continued to spread progressively throughout Africa, first north to the Sudan and subsequently westward, to appear by the mid-1970s in most countries of western Africa. In 1988, the disease was confirmed in Egypt, and in 1989 a single outbreak occurred in Israel, the first report outside the African continent.

Lumpyskin disease is characterized by fever, followed shortly by the development of nodular lesions in the skin which subsequently undergo necrosis. Generalized lymphadenitis and edema of the limbs are common. During the early stages of the disease, affected cattle show lacrimation, nasal discharge, and loss of appetite. The skin nodules involve the dermis and epidermis; they are raised and later ulcerate and may become secondarily infected. Ulcerated lesions may be present in the mouth and nares; postmortem, circumscribed nodules may be found in lungs and alimentary tract. Healing is slow, and affected cattle often remain debilitated for several months.

Morbidity in susceptible herds can be as high as 100%, but mortality is rarely more than 1–2%. The economic importance of the disease relates to the prolonged convalescence, and, in this respect, lumpyskin disease is similar to foot-and-mouth disease; indeed, in South Africa it is regarded as economically more important.

The clinical diagnosis presents few problems to clinicians familiar with it, although the early skin lesions can be confused with generalized skin infections of pseudo-lumpyskin disease, caused by bovine herpesvirus 2 (see Chapter 19).

It is likely that the virus is mechanically transmitted between cattle by biting insects, the virus being perpetuated in a wildlife reservoir host, possibly the African Cape buffalo. Control is by vaccination. Two vaccines are currently available; in South Africa an attenuated live-virus vaccine (Neethling) and in Kenya a strain of sheep/goatpox virus propagated in tissue culture have been used successfully.

Lumpyskin disease has recently shown the potential to spread outside continental Africa. Since it is principally transmitted by insect vectors, the importation of wild ruminants to zoos in different continents could establish new foci of infection, if suitable vectors were available.

DISEASES CAUSED BY SUIPOXVIRUSES

Swinepox is seen sporadically in swine-raising areas throughout the world. Many outbreaks of pox disease in swine have been caused by vaccinia virus, but swinepox virus, which belongs to a different genus, is now the primary cause of the disease. Swinepox is usually a mild disease with lesions restricted to the skin (Fig. 20-5). Lesions may occur anywhere but are most obvious on the belly. A transient low-grade fever may precede the development of papules which, within 1 to 2 days, become vesicles and then umbilicated pustules, 1–2 cm in diameter. The pocks crust over and scab by 7 days; healing is usually complete by 3 weeks. The clinical picture is characteristic; it is seldom necessary to seek laboratory confirmation.

Swinepox is most commonly transmitted between pigs by the bite of the pig louse, *Hematopinus suis*, which is common in many herds; the virus does not replicate in the louse. No vaccines are available for swinepox, which is most easily controlled by elimination of the louse from the affected herd. As with the other poxviruses of farm animals, swinepox virus is being developed as a vaccine vector.

DISEASES CAUSED BY LEPORIPOXVIRUSES

There are five species of viruses in the genus *Leporipoxvirus*, but only myxoma virus is of veterinary importance. It constitutes a serious risk to breeders of European rabbits in California and Europe. It is also important as having provided the most successful example yet of the use

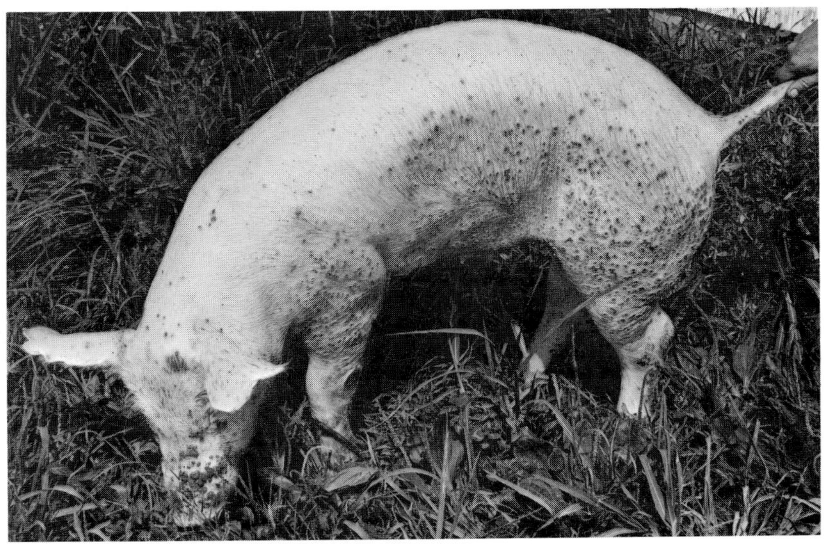

FIG. 20-5. *Swinepox. (Courtesy Dr. R. Miller.)*

of a virus to control a vertebrate pest (i.e., the wild European rabbit in Australia and Europe; see Chapter 4).

Myxomatosis

Myxoma virus causes only a localized benign fibroma in wild rabbits in the Americas (*Sylvilagus* spp.); in contrast, it causes a severe generalized disease in the European rabbit (*Oryctolagus cuniculus*), with a very high mortality (Fig. 20-6). The characteristic early signs of myxomatosis in the European rabbit are blepharoconjunctivitis and swelling of the muzzle and anogenital region, giving the rabbit a leonine appearance. The rabbit is listless, has a high temperature, and often dies within 48 hours of onset of these early signs, an outcome seen especially commonly in infections due to the California strain of myxoma virus. In rabbits that survive longer, subcutaneous gelatinous swellings (hence the name myxomatosis) appear all over the body 2–3 days later. The vast majority of rabbits (over 99%) infected from a wild (*Sylvilagus*) source of myxoma virus die within 12 days of infection. Transmission can occur by droplet infection but is usually due to mechanical transfer of virus by biting arthropods.

Diagnosis of myxomatosis in European rabbits can be made by the clinical appearance or by virus isolation in rabbits, on the chorioallantoic membrane, or in cultured rabbit or chicken cells. Electron microscopy of the exudate or smear preparations of the lesions reveal virions indistinguishable from those of vaccinia virus.

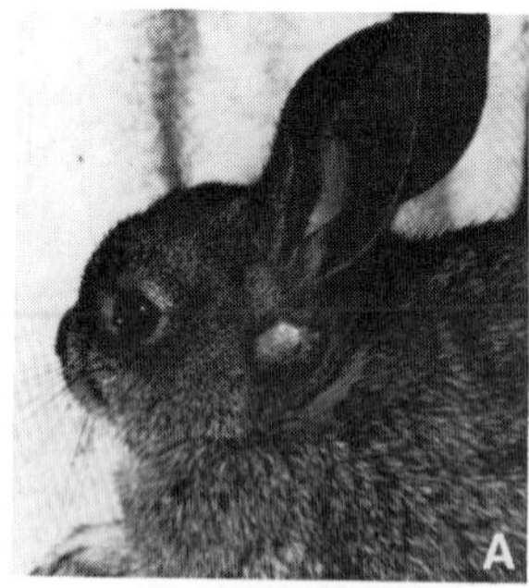

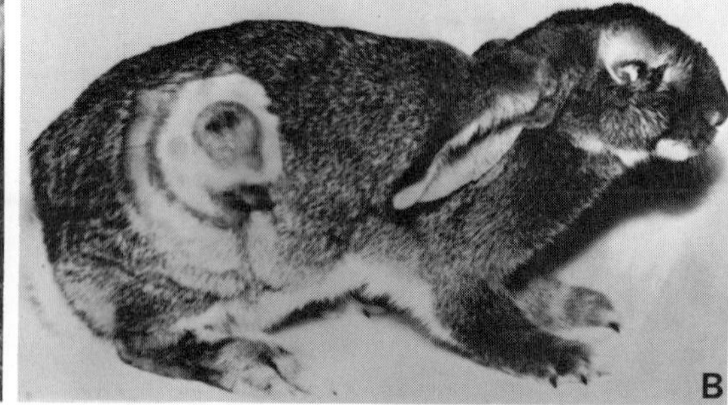

FIG. 20-6. *Myxomatosis. (A) Localized fibroma in* Sylvilagus bachmani. *(B) Severe generalized disease in* Oryctolagus cuniculus, *showing large tumor at site of intradermal inoculation on the flank, generalized lesions, and blepharoconjunctivitis. (A, courtesy Dr. D. Regnery.)*

Laboratory or hutch rabbits can be protected against myxomatosis by inoculation with the related rabbit fibroma virus or with attenuated live-virus vaccines, developed in California and France.

DISEASES CAUSED BY AVIPOXVIRUSES

Poxviruses that are serologically related to each other and specifically infect birds have been recovered from lesions found in all species of poultry and many species of wild birds. Viruses recovered from various species of birds are given names related to their hosts: fowlpox, canarypox, turkeypox, pigeonpox, magpiepox viruses, etc. As judged by their pathogenicity in various avian hosts, there seem to be a number of different species of avian poxvirus, but no systematic analysis of restriction endonuclease patterns of their DNAs has yet been made. Mechanical transmission by arthropods, especially mosquitoes, provides a mechanism for transfer of the virus between a variety of different species of birds.

Fowlpox

Fowlpox is a serious disease of poultry that has occurred worldwide for centuries. Effective vaccines have now reduced the economic loss formerly associated with the disease. There are two forms, probably associated with different modes of infection. The most common, which probably results from infection by biting arthropods, is characterized by small papules on the comb, wattles, and around the beak (Fig. 20-7); occasionally lesions develop on the legs and feet and around the cloaca. The nodules become yellowish and progress to a thick dark scab. Multiple lesions often coalesce. Involvement of the skin around the nares may cause nasal discharge, and lesions on the eyelids can cause excessive lacrimation and predispose poultry to secondary bacterial infections. In uncomplicated cases, healing occurs within 3 weeks.

The second form of fowlpox is probably due to droplet infection and involves infection of the mucous membranes of the mouth, pharynx, larynx, and sometimes the trachea. This is often referred to as the "diphtheritic" form of fowlpox because the lesions, as they coalesce, result in a necrotic pseudomembrane which can cause death by asphyxiation. The prognosis for this form of fowlpox is poor.

Extensive infection in a flock may cause a slow decline in egg production. Cutaneous infection causes little mortality, and these flocks return to normal production on recovery. Recovered birds are immune.

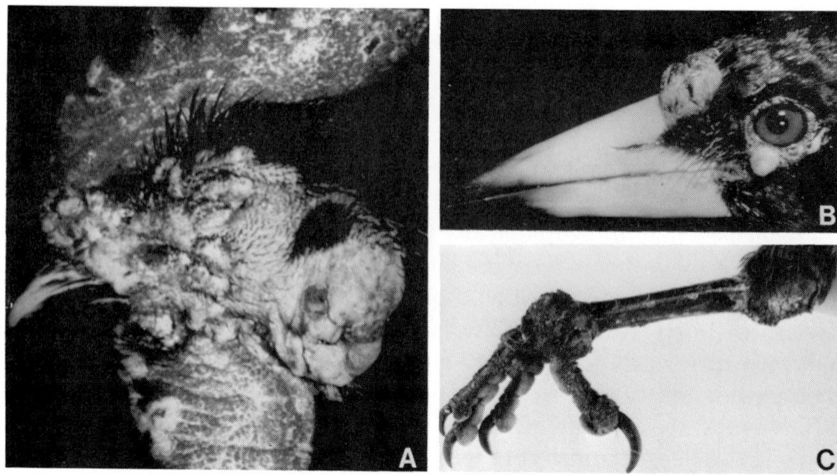

Fig. 20-7. *Avian poxvirus diseases. (A) Fowlpox. (B and C) Poxvirus infection in an Australian magpie. (B) Lesions at the base of the beak and under the eye. (C) Lesions on the foot. (B and C, courtesy K. E. Harrigan.)*

The cutaneous form of fowlpox seldom presents a diagnostic problem. The diphtheritic form is more difficult to diagnose because it can occur in the absence of skin lesions, and it may be confused with vitamin A deficiency and several other respiratory diseases caused by viruses. Electron microscopy can be used to confirm the clinical diagnosis. The virus can be isolated by inoculation of avian cell cultures or the chorioallantoic membrane of the developing chick embryo.

Fowlpox is transmitted within a flock by direct contact with infected birds, by movement of birds into contaminated buildings, and by the mechanical transfer of virus on the mouthparts of mosquitoes, lice, and ticks. If not infected by arthropod vectors, many birds become infected through small abrasions in the skin and possibly by inhalation of virus.

Poultry can be protected by vaccination with pigeonpox virus (another avian poxvirus which is less virulent for chickens), which is applied by light scarification of the skin of the thigh. Attenuated fowlpox vaccines are also available, but they produce a more severe reaction. In Germany fowlpox vaccines have been developed that can be administered in drinking water. In endemically infected flocks, poultry should be vaccinated during the first few weeks of life and again 8–12 weeks later. Recombinant vaccines for poultry are in development using both fowlpox and canarypox as vectors. As discussed in Chapter 13, these vaccines may also have application in mammalian species.

FURTHER READING

Buller, R. M. L. and Palumbo, G. J. (1991). Poxvirus pathogenesis. *Microbiol. Rev.* **55,** 80.

Fenner, F. (1990). Poxvirus. *In* "Fields Virology" (B. N. Fields, D. M. Knipe, R. M. Chanock, M. S. Hirsch, J. L. Melnick, T. P. Monath, and B. Roizman, eds.), 2nd Ed., p. 2113. Raven, New York.

Fenner, F., and Nakano, J. H. (1988). *Poxviridae:* The poxviruses. *In* "Laboratory Diagnosis of Infectious Diseases. Principles and Practice. Volume II, Viral, Rickettsial, and Chlamydial Diseases" (E. H. Lennette, P. Halonen, and F. A. Murphy, eds.), p. 177. Springer-Verlag, New York.

Fenner, F., Henderson, D. A., Arita, I., Jezek, Z., and Ladnyi, I. D. (1988). "Smallpox and Its Eradication." World Health Organization, Geneva.

Fenner, F., Wittek, R., and Dumbell, K. R. (1989). "The Orthopoxviruses." Academic Press, San Diego.

Kitching, R. P. Bhat, P. P., and Black, D. N. (1989). The characterization of African strains of capripoxvirus. *Epidemiol. Infect.* **102,** 335.

Moss, B. (1990). Replication of poxviruses. *In* "Fields Virology" (B. N. Fields, D. M. Knipe, R. M. Chanock, M. S. Hirsch, J. L. Melnick, T. P. Monath, and B. Roizman, eds.), 2nd Ed., p. 2079. Raven, New York.

Moss, B. (1991). Vaccinia virus as a tool for research and vaccine development. *Science* **252,** 1661.

Osterhaus, A. D. M. E., Broeders, H. W., Visser, I. K. G., Teppema, J. S., and Vedder, E. J. (1990). Isolation of an orthopoxvirus from pox-like lesions of a grey seal (*Halichoerus grypus*). *Vet. Rec.* **127,** 91.

Robinson, A. J., and Little, D. J. (1992). Parapoxviruses: Their biology and potential as recombinant vaccines. *In* "Recombinant Poxviruses" (M. M. Binns and G. L. Smith, eds.), p. 285. CRC Press, Boca Raton, Florida.

Turner, P. C., and Moyer, R. W., eds. (1990). Poxviruses. *Curr. Top. Microbiol. Immunol.* **163,** 125.

CHAPTER 21

Iridoviridae and African Swine Fever Virus

Large icosahedral cytoplasmic DNA viruses that used to be grouped together as the family *Iridoviridae* occur in a wide range of animal species, both vertebrate and invertebrate (Table 21-1) In 1984 the species of greatest veterinary importance, African swine fever virus, was removed from the family, because of major differences in the structure of its DNA and its mode of replication, both of which have some resemblances to those of poxviruses; it is currently an "ungrouped" virus.

Although there have been no major epidemics of African swine fever since the early 1980s, it is probably the most serious viral disease threatening the swine industries of developing and industrialized countries. Since its recognition in 1921 in East Africa, the disease has spread to Europe and the Western Hemisphere, causing the death of many hundreds of thousands of domestic swine. African swine fever virus is transmitted by soft ticks of the genus *Ornithodoros;* it is the only DNA virus that can be designated as an arbovirus.

Lymphocystis in fish causes tumorlike lesions on the skin which make affected fish unmarketable. Because lymphocystis virus has been reported to cause disease in more than 90 different species of marine, brackish, and freshwater fish, it is potentially an important pathogen.

TABLE 21-1

Diseases Caused by African Swine Fever Virus and Iridoviruses

Family/Genus	Viruses	Animal species affected	Disease
African swine fever virus group	African swine fever virus	Wild pigs and domestic swine	No disease in warthog (natural host) but severe disease in domestic swine, sometimes with persistent infection
Family *Iridoviridae*			
Ranavirus	Large number of species, principally from frogs	Amphibians	Death in tadpoles but no disease in adult frogs
Lymphocystivirus	Lymphocystis virus	Many species of fish	Tumorlike growths in skin
Iridovirus and *Chloriridovirus*	Two genera which include a large number of viruses	Many species of insects	Affects larvae; large masses of virions produce iridescence

PROPERTIES OF THE VIRUSES

The virions of iridoviruses of vertebrates and of African swine fever virus are morphologically similar (Fig. 21-1). An irregular lipoprotein envelope derived from the plasma membrane gives the virion an irregular spherical shape, about 200–220 nm in diameter. Within the envelope there is an icosahedral capsid which contains a very large number of capsomers, calculated as being either 1892 or 2172. The capsid in turn encloses a lipoprotein membrane which surrounds the DNA-containing core. The genome is a single molecule of dsDNA, 95–190 kbp in size (Table 21-2), which in iridoviruses of the genera *Lymphocystivirus* and

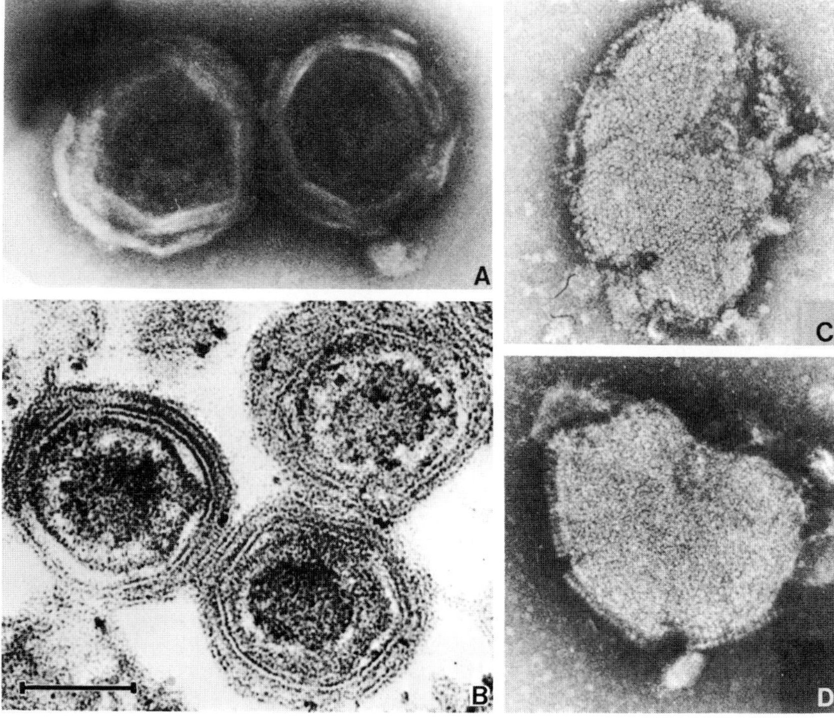

FIG. 21-1. *Virions of African swine fever virus. (A) Negatively stained virions, showing icosahedral capsid and envelope. (B) Thin sections of virions, showing multiple membranes surrounding the core. (C and D) Negatively stained capsids, showing the ordered arrangement of a large number of capsomers. Bar: 100 nm. [From J. L. Carrascosa* et al., Virology **132,** *160 (1984). Courtesy Dr. J. L. Carrascosa.]*

TABLE 21-2
Properties of African Swine Fever Virus and Iridoviruses of Vertebrates

Spherical enveloped virion, 200–220 nm diameter
Icosahedral capsid (1892 or 2172 capsomers) surrounds an internal lipid-containing membrane which encloses the DNA-containing core
Linear dsDNA genome. African swine fever virus: 170–190 kbp, with covalently closed ends and inverted terminal repeats; *Lymphocystivirus*: 95 kbp and *Ranavirus*: 150 kbp, both methylated, circularly permuted and with terminal repeats
African swine fever virus virion contains a virus-coded DNA-dependent RNA polymerase; iridovirus virions lack this enzyme
In both groups, the nucleus is involved in DNA replication
Assembly of capsids in cytoplasm; virions mature by budding from plasma membrane

Ranavirus is methylated, circularly permuted, and contains terminal repeats. In contrast, the African swine fever virus genome resembles that of poxviruses in having covalently closed ends and inverted terminal repeats. The African swine fever virus virion contains, but *Lymphocystivirus* and *Ranavirus* virions lack, a DNA-dependent RNA polymerase. Based on sequence analysis, the thymidine kinase genes of African swine fever virus and poxviruses have about 30% identity, compared with about 25% between the African swine fever virus gene and the thymidine kinase genes of vertebrates. Thus, while African swine fever virus and poxviruses share several important properties, their evolutionary relationship is probably rather distant.

The iridoviruses of vertebrates and African swine fever virus are sensitive to ether, chloroform, and deoxycholate. Infectivity is also sensitive to heat; African swine fever virus is inactivated in 30 minutes at 56°C but survives well, for months and even years, in refrigerated meat. African swine fever virus is also resistant to a wide range of pH, some infectivity surviving for several hours at pH 4 or pH 13; hence, it is not surprising that many common disinfectants are ineffective.

Serotypes have not yet been recognized within either African swine fever virus or lymphocystis virus isolates. However, there are differences in immunogenicity and hemadsorption patterns among different African swine fever virus isolates. Restriction endonuclease analysis of the DNA of isolates of African swine fever virus from Africa, Europe and the Americas permits classification into five groups. All European and American isolates fall within one group, whereas the African isolates show greater variation.

VIRAL REPLICATION

The presence of African swine fever virions of a DNA-dependent RNA polymerase and several other enzymes similar to those present in poxviruses suggests that the early stages of gene expression may be similar to those of poxviruses (see Fig. 20-2). Unlike African swine fever virus, the iridoviruses lack a DNA-dependent RNA polymerase, although their genomes code for several other enzymes.

After penetration by endocytosis, the African swine fever virus virion is uncoated, and the DNA is transcribed in the cytoplasm by the virion-associated RNA polymerase. New mRNA species are transcribed after DNA replication, again by the viral transcriptase. About 50 virus-induced polypeptides have been identified. Synthesis of viral DNA occurs in the cytoplasm, in association with inclusion bodies, and requires a virus-induced DNA polymerase and a functional nucleus in the infected cell. Late in infection, a virus-specific protein appears in the plasma membrane and can be recognized by hemadsorption.

AFRICAN SWINE FEVER

African swine fever virus has probably caused subclinical endemic infection in warthogs in eastern and southern Africa for centuries, but its presence was not detected until the beginning of the twentieth century, when European settlers reported deaths in introduced domestic swine. In 1921 Montgomery described the disease in domestic swine in Kenya as a peracute disease, clinically similar to hog cholera, that commonly caused up to 100% mortality in herds. He showed that the disease was caused by a virus immunologically distinct from hog cholera virus (genus *Pestivirus;* see Chapter 24) and demonstrated that warthogs (*Phacochoerus aethiopicus*) and to a lesser extent bush pigs (*Potamochoerus porcus*) were sources of the infection.

The potential for African swine fever to become a worldwide threat was recognized only when it spread to Portugal in 1957, causing heavy losses, and subsequently to Spain in 1960. African swine fever is now endemic in Spain and Portugal. The numbers of new outbreaks each year vary in cycles, with peaks of several thousand cases occurring in some years. It is from these two countries that further spread of the disease occurred in the 1960s and 1970s to the Caribbean and South America.

Clinical Features

Swine infected with African swine fever virus develop fever (40.5°–42°C) which occurs 5–15 days after exposure and persists for about 4 days. Other clinical signs, usually starting 1 to 2 days after the onset of fever, include inappetence, incoordination, and recumbency. Swine may die at this stage without other clinical signs. In some swine there are cyanotic areas on the ears and limbs. Other clinical signs include dyspnea, vomiting, nasal and conjunctival discharge, and hemorrhage from the nose or anus. Pregnant sows often abort. In East and South Africa, mortality is often 100%, and swine die 4–7 days after onset of fever. Since becoming endemic in domestic swine outside Africa, the virulence of the virus has decreased, the mortality in some herds being no higher than 30%, with most animals suffering from subacute or chronic forms of the disease. Some of the swine that survive are persistently infected.

Pathology and Pathogenesis

In acute fatal cases, gross lesions are most prominent in the lymphatic and vascular systems. Hemorrhages occur widely, and the visceral lymph nodes may resemble blood clots. The spleen is often large and friable, and there are petechial hemorrhages in the cortex of the kidney. The chronic disease is characterized by cutaneous ulcers, pneumonia, pericarditis, pleuritis, and arthritis.

If infection is acquired via the respiratory tract, the virus replicates first in the pharyngeal tonsils and lymph nodes draining the nasal mucosa before being rapidly disseminated throughout the body by a primary viremia, in which virions are associated with both erythrocytes and leukocytes. A generalized infection follows with titers up to 10^9 ID_{50} per milliliter of blood or per gram of tissue. Consequently, all secretions and excretions contain infectious virus.

Experimental studies have shown that African swine fever virus replicates in several cell types within the reticuloendothelial system and causes a severe leukopenia. Infected animals probably die through the indirect effects of viral replication on platelets and complement functions, rather than by the direct cytolytic effect of the virus. Swine that survive may appear healthy or chronically diseased, but both groups may remain persistently infected. Indeed, swine may become persistently infected without ever showing clinical signs. The duration of the persistent infection is now known, but low levels of virus have been detected in tissues over 1 year after exposure. Viremia has been induced in such animals by injection of corticosteroids 6 months after initial infection.

Immunity

The immunologic response of swine to African swine fever virus is puzzling. Virus infection induces antibody detectable by complement fixation, precipitation, immunofluorescence, hemadsorption–inhibition, and ELISA tests; often in chronic infections so much antibody is formed that there is a hypergammaglobulinemia. However, neutralizing antibody has never been demonstrated. For this reason, efforts to produce a vaccine for African swine fever have so far been fruitless.

Diagnosis

The clinical signs of African swine fever are similar to those of several diseases such as erysipelas and acute salmonellosis, but the major diagnostic problem is in distinguishing it from hog cholera. Any febrile disease in swine associated with hemorrhage and death should raise suspicion of African swine fever. Laboratory confirmation is essential, and samples of blood, spleen, and visceral lymph nodes should be collected for virus isolation and for detection of antigen and antibody. Virus isolation is done in swine bone marrow or blood leukocyte cultures, in which hemadsorption to infected cells can be demonstrated and a cytopathic effect is seen within a few days of inoculation; the virus can be adapted to grow in various cell lines such as pig kidney and Vero cells. Antigen detection is done by immunofluorescent staining of tissue smears and frozen sections, or by immunodiffusion using tissue suspensions.

Epidemiology

Two distinct epidemiologic patterns occur: a sylvatic cycle in warthogs in Africa and epidemic and endemic cycles in domestic swine.

Sylvatic Cycle. In its original ecologic niche in southern and eastern Africa, African swine fever virus is maintained in a sylvatic cycle involving asymptomatic infection in wild pigs (warthogs and to a lesser extent bush pigs) and argasid ticks (soft ticks) which occur in the burrows used by these animals. The soft ticks belong to the genus *Ornithodoros*. The tick is a biological vector of the virus (Fig. 21-2). Most tick populations in southern and eastern Africa (Fig. 21-2A) are infected, with infection rates as high as 25%. After feeding on viremic swine, the virus replicates in the gut of the tick and subsequently infects its reproductive system. This leads to transovarial and venereal transmission of the virus between ticks. The virus is also transmitted between developmental stages of the tick (transstadial transmission) and is excreted in tick saliva, coxal fluid,

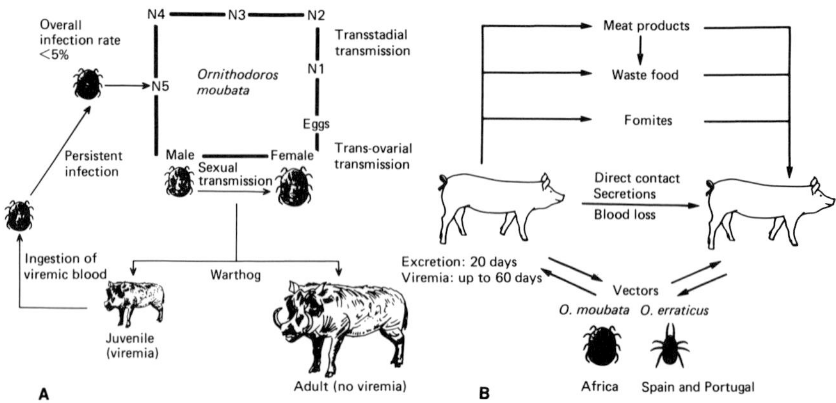

FIG. 21-2. *(A) Transmission cycles of African swine fever virus in warthogs and* Ornithodoros moubata. *(B) Transmission of African Swine fever virus in domestic swine and* Ornithodoros *species. [From P. J. Wilkinson,* Prevent. Vet. Med. **2,** *71 (1984).]*

and Malpighian excrement. Infected ticks may live for several years and be capable of transmitting disease to swine at each feeding.

Serologic studies indicate that many warthog populations in southern and eastern Africa are infected. After primary infection, young warthogs develop viremia sufficient to infect at least some of the ticks feeding on them. Older warthogs are persistently infected but are seldom viremic. It is therefore likely that virus is maintained in a cycle involving young warthogs and ticks.

Domestic Cycle. Primary outbreaks of African swine fever in domestic swine in Africa probably result from the bite of an infected tick, although tissues of acutely infected warthogs, if eaten by domestic swine, can also cause infection.

Introduction of the virus into a previously noninfected country may result in indigenous ticks becoming infected and acting as biological vectors and reservoirs of disease, a feature of great epidemiologic significance. Several species of soft ticks found in association with domestic and feral swine in the Western Hemisphere (the United States and the Caribbean islands) have been shown in experimental studies to be capable of biological transmission of African swine fever virus, although there is no evidence that they have become naturally infected during the epidemics in the Caribbean islands and South America.

Once the virus has been introduced to domestic swine, either by the bite of infected ticks or through infected meat, infected animals form the most important source of virus for susceptible swine (Fig. 21-2B). Disease spreads rapidly by contact and within buildings by aerosol. The mechanical spread of African swine fever virus by people, vehicles, and fomites is possible because of the stability of the virus in blood, feces, and tissues.

The international spread of African swine fever virus has invariably been linked to feeding swine waste food containing scraps of uncooked meat from infected swine. When the virus appeared in Portugal in 1957 and in Brazil in 1978, it was first reported in the vicinity of international airports, among swine fed on food scraps. Virus spread to the Caribbean and Mediterranean islands in 1978 may have arisen from the unloading of infected food scraps from ships.

Prevention and Control

The prevention and control of African swine fever is difficult because of several features: the lack of an effective vaccine, the transmission of virus in fresh meat and some cured pork products, the existence of persistent infection in some swine, the clinical similarity to hog cholera, and the recognition that in some parts of the world soft ticks of the genus *Ornithodoros* are involved in the transmission of the disease.

The presence of the virus in ticks and warthogs in many countries of sub-Saharan Africa makes it impossible to break the sylvatic cycle of the virus. However, domestic swine can be reared in Africa if the management system avoids feeding uncooked waste food scraps and prevents access of ticks and warthogs, usually by double fencing with a wire mesh perimeter fence extending beneath the surface.

Elsewhere in the world, countries that are free of African swine fever maintain their position by prohibiting importation of live swine and swine products from infected countries and by monitoring the efficient destruction of all waste food scraps from ships and aircraft involved in international commerce. If disease does occur in a previously noninfected country, control depends first on early recognition and rapid laboratory diagnosis. The virulent forms of African swine fever cause such dramatic mortality that episodes are quickly brought to the attention of veterinary authorities, but the disease caused by less virulent strains that are now found outside Africa can cause confusion with other diseases, especially hog cholera, and may not be recognized until the virus is well established in the swine population.

Once African swine fever is confirmed in a country that has hitherto been free of disease, its importance necessitates prompt action to first control and then eradicate it. All non-African countries that have become infected have elected to attempt eradication and, in many cases, have received financial assistance from international agencies such as the Food and Agricultural Organization of the United Nations. The strategy for eradication involves slaughter of infected swine and swine in contact with them and disposal of carcasses, preferably by burning. Movement of swine between farms is controlled and feeding of waste food prohibited. Where soft ticks are known to occur, infested buildings are sprayed with acaricides. Restocking of the farm is allowed only if sentinel swine do not become infected.

Using this approach, elimination has been successful in some countries (e.g., France, Malta, and Cuba), but in others (e.g., Spain and Portugal) this has proved difficult, almost certainly because ticks have become infected.

LYMPHOCYSTIS OF FISH

Lymphocystis is not a lethal disease, and the lesions eventually heal. The disease is most noticeable on the skin where papilloma-like lesions are produced by enormously hypertrophied dermal cells (Fig. 21-3), but internal organs and tissues also may be affected. Lymphocystis occurs worldwide and is probably transmitted via abrasions; the virus can be isolated in fish cells grown at a temperature of 23°–25°C. The disease is most commonly seen in brackish water or seawater environments with a slow circulation. Peak incidence is recorded in summer, and local pollution may predispose fish to infection. While currently not an eco-

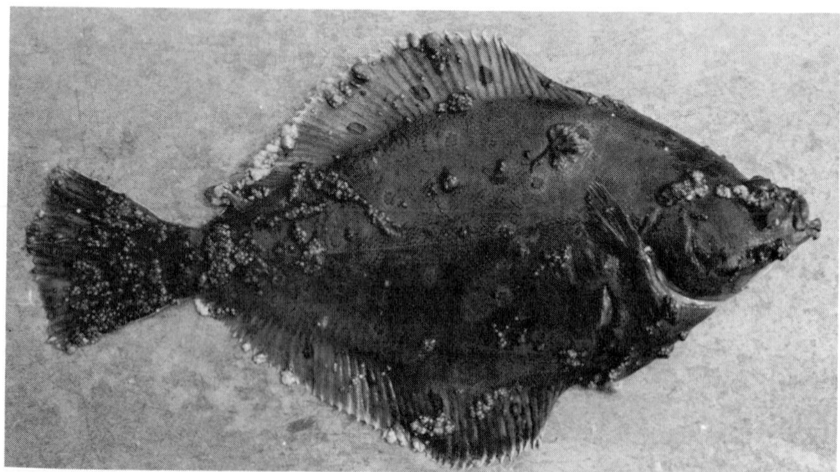

FIG. 21-3. *Lymphocystis in plaice. (Courtesy Dr. P. van Banning.)*

nomically important disease, the fact that the virus can infect a wide range of fish species poses an economic threat to those involved in intensive fish farming, since affected fish are unmarketable.

FURTHER READING

Becker, Y., ed. (1987). "Developments in Veterinary Virology—African Swine Fever." Nijhoff, Boston.

Darai, G., ed. (1990). "Molecular Biology of Iridoviruses," Developments in Molecular Virology Series. Kluwer, Norwell, Massachusetts.

Mebus, C. A. (1988). African swine fever. *Adv. Virus Res.* **35,** 251.

Wardley, R. C., Norley, S. G., Martins, C. V., and Lawman, M. J. (1987). The host response to African swine fever virus. *Prog. Med. Virol.* **34,** 180.

Willis, D. B., ed. (1985). *Iridoviridae. Curr. Top. Microbiol. Immunol.* **116,** 1.

CHAPTER 22

Picornaviridae

Five genera are included in the family *Picornaviridae*, each of which contains viruses causing diseases in domestic or laboratory animals (see Table 22-2). Picornaviruses have played an important role in the history of virology. In 1897, Loeffler and Frosch showed that foot-and-mouth disease was caused by an agent that passed through filters that held back bacteria; this was the first demonstration that a disease of animals was caused by a filterable virus. A century later the same virus was among the first animal viruses to have their structure resolved at the atomic level by X-ray crystallography (see frontispiece).

Many industrialized nations have controlled several of the serious picornaviral diseases of man and animals, such as poliomyelitis and foot-and-mouth disease. Worldwide, however, picornaviruses still create major disease problems in people and animals.

PROPERTIES OF PICORNAVIRUSES

The picornavirus virion is a nonenveloped icosahedron 25–30 nm in diameter (Fig. 22-1). The capsid, appearing smooth and round in outline in electron micrographs, is composed of 60 copies of each of four coat

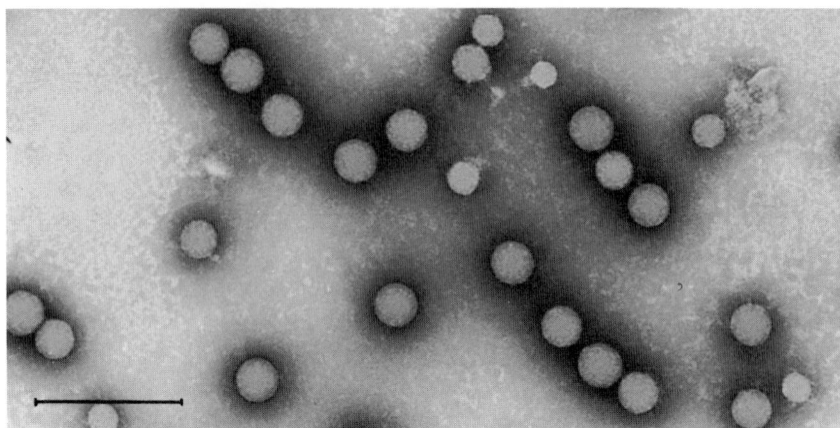

FIG. 22-1. Picornaviridae. *Electron micrograph of negatively stained virions of foot-and-mouth disease virus. Bar: 100 nm. (Courtesy Dr. S. H. Wool.) See frontispiece for a high-resolution picture of the virion of foot-and-mouth disease virus.*

proteins, VP1, VP2, VP3 (each of about 30K), and VP4 (7K–8K). VP1, VP2, and VP3 share a common folding pattern, each containing a conserved core that is an eight-stranded β barrel, but differ in the size of the loops and in the extensions of their amino and carboxy termini (see Fig. 1-4). In the mature virion the cores of VP1, VP2, and VP3 pack to form the continuous icosahedral shell, the connecting loops decorate the outer surface of the particle and contain the major antigenic sites, and the amino-terminal extensions form an intricate network on the inner surface of the protein shell. VP4 is buried in the core, probably in contact with the RNA. For enteroviruses and rhinoviruses the packing together of the cores of VP1, VP2, and VP3 results in the formation of a "canyon"; amino acid residues in the canyon are conserved and are involved in binding the virion to the cell receptor (see Fig. 1-5). However, in foot-and-mouth disease virus there is no canyon, and the receptor-binding amino acid residues are located superficially. Although less immunogenic than intact inactivated virions, preparations of purified VP1 elicit neutralizing antibody, a discovery that has provided a major impetus for the development of recombinant DNA and synthetic peptide vaccines for foot-and-mouth disease (see Chapter 13). Minor polypeptides, of unknown function, have been reported to occur in the virions of many picornaviruses. The foot-and-mouth disease virus virion contains small amounts of a virus-coded component of the RNA-dependent RNA polymerase.

Some properties of the picornaviruses are set out in Table 22-1. The

TABLE 22-1
Properties of Picornaviruses

Nonenveloped icosahedral capsid, 25–30 nm in diameter, 60 capsomers
Linear, plus sense ssRNA genome, 7.5–8.5 kb, protein VPg at 5′ end, polyadenylated at 3′ end, infectious
Virion RNA acts as mRNA and is translated into a polyprotein which is then cleaved to yield 11 individual proteins
Cytoplasmic replication

family *Picornaviridae* is divided into five genera: *Enterovirus, Cardiovirus, Rhinovirus, Aphthovirus,* and *Hepatovirus;* the properties common to members of the family are shown in Table 22-2. The most important differences between viruses of the five genera in their physicochemical properties involved their stability at low pH. The aphthoviruses are unstable below pH 7, the rhinoviruses lose activity below pH 5, and the enterovir-

TABLE 22-2
Disease of Domestic Animals Caused by Picornaviruses

Genus	Virus	Principal species affected	Disease
Enterovirus	Bovine enteroviruses 1–7	Cattle	Mostly subclinical infections
	Porcine enteroviruses 1–11	Swine	Infection frequently subclinical, but porcine enterovirus 1 causes polioencephalomyelitis
	Swine vesicular disease virus	Swine	Swine vesicular disease
	Avian enteroviruses	Chickens	Avian encephalomyelitis
		Ducks	Hepatitis
		Turkeys	Hepatitis
Cardiovirus	Encephalomyocarditis virus	Mammals in contact with rodents	Rarely, encephalomyocarditis in swine
Rhinovirus	Bovine rhinoviruses 1–3	Cattle	Mild rhinitis
Aphthovirus	Foot-and-mouth disease virus, 7 types: A, O, C, SAT1, 2, 3, Asia	Cattle, sheep, goats, and pigs; ruminant wildlife	Foot-and-mouth disease
Hepatovirus	Simian hepatitis A virus	Monkeys	Hepatitis

uses, hepatoviruses, and cardioviruses are stable at pH 3. Another important difference is the presence of a polycytidylic acid tract, of unknown function, in the genome of the apthoviruses and cardioviruses but not in that of either enteroviruses or rhinoviruses.

There are a very large number of picornaviruses, especially in the genera *Enterovirus* and *Rhinovirus,* each antigenically distinct, as determined by neutralization tests.

The stability of picornaviruses to environmental conditions is important in the epidemiology of the diseases they cause and in the selection of methods of disinfection. If protected by mucus and shielded from strong sunlight, picornaviruses are relatively heat-stable at normal ambient temperatures. Enteroviruses may survive several days and often weeks in feces. Aerosols of rhinoviruses and aphthoviruses are less stable, but under conditions of high humidity and low levels of ultraviolet light the viruses may remain viable for several hours. Because of differences in the pH stability, sodium carbonate (washing soda) is effective against the aphthoviruses of foot-and-mouth disease, but it is not a suitable disinfectant against the enterovirus of swine vesicular disease.

VIRAL REPLICATION

Early in the study of viral replication, poliovirus became the primary model for the analysis of the replication of RNA viruses. The work of David Baltimore in particular has provided a detailed description of the poliovirus genome, and of the mechanism of RNA replication, posttranslational proteolytic processing of the polyproteins, and the morphogenesis of a simple icosahedral virus, which serves as a model for picornaviruses in general. The replication of foot-and-mouth disease virus, which has also been studied in considerable detail, parallels that of poliovirus.

The cell receptor for poliovirus is the intercellular adhesion molecule 1 (ICAM-1), and because all serotypes of foot-and-mouth disease virus have a conserved Arg-Gly-Asp motif exposed on their surface and Arg-Gly-Asp peptides block adsorption, it is believed that the foot-and-mouth disease virus receptor is an Arg-Gly-Asp–binding protein. The virion RNA of about 7500 nucleotides has a protein, VPg, linked to the 5′ terminus and a 3′ poly(a) tail. Following adsorption, penetration, and intracellular uncoating, VPg is removed from the virion RNA by cellular enzymes. The virion RNA, acting as mRNA, is translated without interruption into a polyprotein, which is divisible into three regions, P1, P2, and P3, corresponding to the three initial protease cleavage products of the polyprotein (Fig. 22-2). P1 is further cleaved to yield the four structural proteins VP1, VP2, VP3, and VP4. The P2 region codes for three

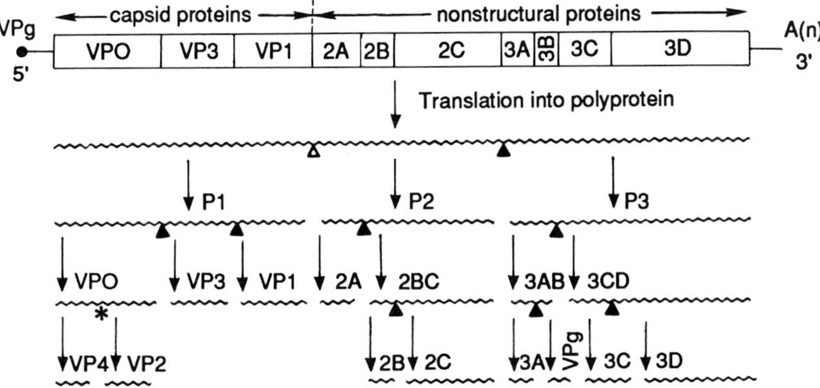

FIG. 22-2. *Poliovirus RNA and the posttranslational processing of the poliovirus polyprotein.* Top: *Poliovirus RNA and its genetic organization. VPg, at the the 5′ terminus, is essential for RNA replication, but the RNA is still infectious if VPg is removed because it can be synthesized from region 3B. The 3′ terminus is polyadenylated, and there are short nontranslated sequences at each end (single lines).* Bottom: *On entry into the cell, the virion RNA acting as messenger is translated into a polyprotein that is rapidly cleaved into polypeptides P1, P2, and P3 by the viral proteases 2A (open triangle) and 3C (closed triangles). P1, P2, and P3 are subsequently cleaved by protease 3C as shown, and polypeptides 2BC, 3AB, and 3CD are further cleaved by protease 3C. VP0 is cleaved into VP4 and VP2 by a third protease during capsid formation, so that VP1, VP2, VP3, and VP4 make up the capsid. The organization of the genome and cleavage patterns are slightly different in different genera of picornaviruses.*

nonstructural proteins including one with protease activity, and the P3 region codes for four proteins including the RNA-dependent RNA polymerase required for RNA replication.

Viral RNA synthesis takes place in a replicative complex which comprises RNA templates and the virus-coded RNA polymerase associated with smooth cytoplasmic membranes. During replication, a replicative form is formed which is completely base-paired to a complementary strand, and there are replicative intermediates consisting of a double-stranded core with nascent single strands of varying lengths. Synthesis of the complementary strand is initiated at the 3′ terminus of the virion RNA and progresses 5′ to 3′. The completed complementary strand serves as a template for the synthesis of virion RNA.

When a cell is doubly infected with two strains of the same species of picornavirus, their genomes sometimes undergo intramolecular recombination, a feature that has been demonstrated with both foot-and-mouth disease virus and poliovirus. In the laboratory, poliovirus/foot-and-mouth disease virus chimeras have been constructed.

APHTHOVIRUSES: FOOT-AND-MOUTH DISEASE

Viruses of the genus *Aphthovirus* cause one disease, foot-and-mouth disease, which is a major world problem. At one time or another, foot-and-mouth disease has occurred in most parts of the world, often causing extensive epidemics in domestic cattle and swine (Table 22-3). Sheep and many species of wildlife are also susceptible. Mortality is low but morbidity is high; convalescence and virus shedding of affected animals may be protracted, and it is these features that make foot-and-mouth disease so important, especially when the virus is introduced into countries previously free of disease.

During the nineteenth century foot-and-mouth disease was widely reported in Europe, Asia, Africa, South America, and North America, and it occurred on one occasion in Australia. From 1880 onward, the control of rinderpest (see Chapter 27) and the improved husbandry in the livestock industries in Europe focused attention on foot-and-mouth disease. Its sequelae were found to be more important than the acute

TABLE 22-3
Geographic Distribution of Foot-and-Mouth Disease

Region	Types	Status
South America	O, A, C	Endemic in most countries but vaccination practiced; not currently seen in Surinam, Guyana, French Guyana, and parts of Chile, Argentina, and Colombia
Europe	O, A, C	Incidence very low in continental Europe where comprehensive vaccination program exists; United Kingdom, Ireland, Sweden, Norway, and Iceland free of infection and no vaccination practiced; vaccination in the European Community discontinued in 1992
Africa	O, A, C, SAT 1, 2, 3	Endemic in most countries; predominance of European types (O, A, C) in north and SAT 1, 2, 3 south of the Sahara; vaccination programs in a few countries only
Asia	O, A, C, Asia 1	Endemic in countries of Near East, Far East, and Central Asia; vaccination programs in some countries; Japan free of infection
North and Central America		Virus-free; last outbreaks: USA, 1929; Canada, 1951; Mexico, 1954
Caribbean		Virus-free; last outbreaks: Curacao, 1961; Guadeloupe, 1964
Oceania		Australia and New Zealand virus-free

illness. In dairy herds, the febrile disease resulted in the loss of milk production for the rest of the lactation period, and mastitis often resulted in a permanent loss of more than 25% of milk production; the growth of beef cattle was retarded. Today, many countries have either eliminated foot-and-mouth disease by compulsory slaughter of infected animals or greatly reduced its incidence by extensive vaccination programs (see Fig. 15-1).

Seven serotypes of foot-and-mouth disease virus have been identified by cross-protection and serologic tests; they are designated O (Oise) and A (Allemagne); C (in anticipation that O and A would be renamed to allow recognition of further types A, B, C, etc.); SAT 1, SAT 2, SAT 3 (South African territories); and Asia 1. Historically, each type has been further subtyped on the basis of quantitative differences in cross-protection and serologic tests. Antigenic variation within a type occurs as a continuous process of antigenic drift without clear-cut demarcations between subtypes. This antigenic heterogeneity has important economic implications for vaccine development and selection, since immunity acquired through infection or use of current vaccines is strictly type-specific and, to a lesser degree, subtype-specific. Difficulty in defining the threshold at which a new isolate should be given subtype status has always been a problem, and current attitudes reflect a pragmatic approach. New strains are now compared with the established vaccine strains of commercial producers, thereby avoiding the complexity of classifying new isolates within a ever-increasing catalog of subtypes, many of which have little relevance to current problems in the field.

Clinical Features

Aphthoviruses infect a wide variety of cloven-hoofed domestic and wild animal species. Although the horse is refractory to infection, cattle, water buffalo, sheep, goats, llamas, camels, and swine are susceptible and develop clinical signs, and more than 70 species of wild mammals belonging to more than 20 families are susceptible. In general, clinical signs are most severe in cattle and swine, but outbreaks have been reported in swine while cattle in close contact with them did not develop clinical disease. Sheep and goats usually experience subclinical infections. Wild animals show a spectrum of responses ranging from inapparent infection to severe disease and even death.

Cattle. After an incubation period of 2–8 days, there is fever, loss of appetite, depression, and a marked drop in milk production. Within 24 hours, drooling of saliva commences, and vesicles develop on the tongue and gums (Fig. 22-3A). The animal may open and close its mouth with

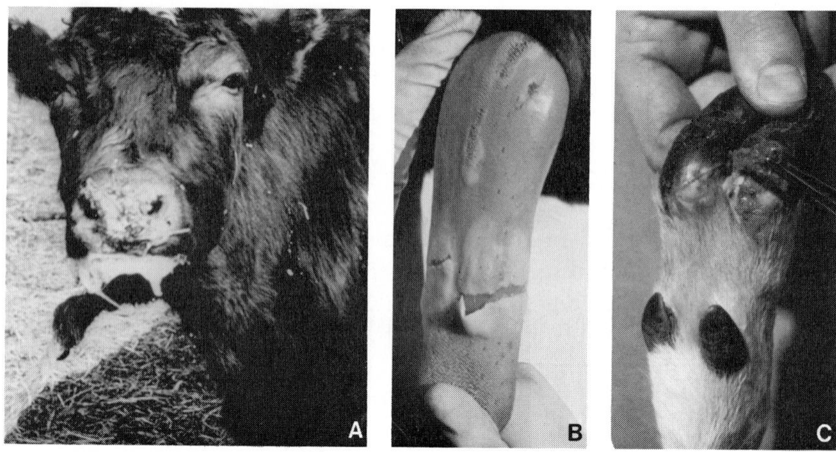

FIG. 22-3. *Foot-and mouth disease. (A) Drooling by a diseased cow. (B) Ruptured vesicles on the tongue of a steer. (C) Vesicular lesions on the foot of a deer.*

a characteristic smacking sound. Vesicles may also be found in the interdigital skin and coronary band of the feet (Fig. 22-3B) and on the teats. The vesicles soon rupture, producing large denuded ulcerative lesions (Fig. 22-3C). Those on the tongue often heal within a few days, but those on the feet and within the nasal cavities often become secondarily infected with bacteria, resulting in prolonged lameness and a mucopurulent nasal discharge. In calves up to 6 months of age, foot-and-mouth disease virus can cause death through myocarditis. The mortality in adult cattle is very low; however, although the virus does not cross the placenta, cattle may abort, presumably as a consequence of fever. Also, affected animals become nonproductive or poorly productive for long periods. They may eat little for a week after the onset of clinical signs and are often very lame; mastitis and abortion further lower milk production. In endemic areas, where cattle may have partial immunity, the disease may be mild or subclinical.

Swine. In swine, lameness is often the first sign. Foot lesions can be severe and may be sufficiently painful to prevent the pig from standing. Denuded areas between the claws usually become infected with bacteria; this causes suppuration and in some cases loss of the claw and prolonged lameness. Vesicles within the mouth are usually less prominent than in cattle, although large vesicles, which quickly rupture, often develop on the snout.

Other Animals. The clinical disease in sheep, goats, and wild ruminants is usually milder than in cattle and is characterized by foot lesions accompanied by lameness.

Pathogenesis

The main route of infection in ruminants is through inhalation of droplets, but ingestion of infected food, inoculation with contaminated vaccines, insemination with contaminated semen, and contact with contaminated clothing, veterinary instruments, etc., can all produce infection. In animals infected via the respiratory tract, initial viral replication occurs in the pharynx, followed by viremic spread to other tissues and organs before the onset of clinical disease. Viral excretion commences about 24 hours prior to the onset of clinical disease and continues for several days. Aerosols produced by infected animals contain large amounts of virus, particularly those produced by swine. Large amounts of virus are also excreted in the milk. The excretion of virus in high titer in droplets and in milk has epidemiologic significance and is important for the control of disease (see below).

Foot-and-mouth disease virus may persist in the pharynx of some animals for a prolonged period after recovery. In cattle, virus may be detectable for periods up to 2 years after exposure to infection, in sheep for about 6 months. Viral persistence does not occur in swine. The carrier state has been observed in wild animals, particularly the African Cape buffalo (*Synceros caffer*), which is commonly found to be infected with more than one of the SAT virus types even in areas where foot-and-mouth disease does not occur in cattle.

The mechanisms by which the virus produces a persistent infection in ruminants are unknown. The virus is present in the pharynx in an infectious form, for pharyngeal fluids inoculated into susceptible animals cause development of foot-and-mouth disease. Attempts to demonstrate that carrier cattle can transmit disease by placing them in contact with susceptible animals have given equivocal results, but transmission of virus from persistently infected African buffalo to cattle has been observed.

Immunity

Recovery from clinical foot-and-mouth disease is correlated with the development of antibody. The early IgM antibodies neutralize the homologous type of virus and may also be effective against heterologous types. In contrast, the IgG produced during convalescence is type-specific and to varying degrees subtype-specific. Little information is available on the role of cell-mediated immunity in recovery from foot-and-mouth disease, but, as in other picornavirus infections, it has been assumed to be of minor importance.

Cattle that have recovered from foot-and-mouth disease are usually immune to infection with the same virus type for 1 year or more, but immunity is not considered lifelong. Recovered animals, however, can be immediately infected with one of the other types of foot-and-mouth disease virus and develop clinical disease.

Laboratory Diagnosis

Rapid diagnosis of foot-and-mouth disease is of paramount importance, especially in countries that are usually free of infection, so that eradication can proceed as quickly as possible. Since three other viruses can produce clinically indistinguishable lesions in domestic animals, confirmation by laboratory diagnosis is essential, although the history of the disease and the involvement of different species can be valuable pointers to the diagnosis (Table 22-4). Foot-and-mouth disease is a notifiable disease in most countries; thus, whenever a vesicular disease of domestic animals is seen, it must be reported immediately to the appropriate government authority.

Specimens for diagnosis are collected by government officials from animals with clinical signs; the exact procedure differs in different countries. Usually, samples include vesicular fluid, epithelial tissue from the edge of ruptured vesicles, blood in anticoagulant, serum, and esophageal/pharyngeal fluids collected with a *cup–probang*. These samples are diluted immediately with an equal volume of tissue culture medium

TABLE 22-4
Differential Diagnosis of Vesicular Diseases Based on Naturally Occurring Disease in Different Domestic Animal Species

		Species[a]			
Disease	Viral family	Cattle	Sheep	Swine	Horse
Foot-and-mouth disease	*Picornaviridae*	S	S	S	R
Swine vesicular disease	*Picornaviridae*	R	R	S	R
Vesicular stomatitis	*Rhabdoviridae*	S	S	S	S
Vesicular exanthema of swine[b]	*Caliciviridae*	R	R	S	R

[a] S, Susceptible by natural exposure; R, resistant by natural exposure.
[b] Now extinct in swine, but virus occurs in marine mammals.

containing 10% fetal calf serum. From dead animals, additional tissue samples may be collected from lymph nodes, thyroid, and heart. Samples should be frozen (preferably at −70°C) and sent immediately to the laboratory in the frozen state. In places where maintenance of the "cold chain" is difficult, duplicate samples should be collected and transported in glycerol buffer at pH 7.6.

A range of diagnostic tests is available for the differentiation of the vesicular diseases, but the ELISA has been standardized whereby, if vesicular fluid or tissues contain adequate amounts of antigen, a diagnosis is available within a few hours. This test can also be used to identify which of the seven types of foot-and-mouth disease virus is the cause of the disease. Sensitive ELISAs are also available for specific antibody determinations.

Cell cultures and, on occasion, cattle are used to isolate virus when the concentration of virus in the vesicular epithelium or fluid is low. Cell cultures are generally used to isolate virus from other tissues, blood, and esophageal or pharyngeal fluids. The isolated virus is identified by the ELISA or the neutralization test.

Epidemiology

The recognition of foot-and-mouth disease as the most important viral disease constraining efficient animal production in many parts of the world has resulted in intensive study of its epidemiology.

Countries Free of Endemic Foot-and-Mouth Disease. In countries where foot-and-mouth disease either has not previously existed or has been eliminated, a "virgin soil" epidemic can rapidly develop from introduction of virus on one farm. Within a short period, often measured in days rather than weeks, the outbreak can extend to so many farms that veterinary authorities have difficulty in controlling its spread (see Fig. 15-1). The reasons for the rapidity of spread are the highly infectious nature of the virus, the production of high-titer virus in respiratory secretions and the large volumes of droplets and aerosols of virus shed by infected animals, the stability of virus in such droplets, the rapid replication cycle with very high virus yields, and the short incubation period.

Foot-and-mouth disease is rapidly spread within a locality by movement of infected animals to market and by mechanical transmission on items such as clothing, shoes, vehicles, and veterinary instruments. The excretion of virus for up to 24 hours prior to onset of clinical signs means that virus dissemination may have occurred from a farm before any suspicion of disease is raised.

It was not until the dramatic epidemic of 1967–1968 in England, in which approximately 634,000 animals were slaughtered before the disease was successfully eradicated, that the importance of long-distance airborne transmission was realized. Long-distance spread is dependent on wind direction and speed, and it is favored by low temperature, high humidity, and overcast skies. Long-distance spread is therefore more likely to occur in temperate rather than tropical climates. So detailed is the knowledge of the characteristics of aerosols of foot-and-mouth disease virus that computer modeling was used in 1981 to predict the likelihood of spread of disease from France across the English Channel to England (Fig. 22-4).

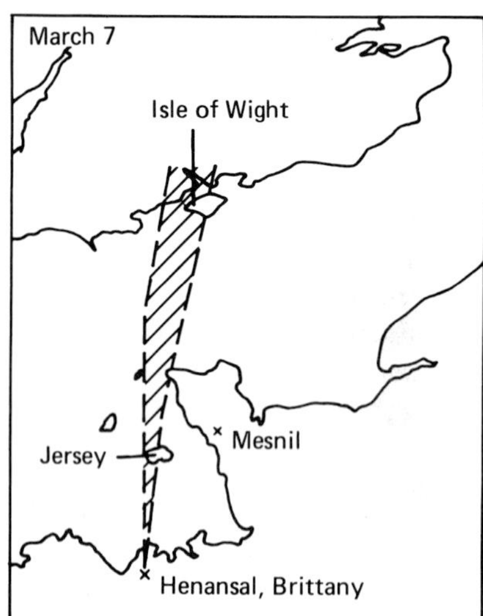

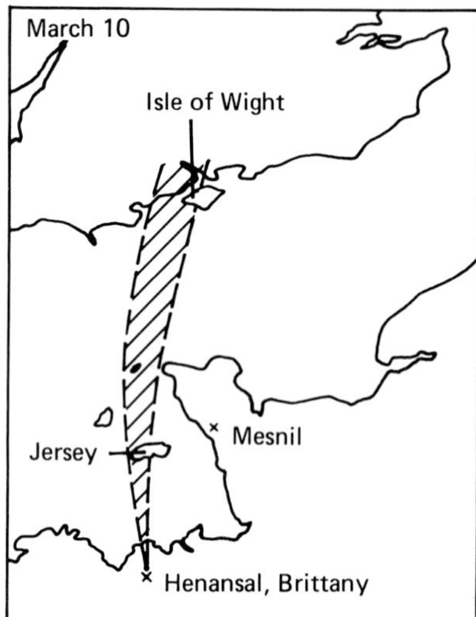

FIG. 22-4. *Airborne spread of foot-and-mouth disease. Between March 4 and 26, 1981, the French veterinary authorities reported 13 outbreaks of foot-and-mouth disease, virus type O, in Brittany. On March 6, a team of meteorologists and virologists in the United Kingdom began analysis to determine whether weather conditions might be favorable for the airborne spread of foot-and-mouth disease virus from France to England. From this analysis it was considered that the risk for the Channel Islands was high, but that it was low in southern England, since the furthest distance previously reported for airborne spread of foot-and-mouth disease virus was approximately 100 km, from Denmark to Sweden in 1966. Single outbreaks were detected in both the areas predicted, on Jersey and on the Isle of Wight. Analysis of wind direction based on data obtained in Jersey revealed that there were two periods, each of 24 hours, on March 7 and 10, which were ideal for transmission of virus from Brittany to Jersey and the Isle of Wight. The distance between Henansal, Brittany, and the Isle of Wight is approximately 250 km. [From A. I. Donaldson* et al., Vet. Rec. **110,** *53 (1982).]*

In contrast to humans, who are generally free to move from country to country without extensive health checks, the international movement of domestic food animals and their products is carefully controlled (see Chapter 15). Nowadays, most introductions of foot-and-mouth disease virus to nonendemic countries can be traced either to meat on the bone being fed to swine or, rarely, to long-distance spread of virus by aerosols.

The use of oligonucleotide fingerprinting of viral RNA and partial sequencing of VP1 to compare an isolate causing disease in one country with a possible source of infection in another country can provide strong evidence to link the two events. Using this approach, scientists investigating the 1981 outbreak in England showed that the outbreaks in England and France were caused by a virus that was identical to a strain used in the preparation of "inactivated" vaccine in France.

Endemic Countries. The introduction of a type not previously present in a country may cause a virgin-soil epidemic because livestock will not have acquired immunity either through natural infection or through vaccination. For example, in 1961, the spread of SAT 1 from Africa through the countries of the Near East, where different types of foot-and-mouth disease virus are endemic, was more dramatic than any recorded spread of this type in Africa.

In some countries, particularly those in the temperate zones with European breeds of cattle, the severity of disease is modified by vaccination. In subtropical and tropical countries, with predominantly local breeds of cattle, the endemic strains produce only mild disease in indigenous cattle but cause severe disease in introduced European breeds. There is a greater variety of antigenic types in Africa and Asia than in Europe and South America, and, in Africa particularly, there is a large wildlife population that can become involved in the epidemiology. The African Cape buffalo (*Synceros caffer*) is believed to be the natural host for the SAT 1, 2, and 3 types of foot-and-mouth disease virus. Transmission of virus occurs between buffaloes, but clinical disease has not been recorded; the African buffalo does not seem to transmit disease readily to domestic cattle.

Control

Foot-and-mouth disease, more than any other disease, has influenced the development of international regulations designed to minimize the risk of introducing animal diseases into a country. Some countries have successfully avoided the introduction of foot-and-mouth disease by prohibiting the importation of all animals and animal products from countries where the disease exists. The United States adopted such a policy from 1929 to 1980; only recently, in the light of improved diagnostic procedures, has it relaxed the embargo to allow small numbers of cattle to be imported for breeding purposes.

For many countries such as Australia, Canada, United Kingdom, and the United States that have a recent history of freedom from foot-and-mouth disease, cost–benefit analyses justify a "stamping out" policy whenever disease occurs or is suspected. This is based on slaughter of affected animals and exposed animals, along with rigid enforcement of quarantine and restrictions on movement. Vaccination is not used. Legislation is in place to support such policies, the most important provision being that foot-and-mouth disease is a notifiable disease. Any suspicion of disease must be brought to the attention of national or state veterinary authorities.

Immunization. In many countries of the world an elimination policy cannot be pursued because of costs, and vaccine is used to reduce the prevalence of disease. Inactivated vaccines that are produced by growing virus in suspended cultures of a baby hamster kidney cell line, inactivated with *N*-acetylethyleneimine, and used with aluminum hydroxide or double oil emulsion as adjuvants are now the only vaccines in general use. By systematic use of inactivated vaccines, many countries in Europe have sufficiently controlled foot-and-mouth disease to discontinue vaccination and adopt an elimination policy whenever clinical disease occurs (see Fig. 15-1). However, it is difficult to produce a vaccine of consistent potency, and much research is in progress with peptide and virus-vectored vaccines.

PORCINE ENTEROVIRUSES

Enteroviruses are ubiquitous and probably occur in all vertebrate species. However, only in swine and poultry do they cause diseases of economic significance.

A number of enteroviruses have been recovered from swine, but only two cause diseases of any importance: an enterovirus that causes swine vesicular disease, the major importance of which is its clinical resemblance to foot-and-mouth disease, and porcine enterovirus 1 which causes porcine polioencephalomyelitis (Teschen/Talfan disease).

The natural history of the porcine enterovirus 1 and of ten other identified porcine enteroviruses (porcine enteroviruses 2–11) is very similar to that of human enteroviruses; that is, porcine enteroviruses are widely distributed, they are transmitted via a fecal–oral cycle, and, in most instances, infections remain confined to the intestinal tract and are subclinical.

Swine Vesicular Disease

Swine vesicular disease was first recognized in Italy in 1966, and since 1972 it has been reported in many other European countries.

Properties of Virus. Swine vesicular disease virus occasionally causes an "influenza-like" illness in man and is closely related serologically and by RNA hybridization tests to human coxsackievirus B5. The virus is stable over a wide pH range, and at neutral pH and 4°C it has been reported to survive for over 160 days without loss of titer. The conditions found on many swine farms are therefore conducive to gross and persistent contamination of the environment.

Clinical Features. Disease is often detected by the sudden appearance of lameness in several swine in a herd. Affected swine have a transient fever, and vesicles appear at the junction between the heel and the coronary band and spread to encircle the digit. In severe cases, the swine are very lame and recovery is protracted. In about 10% of cases, lesions are found on the snout, lips, and tongue. Occasionally, some infected swine develop signs of encephalomyelitis: ataxia, circling, and convulsions. Subclinical infections also occur.

Pathogenesis. Initial infection with swine vesicular disease virus probably occurs through damaged skin, particularly abrasions around the feet. Infection can also occur if swine eat infected garbage, but the titer of virus required to establish infection is higher. Following infection, there is viremia with excretion of large quantities of virus, but persistent infection does not occur. Swine that have recovered from disease develop antibody which protects them from reinfection.

Laboratory Diagnosis. Swine vesicular disease cannot be differentiated clinically from the other vesicular diseases of swine, including foot-and-mouth disease, so that laboratory diagnosis is essential. A variety of rapid laboratory tests is available to distinguish the vesicular diseases. If sufficient vesicular fluid or epithelium is available, the ELISA can be used to detect antigen and establish a diagnosis within 4–24 hours. The virus grows well in cultures of swine kidney cells, producing a cytopathic effect, sometimes as early as 6 hours after inoculation. The virus can also be isolated by intracerebral inoculation of newborn mice, which develop paralysis and die.

Epidemiology. There is no evidence that swine vesicular disease virus exists in any country without clinical disease being reported. Because of its resistance to low pH and ambient temperatures, the virus is easily transmitted between countries in infected meat. Various pork products which are prepared without heat treatment, such as salami, can harbor virus for several months. Fresh pork infected with swine vesicular disease virus can be an additional hazard within a country and delay eradication of disease; infected carcasses may be placed unknowingly in cold storage for months or years, and, when released, such infected meat can give rise to new outbreaks.

Because the virus is so stable, it is extremely difficult to decontaminate infected premises, particularly where swine have been housed on soil. The virus has been isolated from the surface and gut of earthworms collected from soil above burial pits containing carcasses of swine slaughtered because of swine vesicular disease.

Control. Swine vesicular disease is not an economically important disease, but it must be controlled so that diagnostic confusion with foot-and-mouth disease can be avoided. For this reason, swine vesicular disease is a notifiable disease, and most countries have elected to eliminate the virus by a slaughter program, although this may be difficult.

Porcine Enterovirus 1

Porcine polioencephalomyelitis was first recognized in the town of Teschen in Czechoslovakia in 1930. The disease was described as a particularly virulent, highly fatal, nonsuppurative encephalomyelitis in which lesions were present throughout the central nervous system. This severe form of the disease is still recognized, although less severe forms, referred to originally as Talfan disease in the United Kingdom and as endemic posterior paresis in Denmark, are more common and occur worldwide.

Clinical Features. After an incubation period of 4–28 days, the initial signs include fever, anorexia, and depression, followed by tremors and incoordination, usually beginning with the hind limbs. Initially, the limbs may be stiff, then paralysis occurs, leading to prostration followed by convulsions, coma, and death. There may be enhanced responses to touch and sound, paralysis of facial muscles, and loss of voice. In severe outbreaks the mortality may reach 75%. In milder forms of disease the clinical signs are limited to ataxia associated with hind limb paresis from which swine often recover completely in a few days.

Pathogenesis. The pathogenicity of strains of porcine enterovirus 1 varies, and the severity of the disease is also influenced by age, being most severe in young swine. Virus replicates initially in the alimentary tract and associated lymphoid tissues, followed by viremia and invasion of the central nervous system. Histologically the lesions resemble those of other viral encephalomyelitides, with perivascular cuffing, neuronal degeneration, and gliosis. The extent of the lesions parallels the severity of clinical disease and in extreme cases involves the entire spinal cord, brain, and meninges.

Laboratory Diagnosis. Polioencephalomyelitis due to porcine enterovirus 1 must be differentiated from other viral encephalomyelitides including African swine fever, pseudorabies, hemagglutinating encephalomyelitis, rabies, and hog cholera. Virus is readily isolated in porcine cell cultures, neutralization assays being used for typing. Immunofluorescent staining of the infected cell culture is preferred for rapid, definitive diagnosis.

Epidemiology and Control. Infection is acquired by ingestion. Inactivated and attenuated live-virus vaccines, comparable to the Salk and Sabin vaccines for human poliomyelitis, are commercially available. Universal vaccination is not practiced since control in intensive swine units is often satisfactorily achieved by quarantine and hygiene.

Porcine Enteroviruses 2–11

Porcine enteroviruses 2–11 are frequently isolated from the feces of normal swine, and also from swine and diarrhea or pericarditis, and from aborted and stillborn fetuses. In the latter context the viruses were proposed as a cause for a range of reproduction problems to which the acronym SMEDI (for stillbirth, mummification, embryonic death, and infertility) was applied. However, their role in SMEDI and other diseases remains uncertain; porcine parvoviruses are now considered more significant causes of SMEDI (see Chapter 16). Several isolates of porcine enteroviruses 2–11 have been shown to cause encephalomyelitis following experimental infection of swine.

AVIAN ENTEROVIRUSES

Diseases due to enteroviruses occur in chickens, ducks, and turkeys, one species causing encephalomyelitis in chickens and other birds and two others causing hepatitis in ducks and turkeys, respectively. A picornavirus has been associated with avian nephritis, and three other enteroviruses have been associated with runting, and one of these also with diarrhea.

Avian Encephalomyelitis

Avian encephalomyelitis was first described in the New England states of the United States in 1932 and is now recognized worldwide. Its natural history closely parallels that of poliomyelitis of man and polioencephalomyelitis of swine. Avian encephalomyelitis is an important disease of chickens 1–21 days of age, but the virus is not pathogenic in older chickens. When the virus is newly introduced into a flock the mortality rate may exceed 50%. There is only a single antigenic type, but strains vary in virulence. Avian encephalomyelitis virus produces relatively mild encephalomyelitis in quail, turkeys, and pheasants; other avian species are susceptible following experimental infection.

Clinical Features. After an incubation period of 1–7 days, disease occurs which is characterized by dullness, progressive ataxia, tremors particularly of the head and neck, weight loss, blindness, paralysis, and in severe cases prostration, coma, and death. Birds allowed to recover have deficits of the central nervous system and are usually destroyed.

Pathology. No obvious macroscopic lesions are seen postmortem. Histologic lesions typical of viral encephalitis, but not diagnostic of avian encephalomyelitis, are found throughout the central nervous system, with perivascular cuffing, neuronal degeneration, and gliosis.

Laboratory Diagnosis. Clinical signs and histopathology are suggestive, and immunofluorescence is widely used for definitive diagnosis. The virus may be isolated either in cell culture or by inoculating 5- to 7-day-old embryonated hen's eggs obtained from antibody-free hens by the yolk sac route; chicks are allowed to hatch and observed for 7 days for signs of encephalomyelitis. The disease needs to be differentiated from Newcastle disease as well as from a range of nonviral causes of central nervous system disease in chickens.

Epidemiology. High morbidity and mortality occur when avian encephalomyelitis virus is first introduced into a flock. The major mode of transmission is by a fecal–oral route, although transmission via the egg may occur in association with the brief viremic phase of the disease in laying hens. Once established in a flock, losses continue at a greatly reduced incidence, because maternal antibody provides protection for chicks during the critical first 21 days after hatching.

Control. The choice for control is either depopulation or vaccination. Attenuated live-virus vaccines administered in the drinking water are available. The vaccines are administered after chickens reach 10 weeks of age and are designed to provide protection for chicks during the first 21 days after hatching by ensuring that adequate levels of specific antibody are transferred from hens to progeny chicks. Vaccines are not administered to chicks because they are not sufficiently attenuated, nor is there sufficient time to provide protection for chicks hatched into a heavily contaminated environment. Inactivated vaccines are also available and are preferred when immunized birds are housed in close proximity to nonimmunized chickens. Vaccines are also used to control avian encephalomyelitis in quail and turkey.

Duck Hepatitis

Duck hepatitis was first recognized in 1945, among ducks reared on Long Island, New York. There is only one serotype, and the natural history of the virus is similar to that of avian encephalomyelitis virus. Goslings, turkey poults, and chicks of guinea fowl and quail, but not chickens, are susceptible to experimental infection.

Clinical Features. Disease occurs in ducks less than 21 days of age, after an incubation period of 1–5 days. The course of the disease in a clutch of ducklings is often dramatically swift, occurring over a 3-day period with a mortality rate approaching 100%. Affected ducklings tend to stand still with partially closed eyes, fall to one side, paddle spasmodically, and die. There may be some diarrhea. At postmortem, the liver is enlarged, edematous, and mottled with hemorrhages. Histologically there is extensive hepatic necrosis, inflammatory cell infiltration and proliferation of the bile duct epithelium, and encephalitis with neuronal necrosis, gliosis, and perivascular cuffing.

Laboratory Diagnosis. The history, clinical signs, and characteristic postmortem findings are suggestive; immunofluorescence provides rapid, definitive diagnosis. The virus may be isolated in cell culture or by allantoic inoculation of 10-day-old embryonated hen's eggs. Infected eggs, when subsequently candled, often show characteristic greenish discoloration of the embryonic fluids, and most are dead within 4 days after inoculation. Duck hepatitis needs to be differentiated from duck plague (a herpesvirus infection), influenza, and Newcastle disease.

Control. Recovered ducks are immune. Hyperimmune serum has been successfully used to reduce losses during outbreaks. Attenuated egg-adapted live-virus vaccines are used following the same principles as already outlined for avian encephalomyelitis vaccines.

Turkey Hepatitis

Turkey hepatitis was first recognized in 1959 in Canada and the United States. The virus is antigenically related to duck hepatitis virus, and the natural history of the disease resembles that of duck hepatitis.

CARDIOVIRUSES

The genus *Cardiovirus* contains only one species, encephalomyocarditis virus. The natural hosts of the virus are rodents, including the water rat *Hydromys chrysogaster*. The virus is transmitted from rodents to man, monkeys, horses, cattle, and swine. Severe epidemics of myocarditis, with fatalities, have occasionally been reported in swine and other species, such as elephants, notably in Florida and Australia, usually associated with severe mouse or, less commonly, rat infestations.

RHINOVIRUSES

Among domestic animals, rhinoviruses are recognized only in horses and cattle, in which species only a few serotypes are known, compared with over 150 serotypes of human rhinoviruses. The equine and bovine rhinoviruses are antigenically unrelated to each other or to the human rhinoviruses. They cause mild respiratory disease similar to the common cold in man, but they may predispose to more severe forms of respiratory disease. Each is highly host-specific, but man can undergo asymptomatic infection with equine rhinovirus 1.

Three equine rhinovirus serotypes have been identified. In addition to causing respiratory disease, the equine viruses are unusual in that they regularly produce viremia and can be isolated from feces. Three serotypes of bovine rhinovirus have been isolated from cattle with mild respiratory disease.

FURTHER READING

Acharya, R., Fry, E., Stuart, G., Fox, G., Rowlands, D., and Brown F. (1990). The structure of foot-and-mouth disease virus: Implications for its physical and biological properties. *Vet. Microbiol.* **23,** 21.

Acland, H. M., and Littlejohns, I. R. (1986). Encephalomyocarditis. *In* "Diseases of Swine" (A. D. Leman, B. Straw, R. D. Glock, W. L. Mengeling, R. H. C. Penny, and E. Scholl, eds.), 6th Ed., p. 399. Iowa State Univ. Press, Ames.

Barteling, S. J., and Vreeswijk, J. (1991). Developments in foot-and-mouth disease vaccines. *Vaccine* **9,** 75.

Calnek, B. W., Luginbuhl, R. E., and Helmboldt, C. F. (1991). Avian encephalomyelitis (epidemic tremor). *In* "Diseases of Poultry" (B. W. Calnek, ed.), 9th Ed., p. 520. Iowa State Univ. Press, Ames.

Derbyshire, J. B. (1986). Porcine enteroviruses. *In* "Diseases of Swine" (A. D. Leman, B. Straw, R. D. Glock, W. L. Mengeling, R. H. C. Penny, and E. Scholl, eds.), 6th Ed., p. 325. Iowa State Univ. Press, Ames.

Donaldson, A. I., and Kitching, R. P. (1989). Transmission of foot-and-mouth disease by vaccinated cattle following natural challenge. *Res. Vet. Sci.* **46,** 9.

Donaldson, A. I., Gloster, J., Harvey, L. D. J., and Deans, D. H. (1982). Use of prediction models to forecast and analyse airborne spread during the foot-and-mouth disease outbreaks in Brittany, Jersey, and the Isle of Wight in 1981. *Vet. Rec.* **110,** 53.

Jordan, F. W. T., Gooderhan, K. R., and McFerran, J. B. (1990). Diseases associated with *Picornaviridae. In* "Poultry Diseases" (F. T. W. Jordan, ed.), p. 167. Balliere Tindall, London.

Rowlands, D. (1992). Vaccination against foot-and-mouth disease. *In* "Veterinary Vaccines" (S. Hoglund and R. Pandey, eds.), p. 54. Springer-Verlag, Berlin.

Reuckert, R. R. (1990). *Picornaviridae* and their replication. *In* "Fields Virology" (B. N. Fields, D. M. Knipe, R. M. Chanock, M. S. Hirsch, T. P. Monath, and B. Roizman, eds.), 2nd Ed., p. 507. Raven, New York.

Woodcock, P. R., and Fabricant J. (1991). Duck virus hepatitis. *In* "Diseases of Poultry" (B. W. Calnek, ed.), 9th Ed., p. 597. Iowa State Univ. Press, Ames.

CHAPTER 23

Caliciviridae

The family *Caliciviridae* contains one genus, *Calicivirus,* three species of which have been well characterized: vesicular exanthema of swine virus, feline calicivirus, and the virus of rabbit hemorrhagic disease. Vesicular exanthema of swine was first recognized in southern California in 1932 and caused concern because of its similarity to foot-and-mouth disease, but it was eradicated in 1956. Feline calicivirus is one of the two major causes of viral upper respiratory tract disease in cats and has been reported to cause glossitis in dogs. A major new epidemic disease of rabbits, rabbit hemorrhagic disease, first described in 1984, is caused by a calicivirus.

Caliciviruses have been incriminated as causes of two important human diseases, gastroenteritis due to Norwalk virus and water/food-borne hepatitis due to hepatitis E virus. Probable caliciviruses have also been recovered from monkeys, cattle, mink, swine (in addition to vesicular exanthema virus), dog, rabbit, chicken, reptile, amphibian, and insect, but they have not been fully characterized. Those from some species cause gastroenteritis, and a probable strain has been isolated from dogs with vesicular genital disease.

PROPERTIES OF CALICIVIRUSES

The family derives its name from the 32 cup-shaped (*calix* = cup) surface depressions that give the virion its unique appearance (Fig. 23-1). The calicivirus virion is 35–40 nm in diameter, and its icosahedral capsid is constructed from a single, large 67K polypeptide (Table 23-1). A minor 15K polypeptide comprising less than 2% of the total protein has been described, and a third 10K–15K protein that is essential for infectivity is covalently linked to the virion RNA. The virion is relatively resistant to heat and intermediate in its pH stability (>99% inactivated at pH 3).

The plus strand linear ssRNA genome bears a covalently attached protein at its 5′ end; the genome of rabbit hemorrhagic disease virus has been sequenced and comprises 7437 nucleotides. It contains one long open reading frame which in the 5′ region encodes the nonstructural proteins, which include a sequence similar to picornavirus 2C protein, a protease, and RNA polymerase, and at the 3′ end encodes the viral capsid protein. There is a short open reading frame at the extreme 3′ terminus. Sequence comparisons reveal significant homology between regions of the genome of rabbit hemorrhagic disease virus and partial sequences of feline calicivirus and Norwalk virus, as well as with certain amino acid sequence motifs of some picornaviruses.

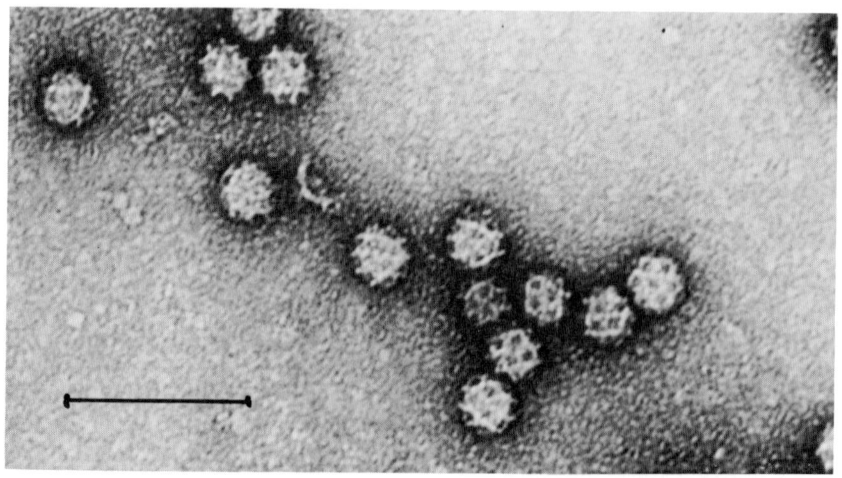

FIG. 23-1. Caliciviridae. *Electron micrograph of negatively stained virions of vesicular exanthema of swine virus. Bar: 100 nm. (Courtesy Dr. S. S. Breese.)*

TABLE 23-1
Properties of Caliciviruses

Nonenveloped spherical virion, 35–40 nm diameter
Icosahedral capsid with 32 cup-shaped depressions, one capsid protein (60K–70K)
Linear plus sense ssRNA genome, 7.4 to 8.2 kb, polyadenylated at 3′ terminus, protein at 5′ terminus essential for infectivity of RNA
Many species have not yet been grown in cultured cells
Cytoplasmic replication; genomic RNA and several subgenomic mRNAs are produced during replication; mature proteins are produced both by processing of polyprotein and translation of subgenomic mRNAs

VIRAL REPLICATION

Caliciviruses replicate in the cytoplasm, and the feline and vesicular exanthema viruses are rapidly cytopathic. They grow well in cell cultures derived from tissues of their respective hosts; vesicular exanthema of swine virus also grows in Vero monkey kidney cells. Of the growing list of probable caliciviruses those from gastroenteritis in pigs and from vesicular genital disease in dogs have been grown in cell cultures, whereas most of the others have proved noncultivable. Virions are found in the cytoplasm either as single scattered particles or as characteristic linear arrays associated with the cytoskeleton, or as paracrystalline arrays.

After infection, calicivirus genomic RNA is translated to form a polyprotein that is cleaved to individual proteins. There is evidence that the subgenomic mRNAs produced in calicivirus-infected cells form a nested set with common 3′ termini, similar to that found in coronavirus-infected cells.

VESICULAR EXANTHEMA OF SWINE

Vesicular exanthema of swine is now an extinct disease, although the virus is still present in marine mammals. It was an acute, febrile contagious disease of swine characterized by the formation of vesicles on the snout, within the oral cavity, and on the feet. First recognized in swine in southern California in 1932, by 1956 it was eradicated from the United States and has not recurred there or been recognized anywhere else. Morbidity was often high but mortality low, and in uncomplicated cases recovery occurred after 1–2 weeks. Its importance derived from the fact that clinically it was indistinguishable from the three other vesicular diseases of swine: foot-and-mouth disease, swine vesicular disease, and vesicular stomatitis (see Chapters 22 and 28). Vesicular exanthema of swine virus showed a remarkable degree of antigenic heterogeneity, at least 13 distinct antigenic types having been identified. Even when recovered concurrently from different swine within a single herd, any two isolates were rarely antigenically identical.

Vesicular exanthema of swine was originally diagnosed as foot-and-mouth disease, and a slaughter policy was implemented; however, sporadic outbreaks continued to occur. When it was established that the virus responsible was not foot-and-mouth disease virus, efforts for eradication diminished. Although there was a clear link between garbage feeding and outbreaks of the disease, ordinances requiring that all garbage fed to swine should be cooked were not rigorously enforced. However, in 1952 it was diagnosed outside California for the first time, initially in Nebraska, and by September 1953 the disease had occurred in 42 states. These experiences led to the rigorous enforcement of garbage cooking laws and a slaughter program which resulted in a rapid decline in the incidence of disease, such that by 1956 it had disappeared.

San Miguel Sea Lion Virus

Although sometimes listed as a separate virus, it is now clear that San Miguel sea lion virus is the same as vesicular exanthema of swine virus and was indeed the source of the disease in swine. It was first isolated in 1972 from material obtained from California sea lions inhabiting San Miguel Island; the animals showed several signs of disease including abortion and vesicular lesions of the flippers. Although serologically distinguishable from the 14 known vesicular exanthema of swine virus serotypes, the virus produced lesions when inoculated into swine. In California, dead carcasses of seals and sea lions washed up on mainland beaches were frequently fed to swine, thus providing the opportunity for infection. Retrospective evidence suggested that the multiple antigenic types of vesicular exanthema of swine virus were generated in the natural hosts of the virus, sea lions, rather than in swine. Thirteen antigenic types of San Miguel sea lion virus have been isolated since 1972, and these have come from a variety of sea mammals including the northern fur seal, northern elephant seal, Pacific walrus, Atlantic bottle nosed dolphin, and northern sea lion as well as from opal eye fish and sea lion liver fluke. In some of these marine mammals the virus has been isolated from vesicular lesions.

FELINE CALICIVIRUS INFECTIONS

Feline calicivirus is one of the two major causes of respiratory disease in cats and produces an acute or subacute disease characterized by conjunctivitis, rhinitis, tracheitis, pneumonia, and vesiculation and ulceration of the oral epithelium. Other common signs are fever, anorexia, lethargy, stiff gait, and sometimes nasal and ocular discharge. Morbidity is high, mortality may reach 30% in very young kittens, and recovery is followed by a prolonged carrier state. Feline calicivirus occurs worldwide, and although all Felidae are probably susceptible, natural infection has been reported only in domestic cats and cheetahs. Economic losses caused by the death of valuable kittens and the costs of providing supportive treatment for sick cats are substantial.

Strains of feline calicivirus vary in virulence. Some strains are associated mainly with subclinical infection or upper respiratory disease; highly virulent strains regularly produce pneumonia, especially in young kittens.

Clinically the disease cannot be differentiated from feline rhinotracheitis caused by feline herpesvirus 1 (see Chapter 19); diagnosis depends on laboratory tests. Both viruses can be readily isolated in cultures of feline cells and may be rapidly differentiated by electron microscopy or lipid solvent sensitivity.

Feline calicivirus can be recovered from about 50% of cats presenting with clinical signs of acute upper respiratory disease. By the age of 1 year virtually all cats have antibodies to it, however, and clinical disease is rare in cats over this age. A high percentage of recovered cats remain persistently infected and shed virus from the oropharynx for several years, possibly for life. When antisera raised in rabbits were used for neutralization assays, feline caliciviruses seemed to show a high degree of antigenic heterogeneity. However, when specific-pathogen-free cat sera were used and a reasonably large collection of viruses analyzed, a pattern of extensive cross-reactions was found, a finding which paved the way for the development of monotypic vaccines. For control, attenuated live-virus and inactivated feline calicivirus vaccines are widely used, usually in combination with feline herpesvirus 1 vaccine.

RABBIT HEMORRHAGIC DISEASE

In 1984 a new, highly infectious disease of the European rabbit, *Oryctolagus cuniculus,* was identified in China. It was characterized by hemorrhagic lesions, particularly affecting the lungs and liver, and has been called rabbit hemorrhagic disease. It killed 470,000 rabbits in the first 6 months and by 1985 had spread throughout China. In 1985 it was reported in Korea, Italy, and then Spain, and by 1988 it had spread throughout Europe and reached North Africa. In December 1988 cases occurred in Mexico City. Both wild and domestic *Oryctolagus cuniculus* were affected, but all other species of mammals except the European hare appear to be resistant to infection. The disease was unknown in Europe before 1984; however, a very similar disease called European brown hare syndrome had been recognized in the early 1980s affecting *Lepus europaeus* and subsequently some other *Lepus* spp. Rabbit hemorrhagic disease is caused by a calicivirus; it appears that a different calicivirus causes the European brown hare syndrome.

Rabbit hemorrhagic disease affects rabbits over 3 months of age, and rabbits less than 2 months old appear to be insusceptible. The disease is often peracute, characterized by sudden death following a 6- to 24-hour period of depression and fever. In acute and subacute forms of the disease rabbits have a serosanguinous nasal discharge and develop a variety of nervous signs. Infection is via the fecal–oral route. Morbidity rates of 100% and mortality rates of 90% are observed in rabbits older than 3 months. At postmortem there is congestion and hemorrhage in the lungs, with accentuated lobular markings, necrosis of the liver, and splenomegaly.

Rabbit hemorrhagic disease virus has not yet been grown in cultured cells, but high concentrations of virus occur in tissues of infected rabbits. The virus hemagglutinates human erythrocytes, and ELISA and immunofluorescence have also been used for diagnosis. Control of entry of virus into commercial rabbitries, either via fomites or via infected wild rabbits, creates a major problem in control. Inactivated vaccines prepared from formalized tissue homogenates provide protection.

FURTHER READING

Berry, E. S., Skilling, D. E., Barlough, J. E., Vedros, N. A., Gage, L. J., and Smith, A. W. (1990). New marine calicivirus serotype infective for swine. *Am. J. Vet. Res.* **51,** 1184.

Carter, M. J. (1990). Transcription of feline calicivirus RNA. *Arch. Virol.* **114,** 143.

Crandell, R. A. (1988). Isolation and characterization of a calicivirus from dogs with vesicular genital disease. *Arch. Virol.* **98,** 65.

Flynn, W. T., and Saif, L. J. (1988). Serial propagation of porcine enteric calici-like virus in primary porcine kidney cell cultures. *J. Clin. Microbiol.* **26,** 206.

Meyers, G., Wirblich, C., and Thiel, H.-J. (1991). Rabbit hemorrhagic disease virus—Molecular cloning and nucleotide sequencing of a calicivirus genome. *Virology* **184,** 664.

Morise, J.-P. (1991). Viral hemorrhagic disease of rabbits and European brown hare syndrome. *Rev. Sci. Tech. Off. Int. Epizoot.* **10,** 263.

Schaffer, F. L. (1979). Caliciviruses. *In* "Comprehensive Virology" (H. Fraenkel-Conrat and R. R. Wagner, eds.), Vol. 14, p. 249. Plenum, New York.

Smith, A. W., and Madin, S. H. (1986). Vesicular exanthemata. *In* "Diseases of Swine" (A. D. Leman, B. Straw, R. D. Glock, W. L. Mengeling, R. H. C. Penny, and E. Scholl, eds.), 6th Ed., p. 358. Iowa State Univ. Press, Ames.

Studdert, M. J. (1978). Caliciviruses. *Arch. Virol.* **58,** 157.

CHAPTER 24
Togaviridae

Early attempts to classify the large number of viruses transmitted by arthropods led to the definition of two major groups, called the Group A and Group B arboviruses. As more was learned about the member viruses, the Group A arboviruses became the family *Togaviridae,* genus *Alphavirus,* and the Group B arboviruses became the family *Flaviviridae,* genus *Flavivirus* (see Chapter 25). Later, rubella virus was placed in the family *Togaviridae* as the only member of the genus *Rubivirus.* The genus *Arterivirus,* which had been part of the family *Togaviridae,* has now been removed and is described as a separate genus in Chapter 34.

There are 30 member viruses of the genus *Alphavirus,* 6 of which cause disease in horses and to a lesser extent in other domestic animals (Table 24-1); these 6 viruses and another 5 cause disease in humans. Alphaviruses exist in particular natural habitats in which specific arthropod and vertebrate hosts play roles in virus survival, geographic extension, overwintering, and amplification (see Chapter 14). The vertebrate reservoir hosts are usually wild mammals or birds; domestic animals and humans are usually not involved in primary transmission cycles in nature, although they may play major roles in geographic extension and amplification events that lead to epidemics. For example, Venezuelan equine encephaltitis virus has a "jungle" endemic transmission cycle in which there is little danger to humans and domestic animals, but when

TABLE 24-1

Alphaviruses That Cause Diseases in Domestic Animals[a,b]

Virus	Mode of transmission	Domestic animal host	Disease	Geographic distribution
Eastern equine encephalitis virus	Mosquito	Horse (human)	Encephalitis	Americas
Western equine encephalitis virus	Mosquito	Horse (human)	Encephalitis	Americas
Highlands J virus	Mosquito	Horse	Encephalitis	Americas
Venezuelan equine encephalitis virus	Mosquito	Horse (human)	Febrile disease, encephalitis	Americas
Getah virus	Mosquito	Horse	Febrile disease	Southeast Asia
Semliki Forest virus	Mosquito	Horse	Febrile disease	Africa

[a] The alphaviruses Chikungunya, O'nyong-nyong, Ross River, Mayaro, and Sindbis cause human disease, often with arthritis.

[b] The other genus in the family *Togaviridae*, *Rubivirus*, contains one virus, rubella virus, that infects only humans.

the amount of virus in an area is amplified via a mosquito–horse–mosquito transmission cycle there can be large epidemics.

PROPERTIES OF TOGAVIRUSES

Virions are spherical, 60–70 nm in diameter, and consist of a tightly adherent lipid bilayer envelope covered with glycoprotein peplomers surrounding an icosahedral capsid (Fig. 24-1). The properties of the togaviruses are summarized in Table 24-2. They are not very stable in the environment and are easily inactivated by disinfectants.

VIRAL REPLICATION

Alphaviruses replicate well and cause cytopathic changes in many kinds of cell cultures, for example, Vero (African green monkey kidney) cells, BHK-21 (baby hamster kidney) cells, and primary chick and duck embryo fibroblasts. They also grow, but do not cause cytopathic changes, in mosquito cells, such as commonly used cell lines derived from *Aedes albopictus*. The viruses also infect and kill newborn mice; in fact, most alphaviruses were first isolated in newborn mice.

Virions are taken up into coated vesicles via receptor-mediated endocytosis; when the coated vesicles become phagolysosomes the low pH causes virions to release viral genomes into the host cell cytoplasm. The

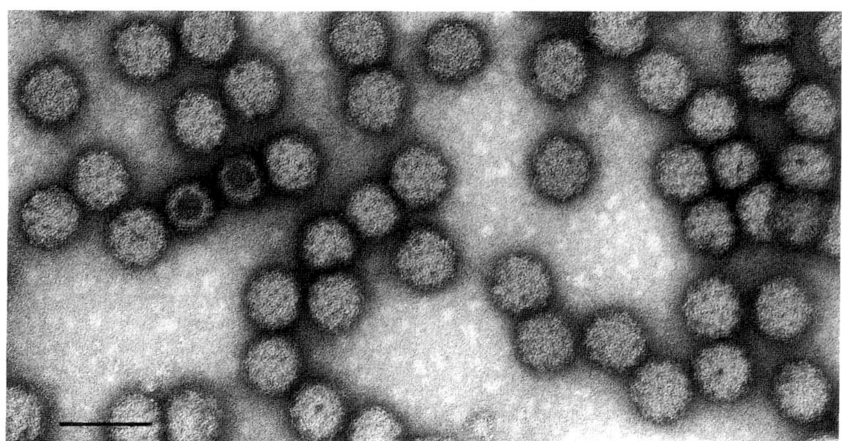

FIG. 24-1. Togaviridae, *genus* Alphavirus. *Negatively stained virions of Semliki Forest virus. Bar: 100 nm. (Courtesy Dr. C.-H. von Bondsdorff.)*

TABLE 24-2
Properties of Togaviruses

Two genera: *Alphavirus,* arthropod-borne viruses; *Rubivirus,* rubella virus (human pathogen)
Spherical virion, enveloped, with peplomers, diameter 60–70 nm
Icosahedral capsid, diameter 35 nm
Linear, plus sense ssRNA genome, 11–12 kb, 5′ end capped, 3′ end polyadenylated, infectious
Genes for nonstructural proteins located at 5′ end of genome
Full-length and subgenomic RNA transcripts; posttranslational cleavage of polyproteins
Two (in some species three) envelope glycoproteins, E1 (45K–53K), E2 (53K–59K), and sometimes E3 (7K–8K), containing virus-specific neutralizing epitopes and alphavirus serogroup and subgroup specificities; one nucleocapsid protein, C (29K–36K), containing broadly cross-reactive alphavirus serogroup specificity
Cytoplasmic replication, budding from plasma membrane

single-stranded plus sense togavirus RNA genome is 11–12 kb in size; its 5′ end is capped and its 3′ end is polyadenylated (Fig. 24-2). During replication, the 5′ two-thirds of the viral RNA genome is translated into a polyprotein, which is cleaved into four nonstructural proteins, two of which form the viral RNA-dependent RNA polymerase. This enzyme directs the transcription of full-length minus sense RNA from which in turn two types of RNA are produced: full-length progeny genomic RNA, and a subgenomic mRNA corresponding to the 3′ one-third of the genomic RNA. The latter is translated into another polyprotein which is cleaved by viral and cellular proteases to yield the four viral structural proteins: the nucleocapsid protein (C), the two (three) peplomer glycoproteins (E1 and E2; in some species E3 also), and the small transmembrane 6K protein. Genomic RNA and nucleoprotein are self-assembled into icosahedral nucleocapsids in the cytoplasm, and these in turn migrate to the plasma membrane. The peplomer structural proteins (E1 and E2) are glycosylated in stepwise fashion as they progress from the endoplasmic reticulum through the Golgi complex to the plasma membrane. Virion assembly takes place via budding of nucleocapsids through the peplomer- and 6K protein-modified plasma membrane.

DISEASES CAUSED BY ALPHAVIRUSES

Alphaviruses cause encephalitis in horses and in man; some of them also cause serious systemic disease (Table 24-1).

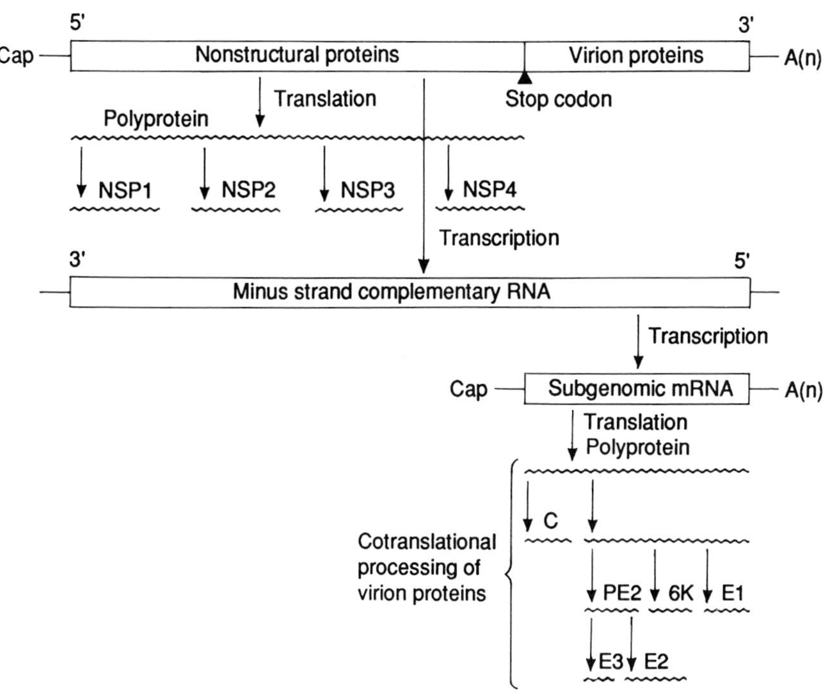

FIG. 24-2. *Diagram of* Alphavirus *genome and its transcription and translation. The plus strand virion RNA is capped and polyadenylated, and there are short nontranslated sequences at each terminus (single lines). The 5′ two-thirds codes for nonstructural proteins and the 3′ one-third for the structural proteins. The portion coding for the nonstructural proteins is translated into a polyprotein which is cleaved into the four nonstructural proteins. Two of these form the RNA polymerase, which transcribes a full-length minus sense copy from the virion RNA, from which in turn two plus sense RNA species, 49 S virion RNA (not shown) and 26 S subgenomic mRNA, are transcribed. The subgenomic 26 S mRNA, which is identical to the 3′ one-third of the virion RNA, is translated into a polyprotein that is then processed into the viral structural proteins E1, E2, E3, 6K, and C.*

Equine Encephalitis

Clinical Features. Infection of horses with Eastern, Western, or Venezuelan equine encephalitis viruses produces a range of clinical manifestations: infection may be subclinical or may present with only fever, anorexia, and depression. Progressive systemic disease often leading to death with only minor neurologic manifestations is most common in

Venezuelan equine encephalitis. Neurologic disease, marked by profound depression (typically with wide stance, hanging head, drooping ears, flaccid lips), is most severe in Eastern equine encephalitis. In horses, the case–fatality rate of Eastern equine encephalitis virus infection is about 90%, Western equine encephalitis virus infection about 20–40%, and Venezuelan equine encephalitis virus infection about 50–80%. Infection leads to long-lasting immunity in survivors.

Pathogenesis. Following the introduction of an alphavirus into an animal via the bite of an arthropod vector, viral replication occurs in cells near the entry site and/or in regional lymph nodes. The resulting primary viremia allows virus to invade specific extraneural tissues and organs, and it may lead to a high-titer secondary viremia, which permits the infection of arthropod vectors. The infection of extraneural organs and tissues, including reticuloendothelial tissues, striated muscle, connective tissue, cardiac muscle, pancreatic epithelium, brown fat, and lymphoid tissues, may directly cause the systemic febrile disease.

Routes of entry of viruses into the central nervous system are discussed in Chapter 6. Encephalitis caused by alphaviruses is probably due to hematogenous spread and subsequent entry of virus by one of several alternative routes: (1) passive diffusion of virus through the endothelium of capillaries in the central nervous system; (2) viral replication in vascular endothelial cells and release of progeny into the parenchyma of the central nervous system; (3) viral invasion of the cerebrospinal fluid with infection of the choroid plexus and ependyma; or (4) carriage of virus in inflammatory or lymphoid cells which may migrate into the parenchyma of the central nervous system. An alternative possibility, supported by recent immunofluorescence studies, is that virus may replicate extensively in the olfactory epithelium, leading to invasion of the brain parenchyma via axonal spread to the olfactory bulbs.

Once virus enters the parenchyma of the central nervous system it spreads throughout the central nervous system. Typical pathologic features include neuronal necrosis with neuronophagia and intense perivascular and interstitial mononuclear inflammatory infiltration. Virus produced in the central nervous system does not reenter the circulation; hence it is not involved in transmission.

Laboratory Diagnosis. Because of the sporadic occurrence and importance of identifying the first seasonal cases of Eastern and Western equine encephalitis, laboratory diagnosis is necessary. Isolation of virus in cell cultures or infant mice is attempted from equine blood and brain tissue, but because viral titers in blood often decline before encephalitis develops, negative results are not helpful. In the face of an outbreak, isolation of virus from mosquitoes collected systematically in the area as part of a comprehensive diagnostic–surveillance program is most helpful.

The diagnosis of Venezuelan equine encephalitis in its endemic foci in South America is important in predicting geographic extension but is often frustrated by the remote location of cases, delays in receiving initial reports, and difficulties in locating sick horses for specimen collection. In the midst of an epidemic, clinical diagnosis may suffice for some purposes, but laboratory confirmation is also needed, based on virus isolation from the blood of early febrile cases and the identification of viral isolates by serologic methods. Serology can also be used for retrospective diagnosis of cases, but because of confusion caused by prior unrecognized infection and immunization, this requires demonstration of IgM antibody or a titer change between paired serum samples.

Epidemiology. The life cycle of virtually every arbovirus is unique, involving variations in arthropod and vertebrate hosts and other ecologic factors. The life cycle of Eastern equine encephalitis virus is used here as an example: In North America this virus is maintained in freshwater swamp habitats by the mosquito *Culiseta melanura* (Fig. 24-3). This mosquito is responsible for amplification of the virus by transmission between wild birds. The infection has no apparent effect on most wild bird species, but there is a high viremia of several days duration in certain species, from which more mosquitoes are infected. It is not clear, however, which of several mosquito species transmit virus to clinically important hosts

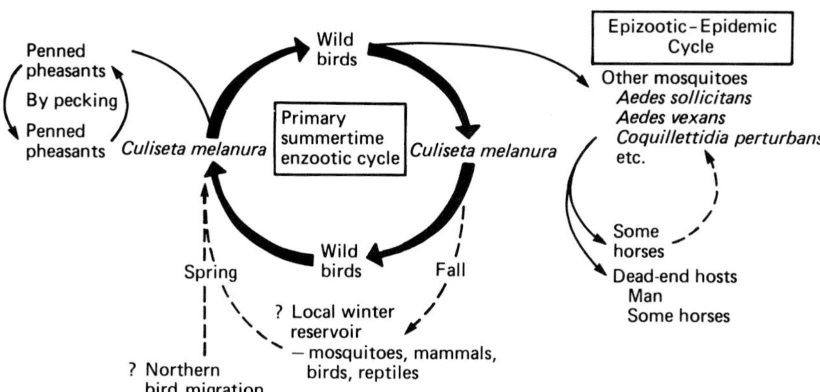

FIG. 24-3. *Features of the transmission cycle of Eastern equine encephalitis virus in the United States. Known parts of the cycle are depicted with solid lines, speculative parts with broken lines. The mode of overwintering is unknown. (Courtesy Dr. T. P. Monath.)*

(horses, humans) because *Culiseta melanura* feeds almost exclusively upon birds. In coastal New Jersey the salt-marsh mosquito *Aedes sollicitans* has been implicated because it feeds on horses as well as birds, but this virus–vector relationship does not operate in other areas. Likewise, the overwintering mechanism of Eastern equine encephalitis virus remains a mystery. Several lines of evidence exclude the possibility that virus is reintroduced from the tropics in Central and South America each year by migrating birds, and there have been repeated failures to demonstrate transovarial transmission of virus in *Culiseta melanura* mosquitoes. Other theories, such as persistent infection of reptiles and amphibians or birds, have not been confirmed.

The mosquito vector involved in epidemic transmission of virus between horses is also a mystery. Occasionally clusters of equine cases occur, suggesting the presence of an efficient vector, but this vector has not been clearly identified. During an outbreak of equine disease in Michigan in 1983, the mosquito *Coquillitidea perturbans* was implicated by virus isolation and by determination of equine and bird blood meal preference, but this mosquito does not inhabit coastal areas.

Highlands J virus, previously thought to be a strain of Western equine encephalitis virus inhabiting the eastern United States, is known to cause encephalitis in horses; this virus is believed to utilize the same vertebrate and arthropod hosts as Eastern equine encephalitis virus, sharing the same unanswered life cycle mysteries. In the western United States, Western equine encephalitis virus is transmitted between birds and to horses and humans by *Culex tarsalis* mosquitoes, which may reach great population densities when climatic conditions or irrigation practices are suitable. For example, in the 1930s equine epidemics of an enormous scale occurred in the western United States, and there were nearly 500,000 associated human cases just between 1937 and 1939.

Control. Immunization of horses with inactivated cell culture vaccines for Eastern, Western, and Venezuelan equine encephalitides, and with an attenuated live-virus vaccine (TC-83) for Venezuelan equine encephalitis, forms the basis of control measures. The inactivated bivalent or trivalent vaccines are given annually in the spring, in two doses 7–10 days apart. The attenuated live-virus Venezuelan equine encephalitis vaccine produces long-lasting immunity, but for practical reasons it also is given annually. In many areas, mosquito larviciding programs are in place; in short-term emergency situations, such as during an outbreak or when sentinel surveillance indicates the likelihood of an outbreak, such programs are supplemented by aerial spraying with ultra-low volume insecticides, such as malathion or synthetic pyrethrins. Prohibition of the movement of horses is also used in the face of outbreaks.

In an unprecedented event in the history of veterinary medicine, an epidemic of Venezuelan equine encephalitis, which had started in northern South America in 1969 and by 1971 had resulted in the deaths of hundreds of thousands of horses throughout Central America, Mexico, and Texas, was brought to a complete halt by an integrated international disease control program. This program included (1) a surveillance system to target control activities, (2) widespread use of the then experimental attenuated live-virus equine vaccine (TC-83), and (3) widespread use of ultra-low volume aerial spraying of insecticides. With the end of the 1971 vector season, the epidemic strain of the virus disappeared from Central and North America. This control program was extremely expensive and demanding of human resources; however, much was learned which should allow an earlier and perhaps less expensive response to any future reemergence of the virus from its still unknown interepidemic ecologic niche on northern South America.

Infections of Pheasants and Whooping Cranes. In eastern North America, many outbreaks of Eastern equine encephalitis virus infection have occurred in pheasants, resulting in a mortality rate in flocks of 5–75%. The virus is introduced into flocks via mosquitoes and is spread when healthy birds peck on sick, viremic birds. Mortality has also been observed in other domestic fowl, such as Pekin ducks. Prevention has been attempted by use of insecticides on premises and vaccine (equine vaccine) in valuable birds, but because of the sporadic occurrence of the disease, usually nothing is done systematically to prevent loss. The occurrence of Eastern equine encephalitis virus infection in whooping cranes, an endangered species, has been successfully dealt with by the use of vaccine.

Human Infections. The equine encephalitis viruses are zoonotic and cause significant human disease. Eastern equine encephalitis virus causes sporadic, severe, often fatal cases of neurologic disease, often with sequelae in survivors. The overall case–fatality rate among clinical cases is about 30%. Western equine encephalitis virus is usually less severe and has a case–fatality rate of about 3%. Venezuelan equine encephalitis virus causes a systemic febrile illness, and about 1% of those affected develop clinical encephalitis. In the absence of adequate medical care, case–fatality rates as high as 24–30% have been reported in young children with encephalitis. The risk posed for veterinarians by these viruses is small, but care should be taken to avoid penetration of the skin when working with sick horses or performing equine necropsies when there is suspicion of these infections.

FURTHER READING

Calisher, C. H., and Monath, T. P. (1988). *Togaviridae* and *Flaviviridae:* The alphaviruses and flaviviruses. *In* "Laboratory Diagnosis of Infectious Diseases, Principles and Practices" (E. H. Lennette, P. Halonen, and F. A. Murphy, eds.), Vol. 2, p. 414. Springer-Verlag, New York.

Karabatsos, N., ed. (1985). "International Catalogue of Arboviruses," 3rd Ed. American Society of Tropical Medicine and Hygiene, San Antonio, Texas.

Koblet, H. (1990). The "merry-go-round": Alphaviruses between vertebrate and invertebrate cells. *Adv. Virus. Res.* **38,** 343.

Monath, T. P., ed. (1988). "The Arboviruses: Epidemiology and Ecology." CRC Press, Boca Raton, Florida.

Peters, C. J., and Dalrymple, J. M. (1990). Alphaviruses. *In* "Fields Virology" (B. N. Fields, D. M. Knipe, R. M. Chanock, M. S. Hirsch, J. L. Melnick, T. P. Monath, and B. Roizman, eds.), 2nd Ed., p. 713. Raven, New York.

Schlesinger, S., and Schlesinger, M. J. (1990). Replication of togaviruses and flaviviruses. *In* "Fields Virology" (B. N. Fields, D. M. Knipe, R. M. Chanock, M. S. Hirsch, J. L. Melnick, T. P. Monath, and B. Roizman, eds.), 2nd Ed., p. 697. Raven, New York.

Scott, T. W., and Weaver, S. C. (1989). Eastern equine encephalitis virus: Epidemiology and evolution of mosquito transmission. *Adv. Virus Res.* **37,** 277.

CHAPTER 25

Flaviviridae

As noted in the preceding chapter, one of the two original major groups of arthropod-borne viruses, the Group B arboviruses, has become the family *Flaviviridae*, genus *Flavivirus* (the other, the Group A arboviruses, became the family *Togaviridae, genus Alphavirus*). Non-arthropod-borne viruses with physicochemical and molecular biological characteristics similar to those of the arthropod-borne flaviviruses have also been placed in the family *Flaviviridae*, in the genus *Pestivirus* (bovine virus diarrhea virus, hog cholera virus, border disease virus) and a genus for human hepatitis C virus for which the name *Hepatovirus* has been proposed.

There are over 80 recognized member viruses in the genus *Flavivirus;* of these about 30 cause disease in humans, varying from febrile illnesses, sometimes with rashes, to life-threatening hemorrhagic fevers, encephalitis, and hepatitis. About 10 of these viruses are of veterinary importance, the most important being louping ill, Wesselsbron, and Japanese encephalitis viruses (Table 25-1).

The pestiviruses occur worldwide as economically important animal pathogens. Experimentally, the viruses have an overlapping host spectrum: hog cholera virus can be transmitted to cattle, and bovine virus diarrhea virus can infect pigs, sheep, and goats as well as a wide range of ruminants. However, in nature these viruses are species-specific. Hog

TABLE 25-1

Flaviviruses That Cause Diseases in Domestic Animals

Genus/virus	Mode of transmission	Animal host	Disease	Geographic distribution
Flavivirus[a]				
Louping ill	Tick	Sheep	Encephalitis	Europe
Wesselsbron	Mosquito	Sheep	Generalized infection, abortion	Africa
Japanese encephalitis	Mosquito	Swine	Abortion, neonatal disease	Asia
Pestivirus				
Bovine virus diarrhea virus	Contact	Cattle	Mostly inapparent	Worldwide
	Congenital	Calves	Congenital disease: generalized, persistent infection, mucosal disease (acute, chronic)	
Border disease virus	Contact	Sheep	Mostly inapparent	Worldwide
	Congenital		Congenital disease (hairy shaker disease)	
Hog cholera virus	Contact	Swine	Respiratory disease	Worldwide, but eradicated in some countries
			Congenital disease, generalized infection	

[a] Many other members of the genus *Flavivirus* cause important human diseases, including yellow fever virus, the four dengue viruses, Japanese encephalitis virus, Murray Valley encephalitis virus, West Nile virus, St. Louis encephalitis virus, Russian spring–summer encephalitis virus, Omsk hemorrhagic fever virus, Central European tick-borne encephalitis virus, and Kyasanur Forest virus. Hepatitis C virus, an important cause of human hepatitis, is probably a member of the family *Flaviviridae*.

cholera was first recognized in Ohio in 1833, and there is speculation that it might have emerged as a new pathogen of swine at that time and place, perhaps via a novel host–range mutation of bovine virus diarrhea virus.

PROPERTIES OF FLAVIVIRUSES

Flavivirus virions are spherical, 40–50 nm in diameter, and consist of a tightly adherent lipid bilayer envelope covered with glycoprotein peplomers surrounding an icosahedral capsid (Fig. 25-1). Pestiviruses (Latin: *pestis* = plague) are similar in size and appearance (Table 25-2). Flaviviruses and pestiviruses are not very stable in the environment and are easily inactivated by heat and by disinfectants containing detergents or lipid solvents. However, the stability of hog cholera virus in meat products and offal for weeks or even months has contributed importantly to the spread of the virus and to its reintroduction into virus-free areas.

VIRAL REPLICATION

Flaviviruses replicate well and cause cytopathic changes in many kinds of cell cultures, for example, Vero (African green monkey kidney) cells, BHK-21 (baby hamster kidney) cells, and primary chick and duck embryo fibroblast cells; they also grow, but do not cause cytopathic changes, in

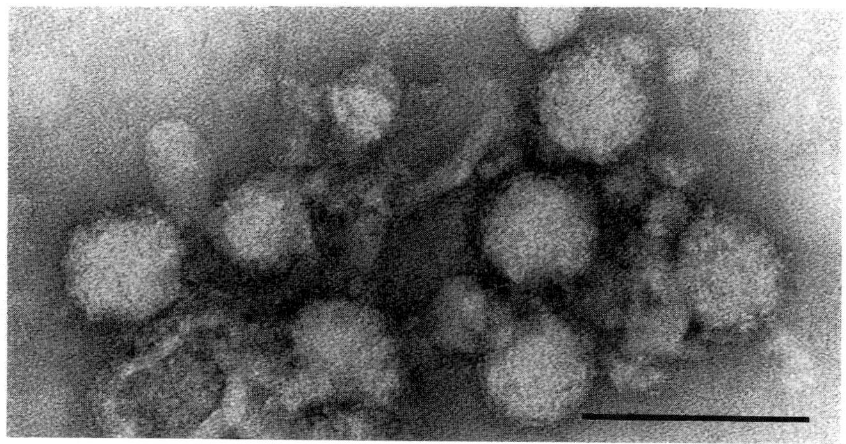

FIG. 25-1. Flaviviridae, *genus* Flavivirus. *Negatively stained virions of St. Louis encephalitis virus. Bar: 100 nm.*

TABLE 25-2
Properties of Flaviviruses

Genera: *Flavivirus:* mostly arthropod-borne viruses
Pestivirus: non-arthropod-borne, several veterinary pathogens
Unnamed proposed genus: human hepatitis C virus
Spherical virion, enveloped with peplomers, diameter 40–50 nm
Icosahedral capsid, diameter 25–30 nm
Linear plus sense ss RNA genome, 11–12 kb, 5′ end capped, but 3′ end usually not polyadenylated, infectious; genes for structural proteins located at 5′ end of genome
Flaviviruses: Structural proteins comprise one envelope glycoprotein, E (50K–60K), containing neutralizing epitopes, one nonglycosylated envelope protein, M (8K), and one nucleocapsid protein, C (14K)
Pestiviruses: Structural proteins comprise three envelope glycoproteins (gp48, gp25, and gp53), one of which (gp53) contains neutralizing epitopes, and one nucleocapsid protein, C (20K)
Cytoplasmic replication; polyproteins translated from genomic RNA are cotranslationally cleaved to yield several nonstructural proteins and three or four structural proteins; maturation occurs on intracytoplasmic membranes without evidence of budding

mosquito cells, such as commonly used cell lines derived from *Aedes albopictus*. Flaviviruses also infect and kill newborn mice; in fact, most of these viruses were first isolated in newborn mice. The pestiviruses replicate in primary and continuous cell cultures derived from the principal host species: bovine virus diarrhea virus in bovine embryonic fibroblast or kidney cells and hog cholera virus in porcine lymphoid or kidney cells. Pestiviruses isolated from naturally infected animals are often noncytopathic in cell culture but yield cytopathic variants during passage: however, cytopathic strains of bovine virus diarrhea virus may be isolated directly from cattle with mucosal disease.

The Genus *Flavivirus*. Flaviviruses enter cells via receptor-mediated endocytosis, and replication takes place in the cytoplasm. Replication is rather slow, and titers of virus produced in cultured cells and *in vivo* in experimental animal tissues (e.g., suckling mouse brain) are in some cases low and fleeting. These viruses only partially shut off protein and RNA synthesis of mammalian host cells and do not shut off these activities in mosquito cells at all. The flavivirus genome consists of a single molecule of plus sense ssRNA, 11 kb in size, which is infectious (Fig. 25-2). The genomic RNA is capped at its 5′ end; its 3′ end is usually not polyadenylated, but some flaviviruses have a short poly(A) tail. Replication involves the synthesis of complementary, minus strand molecules which in turn serve as template for the synthesis of more plus strand molecules which are encapsidated. During infection, plus strand synthe-

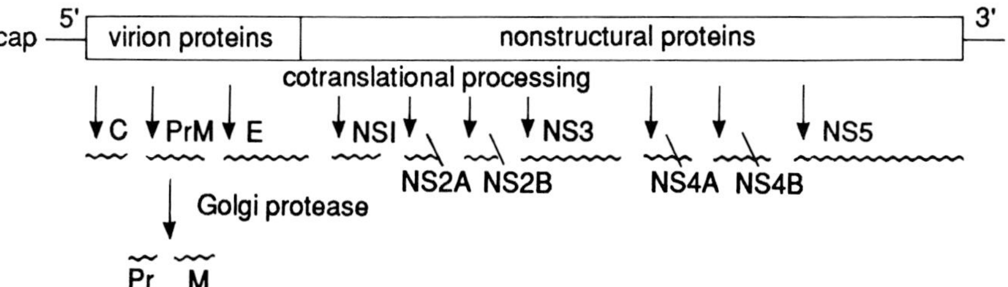

FIG. 25-2. *Structure and translation of the flavivirus genome. The regions of the genome encoding the structural and nonstructural proteins are shown at top; the RNA is capped at 5′ end but is not polyadenylated. There are short nontranslated sequences at each terminus (single lines). The coding region is cotranslationally cleaved by viral and cellular proteases to form the structural proteins C, M, and E and seven nonstructural proteins.*

sis is favored, suggesting complex regulatory mechanisms involving host cell constituents.

The incoming genomic RNA serves directly as messenger; it contains one large open reading frame of over 10 kb and is translated completely from its 5′ end to produce one large precursor polyprotein which is then cleaved and modified to produce individual viral proteins. About one-third of the length of the genomic RNA from the 5′ end encodes the three structural proteins (C, the nucleocapsid protein; PrM, a glycosylated precursor which is cleaved into M, the transmembrane protein; and E, the major peplomer glycoprotein), and the remaining two-thirds encodes a number of nonstructural proteins (NS1, which is involved in viral synthesis and virion assembly and release, NS2A, NS2B, NS3, and NS5, which comprise parts of the RNA polymerase, NS4A, and NS4B). Virion assembly occurs in vertebrate cells on membranes of the endoplasmic reticulum and in mosquito cells on the plasma membrane also, but preformed capsids and budding are not seen. Instead, fully formed virions appear within cisternae of the endoplasmic reticulum and are released via cell lysis.

The Genus *Pestivirus*. The pestivirus genome is a single molecule of single-stranded plus sense RNA, 12 kb in size, which is infectious. Complete genome sequencing of several of the viruses indicates that there is one large open reading frame spanning almost the entire molecule. Thus, pestivirus replication and transcription probably resemble the schemes employed by the flaviviruses. Hog cholera virus is composed of four structural proteins: a nucleocapsid protein (C) and three glycoproteins (gp48, gp25, and gp53). There are about eight nonstructural proteins associated with virus replication. Little information is available on virion assembly; mature virions appear on membranes of the endoplasmic reticulum of infected cells, but preformed capsids and budding are not seen. Virions are released via exocytosis and cell lysis.

DISEASES CAUSED BY MEMBERS OF THE GENUS *FLAVIVIRUS*

Of the more than 80 recognized flaviviruses, about 15 cause important diseases in man, including yellow fever virus, four serotypes of dengue virus, and several viruses causing encephalitis (e.g., St. Louis, Japanese, and Russian spring–summer encephalitis viruses). However, only three members of the genus *Flavivirus* cause diseases of veterinary importance, namely, louping ill, Wesselsbron, and Japanese encephalitis viruses (see Table 25-1). On the other hand, the pestiviruses are important veterinary pathogens, causing bovine virus diarrhea, hog cholera, and border disease of sheep.

Louping Ill

Louping ill is an infectious encephalomyelitis of sheep that occurs in the British Isles and the Iberian peninsula. Louping ill virus is a member of a serocomplex of 14 related tick-borne viruses that includes Russian spring–summer encephalitis virus, Central European encephalitis virus, Omsk hemorrhagic fever virus, and Powassan virus. The viral life cycle involves transmission between sheep by the tick *Ixodes ricinus,* with occasional involvement of horses, cattle, deer, and grouse. The disease occurs in spring and summer. Infected sheep develop a prolonged viremia and a biphasic febrile response, the second peak of which coincides with the development of nervous system dysfunction: cerebellar ataxia, tremors, hyperexcitability, and paralysis. The disease gains its name from the peculiar leaping gait of ataxic sheep. Few animals that develop neurologic signs survive, and most of those that do exhibit neurologic deficits as sequelae. Control of the disease involves immunization of lambs with an inactivated, concentrated virus vaccine produced in cell cultures, dipping all sheep with residually active acaricides, and environmental control of ticks. Louping ill virus is zoonotic, being transmitted to humans by ticks or occupationally by contact with infected sheep tissues. The human disease is biphasic; the first phase is influenza-like, and the second phase is a menigoencephalitic syndrome that resolves without sequelae in 4–10 days.

Wesselsbron Disease

Wesselsbron virus is the cause of an important disease of sheep found in many parts of sub-Saharan Africa. The clinical disease and its epidemiology resemble Rift Valley fever. The most susceptible species is the sheep, in which infection is marked by fever, depression, hepatitis with jaundice, and subcutaneous edema. Abortions are frequent, and mortality is high in pregnant ewes and newborn lambs. Cattle, horses, and swine are infected subclinically. The virus is transmitted in summer and fall by various *Aedes* mosquitoes; the disease is a particular problem in low-lying humid areas where mosquito density is greatest. Control involves immunization of lambs with an attenuated live-virus vaccine which is often combined with Rift Valley fever vaccine. Wesselsbron virus is zoonotic, causing in man a febrile disease with headache, myalgia, and arthralgia.

Japanese Encephalitis

Japanese encephalitis virus is a member of a serocomplex containing three other viruses; St. Louis encephalitis virus, Murray Valley encephalitis virus, and West Nile virus. Each represents an important human disease problem in a different part of the world, but only Japanese encephalitis causes significant disease in domestic animals. Japanese encephalitis virus is the most important mosquito-borne human pathogen in Japan, China, Korea, Thailand, and other countries of southeastern Asia, and it has recently extended its range westward into India, Nepal, and Sri Lanka and eastward into the Pacific islands of Saipan and the northern Marinas.

The mosquito *Culex tritaeniorynchus,* which breeds in freshwater habitats and irrigated rice fields, and feeds on birds, swine, and humans, is the most common vector. Swine are the most abundant species of domestic animal in many parts of Asia; they have a short life span and continuously provide generations of susceptible hosts. The mosquito–swine–mosquito transmission cycle serves as an efficient mode of virus amplification.

In several Asian countries, Japanese encephalitis infection in swine causes considerable losses because of a high abortion rate in sows and a high neonatal mortality rate. Adult swine, horses, cattle, and sheep usually do not manifest clinical disease, but they may serve as virus amplifiers. In Japan, control of the human and swine diseases has been very successful; a national program is based on immunization of children and swine with different inactivated virus vaccines produced in mice.

Attenuated live-virus vaccines for human and animal use are under development; these vaccines offer the possibility of lower costs and may be suitable for use in large areas of southeastern Asia.

DISEASES CAUSED BY MEMBERS OF THE GENUS *PESTIVIRUS*

Bovine Virus Diarrhea

Bovine virus diarrhea and mucosal disease are clinically dissimilar disease syndromes, and were originally described as separate diseases, but they are now known to have a common viral etiology. There is a consensus that the disease, overall, should be called bovine virus diarrhea, that the term mucosal disease should be reserved for the chronic disease syndrome associated with persistent infection, and that the causative agent should be called bovine virus diarrhea virus (family *Flaviviridae*, genus *Pestivirus*). The disease is an important cause of morbidity and mortality worldwide in dairy and beef cattle.

Clinical Features and Pathogenesis. The acute infection of fully susceptible cattle (bovine virus diarrhea) may occur at any age and is usually a trivial illness lasting a few days. The prerequisite for the development of mucosal disease is a persistent infection, acquired *in utero* and characterized by high mortality and low morbidity rates, specific immune tolerance, and immunosuppression. Mucosal disease is recognized clinically in a herd by fever, anorexia, watery diarrhea, and erosive stomatitis, sometimes complicated by lameness and pneumonia, usually in only a few animals.

The clinical and pathologic manifestations of infection in individual cattle vary with age and pregnancy status. Three situations are considered; postnatal infection of nonpregnant cattle, infection of pregnant cows, and persistently infected cattle.

Postnatal Infection of Nonpregnant Cattle. After an incubation period of 5 to 7 days there is fever and leukopenia, but otherwise the infection is usually subclinical. Some cattle in a susceptible herd may exhibit diarrhea, which may be explosive in character, some may have a nasal and ocular discharge and an erosive stomatitis, and in dairy cows there may be a considerable drop in milk yield. This disease is referred to as bovine virus diarrhea. Because of immunosuppression associated with infection, the disease in calves may be manifested by increased problems with opportunistic respiratory and intestinal infections. When infection of susceptible cows occurs via infected semen from a persistently infected bull, there is usually embryo death and transient repeated breeding problems, often not recognized in usual husbandry systems.

Infection of Pregnant Cows. As described above, infection of adult cattle is usually of little consequence, except that there is a high frequency of transplacental spread of virus to the fetus (Fig. 25-3). This may result in any one of several outcomes. Depending on the age (immunologic maturity) of the fetus and the strain of virus, infection may result in fetal death and mummification or abortion, congenital anomalies, the birth of a weak undersized calf ("weak calf syndrome"), or the birth of a clinically normal calf. Infection before 100 days of gestation usually causes destructive lesions and retardation in growth of organs and tissues, resulting in death or low birth weight. Between 100 and 150 days of gestation infection often affects organogenesis of the eye and central nervous system, seen as cerebellar hypoplasia, cavitation of the cerebrum, and retinal dysplasia. Surviving calves that have been infected *in utero* before the development of immunologic competence remain infected for life. They never mount an effective immune response to the virus; this is persistent tolerant infection. Such calves, which remain seronegative to all tests,

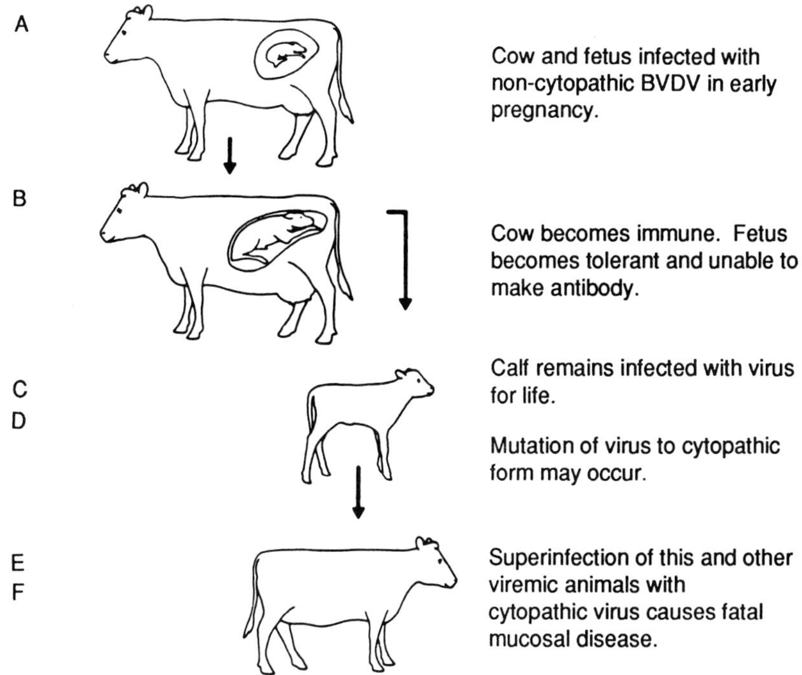

FIG. 25-3. *Pathogenesis of mucosal disease in cattle. (A)* In utero *infection. (B) Immune tolerance. (C) Persistent viremia. (D) Mutation. (E) Superinfection leading to (F) mucosal disease. [Modified from J. Brownlie,* Vet. Microbiol. **23,** *371 (1990).]*

shed large amounts of virus in all body secretions and excretions and are very efficient in transmitting virus to susceptible animals in the herd. These animals also have a high probability of developing clinical mucosal disease. Fetuses that are infected *in utero* after the development of immune competence (at about 125 days of gestation) and survive, whether manifesting pathologic damage or not, usually develop neutralizing antibody and eliminate the virus.

Persistently Infected Cattle. In susceptible herds to which the virus has been recently introduced, a high proportion of calves born in the next calving season may be persistently infected. Mortality in these calves often reaches 50% in the first year of life, owing to the various manifestations of mucosal disease. The full complexity of the pathogenesis of mucosal disease has only recently begun to emerge. Although the precise immunologic mechanisms are still obscure, it appears that mucosal disease only occurs when persistently infected calves are exposed to a second biotype of bovine virus diarrhea virus. There is chronic fever, anorexia, profuse watery diarrhea, nasal discharge, and erosive or ulcerative stomatitis, with dehydration and emaciation, and death usually follows in a few weeks to a few months. Pathologically, there are multiple erosions with little surrounding inflammation, occurring from the mouth to the abomasum. In the intestine, discoloration of mucosal folds due to mucosal hyperemia and hemorrhage may occur, giving a striped appearance to the luminal surface. Histologic examination confirms the epithelial necrosis seen visibly and also indicates a massive destruction of lymphoid tissue.

Epidemiology. The virus is transmitted easily from animal to animal and from herd to herd by indirect means through feed contaminated with urine or oral/nasal secretions, feces, or aborted fetuses and placentas. The virus is transmitted directly to susceptible hosts, rather poorly from acutely affected cattle and very efficiently from persistently infected animals. Some persistently infected females survive to breeding age and may give birth to persistently infected offspring, thereby perpetuating the transmission pattern. Where infection has been present in a herd for some time and the majority of cattle are immune, the introduction of susceptible animals, typically heifers, results in sporadic losses, often continuing over a period of years if husbandry practices remain unchanged. Where infection is absent in a herd, the introduction of a persistently infected animal is often followed by dramatic losses. Since the infection also occurs in sheep and goats, as well as swine, deer, bison, and other wild ruminants, these species may also be sources of virus for the initiation of infection in cattle herds.

Diagnosis. A presumptive diagnosis of bovine virus diarrhea can be made on the basis of clinical history, examination of herd reproduction records, clinical signs, and gross and microscopic lesions. When present, oral lesions are especially suggestive of the disease. Laboratory diagnosis is based on virus isolation in cell culture, viral antigen detection in tissues, detection of viral RNA in tissues by *in situ* hybridization or the polymerase chain reaction, and serology. Specimens for virus isolation include feces, nasal exudates, blood and tissues collected at necropsy, and aborted fetuses. Immunofluorescence may be used to detect viral antigen in cell cultures and tissues. Also, paired acute and convalescent sera may be examined serologically, usually by a neutralization test, but caution must be used in the interpretation of negative results because of the seronegativity of persistently infected, tolerant animals.

Prevention and Control. The economic importance of bovine virus diarrhea is clear, especially in feedlots and in dairy herds; there is no treatment, however, and control is far from satisfactory. The major objective of control measures is to prevent the further occurrence of persistently infected cattle in the herd. This requires the identification and elimination of such animals and the avoidance of further introductions by quarantine, a process that is economically burdensome but is increasingly practiced. An alternative is to allow the introduction into the herd of immune animals only.

In most areas, immunization is the only control strategy used, but vaccines have several drawbacks. Inactivated virus vaccines, containing detergent-"split" virus produced in cell cultures, have met with only limited success. Attenuated live-virus vaccines, also produced in cell cultures, are more widely used, but there is concern that they may induce mucosal disease. There is great need for a safe, efficacious vaccine.

Border Disease

A pestivirus very similar to that which causes bovine virus diarrhea in cattle (perhaps just a host-variant virus) also infects sheep worldwide. The disease in sheep was first described on farms in border areas between England and Wales; hence the ovine disease is known as border disease, and also, because of its clinical signs, "hairy shaker disease." Where the disease has been recognized, its incidence is low, and it is not a significant economic problem. In adult sheep the infection is always subclinical, but infection of pregnant ewes results in the delivery of dead or deformed lambs. Newborn lambs are characterized by excessive hairiness of the birth coat, poor growth rate, and neurologic disease evidenced by erratic gait and continuous trembling of limbs. These signs are due to defective myelination of nerve fibers in the central nervous system. In some lambs an immune response to the virus starts *in utero,* while in others there is infection of the lymphoreticuloendothelial system resulting in immunosuppression and permanent seronegativity. The latter animals, whether exhibiting clinical signs of infection or not, may be carriers and shed virus continuously in all body secretions. Control has been attempted in an investigational setting using either inactivated or attenuated live-virus bovine virus diarrhea vaccines, but in the practical setting no control measures are economically worthwhile.

Hog Cholera

Hog cholera, also called European swine fever, is economically the most important contagious disease of swine worldwide. Where the disease is present losses are severe, and where immunization and eradication programs are in place there are large costs for maintenance of public disease control agencies. The name "swine fever," used as a vernacular term in Europe ever since the disease was first recognized in the nineteenth century, was changed to "European swine fever" in the 1970s to distinguish it from African swine fever. However, in the rest of the world and in the scientific literature the disease is called hog cholera, and its etiologic agent is called hog cholera virus (family *Flaviviridae,* genus *Pestivirus*). The virus is serologically related to bovine virus diarrhea virus.

Clinical Features. In its classic form, hog cholera is an acute infection accompanied by high fever, depression, anorexia, and conjunctivitis. These signs appear after an incubation period of 2–4 days and are followed by vomiting, diarrhea and/or constipation, opportunistic bacterial pneumonia, and nervous system dysfunctions such as paresis, paralysis, lethargy, circling tremors, and occasionally convulsions. Light-skinned swine exhibit a diffuse hyperemia and purplish discoloration of the skin on the abdomen and ears. There is severe leukopenia, occurring early and reaching levels unmatched in any other disease of swine. In a susceptible herd, clinical signs are usually seen first in a few pigs, often when they huddle and pile up, as if they were cold. Then over the course of about 10 days nearly all animals in the herd become sick. Young swine may die peracutely without clinical signs; older pigs may die within 1 week of onset from the effects of the viral infection or later from the added effects of opportunistic bacterial superinfection. The herd mortality rate may reach 100%.

Less dramatic subacute or chronic forms of disease have been recognized in which there is a prolonged incubation period and an extended period of clinical disease with death occurring weeks or months afterward. These forms of disease have been associated with viruses of low or moderate virulence. When such viruses are inoculated into susceptible swine they may cause subclinical infection with the development of immunity or nonlethal disease with sequelae. Often there is a transient recovery phase of 2–6 weeks which is then followed by a relapse with emaciation, dermatitis, purpura, and death.

Pathology. In peracute cases there may be no gross changes noted at necropsy; in acute cases there are submucosal and subserosal petechial hemorrhages which are most evident under the capsule of the kidney, in intestinal serosa, and in the cortex of lymph nodes. There is congestion and infarction in the spleen, liver, bone marrow, and lungs. These lesions are caused by viral infection of the endothelium of small vessels.

In subacute or chronic cases there is necrotic ulceration of the mucosa of the large intestine and evidence of opportunistic bacterial pneumonia and enteritis. This syndrome is associated with a high incidence of abortion, fetal death and mummification, and congenital anomalies. Liveborn piglets, whether healthy or abnormal, are persistently infected, immunologically tolerant, and life-long virus shedders.

Laboratory Diagnosis. A positive diagnosis of hog cholera is difficult to make without laboratory confirmation. This is particularly true of the subacute and chronic forms of the disease. An acute highly infectious, hemorrhagic disease with a high mortality rate should always arouse suspicion of hog cholera, no matter what the herd vaccination status or the area or national eradication program status. When hog cholera is suspected, disease control authorities must be notified, and tissue specimens (pancreas, lymph nodes, tonsil, spleen, blood) must be submitted to an authorized laboratory. Immunofluorescence and ELISA techniques allow rapid detection of viral antigens in tissues (tonsils, lymph nodes, spleen, parotid gland). Virus isolation and neutralizing antibody assays are done in swine cell cultures, but because the virus is not cytopathic such assays are complex, employing immunofluorescence to detect the presence of virus. Where specific, sensitive, and rapid diagnostic techniques are not available, tissues are fixed in 10% formalin for histologic diagnosis.

Epidemiology. Hog cholera is transmitted by close contact with infected swine, or indirectly via excretions and secretions of infected swine. Shoes, clothing, and vehicles have been incriminated in the transportation of virus between herds. Carriage of virus between herds by inapparently infected carrier pigs is also important. Garbage and kitchen scrap feeding was at one time an important mode of virus transmission between herds; this was especially important because many pigs were slaughtered when they showed the first signs of disease, and pork scraps containing high titers of virus were then fed to swine. Garbage cooking regulations now in place in many countries have stopped this and several other similar disease problems.

Prevention, Control, and Eradication. For many years, control of hog cholera involved quarantine and immunization. The first immunization schemes employed virulent virus inoculated together with enough immune serum to prevent clinical disease. Later, in the 1960s, attenuated live-virus vaccines prepared in rabbits were widely used in many countries. In many developed countries this control strategy has given way in recent years to the strategy of eradication; by use of "test and slaughter," hog cholera has been eradicated from the United States, Canada, Australia, and many European countries.

Eradication programs have been extremely expensive, but very successful. Several factors have contributed to their success. (1) Hog cholera virus infection is restricted to domestic swine, and the virus has not been transmitted to any important extent by feral swine or wild pig species; therefore, reintroduction of virus from uncontrollable sources has not been a problem. (2) Effective herd immunity induced by vaccines reduced the incidence of infection to a level where the amount of slaughtering needed to complete the eradication of the virus was economically feasible. (3) The system for surveillance of the swine population was supported by good diagnostic techniques and reliable clinical diagnosis. (4) It was clear that persistent infections with chronic virus shedding, masked by the presence of vaccine viruses, would always lead to disease and economic losses whenever herd immunity waned. (5) There was good support from the swine industries in all countries where eradication programs were introduced.

FURTHER READING

Brownlie, J. (1990). Pathogenesis of mucosal disease and molecular aspects of bovine virus diarrhoea virus. *Vet. Microbiol.* **23,** 371.

Brownlie, J., and Clarke, M. C., eds. (1990). "Bovine Virus Diarrhea." *Off. Int. Epizoot. Sci. Tech. Rev.* **9.**

Callis, J. J., Dardiri, A. H., Ferris, D. H., Gay, G. J., Mason, J., and Wilder, F. W. (1982). "Illustrated Manual for the Recognition and Diagnosis of Certain Animal Diseases." United States Department of Agriculture, Washington, D.C.

Chambers, T. J., Hahn, C. S., Galler, R., and Rice, C. M. (1990). Flavivirus genome organization, expression and replication. *Annu. Rev. Microbiol.* **44,** 649.

Collett, M. S., Moennig, V., and Horzinek, M. C. (1989). Recent advances in pestivirus research. *J. Gen. Virol.* **70,** 253.

Duffel, S. J., and Harkness, J. W. (1985). Bovine virus diarrhea–mucosal disease infection in cattle. *Vet. Rec.* **117,** 240.

Harkness, J. W. (1985). Classical swine fever and its diagnosis: A current view. *Vet. Rec.* **116,** 288.

Moennig, V. (1990). Pestiviruses: A review. *Vet. Microbiol.* **23,** 35.

Moennig, V., and Plagemann, P. G. W. (1991). The pestiviruses. *Adv. Virus Res.* **41,** 53.

Monath, T. P., ed. (1988). "The Arboviruses: Epidemiology and Ecology." CRC Press, Boca Raton, Florida.

Monath, T. P. (1990). Flaviviruses. *In* "Fields Virology" (B. N. Fields, D. M. Knipe, R. M. Chanock, M. S. Hirsch, J. L. Melnick, T. P. Monath, and B. Roizman, eds.), 2nd Ed., p. 763. Raven, New York.

Rice, C. M., Lenches, E. M., Eddy, S. R., Shin, S. J., Sheets, R. L., and Strauss, J. H. (1985). Nucleotide sequence of yellow fever virus; implications for flavivirus gene expression and evolution. *Science* **229,** 726.

Terpstra, C. (1985). Border disease: A congenital infection of small ruminants. *Prog. Vet. Microbiol. Immunol.* **1,** 175.

CHAPTER 26

Coronaviridae

The coronaviruses are single-stranded RNA viruses that infect a wide range of mammalian and avian species; they are important causes of respiratory and enteric disease, encephalomyelitis, hepatitis, serositis, and vasculitis in domestic animals (Table 26-1). In humans, coronaviruses are one of several groups of viruses that cause the common cold.

Most coronaviruses show a pronounced tropism for epithelial cells of the respiratory and the intestinal tract. In general, coronaviruses cause mild or inapparent infections in adults but severe diseases in newborn or young animals.

PROPERTIES OF CORONAVIRUSES

The coronaviruses were so named because the unusually large club-shaped peplomers projecting from the envelope give the particle the appearance of a solar corona (Fig. 26-1). Though typically about 100 nm in diameter, the virion is pleomorphic and can range in size from 75 to 160 nm (Table 26-2). The helical ribonucleoprotein, difficult to discern in electron micrographs, is composed of the genomic RNA and the phosphorylated nucleocapsid protein N (50K–60K). The envelope includes a lipid bilayer derived from intracellular membranes of the host cell and three types of glycoproteins, M (E1, 23K–29K), HE (E3, 62K–65K,

TABLE 26-1

Antigenic Groups and Diseases Caused by Coronaviruses[a]

Antigenic group	Virus	Disease
I (mammalian)	Human coronavirus 229 E	Common cold
	Transmissible gastroenteritis virus of swine	Gastroenteritis
	Feline infectious peritonitis virus	Peritonitis, pneumonia, meningoencephalitis, panophthalmitis, wasting
	Canine coronavirus	Enteritis
II (mammalian)	Human coronavirus OC43	Common cold
	Mouse hepatitis virus (many serotypes)	Hepatitis, encephalomyelitis, enteritis
	Bovine coronavirus	Gastroenteritis
	Porcine hemagglutinating encephalomyelitis virus	Vomiting, wasting, and encephalomyelitis
III (avian)	Infectious bronchitis virus of chickens (at least eight serotypes)	Tracheobronchitis, nephritis
IV (avian)	Bluecomb disease virus of turkeys	Enteritis

[a] Coronaviruses have been associated with infections of the respiratory and enteric tracts and with central nervous system disease in monkeys, rats, rabbits, and other species.

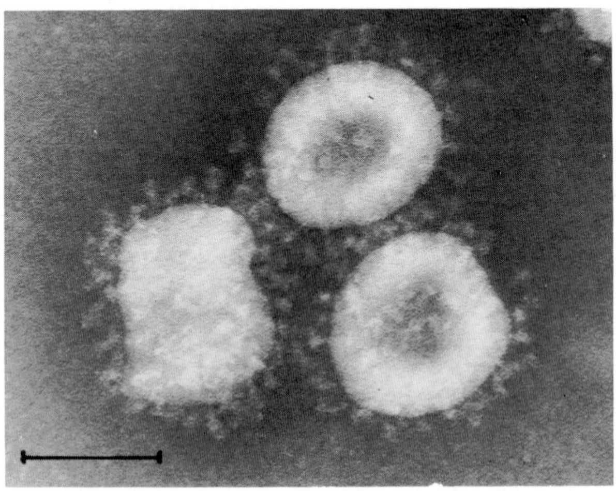

FIG. 26-1. Coronaviridae. *Negatively stained preparation of virions. Bar = 100 nm.*

TABLE 26-2
Properties of Coronaviruses

Pleomorphic spherical virion, 75–160 nm (average 100 nm) in diameter
Envelope with large, widely spaced, club-shaped peplomers
Tubular nucleocapsid with helical symmetry, 10–20 nm in diameter
Linear plus sense ssRNA genome, 27–33 kb, capped and polyadenylated, infectious
Three or four structural proteins: peplomer glycoprotein S (E2, 180K–220K), transmembrane glycoprotein M (E1, 23K–29K), nucleocapsid phosphoprotein N (50K–60K); some viruses have peplomers with hemagglutinin plus acetylesterase activity, HE (E3, 62K–65K)
Replicates in cytoplasm; full-length minus sense RNA strand is transcribed from the virion RNA, from which a nested set of mRNAs is produced with unique sequences at their 5′ ends, which are translated; maturation is by budding into endoplasmic reticulum and Golgi cisternae, with virions released by exocytosis

absent in some coronaviruses), and S (E2, 170K–220K). M (E1) is a transmembrane protein that performs the role filled by the matrix protein in other enveloped viruses. The large peplomers are composed of S (E2) which binds to cellular receptors, causes membrane fusion, and induces the production of neutralizing antibodies. HE (hemagglutinin esterase, E3), which is found particularly in the antigenic group II coronaviruses, binds to erythrocytes of some species and has receptor-destroying (acetylesterase) activity.

The genome consists of a single linear molecule of plus sense ssRNA, 27–33 kb (the largest of all RNA virus genomes), which is capped and polyadenylated. Viral RNA is infectious.

The family contains one genus, *Coronavirus,* which has been divided into four antigenic groups (Table 26-1). Viruses within each group show some antigenic cross-reactivity, and there may be a number of serotypes within one virus species. Animals immune to one serotype are susceptible to infection with different serotypes of the same coronavirus.

VIRAL REPLICATION

The whole of the replication cycle occurs in the cytoplasm and is relatively slow. Following adsorption, penetration, and uncoating, the input virion RNA molecule is translated directly, one of the products being an RNA polymerase which then transcribes a full-length minus sense RNA, from which is transcribed a 3′-coterminal "nested set" of subgenomic mRNAs (Fig. 26-2). The nested set comprises five to seven overlapping species of mRNAs which extend for different lengths from a common 3′ terminus. The genomic RNA and all mRNAs have an identical 5′

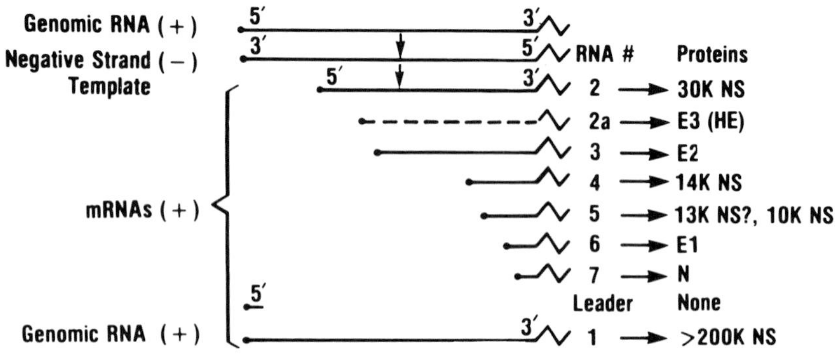

FIG. 26-2. *Coronavirus transcription and translation. After release of the (+) strand genomic RNA in the cytoplasm, an RNA-dependent RNA polymerase is synthesized, which transcribes a full-length (−) strand RNA, from which are synthesized (a) new genomic RNA, (b) an overlapping series of subgenomic mRNAs, and (c) leader RNA. The genomic RNA and mRNAs are capped and polyadenylated (zigzag line) and form a "nested set" with common 3′ ends and a common leader sequence on the 5′ end. Only the unique sequence of the mRNAs toward the 5′ end is translated, to produce several nonstructural proteins (NS) and four structural proteins: M (E1), transmembrane glycoprotein; S (E2), peplomer glycoprotein; N, nucleoprotein; and in some coronaviruses HE (E3), hemagglutinin–esterase glycoprotein. Maturation and assembly occur in the rough endoplasmic reticulum and the Golgi, and virions are released by exocytosis. [Modified from K. V. Holmes,* In *"Fields Virology" (B. N. Fields* et al., *eds.), 2nd Ed., p. 847. Raven, New York, 1990.]*

leader sequence of about 72 nucleotides. Accordingly, the nested set of mRNAs is formed by the unusual mechanism of joining two noncontiguous RNAs. The joining of the 5′ leader sequence to the remaining part of each mRNA occurs during transcription. Probably multiple copies of the 5′ leader RNA are synthesized independently, following which they bind to complementary intragenic initiation sites on the (−) strand RNA where they are linked to form each member of the nested set. Only the unique sequence toward the 5′ end, which is not shared with the next smallest mRNA in the nested set, is translated, each product therefore being a unique protein.

The translation of the structural proteins M, S, and N is associated with maturation of virions by budding into vesicles formed from the rough endoplasmic reticulum and Golgi apparatus. The S protein, which is glycosylated cotranslationally, and the M protein, which is glycosylated in the Golgi apparatus, become inserted in the vesicle membrane and serve as sites for association with nucleocapsid. Virions are released by exocytosis when the virion-filled vesicles fuse with the plasma membrane.

DISEASES CAUSED BY CORONAVIRUSES

Bovine Coronavirus Diarrhea

Rotaviruses are the major cause of viral diarrhea in the young calf, but coronaviruses are also important. Coronaviruses were first reported as a cause of diarrhea in calves in the United States in 1973, and since then the virus has been recognized worldwide. Initially, diagnosis was based on detection of virus by electron microscopy, but subsequently the addition of trypsin to the culture medium was shown to facilitate the isolation of virus in cell culture. For several virus strains a variety of bovine cell cultures and human HRT-18 cells are susceptible, and viral growth can be recognized by hemadsorption.

The pathogenesis is similar to that of rotavirus diarrhea (see Chapter 9). Disease is most commonly seen in calves at about 1 week of age, the time when antibody in the dam's milk has fallen to a low level. The diarrhea usually lasts for 4 or 5 days. The destruction of the absorptive cells of the intestinal epithelium of the small intestine, and to a lesser extent those of the large intestine, leads to the rapid loss of water and electrolytes. Glucose and lactate metabolism is affected; hypoglycemia, lactic acidosis, and hypervolemia can lead to acute shock, heart failure, and death, although coronavirus diarrhea is generally less severe than that caused by rotaviruses. Bovine coronaviruses may cause diarrhea in humans.

Available vaccines are not effective, because they do not appear to contain sufficient antigenic mass and cannot be given early enough. Alternatives to vaccinating calves are to immunize the dam to promote elevated antibody levels in the colostrum or to feed antibody directly to the calf in colostrum. Monoclonal (mouse) antibody to control *E. coli* infections in calves is available commercially; similar preparations could be used to control coronavirus and rotavirus diarrhea.

Winter dysentery is a sporadic acute disease of adult cattle that occurs in many countries throughout the world, and it is believed to be caused by coronaviruses. The clinical syndrome is characterized by bloody diarrhea accompanied by decreased milk production, depression, and anorexia.

Transmissible Gastroenteritis of Swine

Transmissible gastroenteritis of swine was first recognized in the United States in 1964, but it is now seen in Europe and several other countries. It usually occurs in the winter months and is characterized by an explosive outbreak of vomiting and profuse diarrhea. Transmissible gastoenteritis is one of the major causes of death in young piglets in the midwestern United States. Mortality is high, vaccines are of limited efficacy, and it appears to be difficult to prevent the introduction of the virus into herds.

Clinical Features. The disease is usually recognized at farrowing time. The incubation period is short, usually 1–3 days, and all litters within the farrowing house are commonly affected at the same time. The clinical signs in piglets are vomiting followed by a watery diarrhea and rapid loss of weight. The diarrhea is profuse, with an offensive odor, and often contains curds of undigested milk. Piglets infected when under 7 days of age generally die within 2 to 7 days of the onset of signs; piglets over 3 weeks of age usually live but may be unthrifty for several weeks. In growing, finishing, and adult swine the disease is commonly associated with inappetence and diarrhea of a few days' duration, and may even go unnoticed. Sows infected late in pregnancy may develop pyrexia, but they are otherwise normal and rarely abort.

Diagnosis. A presumptive diagnosis of transmissible gastroenteritis can be made from the sudden appearance of a rapidly spreading and often fatal disease of young piglets accompanied by vomiting and diarrhea. The clinical diagnosis can be confirmed by a range of techniques: demonstration of specific antigen by immunofluorescence, isolation of virus in a range of cell types, and demonstration of rising antibody titers in paired sera from sows with affected litters or from pigs that have recovered from the disease.

Epidemiology and Control. Transmissible gastroenteritis occurs most commonly in the winter months (in North America between November and April), but its source is unknown. Its presence becomes apparent only when large numbers of piglets are born at a time when weather conditions favor transmission. Control is difficult, although good management of the farrowing house can reduce the risk. The most widely used vaccination regimen involves vaccinating the sow with an attenuated vaccine 3 weeks before farrowing, thus providing piglets with high levels of protective antibody in the colostrum during the critical first few days of life.

A "respiratory variant" of transmissible gastroenteritis, with a definite tropism for the respiratory tract, is widespread in Europe. It usually causes inapparent infection but can interfere with the serodiagnosis, although certain glycoprotein-specific monoclonal antibodies can be used to differentiate between the two viruses.

Porcine Hemagglutinating Encephalomyelitis Virus

The disease caused by porcine hemagglutinating encephalomyelitis virus was first reported in Canadian swine in 1958, but it has now been recognized in the United States and Europe. Many of its clinical and pathologic features are indistinguishable from those of porcine polioencephalomyelitis, which is caused by a picornavirus. The disease, which is seen principally in piglets under 2 weeks of age, is characterized by anorexia, hyperesthesia, muscle tremors, paddling of the legs, vomiting, and depression, often leading to emaciation and death. In contrast to transmissible gastroenteritis, diarrhea is not commonly seen. Mortality in young piglets is high; older litters often survive, but the pigs remain permanently stunted. Serologic surveys indicate that the virus is present in many swine herds, in many of which clinical disease has not been recorded.

The virus infects pigs via the upper respiratory tract and pharynx, from where it spreads to the brain via peripheral nerves. In the central nervous system, virus is first detected in the sensory nuclei of the trigeminal and vagal nerves, with subsequent spread to the brain stem, cerebral hemispheres, and cerebellum. The infection of other organs does not contribute significantly to the pathogenesis of the disease.

A clinical diagnosis of porcine hemagglutinating virus encephalomyelitis can be confirmed by the isolation of virus in primary cultures of porcine cells, growth of the virus being detected by hemagglutination. Since no vaccines are available, good husbandry is essential for the prevention and control of the disease.

Porcine Epidemic Diarrhea

A porcine coronavirus (CV 777), causing acute diarrhea in swine of all ages, including suckling piglets, has been described in several countries of Western Europe. Antigenically this virus is not related to the established groups of coronaviruses. The main clinical sign in piglets is watery diarrhea, sometimes preceded by vomiting. In adult pigs the infection may remain subclinical, or the disease signs may be limited to depression, anorexia, and vomiting. The mortality rates in piglets is usually about 50% but may be as high as 90%. Older pigs recover after about 1 week. A diagnosis can be made either by direct demonstration of the virus in the feces of affected animals or by demonstration of antibodies. Vaccines are not available.

Canine Coronavirus Diarrhea

Canine coronavirus usually produces a mild gastroenteritis from which the dog recovers. Although originally described before the first occurrence of canine parvovirus enteritis in 1978 (see Chapter 16), it now commonly occurs in association with canine parvovirus infection, which causes a more severe and sometimes fatal diarrhea. The virus commonly infects pups and is probably worldwide in distribution. Epidemics of coronavirus enteritis have been recorded in wild dogs. The disease is similar in progression to that caused by enteric coronavirus infections in other species, such as calf coronavirus disease. Serologically, canine coronavirus is closely related to transmissible gastroenteritis virus of swine. Although canine coronavirus does not infect pigs, transmissible gastroenteritis virus produces a subclinical infection in dogs.

Since there are many causes of diarrhea in dogs, clinical suspicion of canine coronavirus infections should be confirmed by electron microscopy or virus isolation in primary canine cell culture. Detection of antibody to canine coronavirus in the sera of pups is of limited value, since it may be of maternal origin and unrelated to the cause of the diarrhea. An inactivated vaccine is available for the control of canine coronavirus infection.

Feline Infectious Peritonitis

Feline infectious peritonitis is an important disease that occurs in cats of all ages and in all parts of the world. Serologic surveys have established that the virus is widely distributed in wild and domestic cats. For example, in catteries it is not unusual to find over 90% of cats with antibody to the virus. However, the incidence of clinical disease is much lower (<10%), indicating that subclinical infections are common.

Feline infectious peritonitis often occurs in association with other diseases, particularly those likely to cause immunosuppression, such as feline leukemia, feline immunodeficiency, feline panleukopenia, and feline syncytial virus infections. A second feline coronavirus that causes diarrhea may be a variant of infectious peritonitis virus with a tropism for the epithelial cells of the intestine.

Clinical Features. The clinical onset of feline infectious peritonitis is insidious; the cat loses its appetite, is depressed, and may have a fever. Progressive debility follows, and in the classic ("wet") form of the disease, abdominal distention is seen as a result of the peritonitis, although only a proportion of clinically diseased cats develop peritonitis. Pleuritis causing dyspnea is observed in some cats, and there are reports of neurologic and ocular disease occurring in others. Affected cats die within 1 to 8 weeks. Peritoneal fluid from cats with peritonitis clots, contains high concentrations of protein, and is often flecked with fibrin.

Pathogenesis and Pathology. Most cats with feline infectious peritonitis have antibody to the virus, often to very high titer, and immune complexes have been demonstrated in the renal glomeruli. It is also clear from studies with experimental vaccines that preexisting antibody may complex with virus and, without destroying or neutralizing its infectivity, may enhance its uptake by macrophages via Fc-mediated endocytosis. These and other observations support the concept that at least some of the pathology of feline infectious peritonitis is immunologically mediated. Until recently, it had been assumed that antibody to coronaviruses in cats was due exclusively to prior exposure to feline infectious peritonitis virus. It is now realized that transmissible gastroenteritis virus of swine produces subclinical infection in cats and, further, that cats can be infected with feline enteric coronavirus, which has not yet been fully characterized and has been described only in California. The immune response of cats following infection with either of these viruses can "sensitize" them to feline infectious peritonitis virus and induce the rapid onset of clinical disease if infection occurs.

Diagnosis. Clinical diagnosis of the classic ("wet") form of feline infectious peritonitis is not difficult. When doubt exists, virus isolation from peritoneal exudates, blood, and homogenates of abdominal and thoracic organs can be attempted in feline embryonic lung cultures. Antibody can be detected in sera by several techniques, but in view of the frequency of inapparent infections with infectious peritonitis virus, interpretation of such data is difficult. A polyclonal hypergammaglobulinemia in the presence of appropriate clinical signs can aid diagnosis.

Epidemiology and Control. Under natural conditions, feline infectious peritonitis virus probably spreads by aerosol from clinically diseased cats. The roles of fecal excretion of the virus and subclinically infected cats in the epidemiology of the disease have not been critically examined. The fact that some cats with actively or passively acquired antibody develop a more rapidly progressive form of the disease than seronegative cats inoculated with the same dose of virus represents a major hurdle to the development of effective vaccines. Control of feline infectious peritonitis depends on segregation of infected cats. Any cat with antibody to the virus must be regarded as persistently infected.

Avian Infectious Bronchitis

Avian infectious bronchitis (gasping disease) was first shown to be of viral etiology in the United States in the 1930s. It has now been found in almost every country of the world and is one of the most important viral diseases of chickens. The causative virus, the first coronavirus to be recognized, is responsible for an acute respiratory disease which can produce very high mortality rates in young chicks.

Clinical Features. Outbreaks of infectious bronchitis are explosive, the virus spreading rapidly to involve the entire flock within a few days. Chicks between 1 and 4 weeks of age show the most severe disease, which is recognized initially by coughing, sneezing, nasal discharge, and respiratory distress (Fig. 26-3A). Mortality in young chicks is usually 25–30% but in some outbreaks can be as high as 75%. In older birds the disease often goes unnoticed, but in laying hens there is a marked drop

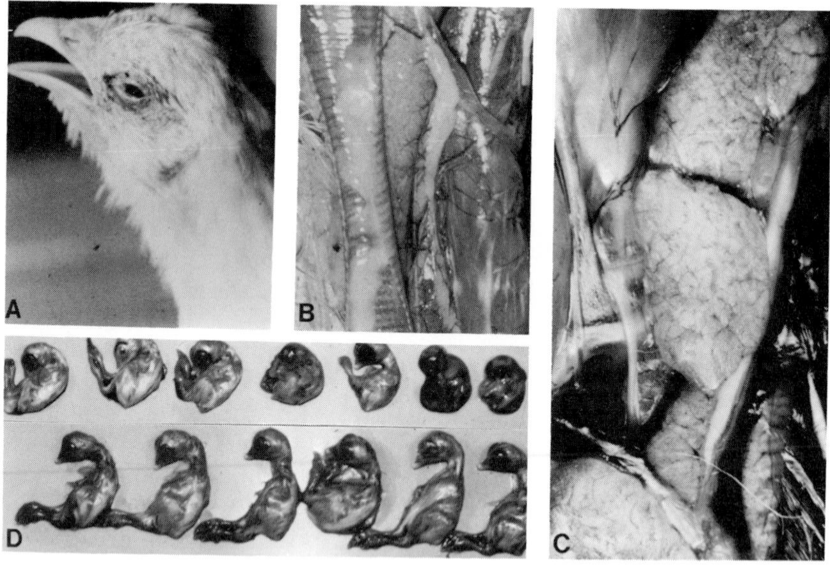

FIG. 26-3. *Avian infectious bronchitis. (A) One synonym for the disease is "gasping disease." (B) Thick mucopurulent exudate in the trachea. (C) Nephrosis. The kidney is pale and enlarged to about five times normal size. (D) Embryos from hen's eggs inoculated via the allantoic cavity with serial dilutions of virus when 9 days old, and examined 11 days later. Amounts of virus diminish in pairs from right to left in the top row and from left to right in the bottom row. (Courtesy R. J. H. Wells.)*

in egg production, with many soft-shelled and malformed eggs being laid.

Pathology and Pathogenesis. The course of the disease in young chicks is from 7 to 21 days depending on the severity of the disease. Necropsy of young chicks dying from infectious bronchitis shows sinusitis, catarrhal tracheitis (Fig. 26-3B), bronchitis, and congestion and edema of the lungs. Caseous plugs may be present in the bronchi. The primary target for viral replication is the trachea, but the virus also replicates in the lungs, ovaries, and lymphoid tissue. Infectious bronchitis virus can establish persistent infection in some chickens, which results in shedding of virus in the feces for several months after initial exposure to the virus. When virus persists in the presence of high levels of antibody, severe nephritis can occur, which possibly reflects an immune complex-mediated disease (Fig. 26-3C).

Laboratory Diagnosis. In contrast to several of the coronaviruses, infectious bronchitis virus can be easily isolated by the allantoic inoculation of 9- to 12-day-old embryonated eggs obtained from seronegative hens. The virus rarely causes embryonic death in the first passage, but egg-adapted strains kill the embryo within 48 hours. Infected embryos are to a variable degree stunted or curled tightly (Fig. 26-3D). A range of cell and organ cultures can also be used for virus isolation. At least eight serotypes of infectious bronchitis virus exist and fall into two major groups; virus isolates of widely differing pathogenicity occur within each antigenic group.

Epidemiology and Control. Infectious bronchitis virus spreads between birds by aerosol and by ingestion of food contaminated with feces. Outbreaks of infectious bronchitis have declined in recent years owing to the wide use of vaccines; however, it may occur even in vaccinated flocks following the introduction of infected replacement chicks from another farm. To minimize this risk, most poultry farms purchase only 1-day-old chicks and rear them in isolation.

Attenuated vaccines, administered in the drinking water or as aerosols, are widely used to protect chicks and are usually given between 7 and 10 days, and again at 4 weeks. Vaccination earlier than 7 days may be unsuccessful because most chicks have passive immunity up to this age. The presence of several serotypes would at first appear to make vaccine formulation difficult; however, no correlation between serotypic variation and resistance to infection has been shown. Local immunity in the respiratory system is critical for protection and can be generated by heterotypic vaccine strains. Control of infectious bronchitis is difficult because of the presence of persistently infected chickens in many flocks; vaccination programs should be tailored to the type of poultry operation and the strains of virus prevalent in the area.

Bluecomb Disease

Bluecomb was first recognized in domestic turkeys in the United States in 1951 and has now been recorded in other countries. The disease affects turkeys of all ages but is most severe in 1- to 6-week-old poults. The onset is characterized by loss of appetite, constant chirping, diarrhea, weight loss, and depression. The skin of the head and neck may become cyanosed. The lesions in the digestive tract are very similar to those seen in coronavirus infections in mammals, and younger poults may die. Some turkeys may shed virus in their feces for several months.

Only one serotype of bluecomb virus is recognized; the virus can be isolated in embryonated eggs of turkeys and chickens or in turkey embryo intestinal organ culture. An inactivated vaccine is available, but it is generally considered to be ineffective.

Mouse Hepatitis

Mouse hepatitis virus, first isolated in 1949 and later classified as a coronavirus, is a highly contagious and common virus of laboratory mice, which is endemic in many mouse colonies throughout the world. It is of major concern to mouse breeders and has served as a model system for coronavirus research. Though often subclinical, it can cause severe disease, and even subclinical mouse coronavirus infection may greatly distort experimental results.

Many strains of mouse hepatitis virus have been isolated. All share cross-reacting antigens, but each possesses strain-specific antigenicity, with considerable overlap. However, serologic or genetic relatedness is not a reliable predictor of biological behavior. Infection with different serotypes of the virus can cause hepatitis, encephalomyelitis, enteritis, and nephritis, the type and severity of the disease being dependent on the strain of virus and the age and strain of the mouse.

Except in the athymic nude mouse, infections appear to be subclinical or acute and self-limiting, without viral persistence or a carrier state. Maintenance of infection in a mouse population therefore requires continual exposure of new, susceptible mice, either by introduction from outside or by breeding. If neonatal mice are brought into endemically infected mouse rooms, they suffer high mortality, but if introduced as weanlings they usually sustain subclinical infections, which maintain the endemic situation.

The various serotypes of mouse coronavirus can be grown in several lines of mouse cells, the characteristic cytopathic effect being the formation of syncytia.

Since mouse hepatitis virus causes acute, nonpersistent infections, control is achieved by breaking the infectious cycle by cessation of breeding or quarantine without the introduction of new mice. However, it is very difficult to prevent the reentry of virus into facilities receiving mice from outside sources. Because of the multiplicity of serotypes, vaccination is impractical.

FURTHER READING

Andries, K. (1990). Hemagglutinating encephalomyelitis virus. *In* "Virus Infections of Porcines" (M. B. Pensaert, ed.), p. 177. Elsevier, Amsterdam.

Appel, M. (1987). Canine coronavirus. *In* "Virus Infections of Carnivores" (M. Appel, ed.), p. 115. Elsevier, Amsterdam.

Bohl, E. H., and Pensaert, M. B. (1989). Transmissible gastroenteritis virus (classical enteric variant) and transmissible gastroenteritis variant (respiratory variant). *In* "Virus Infections of Porcines" (M. B. Pensaert, ed.), p. 139. Elsevier, Amsterdam.

Holmes, K. V. (1990). Coronaviridae and their replication. *In* "Fields Virology" (B. N. Fields, D. M. Knipe, R. M. Chanock, M. S. Hirsch, J. L. Melnick, T. P. Monath, and B. Roizman, eds.), 2nd Ed., p. 841. Raven, New York.

Mebus, C. A. (1990). Neonatal calf diarrhea virus. *In* "Virus Infections of Ruminants" (Z. Dinter and B. Morein, eds.), p. 295. Elsevier, Amsterdam.

Pensaert, M. B. (1989). Porcine epidemic diarrhea virus. *In* "Virus Infections of Porcines" (M. B. Pensaert, ed.), p. 167. Elsevier, Amsterdam.

Saif, L. J., Brock, K. V., Redman, D. R., and Kohler, E. M. (1991). Winter dysentery in dairy herds: Electron microscopic and serological evidence for an association with coronavirus infection. *Vet. Rec.* **128,** 447.

Sparks, A. H., Gruffydd, T. J., and Harbour, D. A. (1991). Feline infectious bronchitis: A review of clinico-pathological changes in 65 cases, and a critical assessment of their diagnostic value. *Vet. Rec.* **129,** 209.

CHAPTER 27

Paramyxoviridae

Paramyxoviruses and orthomyxoviruses were originally grouped together as the "myxoviruses" because of the morphologic similarity of the virions and the fact that the prototype viruses, Newcastle disease virus and influenza virus, each carry a hemagglutinin and a neuraminidase. However, it was later realized that the viruses of each group differ in such basic properties as genome structure and mode of replication; hence they were separated into two families.

The family *Paramyxoviridae* contains three genera, *Paramyxovirus, Morbillivirus,* and *Pneumovirus,* and includes some of the most important pathogens of domestic animals and humans (Table 27-1). Of the diseases caused by the member viruses, the most significant economic losses are caused by Newcastle disease virus, rinderpest virus, and bovine respiratory syncytial virus.

PROPERTIES OF PARAMYXOVIRUSES

The virions are pleomorphic, usually roughly spherical or filamentous, with a diameter of 150 nm or more (Table 27-2). They consist of a nucleocapsid of helical symmetry, 13–18 nm in diameter, which is surrounded

TABLE 27-1

Diseases of Domestic Animals Caused by Paramyxoviruses

Virus	Animal species affected	Disease
Paramyxovirus		
Parainfluenzavirus 1 (Sendai)	Mouse, rat, rabbit	Severe respiratory disease in laboratory rats and mice
Parainfluenzavirus 2 (SV5)	Dog	Respiratory disease
Parainfluenzavirus 3	Cattle, sheep, other mammals	Respiratory disease in cattle and sheep
Paramyxovirus	Pigs	Encephalitis, reproductive failure, corneal opacities
Newcastle disease virus (avian paramyxovirus 1)	Domestic and wild fowl	Severe generalized disease with central nervous system signs
Morbillivirus		
Rinderpest virus	Cattle, wild ruminants	Severe generalized disease
Peste des petits ruminants virus	Sheep, goats	Like rinderpest
Canine distemper virus	Canidae, Procynoidae, Mustelidae	Severe generalized disease; central nervous system signs
Phocine distemper virus	Different seal species	Like canine distemper
Pneumovirus		
Bovine respiratory syncytial virus	Cattle, sheep	Respiratory disease
Turkey rhinotracheitis virus	Turkey, chicken	Severe respiratory disease in turkeys, swollen head syndrome of chickens

TABLE 27-2

Properties of Members of the Family Paramyxoviridae

Three genera: *Paramyxovirus, Morbillivirus, Pneumovirus*

Pleomorphic virion, some roughly spherical, 150 nm or more in diameter, filamentous forms common

Envelope derived from the cell membrane, incorporating 2 viral glycoproteins and 1 or 2 nonglycosylated proteins

Helical nucleocapsid, 18 nm diameter (*Paramyxovirus, Morbillivirus*) or 13 nm diameter (*Pneumovirus*)

Linear, minus sense ssRNA genome, 15 to 16 kb, with 7–8 open reading frames encoding 10–12 polypeptides, including NP (or N), P, M, F, L, and HN (or H or G), which are common to all genera

Cytoplasmic replication, with budding from the plasma membrane

Syncytium formation, intracytoplasmic and intranuclear (morbillivirus) inclusion bodies by an envelope derived from the cell surface membrane. The envelope possesses two types of glycoproteins, 8–12 nm in length, exposed as projections at the viral surface, and one or two unglycosylated proteins. The envelope is very fragile, rendering the virion vulnerable to destruction by storage, freezing, or even preparation for electron microscopy, so that it may rupture and reveal the nucleocapsid, which occurs as a single helix about 1 μm long (Fig. 27-1).

The genome is of minus sense ssRNA and 15–16 kb in length, containing a set of 6 or more genes, covalently linked in tandems (Fig. 27-2). It

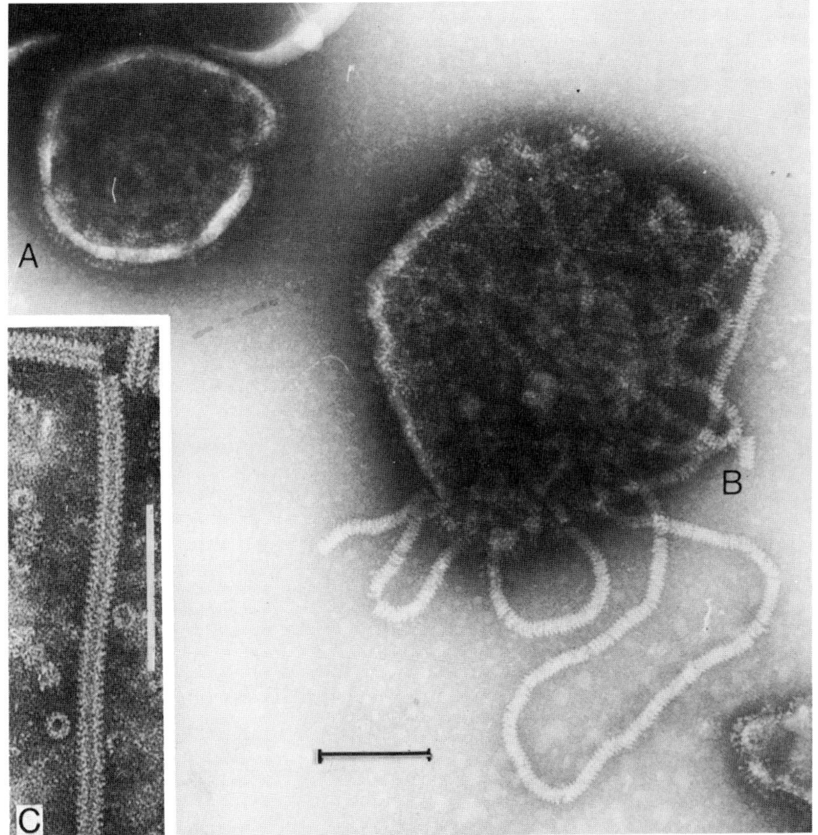

FIG. 27-1. *Negatively stained virions of a paramyxovirus. (A) Intact virion, with peplomers visible at lower edge. (B) Partially disrupted virion, showing nucleocapsid. (C) Enlargement of a portion of the nucleocapsid, in longitudinal and cross section. Bars: 100 nm. (Courtesy Dr. A. J. Gibbs.)*

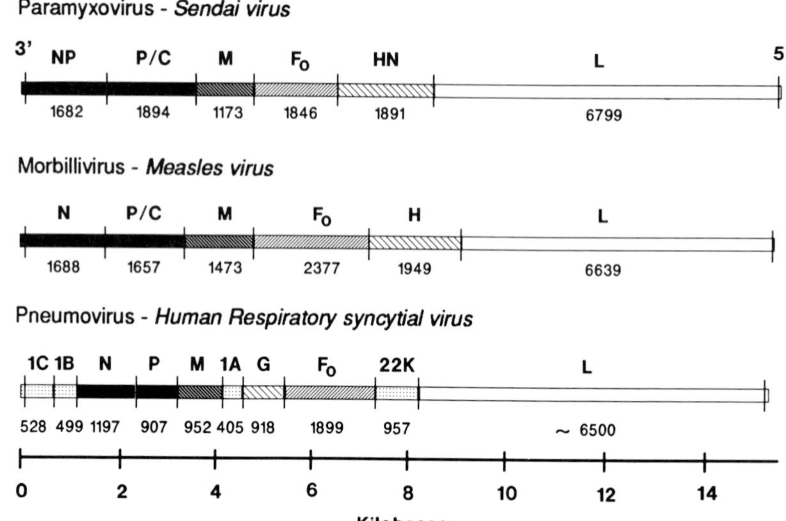

FIG. 27-2. *Genetic map of a typical member of each paramyxovirus genus. Homologous genes are indicated by the style of shading, and the number beneath each gene is its length in bases. [From D. W. Kingsbury,* In *"Fields Virology" (B. N. Fields,* et al., *eds.), 2nd Ed., p. 935. Raven, New York, 1990.]*

encodes 7–10 structural and 1 or more nonstructural proteins. The gene coding for the nucleoprotein (NP/N) is located at the 3′ terminus or near the 3′ end (*Pneumovirus*) of the genome. Auxiliary nucleocapsid proteins, such as a phosphoprotein (P) and a large putative polymerase protein (L) needed for replication and transcription, are associated with the nucleoprotein. They possess various enzyme activities: transcriptase, polyadenylate transferase, and methyltransferase. In the initial step of replication HN (or H or G) protein-mediated attachment is coordinated with F protein-mediated fusion of the virion envelope and host cell membrane. The glycoproteins are HN (hemagglutinin–neuraminidase), H or G (mediates viral attachment), and F (fusion) (Table 27-3). The F protein mediates fusion of the viral envelope with the cellular membrane and also assists in viral attachment, but in addition it mediates cell–cell fusion and allows infection to spread without virus release even in the presence of antibodies. There is no detectable neuraminidase activity in morbilliviruses and no detectable hemagglutinin or neuraminidase activity in pneumoviruses, but in each case virion attachment is carried out by analogous proteins.

To acquire biological activity the F protein must be cleaved by a cellular

TABLE 27-3
Functions and Terminology of Virion Proteins in Paramyxoviruses

Function	Genus		
	Paramyxovirus	*Morbillivirus*	*Pneumovirus*
Attachment protein: hemagglutinin, induction of productive immunity	HN	H	G[a]
Neuraminidase: virion release, destruction of mucin inhibitors	HN	None	None
Fusion protein: cell fusion, virus penetration, cell–cell spread, contribution to induction of protective immunity	F	F	F
Nucleoprotein: protection of genome RNA	NP	N	N
Transcriptase: RNA genome transcription	L and P	L and P	L and P
Matrix protein: virion core stability	M	M	M
Other: functions unknown	SH	—	SH, 22K

[a] No hemagglutinating activity.

protease into two disulfide-linked polypeptides, F1 and F2; when a host cell does not contain appropriate proteases, the virus formed is not infectious. Since the F protein is essential for viral penetration and for direct intracellular spread by cell-to-cell fusion, it plays a key role in the pathogenesis of paramyxovirus infections, including persistent infections. Paramyxovirus vaccines, to be maximally effective, must elicit antibodies against the F protein as well as against the attachment protein.

In contrast to the antigenic variability of the envelope glycoproteins of the orthomyxoviruses (see Chapters 4 and 29), the peplomers of paramyxoviruses are antigenically remarkably stable, geographically and over time.

VIRAL REPLICATION

Several different cell types are used to grow different paramyxoviruses. Cell cultures derived from homologous species are usually used for morbilliviruses and pneumoviruses; however, these viruses are not readily cultivated, and adaptation by passage is usually necessary. Viral replication in cell cultures is usually lytic, but carrier cultures readily arise in many virus–host cell systems. Syncytium formation in cell cultures and *in vivo* is a characteristic feature of the cytopathology, as is the formation of acidophilic inclusions in the cytoplasm. Even though their replication is entirely cytoplasmic, morbilliviruses also produce acidophilic intranuclear inclusions. Hemadsorption is readily demonstrated with parainfluenzaviruses and some morbilliviruses, but not with pneumoviruses.

The minus sense of ssRNA genome of paramyxoviruses is transcribed by a virion-associated RNA-dependent RNA polymerase (transcriptase) into six or ten discrete unprocessed plus sense mRNAs by sequential interrupted synthesis from a single promoter. Full-length plus sense RNA is also synthesized and serves as template for the replication of minus sense viral genomic RNA. Control of these processes is mainly at the level of transcription. Virion maturation involves (1) the incorporation of viral glycoproteins into the host cell plasma membrane, (2) the association of matrix protein (M) and other nonglycosylated proteins with the altered host cell membrane, (3) the alignment of nucleocapsid (RNA plus NP plus L plus P) beneath the M protein, and (4) the formation and release via budding of mature virions from the sites of modified plasma membrane.

DISEASES CAUSED BY MEMBERS OF THE GENUS *PARAMYXOVIRUS*

Mammalian parainfluenza viruses 1, 2, and 3 and Newcastle disease virus (avian paramyxovirus 1) cause important infections of domestic animals (see Table 27-1).

Mammalian Parainfluenzaviruses

Mammalian parainfluenzaviruses occur worldwide in many species of mammals including humans. They are associated with local infections of the respiratory tract, which are usually subclinical unless associated with secondary bacterial infections. The three serotypes that affect domestic animals have a wide host range.

Parainfluenzavirus 1 Infections. Parainfluenzavirus 1, also known as Sendai virus, produces natural infections in humans, monkeys, guinea pigs, rabbits, rats, and mice. Whereas in most species infection remains subclinical, severe respiratory disease with high mortality can occur in breeding colonies of laboratory mice and rats. It is a significant disease in laboratory rodents used for biomedical research, and it is difficult to control or eliminate because cross-infection occurs between different rodent species.

Parainfluenzavirus 2 Infections. Parainfluenza virus 2, also known as simian virus 5 (SV5), infects humans, monkeys, and dogs, and probably cattle, sheep, swine, and cats. A virus antigenically related to SV5 has been isolated from chickens. Parainfluenzavirus 2 infections play a role in the kennel cough syndrome of dogs. Infections of dogs with parainfluenzavirus 2 alone are common and either cause mild clinical signs or remain subclinical. More serious disease develops when additional microbial or viral agents, poor hygiene, or stress complicate parainfluenzavirus 2 infections, which is characterized by the sudden onset of serous nasal secretion, cough, and fever, lasting for 3 to 14 days. In severe cases (mostly in malnourished or young dogs) there are also conjunctivitis, tonsillitis, anorexia, and lethargy. Since a number of other infections can induce similar clinical signs, definitive diagnosis depends on virus isolation from nasal or throat swabs. Vaccines are available for the control of parainfluenza 2 infections in dogs.

Parainfluenzavirus 3 Infections. Antibodies to parainfluenzavirus 3 have been demonstrated in humans, cattle, sheep, water buffaloes, deer, pigs, dogs, cats, monkeys, guinea pigs, and rats. The seroprevalence in cattle varies between 60% and 90%. Parainfluenzavirus 3 causes clinical disease in cattle and sheep independently of its role of predisposing animals to secondary bacterial infections of the respiratory tract. In calves and lambs infection is marked by fever, lacrimation, serous nasal discharge, depression, dyspnea, and coughing. Many animals exhibit minimal clinical signs, but some may develop interstitial pneumonia, in which inflammatory consolidation is usually present only in the anterior lobes of the lungs. Because of the variety of agents that can cause this kind of clinical and pathologic manifestations, etiologic diagnosis can only be achieved by virus isolation from nasal swabs or postmortem material. Virus isolation is done in cell cultures of bovine origin, and virus is identified serologically (by immunofluorescence, hemagglutination inhibition, or virus neutralization).

The uncomplicated respiratory infection caused by parainfluenzavirus 3 runs a clinical course of 3 to 4 days, with complete recovery the rule. However, the true importance of the infection in cattle and sheep derives from its role in endemic pneumonia, which in cattle in many countries is called "shipping fever." In this case the viral respiratory infection alone or in concert with other viral infections (adenovirus, infectious bovine rhinotracheitis, bovine respiratory syncytial virus infections) predisposes to secondary bacterial invasion, especially by *Pasteurella haemolytica*. Poor hygiene, crowding, transport, harsh climatic conditions, and other causes of stress exacerbate parainfluenza 3 infections and associated bacterial infections (see Chapter 9).

Antibiotics, which help control secondary bacterial infections, and immunization are used to control shipping fever. Attenuated live-virus and inactivated parainfluenzavirus 3 vaccines are available, usually given combined with other antigens, for example, infectious bovine rhinotracheitis virus, bovine adenovirus, and bovine virus diarrhea virus vaccines.

A paramyxovirus has been isolated from numerous outbreaks of a disease in young pigs in Mexico that is characterized by encephalomyelitis, reproductive failure, and corneal opacity, which may be the only clinical sign in older pigs, hence the common name for the disease, "blue eye." There is no serologic cross-reactivity with any other paramyxovirus, but analysis of the genome suggests that it is most closely related to mumps virus.

Newcastle Disease

Nine serotypes of avian paramyxoviruses are recognized, but only avian paramyxovirus 1, Newcastle disease virus, is associated with a clearly defined disease. Newcastle is a highly contagious infection of many avian species. It was first observed in Java in 1926, and in autumn of that year the virus spread to England, where it was first recognized in Newcastle, hence the name. Later observed in many parts of the world, Newcastle disease has caused devastating epidemics in poultry in many countries. The disease represents a serious threat to chicken and turkey industries in countries free of virulent strains of the virus, and where virulent strains are endemic Newcastle disease is a major cause of economic loss. Acute disease due to Newcastle disease virus has also been observed in pigeons, mainly in Europe.

Newcastle disease outbreaks vary in clinical severity and transmissibility. In some outbreaks, especially in adult chickens, clinical signs may be minimal. The virus causing this form of disease is termed lentogenic. In other outbreaks the disease may have a mortality rate of up to 25%, often higher in young birds; this virus is termed mesogenic. In yet other outbreaks there is a very high mortality rate, sometimes approaching 100%, caused by velogenic viruses. Cleavability of the F protein is the main factor influencing virulence.

The acute clinical disease is associated with respiratory distress, circulatory disturbances, and severe diarrhea. Central nervous system signs dominate in chronic cases. Economic consequences arise from the high mortality associated with the infection by velogenic viruses, as well as from the reduced weight gains and production losses in survivors of any form of the disease. In most countries with developed poultry industries the lentogenic form is most common and the velogenic form considered exotic. Although Newcastle disease lost some of its importance during the 1980s owing to the success of strict control measures, it remains a threatening disease in industrialized countries and the cause of substantial losses in developing countries.

Properties of Newcastle Disease Virus. There is only one serotype, but minor antigenic variations have been found using monoclonal antibodies. Individual virus strains vary considerably in virulence. Besides mean death time in embryonated fowl eggs, intracerebral pathogenicity index in 1-day-old chicks and plaque formation in chick embryo cells in the presence or absence of trypsin, which relates to whether or not posttranslational cleavage of the F polypeptide precursor occurs in the host system, can be used as markers for virulence.

Compared with most paramyxoviruses, Newcastle disease virus is relatively heat-stable, a feature of great importance in relation to its epidemiology and control. It remains infectious in bone marrow and muscles of slaughtered chickens for at least 6 months at −20°C and for up to 4 months at refrigerator temperature. Infectious virus may survive for months at room temperature in eggs laid by infected hens and for over 1 year at 4°C. Similar survival times have been observed for virus on feathers, and virus may remain infectious for long periods in contaminated premises. Quaternary ammonium compounds, 1–2% Lysol, 0.1% cresol, and 2% formalin are used for disinfection.

Clinical Features. The incubation period in natural infections is 4–6 days. Variability in virulence determines the course of disease. Peracute disease associated with velogenic virus strains is usually lethal. Acute and subacute disease associated with mesogenic and lentogenic virus strains are most common in developed countries with modern poultry industries. Disease commences with anorexia, elevated temperature up to 43°C (normal 40°–41°C), dullness, and thirst, along with ruffled feathers, a hemorrhagic comb, closed eyes, and dry larynx and pharynx. Sick birds sneeze and show respiratory distress, and they have watery diarrhea. A drop in egg production can last up to 8 weeks. Eggs laid during this phase are small and soft-shelled, and the albumen is watery. Surviving birds may exhibit central nervous system signs, characterized by paresis of limbs, ataxia, torticollis, and circling movements, or by myoclony and tremors. In turkeys clinical signs are similar to those in chickens, whereas in pheasants, ducks, and geese mainly central nervous system involvement is observed. In pigeons a severe, rapidly spreading disease occurs with anorexia, diarrhea, polyuria, conjunctivitis, edema, and central nervous system signs including paresis of legs and wings.

Pathogenesis and Immunity. Initially the virus replicates in the mucosal epithelium of the upper respiratory and intestinal tracts; shortly after infection virus spreads via the blood to the spleen and bone marrow, producing a secondary viremia. This leads to infection of other target organs: lung, intestine, and the central nervous system. Respiratory distress and dyspnea result from congestion of the lungs and damage to the respiratory center in the brain. Gross pathologic findings include ecchymotic hemorrhages in the larynx, trachea, esophagus, and throughout the intestine. The most prominent histologic lesions are necrotic foci in the intestinal mucosa and lymphatic tissue and hyperemic changes in most organs, including the brain.

Antibody production is rapid. Hemagglutination-inhibiting antibody can be detected within 4 to 6 days of infection and persists for at least 2 years. The level of hemagglutinating-inhibiting antibody is a measure of immunity. Maternal antibodies protect chicks for 3 to 4 weeks after hatching. IgG confined to the circulation does not prevent respiratory infection but blocks viremia; locally produced IgA antibodies play an important role in protection in both the respiratory tract and the intestine.

Laboratory Diagnosis. Since the signs are relatively nonspecific, diagnosis must be confirmed by virus isolation and serology. The virus may be isolated from spleen, brain, or lungs by allantoic inoculation of 10-day-old embryonated eggs, the virus being differentiated from other viruses by hemadsorption–inhibition and hemagglutination–inhibition tests. Determination of virulence is essential for field isolates. In addition to the neuropathic index and the mean death time of chicken embryos, plaque formation in the presence or absence of trypsin in chicken cells is used. The hemagglutination–inhibition test is used for the diagnosis and surveillance of chronic Newcastle disease in countries where this form of the disease is endemic.

Epidemiology. The host spectrum of Newcastle disease virus includes gallinaceous birds (domestic chicken, turkey, guinea fowl, peacock) and pheasants, quail, partridges, and pigeons. Geese and ducks rarely develop disease. Wild birds represent a potentially important but unknown reservoir, virus having been isolated from a wide range of species. Occasional human infections occur, as an occupational disease with conjunctivitis and sometimes laryngitis, pharyngitis, and tracheitis.

In birds that survive, virus is shed in all secretions and excretions for at least 4 weeks. Trade in infected avian species and products plays a key role in the spread of Newcastle disease from infected to noninfected areas, and importation of the virus to various countries in frozen chickens has occurred. Virus may also be disseminated with uncooked kitchen refuse, foodstuffs, bedding, manure, and transport containers. By comparison, the epidemiologic role of live vectors such as wild birds or possibly mites is less important, although the former may carry virus into previously uninfected countries. Transmission occurs by direct contact between birds by the airborne route via aerosols and dust particles, and via contaminated feed and water. Mechanical spread between flocks is favored by the relative stability of the virus and its wide host range. With lentogenic strains transovarial transmission is important, and virus-infected chicks may hatch from virus-containing eggs.

DISEASES CAUSED BY MORBILLIVIRUSES

The close relationships between the three major morbilliviruses, measles, canine distemper, and rinderpest viruses, including their antigenic cross-reactivities, are reflected in the very similar pathogeneses of the diseases that they cause in humans, dogs, and cattle, respectively.

Rinderpest

Rinderpest virus has caused catastrophic losses in cattle in many parts of the world for centuries. The disease was first described in the fourth century and was not eliminated from Europe until the nineteenth century; today it is still the cause of great economic loss in Africa, the Middle East, and parts of Asia. It has been suggested on the basis of genetic studies that rinderpest virus is the archetype morbillivirus, having given rise to canine distemper and human measles viruses some 5000–10,000 years ago.

Rinderpest is a highly infectious acute or subacute systemic disease of cattle which is characterized by necrosis and erosions of the mucosa in the respiratory and digestive tracts. Early constipation, usually preceeded by dehydration and prostration, is followed by diarrhea. Owing to the high mortality, the disease can cause catastrophic economic losses.

Properties of Rinderpest Virus. There is only one serotype, which is antigenically stable and exhibits extensive cross-reactivity with the other morbilliviruses. The virus is labile and is rapidly inactivated in decaying carcasses, within a few hours under tropical conditions. In manure the virus remains infectious for about 48 hours, whereas meat, spleen, and lymph nodes at 5°C remain infectious for 2 to 3 days. For disinfection, sodium hydroxide, detergents, and all commercial disinfectants are effective.

Clinical Features. Clinical signs are variable depending on the susceptibility of the breed or species or ruminants and the immune status of the animal. After an incubation period of 4 to 15 days, the temperature rises to 41°C, and anorexia, weakness, and depression develop. There is increased lacrimal and nasal secretion, accompanied by salivation. Focal necrosis, superficial erosions, and petechiae appear in the mucosae of the mouth. Dyspnea, coughing, and diarrhea occur between days 4 and 7 of fever. Feces are watery and contain blood and sloughed mucosa; dehydration develops in severe cases. Death usually occurs between 6 and 12 days after the onset of the clinical signs. In highly susceptible cattle populations, all infected animals become sick, and a mortality rate of up to 90% has been observed. Indigenous breeds in Africa have a lower mortality, up to 50%. Surviving cattle recover 4–5 weeks after the onset of disease and are immune for life; there is no carrier state.

Pathogenesis and Immunity. After intranasal infection, virus replicates and viral antigen can be demonstrated in tonsils and mandibular and pharyngeal lymph nodes 24 hours after infection. Viremia develops 2–3 days after infection and 1–3 days before the animal becomes febrile. After systemic spread, virus can be demonstrated in lymph nodes, spleen, bone marrow, and mucosae of the upper respiratory tract, lung, and the digestive tract. Thereafter it replicates in the nasal mucosa, causing necrosis, erosions, and fibrinous exudation. Cattle that survive rinderpest have a lifelong immunity. Neutralizing antibodies appear 6–7 days after the onset of clinical signs, and maximum titers are reached during the third and fourth weeks.

Laboratory Diagnosis. In countries where rinderpest is endemic, clinical diagnosis is usually sufficient. In countries free of the disease but subject to importations, rinderpest can be confused with other diseases affecting the mucosa, such as bovine virus diarrhea and malignant catarrhal fever, and, in the early stages, differentiation from infectious bovine rhinotracheitis and foot-and-mouth disease is difficult. The virus infects a wide range of cells, but isolation for laboratory diagnosis is routinely carried out in bovine kidney cell cultures. The neutralization test and an ELISA are used for serologic diagnosis.

Epidemiology. The host range includes domestic cattle, water buffaloes, sheep, and goats. Camels are susceptible but do not play an important role in the epidemiology of the disease. Domestic pigs can develop clinical signs and are regarded as an important virus reservoir in Asia. Among wild animals, all species of the genus *Artiodactyla* are susceptible.

In endemic areas the disease spreads from animal to animal by contact, infection occurring through aerosol droplets. Virus is shed in secretions from the nose, throat, and conjunctiva as well as in feces, urine, and milk. Infected cattle excrete virus during the incubation period, before clinical signs occur, and in Africa and Asia such animals are the most important source for the introduction of rinderpest into disease-free areas. Because the virus is thermolabile, indirect spread via fresh meat and meat products, food, and transport vehicles is unusual.

Prevention and Control. In rinderpest-free countries, veterinary public health measures are designed to prevent introduction of the virus. Importation of uncooked meat and meat products from infected countries is forbidden, and zoo animals must be quarantined before being transported to such countries. In countries with endemic rinderpest, or where the disease has a high probability of being introduced, attenuated live-virus vaccines are used.

The vaccine is based on a strain of virus adapted to rabbits and then serially passaged in calf kidney cells, resulting in a vaccine that is safe because it is not excreted from recipients, efficacious because it induces lifelong immunity, and inexpensive to produce. It is one of the best vaccines available for any animal disease, but the currently used vaccine is thermolabile and requires a well-maintained "cold chain," a difficult practical problem in many areas where rinderpest occurs. With the attenuated live-virus vaccine grown in cell culture, antibody can be first detected 7–17 days after vaccination, and neutralizing antibodies persist for life.

Peste des Petits Ruminants

Peste des petits ruminants is a highly contagious, systemic disease of goats and sheep very similar to rinderpest and caused by a closely related morbillivirus. Unlike rinderpest, however, many infections are subclinical. It occurs mainly in West Africa, although outbreaks have also been described elsewhere. After an incubation period of 5 or 6 days, clinical signs develop, including fever, anorexia, a necrotic stomatitis with gingivitis, and diarrhea. The course of the disease may be peracute, acute, or chronic; however, the virus does not persist. Peste des petits ruminants has economic consequences, in that mortality in goats can reach 95% and in sheep only slightly less. Transmission of the virus is similar to that of rinderpest. Wild animals are not believed to play a role in viral spread. Control depends on vaccination. Because of the close antigenic relationship to rinderpest virus, rinderpest virus vaccines are employed, and they protect sheep and goats for at least 1 year.

Canine Distemper

Canine distemper is the most important viral disease of dogs, producing high morbidity and mortality in unvaccinated populations worldwide. It is a highly infectious, acute or subacute, febrile disease of dogs and other carnivores, which has been known since 1760. Edward Jenner first described the course and clinical features of the disease in 1809; its viral etiology was demonstrated in 1909. It is now comparatively rare in many industrialized countries, being well controlled by vaccination.

Properties of Canine Distemper Virus. There is only one serotype of the virus, but strains vary in virulence. Growth of the virus in cell cultures from dog, ferret, monkey, and human, or in embryonated hen's eggs, is possible only after adaptation. Inactivation is rapid at 37°C and occurs after a few hours at room temperature. Disinfectants readily destroy viral infectivity.

Clinical Features. Peracute cases with sudden onset of fever and sudden death are rare, but the acute disease is common. After an incubation period of 3–7 days, infected dogs develop a biphasic rise of temperature up to 41°C. Anorexia, catarrh, conjunctivitis, and depression are common during this stage. Some dogs show primarily respiratory signs, others intestinal signs. The first signs of the pulmonary form are a catarrhal inflammation of the larynx and bronchi, tonsillitis, and a cough. Later bronchitis or catarrhal bronchopneumonia develop, and sometimes pleuritis. Gastrointestinal signs include severe vomiting and watery diarrhea. After the onset of the disease, central nervous system signs are observed in some dogs, characterized by behavioral changes, forced movements, local myoclony, tonic–clonic spasms, epileptoid attacks, ataxia, and paresis. The duration of disease varies, depending on complications caused by secondary bacterial infections. The mortality rate ranges between 30% and 80%, but surviving dogs often have permanent central nervous system sequelae. In old dogs, an unusual encephalitis may occur as a late complication of distemper (see Chapters 9 and 10). Another late complication is "hard-pad" disease, in which hyperkeratosis of foot pads and the nose occurs; this syndrome usually leads to death. Elevated levels of antibodies to canine distemper virus have been found in dogs with rheumatoid arthritis.

Pathogenesis and Immunity. The pathogenesis of canine distemper was described in Chapter 9 (see Fig. 9-4). Briefly, it is a generalized infection in which, after initial viral replication in the oropharyngeal lymphoid tissue, cell-associated viremia occurs with virus becoming distributed throughout the body. Some dogs develop an early immune response and recover quickly; in others viral infection of the respiratory, intestinal, and urogenital tracts leads to death. Some dogs develop a demyelinating encephalomyelitis about 1 month after infection, very rarely virus persists in the brain to cause old dog encephalitis years later. Dogs surviving distemper have lifelong immunity to reinfection. Antibodies can first be demonstrated after 6 to 9 days and reach their peak 2–4 weeks after infection, persisting with unchanged titers for about 2 years. Neutralizing antibodies are transferred to offspring in colostrum.

Laboratory Diagnosis. Clinical signs of canine distemper are no longer considered pathognomonic where vaccination is widely practiced, since the disease is so rare; hence, laboratory diagnosis is necessary to exclude infectious canine hepatitis, canine parvovirus disease, leptospirosis, toxoplasmosis, and rabies. The most useful diagnostic method is the demonstration by immunohistologic methods of antigen in impression smears of the conjunctiva or in peripheral blood lymphocytes (antemortem), or in lung, stomach, intestinal, and bladder tissues (postmortem).

Epidemiology. The host range of canine distemper virus embraces all species of the families Canidae (dog, dingo, fox, coyote, jackal, wolf), Procyonidae (raccoon, panda), and Mustelidae (weasel, ferret, mink, skunk, badger, marten, otter).

Canine distemper virus is shed with all secretions and excretions from the fifth day after infection, which is before the onset of clinical signs, sometimes for weeks. Transmission is mainly via direct contact and droplet infections. Young dogs are more susceptible than old ones, the highest susceptibility occurring between the ages of 4 and 6 months, after they have lost maternal antibody.

There are differences between urban and isolated dogs with respect to epidemiology. Infections are frequent in urban dogs, in kennels, and in other situations where close contact between dogs occurs. Serologic investigations show that 80% of all puppies born to vaccinated urban bitches have antibodies to distemper virus up to the age of 8 weeks. This rate decreases to 10% by the age of 4 or 5 months, after which the percentage with antibodies slowly increases again, reaching 85% at the age of 2 years. In rural areas the number of dogs is too small to support a continuing chain of infection, so that highly susceptible dog populations develop, a situation which leads to catastrophic epidemics affecting dogs of all ages.

Prevention and Control. Immunization is effective in controlling distemper, using attenuated live-virus vaccines at the age of 8 weeks and again at 12 to 16 weeks. Annual revaccination is usually recommended by vaccine manufacturers. Neutralizing antibodies are detectable 6 days after immunization, reaching a peak 3–5 weeks later. For treatment, hyperimmune serum or immune IgG can be used prophylactically immediately after exposure. Antibiotic therapy generally has a beneficial effect by lessening the effect of secondary opportunistic bacterial infections.

Phocine Distemper

A disease similar to canine distemper occurred in 1988 in harbor seals and to lesser extent in gray seals in the North Sea and the Baltic Sea and in Lake Baikal seals 1 year earlier. The mortality rate was very high and exceeded 80% in certain areas. The causative agent, called phocine distemper virus, was found to be closely related to canine distemper virus, but the epidemiology of the outbreaks remains obscure.

DISEASES CAUSED BY PNEUMOVIRUSES

Respiratory Syncytial Virus Infections

Respiratory syncytial virus disease seems to be an "emerging disease," the cause of more and more pneumonia, interstitial pulmonary edema, and emphysema, especially in recently weaned calves and young cattle. Sheep are also susceptible to bovine respiratory syncytial virus. The virus was first detected in Japan, Belgium, and Switzerland in 1970, and it was isolated a little later in England and the United States. It probably occurs worldwide.

Clinical Features. Respiratory syncytial virus disease is particularly important in recently weaned calves and young cattle, especially when they are maintained in closely confined conditions. Infection is characterized by sudden onset of fever, hyperpnea, lethargy, rhinitis, and cough. Bronchiolitis and multifocal and interstitial pneumonia may be associated with interstitial endema and emphysema, and cases progressing to severe bronchopneumonia may end in death. The highest mortality often occurs in calves on a high plane of nutrition, leading to the speculation that certain feedstuffs such as corn silage may predispose cattle to the effect of infection. In general, in outbreak situations morbidity is high but mortality low.

Pathogenesis and Pathology. In calves infected experimentally, the virus causes complete loss of the ciliated epithelium 8–10 days after infection so that pulmonary clearance is compromised, with consequent secondary infections (see Chapter 9). At necropsy, subpleural and interstitial emphysema may be seen in all lobes of the lungs; if secondary bacterial infection if present there may be areas of consolidation. A characteristic finding is the presence of syncytial cells in the lungs, which are usually larger than those associated with parainfluenzavirus 3 infection.

Laboratory Diagnosis. Bovine respiratory syncytial virus grows in a variety of bovine cell cultures, best in those derived from respiratory tract cells. The cytopathic effect is similar to that of parainfluenzavirus 3; syncytia and intracytoplasmic inclusions are prominent. However, since viral infectivity is thermolabile and sensitive to freeze–thaw cycles, virus isolation is difficult. Immunofluorescent detection of viral antigen in lung tissue from early cases of the disease is sensitive and reliable.

Epidemiology and Control. Most commonly, the infection occurs during the winter months when cattle and sheep are housed in confined conditions. However, there have been important outbreaks in cow–calf operations in summer as well. The virus spreads rapidly, probably through aerosols or droplets of respiratory tract excretions. Reinfection of the respiratory tract is not uncommon in calves with antibody. Preexisting antibody, whether derived passively from maternal transfer or actively by prior infection or vaccination, does not prevent viral replication and excretion, although clinical signs may be mild or inapparent if the antibody titer is high. Even then, the stress of transport, etc., may result in acute disease if virus is reintroduced.

The role of respiratory syncytial virus in endemic pneumonia ("shipping fever") in cattle and sheep is not clearly understood. The virus has been isolated from the respiratory tract of sick calves and lambs after arrival in the feedlot, and antibody prevalence studies have indicated that infection at this time is widespread; the virus is probably endemic in this environment, along with other viral respiratory tract pathogens. The unresolved question is whether or how often infection leads to fibrinous pheumonia caused by *Pasteurella haemolytica,* the true end event in shipping fever (see Chapter 9).

For control, it should be kept in mind that clinical disease of the respiratory tract is often caused by several factors acting together. Therefore, careful diagnosis is needed before control measures are applied. A commercial attentuated live-virus vaccine is available for use in cattle.

Turkey Rhinotracheitis

First described in South Africa in 1978, turkey rhinotracheitis has now been recognized in Europe and Israel and is caused by a pneumovirus. In turkeys it causes catarrhal infections of the upper respiratory tract, foamy conjunctivitis, and sinusitis in young poults, the signs probably being exacerbated by secondary infections. In laying birds a drop in egg production is associated with slight respiratory distress. Morbidity is often 100%; mortality ranges from 0.4% to 90% and is highest in young poults. A milder form of the disease occurring in chickens is "swollen head syndrome."

Virus isolation is difficult but can be achieved by serial passage in 6- to 7-day-old turkey or chicken embryos or in chicken embryo tracheal organ cultures. Antibodies can be measured by ELISA. Attenuated live-virus vaccines are available commercially.

FURTHER READING

Al-Darraji, A. M., Cutlip, R. C., Lehmkuhl, H. D., Graham, D. L., Kluge, J. P., and Frank, G. H. (1982). Experimental infection of lambs with bovine respiratory syncytial virus and *Pasteurella haemolytica:* Clinical and microbiological studies. *Am. J. Vet. Res.* **43,** 236.

Alexander, D. J. (1988). "Newcastle Disease." Kluwer Academic Publ., Boston.

Alexander, D. J. (1991). Pneumovirus infections (turkey rhinotracheitis and swollen head syndrome of chickens). *In* "Diseases of Poultry" (B. W. Calnek, ed.), 9th Ed., p. 669. Wolfe Publ., London.

Appel, M. J., ed. (1987). "Virus Infections of Carnivores." Elsevier, Amsterdam.

Diallo, A. (1990). Morbillivirus group: Genome organisation and proteins. *Vet. Microbiol.* **23,** 155.

Dinter, Z., and Morein, B., eds. (1990). "Virus Infections of Ruminants." Elsevier, Amsterdam.

Kingsbury, D. W. (1990). *Paramyxoviridae* and their replication. *In* "Fields Virology" (B. N. Fields, D. M. Knipe, R. M. Chanock, M. S. Hirsch, J. L. Melnick, T. P. Monath, and B. Roizman, eds.), 2nd Ed., p. 935. Raven, New York.

Nagai, Y., Hamaguchi, M., and Toyoda, T. (1989). Molecular biology of Newcastle disease virus. *Prog. Vet. Microbiol. Immunol.* **5,** 16.

Osterhaus, A. D. M. E., Groen, J., Spijkers, H. E. M., Broeders, H. W. J., UytdeHagg, F. G. C. M., de Vries, P., Teppema, J. S., Visser, I. K. G., van de Bildt, M. W. G., and Vedder, E. J. (1990). Mass mortality in seals caused by a newly discovered virus-like morbillivirus. *Vet. Microbiol.* **23,** 343.

Stephan, H. A., Gay, G. M., and Ramirez, T. C. (1988). Encephalomyelitis, reproductive failure and corneal opacity (blue eye) in pigs, associated with a paramyxovirus infection. *Vet. Rec.* **122,** 6.

CHAPTER 28

Rhabdoviridae

The family *Rhabdoviridae* encompasses more than 150 viruses of vertebrates, invertebrates (mostly arthropods), and plants, the virions of each having a distinctive bullet-shaped morphology. Important animal pathogens occur throughout the family: the genus *Vesiculovirus* (vesicular stomatitis viruses and others), the genus *Lyssavirus* (rabies virus, rabies-related viruses, bovine ephemeral fever virus, bovine ephemeral fever-related viruses, and others), viruses in serogroups that have not as yet been placed in a genus, and certain ungrouped viruses. Important rhabdoviruses of fish occur in each of the established genera, and others remain to be placed.

Rabies virus is the cause of one of the oldest and most feared diseases of man and animals and was recognized in Egypt before 2300 B.C. and in ancient Greece, where it was well described by Aristotle. Perhaps the most lethal of all infectious diseases, rabies also has the distinction of having stimulated one of the great early discoveries in biomedical research. In 1885, before the nature of viruses was comprehended, Louis Pasteur developed, tested, and applied a rabies vaccine, thereby opening the modern era of infectious disease prevention by vaccination.

Vesicular stomatitis of horses, cattle, and swine was first recognized as distinct from foot-and-mouth disease early in the nineteenth century, and thereafter it was found to cause periodic epidemics throughout the Western hemisphere. The disease was a significant problem in artillery and cavalry horses during the American Civil War. Bovine ephemeral fever was first recognized in Africa in 1867 and is now known to be endemic or the cause of periodic epidemics in Africa, most of Southeast Asia, Japan, and Australia. Several fish rhabdoviruses are the cause of serious losses in the expanding aquaculture industries of North America, Europe, and Asia.

PROPERTIES OF RHABDOVIRUSES

Rhabdoviruses are approximately 70 nm wide, 170 nm long (although some species are longer, some shorter) and consist of a lipid-containing bilayer envelope with glycoprotein peplomers surrounding a helically wound nucleocapsid, which gives the viruses their distinctive bullet-shaped or conical morphology (Fig. 28-1). The viruses contain a single linear molecule of minus sense ssRNA, 11–12 kb in size. During rhabdovirus replication, defective interfering (DI) virus particles are commonly formed. These are shorter and have a smaller RNA molecule than normal infectious particles, with complex deletion mutations in their genome (see Chapter 4). Rhabdovirus virions contain five proteins (Table 28-2) (all molecular mass values are for vesicular stomatitis–Indiana virus):

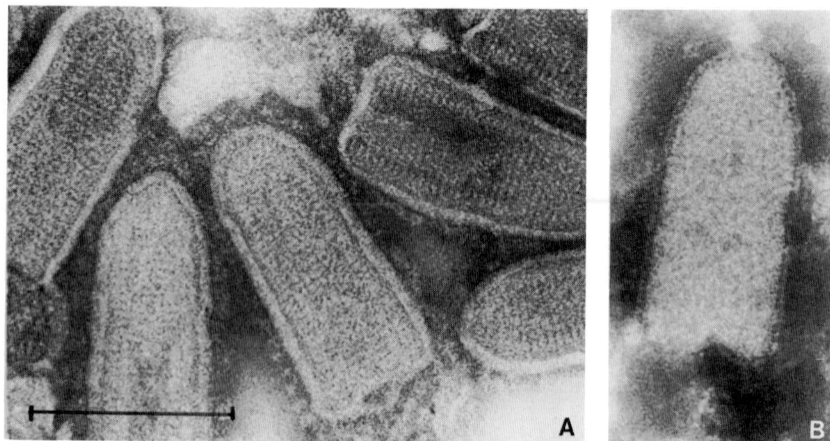

FIG. 28-1. Rhabdoviridae. *Negatively stained virions of (A) vesicular stomatitis–Indiana virus and (B) rabies virus. Bar: 100 nm.*

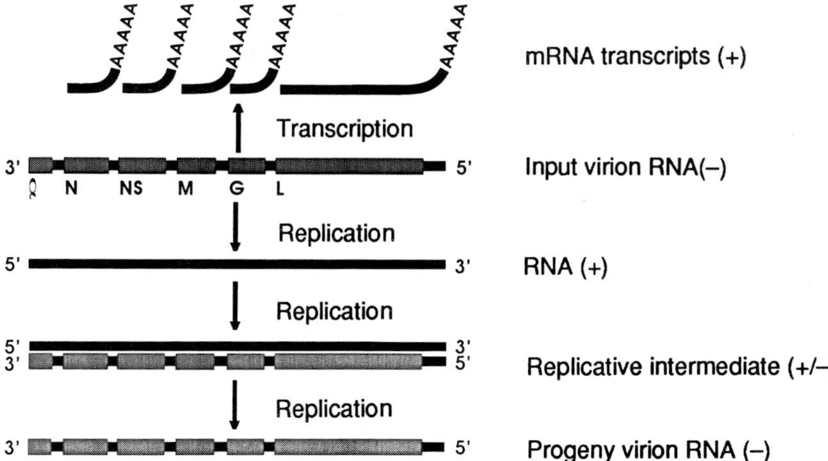

FIG. 28-2. *Genome structure of vesicular stomatitis virus and its mode of replication. Wide bars indicate genes and their relative sizes; narrow bars indicate noncoding nucleotides, and the long narrow bar indicates (+) strand complementary RNA. The N protein-RNA core plus the NS and L proteins comprise the transcription complex. Polyadenylation occurs by a "stuttering" mechanism signaled by an 11-base sequence at the end of each gene except the leader gene. RNA replication occurs through a replicative intermediate (+/–) dsRNA. l, leader; N, nucleoprotein; NS, nonstructural protein; M, matrix protein; G, peplomer glycoprotein, L, with NS, RNA polymerase.*

transcriptase L (150K), glycoprotein G (70K–80K), nucleoprotein N (50K–62K), nonstructural protein NS (40K–50K), and matrix protein M (20K–30K) (for rabies virus: NS/M = M_1, M_2). The glycoprotein forms the surface peplomers and contains neutralizing epitopes, which are the targets of immunoprophylaxis and immunotherapy; it and the nucleoprotein have epitopes involved in cell-mediated immunity.

Classification

Based on the properties of the virions and on serologic relationships, two genera, *Vesiculovirus* and *Lyssavirus*, have been defined among the rhabdoviruses of animals (Table 28-1). The genus *Vesiculovirus* contains about 35 serologically distinct viruses, only 7 of which cause vesicular disease in horses, cattle, and swine. Several fish and eel rhabdoviruses are also members of this genus.

The genus *Lyssavirus* contains rabies virus and three rabieslike viruses from Africa, namely, Mokola, Lagos bat, and Duvenhage viruses. Duvenhage virus has also been isolated on many occasions from bats in northern

TABLE 28-1
Rhabdoviruses That Affect Domestic Animals

Virus	Geographic distribution
Vesiculovirus	
Vesicular stomatitis–Indiana	North, Central, and South America
Vesicular stomatitis–New Jersey	North, Central, and South America
Cocal	Trinidad, Brazil
Alagoas	Argentina, Brazil
Piry	Brazil
Chandipura	India, Nigeria
Isfahan	Iran
Many other vesiculoviruses not associated with disease in domestic animals or humans	Worldwide
Lyssavirus	
Rabies	All continents except Australia
Rabieslike viruses	
Mokola	Central Africa
Lagos bat	Central and South Africa
Duvenhage	South Africa
Duvenhage/European bat virus	Europe
Other rhabdoviruses of mammals	
Bovine ephemeral fever	Asia, Africa, Australia
Many other viruses possibly associated with bovine ephemeral fever-like disease in animals	Worldwide
Many other rhabdoviruses not associated with disease in domestic animals or humans	Worldwide

Europe. Each of these viruses must be considered capable of causing rabieslike disease in animals and humans. In addition to these viruses, the genus also contains bovine ephemeral fever virus and many other serologically distinct viruses, including many bovine ephemeral fever-like viruses. Five important fish rhabdoviruses, including infectious hematopoietic necrosis virus, hirame rhabdovirus, and viral hemorrhagic septicemia virus, are also members of this genus.

VIRAL REPLICATION

"Fixed" (laboratory-adapted) rabies virus and vesicular stomatitis viruses replicate well in many kinds of cell cultures, for example, Vero (African green monkey kidney) cells, BHK-21 (baby hamster kidney) cells which are the most common substrate for animal rabies vaccines, chick embryo fibroblasts which are also a common substrate for vaccines, and human diploid fibroblasts (WI-38, MRC 5) which are the substrate for modern human vaccines. Laboratory-adapted ("fixed") rabies virus and vesicular stomatitis viruses, as well as wild-type ("street") rabies virus and bovine ephemeral fever virus (after adaptation), replicate to high titer in suckling mouse and suckling hamster brain.

Viral entry into its host cell occurs via fusion of the viral envelope with the cell membrane; all replication steps occur in the cytoplasm. Using virion RNA as template, viral transcriptase (L + NS) transcribes five subgenomic mRNA species, which are translated into the five viral proteins (Fig. 28-2). Replication of genomic RNA and attachment of nucleoprotein molecules to it lead to the formation of helically wound nucleocapsids. These in turn are formed into mature virions by budding through cell membranes modified by the insertion of viral glycoprotein. Vesicular stomatitis virus replication usually causes rapid cytopathology, but the replication of rabies and bovine ephemeral fever viruses is usually noncytopathic because these viruses do not shut down host cell protein and nucleic acid synthesis.

RABIES

Rabies virus can infect all warm-blooded animals, and in nearly all instances the infection ends in death. Cattle rabies is important in Central and South America, where it is estimated that more than 1 million cattle die each year. Dog rabies is still important in many parts of the world; virus in the saliva of infected dogs causes most of the estimated 75,000 human rabies cases that occur each year worldwide. In many countries of Europe, and in the United States and Canada, wildlife rabies has become of increasing relative importance. Rabies is present throughout

TABLE 28-2
Properties of Rhabdoviruses

Bullet-shaped enveloped virion, 70 × 170 nm, with glycoprotein peplomers on virion surface and matrix protein under lipoprotein envelope
Nucleocapsid with helical symmetry
Linear minus sense ssRNA genome, 11–12 kb
Cytoplasmic replication; viral transcriptase transcribes five subgenomic mRNAs which are translated into five proteins: transcriptase (150K), nucleoprotein (50K–62K), matrix protein (20K–30K), glycoprotein peplomer (70K–80K), and nonstructural protein (40K–50K); maturation by budding through plasma membrane
Some species cause rapid cytopathology; others, such as rabies virus, are noncytopathogenic

the world, with the exception of Australia, Japan, Great Britain, and many smaller islands such as Hawaii and most of the islands of the Caribbean basin.

Clinical Features

The clinical features of rabies are similar in most species, but there is great variation between individuals. Following the bite of a rabid animal the incubation period is usually between 14 and 90 days, but may be considerably longer. An incubation period of 2 years has been reported in a cat, and four human cases have been described in industrialized countries with incubation periods proven to be from at least 11 months to at least 6 years. In each of the human cases the virus was shown to be a dog genotype from a developing country.

There is a prodromal phase prior to overt clinical disease, which often is overlooked in animals or is recalled only in retrospect as a change in temperament. Two clinical forms of the disease are recognized: furious and dumb or paralytic. In the furious form, the animal becomes restless, nervous, aggressive, and often dangerous as it loses all fear of man and bites at anything that gains its attention. The animal often cannot swallow water, giving rise to the synonym for the disease, "hydrophobia." There is often excessive salivation, exaggerated responses to light and sound, and hyperesthesia. As the encephalitis progresses, fury gives way to paralysis, and the animal presents the same clinical features as seen in the dumb form of the disease. Terminally, there are often convulsive seizures, coma, and respiratory arrest, with death occurring 2 to 7 days after the onset of clinical signs. A higher proportion of dogs, cats, and horses exhibit fury than is the case for cattle or other ruminants or laboratory animal species.

Pathogenesis and Immunity

Rabies virus enters the body in the bite or occasionally the scratch of a rabid animal or when virus-laden saliva from a rabid animal enters an open wound. Virus may gain direct entry into nerve endings present in the bite site, or virus may replicate and be amplified in the bite site, in muscle, after which it invades peripheral nerve endings. The viral genome then moves centripetally in the cytoplasm of the axons of the peripheral nervous system until it reaches the central nervous system, usually in the spinal cord (see Chapter 9). Viral entry into the spinal cord and then the brain (particularly the limbic system) is associated with clinical signs of neuronal dysfunction. Usually, at about the same time that central nervous system infection causes fury, virions are also shed from the apical end of mucus-secreting cells in the salivary glands and are delivered in high concentrations into saliva (see Fig. 9-5B). In some cases, virus is excreted into the saliva several days (rarely up to 14 days) before clinical signs develop; in other cases virus may never be present in the saliva, even at the terminal stages of the disease.

Throughout the course of rabies, host inflammatory and specific immune responses are only minimally stimulated, probably because the infection is noncytopathic in muscle and in nerve cells and because the infection is largely confined to the immunologically sequestered environment of the nervous system. At death, except for a moderate mononuclear inflammatory cell infiltration in the nervous system, there is little histologic evidence of a host response to infection. Further, in experimentally infected animals neutralizing antibody reaches significant levels only as death approaches, when it is too late to be of help, and may contribute to immunopathologic disease.

Laboratory Diagnosis

It is important that the laboratory diagnosis of rabies in animals be undertaken in approved laboratories by qualified, experienced personnel, since in many cases decisions on human treatment and/or animal indemnification are involved. If there is human exposure or suspected animal-to-animal transmission, or if clinical observation suggests rabies, the animal must be killed and brain tissue collected for testing. Postmortem diagnosis involves direct immunofluorescence of touch impressions of brain tissue (medulla, cerebellum, and hippocampus) from the suspect animal (see Fig. 12-5). When necessitated by circumstances, postmortem diagnosis can also be performed using the polymerase chain reaction (PCR) with primers that amplify both genomic RNA and viral mRNA sequences from nervous system tissues of suspect cases. From antemortem diagnosis, immunofluorescence or PCR assays on skin biopsy, corneal impression, or saliva specimens can be used. Only positive results are of diagnostic value, since the lack of sensitivity of these procedures does not exclude an infection. A comprehensive algorithm is available to guide the public health worker and physician in deciding on the course of human postexposure treatment (Table 28-3).

Epidemiology, Prevention, and Control

Rabies virus is not stable in the environment and in usual circumstances is only a risk when transmitted by the bite or scratch of a rabid animal. In bat caves, however, where the amounts of virus may be very high, it can be transmitted via aerosol.

TABLE 28-3

Rabies: Guide for Human Postexposure Prophylaxis

Animal species	Condition of animal at time of attack	Treatment of exposed person[a]
Domestic animals		
Dog, cat	Healthy and available for 10 days of observation	None, unless animal develops signs of rabies[b]
	Rabid or suspected rabid	Immediate rabies immune globulin[c] and vaccine[d]
	Unknown (escaped)	Consult public health official; if treatment is indicated, give rabies immune globulin and vaccine
Wild animals		
Skunk, bat, fox, coyote, raccoon, bobcat, woodchuck, and other carnivores	Regard as rabid unless proved negative by laboratory tests[e] or from geographic area known to be rabies-free	Rabies immune globulin[c] and vaccine[d]
Other		
Livestock, rodents, lagomorphs (rabbits, hares)	Consider individually	Public health officials should be consulted about the need for rabies prophylaxis; bites of squirrels, hamsters, guinea pigs, gerbils, chipmunks, rats, mice, other rodents, rabbits, and hares almost never call for antirabies prophylaxis

[a] In applying these recommendations, take into account the animal species involved, the circumstances of the bite or other exposure, the vaccination status of the animal, and presence of rabies in the region. Public health officials should be consulted if questions arise about the need for rabies prophylaxis. All bites and wounds should immediately be thoroughly cleansed with soap and water. If antirabies treatment is indicated, both rabies immune globulin and vaccine should be given as soon as possible, regardless of the interval from exposure.

[b] If during the 10-day observation period a dog or cat should exhibit clinical signs of rabies, it should be immediately killed and tested, and treatment of the exposed individual with serum and vaccine should be started.

[c] If rabies immune globulin is not available, use antirabies serum (equine). Do not use more than the recommended dosage. Anticipate possible need to treat for serum sickness.

[d] Five 1-ml intramuscular doses to be given on days 0, 3, 7, 14, and 28. WHO recommends an optimal sixth dose at 90 days. Local reactions to vaccines are common and do not contraindicate continuing treatment. Discontinue vaccine if fluorescent antibody tests of the animal are negative.

[e] The animal should be killed and tested as soon as possible; holding for observation is not recommended.

The control of rabies in different countries of the world poses very different problems, depending on whether they are free of the disease, whether they are industrialized or developing countries, and whether vampire bat rabies is a problem.

Rabies-free Countries. Rigidly enforced quarantine of dogs and cats for 6 months has been effectively used to exclude rabies from Australia, Japan, New Zealand, Hawaii, and several other islands. Rabies did not become endemic in wildlife in the United Kingdom and was eradicated from dogs in that country in 1902, and again in 1922, after its reestablishment in the dog population in 1918.

Developing Countries. In most countries of Asia, Latin America, and Africa, endemic dog rabies is a serious problem, marked by significant domestic animal and human mortality. In these countries, large numbers of doses of human vaccines are used, and there is a need for comprehensive, professionally organized, and publicly supported agencies in the following areas: (1) stray dog and cat elimination and control of the movement of pets (quarantine may be called for in emergencies); (2) immunization of dogs and cats, so as to break the chains of virus transmission; (3) laboratory diagnosis, to confirm clinical observations and obtain accurate incidence data; (4) surveillance, to measure the effectiveness of all control measures; and (5) public education programs to assure cooperation.

Industrialized Countries. Fox rabies is endemic in several countries of western Europe (Fig. 28-3). Varying patterns of endemic wildlife rabies are recognized in the United States and Canada (Fig. 28-4). Fox rabies is a problem in the Appalachian mountain regions of the United States, in Ontario, Canada, in many European countries, and in polar areas inhabited by the arctic fox. Skunk rabies is common in central North America, from Texas to Saskatchewan, where it is the principal cause of rabies in cattle. Raccoon rabies in the United States began a gradual northern movement from Florida in the 1950s, reaching Georgia in the 1960s, and then causing an explosive epidemic in Virginia, Maryland, Pennsylvania, and the District of Columbia in the 1980s and in New Jersey, New York, and Connecticut in the 1990s. This northern movement started with the importation of raccoons, for sporting purposes, from rabies-infected areas in the south. Studies with monoclonal antibodies have shown that raccoon isolates from newly affected northern areas are the same as older isolates from Florida and Georgia. Historically, rabies control in wildlife has been based on animal population reduction by trapping and poisoning, but in the past few years, fox immunization, by the distribution of baits containing an attenuated live-virus rabies

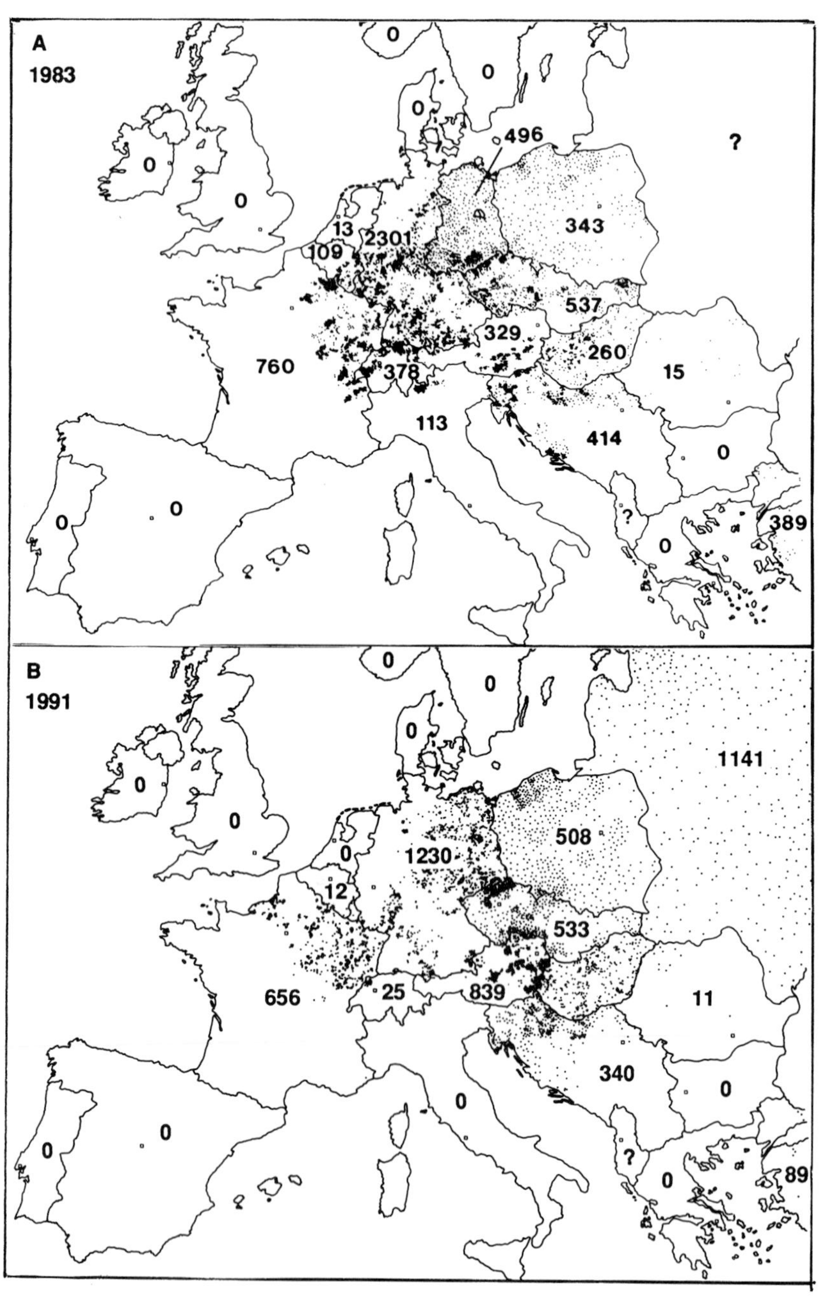
A
1983
0
0
0
0
0
496
?
343
13
2301
109
537
329
260
15
760
378
113
414
0
0
0
?
389
0
B
1991
0
0
0
0
0
1141
508
0
1230
12
533
656
25
839
11
340
0
0
0
0
?
89
0

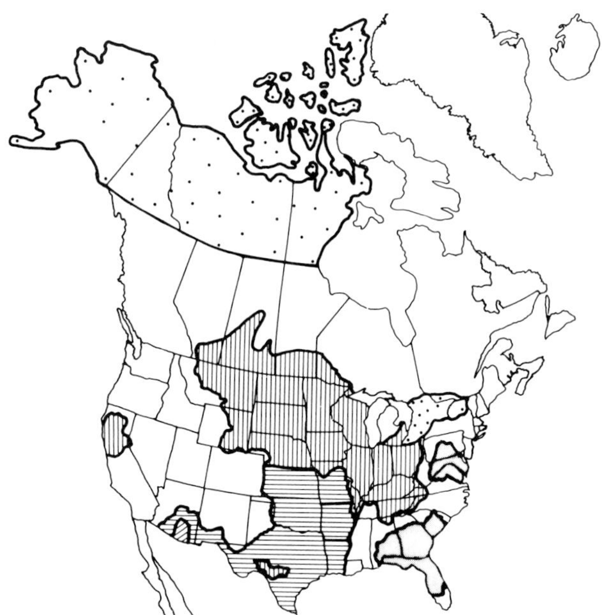

Fig. 28-4. *Distribution of antigenic variants of rabies in the United States and Canada. Vertical lines, skunk (north central states and California) and gray fox (Texas); horizontal lines, skunk (south-central states); close stipple, raccoon; large dots, red fox and Arctic fox; diagonal lines, gray fox (Arizona). [From J. S. Smith,* Adv. Virus Res. **36,** *215 (1989).]*

vaccine, appears to have been highly successful in reducing transmission in Switzerland and Germany (compare data for 1983 and 1991, Fig. 28-3). The question of whether immunization of other wildlife species will be useful, especially in more complex ecosystems, will depend on population density of the target species, on further research on the safety and efficacy of orally ingested wildlife vaccines, on development of delivery systems appropriate for each reservoir host species, and on solution of legal and jurisdictional problems. Many of these problems are now being

---

Fig. 28-3. *Occurrence of fox rabies in Europe during the last quarter of 1983 and the first quarter of 1991. Note the decline in cases in Switzerland and what was West Germany, where active campaigns of fox vaccination have been pursued. (Courtesy of the World Health Organization Collaborating Centre for Surveillance of Rabies, Tübingen, Germany.)*

solved, and comprehensive field studies are in progress, including trials with a vaccinia virus–rabies glycoprotein recombinant.

Latin America. In several countries of Latin America vampire bat rabies is a problem to livestock industries (and to humans). Here control efforts have depended on the use of bovine vaccines and more recently on the use of anticoagulants such as diphenadione and warfarin. When vampire bats feed on the blood of treated cattle, they suffer fatal hemorrhages in their wing capillaries.

Vaccination. Animal rabies vaccines, produced in cultured cells as inactivated or in some countries as attenuated live-virus vaccines, are efficacious and safe. An update of indications and contraindications for the use of each licensed animal rabies vaccine is published annually in the United States (see Further Reading).

Veterinarians and other individuals occupationally or otherwise at risk of rabies should be prophylactically immunized. Because of several variables in the level and nature of risk, the immediate availability of postexposure booster vaccination, etc., a comprehensive set of recommendations for prophylactic vaccine use has been produced and is updated each year (Table 28-4).

VESICULAR STOMATITIS

Originally, vesicular stomatitis was considered of interest only because of its role in the differential diagnosis of foot-and-mouth disease in cattle and the debilitating lameness it can cause in horses. More recently, however, the disease has been recognized as the cause of economically important losses in conditioning and milk production in cattle, especially as more dairying is undertaken in warmer climates.

Clinical Features

The clinical features of vesicular stomatitis infection vary greatly among animals in a herd. Lesions develop quickly after an incubation period of 1–5 days. Excess salivation and fever often are the first signs of infection in cattle and horses, and lameness is often the first sign in swine. Vesicular lesions on the tongue, the oral mucosa, teats, and coronary bands of cattle may progress to total epithelial denudation with secondary bacterial infection. Lesions may cause profuse salivation and anorexia, lameness, and rejection of the suckling calf. In horses, tongue lesions are most pronounced, often progressing to complete sloughing of the epithelium. In swine, vesicular lesions are most common on the

TABLE 28-4

Rabies: Criteria for Human Preexposure Immunization[a]

Risk category	Nature of risk	Typical population	Preexposure regimen
Continuous	Virus present continuously, often in high concentrations; aerosol, mucous membrane, bite, or nonbite exposure; specific exposure may go unrecognized	Rabies research laboratory workers,[b] rabies biologics production workers	Primary preexposure immunization course; serologic testing every 6 months; booster immunization when antibody level falls below acceptable level[c]
Frequent	Exposure usually episodic, with source recognized, but exposure may also be unrecognized; aerosol, mucous membrane, bite, or nonbite exposure	Rabies diagnostic laboratory workers,[b] spelunkers, workers, veterinarians and staff, animal control and wildlife workers in rabies-enzootic areas; travelers visiting areas of enzootic rabies	Primary preexposure immunization course; serologic testing or booster immunization every 2 years[c]
Infrequent (but greater than population at large)	Exposure nearly always episodic with source recognized; mucous membrane, bite, or nonbite exposure	Veterinarians and animal control and wildlife workers in areas of low rabies enzoocity; veterinary students	Primary preexposure immunization course; no serologic testing or booster immunization
Rare (the population at large)	Exposure always episodic; mucous membrane or bite exposure with source recognized	Population at large in countries with animal rabies, including persons in rabies-epizootic areas	No vaccination necessary

[a] Preexposure immunization consists of three doses of modern cell-culture vaccine, 1.0 ml intramuscularly, one each on days 0, 7, and 28. Administration of routine booster doses of vaccine depends on exposure risk category as noted above. Preexposure immunization of immunosuppressed persons is not recommended.

[b] Judgment of relative risk and extra monitoring of immunization status of laboratory workers are the responsibilities of the laboratory supervisor in most countries.

[c] Minimum acceptable antibody level is complete virus neutralization at a 1:5 serum dilution by WHO standard RFFIT test. Booster immunization should be given when the titer falls below this level.

snout and coronary bands. Lesions usually heal within 7 to 10 days, and there are no sequelae.

Pathogenesis and Immunity

The virus probably enters the body through breaks in the mucosa and skin, owing to the minor abrasions caused, for example, by rough forage, or via the bites of arthropods. There does not seem to be a systemic, viremic phase of infection except in swine and small laboratory animals. Local vesiculation and epithelial denudation follow epithelial cell destruction and interstitial edema, which separates the epithelium from underlying tissues. Spread of such lesions occurs by extension, such that it is common for the entire epithelium of the tongue or teat to be sloughed. High titers of infectious virus are present, usually for a short time, in vesicular fluids and in tissues at the margins of lesions, and virus may be transmitted by fomites, such as contaminated food, milking machines, and restraint devices. The virus may also be transmitted mechanically by arthropods. Despite the extent of the epithelial damage, healing is usually rapid and complete. Although infection results in solid homologous immunity for a limited time, immunity is not lifelong, and animals may become reinfected. There is no serologic cross-reactivity between vesicular stomatitis–New Jersey and vesicular stomatitis–Indiana viruses.

Laboratory Diagnosis

Virus can be recovered from vesicular fluids and tissue scrapings by standard virus isolation techniques in cell culture (or in embryonated eggs, or in suckling mice by intracerebral inoculation). Virus isolates are identified by conventional serologic methods; modern rapid methods have not yet been applied. Because diagnosis may involve differentiation from foot-and-mouth disease, these procedures should be carried out in an authorized reference laboratory.

Epidemiology

Vesicular stomatitis viruses can be stable in the environment for days, for example, on milking machine parts where transmission results in teat and udder lesions and in cool water, in soil, and on vegetation where transmission results in mouth lesions. In some tropical and subtropical areas, there is evidence for transmission of vesicular stomatitis viruses by sandflies (*Lutzomyia* spp.), with transovarial transmission in sandflies contributing to the perpetuation of the viruses in endemic foci.

Throughout the Americas, vesicular stomatitis of cattle, horses, and swine is a recurring disease problem, appearing annually or at intervals of 2 or 3 years in tropical and subtropical countries and at intervals of 5 to 10 years in the temperate zones of both North and South America.

The genome of vesicular stomatitis viruses has been shown to accumulate mutations rapidly and randomly during passage in the laboratory. The question is now being asked how this high capacity for "drift" relates to genetic stability or diversity in nature. Genomic analysis of large numbers of vesicular stomatitis–New Jersey and vesicular stomatitis–Indiana isolates has indicated that temperate zone epidemics are caused by a single viral genotype, suggesting spread from a common origin. For example, all vesicular stomatitis–Indiana isolates from the United States and Mexico derive from a recent common ancestor. Epidemic isolates from different geographic areas, such as the temperate zones of North and South America, have been shown to be distinct, indicating spatial genetic isolation. Isolates from different endemic foci in the tropics are also distinct, but they reflect a more complex genetic diversity including multiple phylogenetic lineages. For example, multiple genotypes of vesicular stomatitis–Indiana virus coexist in Costa Rica, Panama, and adjacent countries of South America. Within even small endemic foci these variants may be maintained over an extended period of time.

Even though the geographic range of the vesicular stomatitis viruses is large, disease problems are restricted to favorable habitats. For example, in the upper Mississippi valley in the United States, disease appears regularly in aspen parklands, a narrow zone separating hardwood forest from open prairies. In the western mountainous regions of the United States, disease seems to move up and down valleys, rarely reaching higher pastures. Seasonally, the disease may appear almost simultaneously over large areas, or in multiple spreading foci, suggesting that the virus might be arthropod-borne, although in studies over many years few virus isolates have been made from arthropods. In a large epidemic of vesicular stomatitis–New Jersey that occurred in the western United States in 1982, many virus isolates were made from flies, mostly from the common housefly, *Musca domestica,* but it is not clear how flies, including biting flies, might fulfill known patterns of virus transmission between herds and between individual animals. The manner by which vesicular stomatitis viruses are transmitted over long distances also remains controversial despite years of study. Arthropod involvement is also suggested here.

Prevention and Control

Outbreaks of disease may be explosive, so avoidance of pasturages known as sites of transmission may help to avoid infection, but in general little is usually done even in the face of an epidemic. In temperate zones epidemics occur at such infrequent intervals that the index of suspicion falls to a low level during interepidemic periods. Both inactivated and attenuated live-virus vaccines are available, but neither are much used.

Human Disease

Vesicular stomatitis viruses are zoonotic, being transmissible to man (typically, farmers and veterinarians) from vesicular fluids and tissues of infected animals, but there are no practical measures for preventing occupational exposure. The disease in man resembles influenza, presenting with an acute onset of fever, chills, and muscle pain. It resolves without complications within 7–10 days. Human cases are not uncommon during epidemics, but because of lack of awareness, few cases are reported.

BOVINE EPHEMERAL FEVER

Bovine ephemeral fever, also called three-day sickness, is a widespread disease of cattle, spanning tropical and subtropical zones of Africa, Australia, and Asia. From these endemic sites the disease extends intermittently into temperate zones in major or minor epidemics. The disease has never been reported in North or South America or Europe.

Clinical Features

Clinical features in cattle are characteristic, but all are not seen in an individual animal. Onset is sudden; the disease is marked by a biphasic or polyphasic fever with an immediate drop in milk production. Other clinical signs are associated with the second and later febrile phases: these include depression, muscle stiffness, lameness, and less often nasal and ocular discharges, cessation of rumination, and constipation. Infrequently there is diarrhea and temporary or permanent paresis. Usually, recovery is dramatic and complete in 3 days (range 2–5 days). Morbidity rates often approach 100%, and the mortality rate in an outbreak is usually 1–2% but can reach 10–20% in mature well-conditioned beef cattle and high producing dairy cattle. Subclinical cases do occur, but their relative rate is unknown because antibody testing is confounded by intercurrent infections in the same areas by related but nonpathogenic rhabdoviruses.

Pathogenesis and Immunity

The pathogenesis of the disease is complex; it seems clear that pathophysiologic and immunologic effects on the host inflammatory response, mediated by the release of lymphokines, are involved in the expression of disease. There is no evidence that the virus causes widespread tissue destruction. In all cases there is an early neutrophilia with an abnormal level of immature neutrophil polymorphonuclear cells in the circulation ("left shift"). There is a rise in plasma fibrinogen and a significant drop in plasma calcium. Therapeutically, there is a dramatic response to non-steroid anti-inflammatory drugs and often to calcium infusion. Infection results in solid immunity; because outbreaks tend to involve most animals in a herd, repeat clinical episodes usually involve young animals born since previous outbreaks.

Laboratory Diagnosis

Laboratory diagnosis is difficult; the "gold standard" is virus isolation by blind passage in mosquito (*Aedes albopictus*) cells or suckling mouse brain. Detection of a rise in antibody is the most practical diagnostic technique available; this is done by ELISA or neutralization assays which are virus specific, or by immunofluorescence or agar gel precipitin tests which are cross-reactive with related rhabdoviruses.

Epidemiology and Control

Bovine empheral fever virus is transmitted by two types of arthropod vectors, *Culicoides* and culicine and anopheline mosquitoes; endemic and epidemic spread is limited to the distribution of vectors. There is epidemiologic evidence that more arthropod vector species remain to be identified. Prevention by vector control is impractical in the areas of the world where this disease is prevalent. In Japan, South Africa, and Australia inactivated and attenuated live-virus vaccines have been used. Problems with conventional vaccines stem from lack of potency; inactivated vaccines require more antigenic mass than it has been possible to achieve, and attenuated live-virus vaccines suffer from a loss in immunogenicity linked with the attenuation process. A recombinant DNA-derived G protein vaccine is under development.

FISH RHABDOVIRUSES

At least nine serologically distinct rhabdoviruses cause economically important diseases in fish (Table 28-5), fish rhabdoviruses being very similar to those of mammals. The protein profiles of infectious hematopoietic necrosis virus, viral hemorrhagic septicemia virus, hirame rhabdovirus, and eel rhabdovirus 2 resemble those of members of the genus *Lyssavirus;* those of spring viremia of carp virus, pike fry rhabdovirus, and eel rhabdovirus 1 resemble those of the members of the genus *Vesiculovirus*. All of these fish rhabdoviruses are antigenically distin-

TABLE 28-5

Rhabdoviruses of Fish

Virus	Species affected	Geographic distribution	Growth temperature[a] (°C)	
			Range	Optimum
Viral hemorrhagic septicemia virus (Egtved virus)	Salmonids, pike, sea bass, turbot, Pacific and Atlantic cod	Europe, west coast of United States	6–20	10–15
Infectious hematopoietic necrosis virus	Salmonids	Western North America, France, Italy, Japan, China, Taiwan	4–20	13–18
Hirame rhabdovirus	Japanese flounder	Japan	5–20	15–20
Spring viremia of carp virus	Cyprinids	Europe	4–32	Variable[b]
Pike fry rhabdovirus	Northern pike, guppies, cyprinids, pike	Europe, including Russia	10–31	21–28
Eel rhabdovirus	American, European eels, rainbow trout fry[c]	Japan and Europe	15–20	15
Perch rhabdovirus	Perch	Europe	10–20	15
Rio Grande cichlid rhabdovirus	Rio Grande cichlid	United States	23–30	—
Ulcerative syndrome and snakehead rhabdovirus	Snakehead	Southeast Asia	18–35	24–30

[a] Measured in cultured piscine cells.
[b] Depends on cell line.
[c] Experimental infections only.

guishable by neutralization tests. The viruses may be propagated in a variety of piscine cell lines and also in mammalian, avian, and reptilian cells, the optimal growth temperatures and the temperature range for growth differing from one virus to another.

Viral Hemorrhagic Septicemia of Trout

Viral hemorrhagic septicemia of trout causes losses in European countries, and it has recently been found in salmonids and Pacific cod in Washington and Alaska, respectively. It is more severe when the water temperature falls below 15°C, and mortality may reach 80% when the virus is introduced into a new area. The acute disease is marked by lethargy, darkened pigmentation, hemorrhages into visceral organs, muscle, and swim bladder, and death. The chronic infection may be inapparent, or there may be continuing mortality. Diagnostic tests (fluorescent antibody, immunodiffusion, or neutralization) are available. Control involves avoidance of contamination of premises (via use of certified viral hemorrhagic septicemia-free stock), eradication by slaughter, and disinfection when disease is found; in some cases, raising the water temperature may reduce losses. Vaccination has shown promise in pilot experiments in Denmark and France.

Infectious Hematopoietic Necrosis

Infectious hematopoietic necrosis disease of salmonids is caused by a group of serologically related viruses, each infecting particular species of salmon or trout. The disease causes frequent losses in hatcheries along the Pacific coast of North America from Alaska to northern California, in France and Italy, and in Japan and Taiwan. Epidemics usually involve juvenile fish at water temperatures below 15°C; mortality may reach 50–90%. Survivors become lifelong carriers and shed large amounts of virus in urine and feces and in ovarian and seminal fluids at spawning. Acutely infected fish are dark in color, lethargic, and show anemia, exophthalmia, distention of the abdomen, and hemorrhages at the base of fins. Control measures center on isolation of premises and are similar to those for viral hemorrhagic septicemia. Elevation of water temperature to at least 18°C is very effective in controlling the disease but is usually not economically feasible. Inactivated and attenuated live-virus vaccines have been developed, but the most promising control measure for the future is selective breeding for resistance.

Spring Viremia of Carp

Spring viremia of carp occurs in European countries when the water temperature rises in spring. Diseased fish excrete large amounts of virus, and the virus can be spread by a blood-sucking ectoparasite, *Argulus*. Infected fish become lethargic and have abdominal swelling indicative of visceral organ edema and hemorrhages. Control is possible by isolation of premises. A vaccine has been developed, but it must be injected.

Other Rhabdovirus Diseases of Fish

Pike fry rhabdovirus causes a disease similar to spring viremia of carp virus in hatchery-reared pike fry in The Netherlands, where it is controlled primarily by isolation and by iodophor treatment of eggs to remove surface virus contamination. Rhabdoviruses with serologic properties similar to those of the pike fry rhabdovirus have been found in several species of cyprinids including the grass carp. Five rhabdoviruses have been isolated from eels that are serologically distinct from other known fish rhabdoviruses. None of the eel viruses has been demonstrated to cause disease in the freshwater stages of eel, but certain isolates are pathogenic for rainbow trout fry, inducing disease with hemorrhagic septicemia in salmonid fish. The hirame rhabdovirus causes serious losses among cultured Japanese flounder, which suffer a hemorrhagic disease with pathologic characteristics resembling viral hemorrhagic septicemia and infectious hempoietic necrosis in salmonids. The perch and Rio Grande cichlid rhabdoviruses have been isolated from fish cell lines and induce clinical diseases similar to those occurring naturally. The perch rhabdovirus appears to be serologically distinct from any known fish rhabdoviruses. Rhabdoviruses belonging to both *Lyssavirus* and *Vesiculovirus* have been isolated from snakeheads, an important food fish in Thailand; however, it has yet to be demonstrated whether they have a role in the chronic ulcerative syndrome often suffered by this species.

FURTHER READING

Advisory Committee on Immunization Practices, Centers for Disease Control. (1991). Rabies prevention—United States, 1991. *MMWR Rec. Rep.* **40,** 1.

Baer, G. M., ed. (1991). "The Natural History of Rabies," 2nd Ed. CRC Press, Boca Raton, Florida.

Baer, G. M., Birdbord, K., Hui, F. W., Shope, R. E., and Wunner, W. H., eds. (1988). Research toward rabies prevention. *Rev. Infect. Dis.* **10,** (Suppl. 4).

Bilsel, P. A., and Nichol, S. T. (1990). Polymerase errors accumulating during natural evolution of the glycoprotein gene of vesicular stomatitis–Indiana serotype isolates. *J. Virol.* **64,** 4873.

Bishop, D. H. L., ed. (1979–1980). "Rhabdoviruses," Vols. 1–3. CRC Press, Boca Raton, Florida.

Brochier, B., Kieny, M. P., Costy, F., Coppens, P., Bauduin, B., Lecocq, J. P., Languet, B., Chappuis, G., Desmettre, P., Afiademanyo, K., Libois, R., and Pastoret, P.-P. (1991).

Large-scale eradication of rabies using recombinant vaccinia–rabies vaccine. *Nature (London)* **354,** 520.
Calisher, C. H., Karabatsos, N., Zeller, H., Digoutte, J.-P., Tesh, R. B., Shope, R. E., Travasoos da Rosa, A. P. A., and St. George, T. D. (1989). Antigenic relationships among rhabdoviruses from vertebrates and hematophagous arthropods. *Intervirology* **30,** 241.
Leong, J.-A., and Munn, C. B. (1991). Potential uses of recombinant DNA in the development of fish vaccines. *Bull. Eur. Assoc. Fish Pathol.* **11,** 30.
National Association of State Public Health Veterinarians. (1990). Compendium of animal rabies control. *J. Am. Vet. Med. Assoc.* **196,** 36.
Pastoret, P.-P., Brochier, B., Blancou, J., Artois, M., Aubert, M., Kieny, M.-P., Lecocq, J.-P., Languet, B., Chappuis, G., and Desmettre, P. (1992). Development and deliberate release of a vaccinia-rabies recombinant virus for the oral vaccination of foxes against rabies. *In* "Recombinant Poxviruses" (M. M. Binns and G. L. Smith, eds.), p. 163. CRC Press, Boca Raton, Florida.
St. George, T. D. (1988). Bovine ephemeral fever. *In* "The Arboviruses: Epidemiology and Ecology" (T. P. Monath, ed.), Vol. 2, p. 71. CRC Press, Boca Raton, Florida.
Smith, J. S. (1989). Rabies virus epitopic variation: Use in ecologic studies. *Adv. Virus Res.* **36,** 215.
Smith, J. S. (1991). Rabies virus. *In* "Manual of Clinical Microbiology," 5th Ed., p. 936. American Society of Microbiology, Washington, D. C.
Wolf, K. (1988). "Fish Viruses and Fish Viral Diseases." Comstock Publ. Associates (Cornell Univ. Press), Ithaca, New York.
World Health Organization. (1984). WHO Expert Committee on Rabies. Seventh Report. WHO Tech. Rep Series 709. World Health Organization, Geneva.
Yuill, T. M. (1983). Vesicular stomatitis. *In* "CRC Handbook Series in Zoonoses" (H. Steele, ed.), p. 125. CRC Press, Boca Raton, Florida.

CHAPTER 29

Orthomyxoviridae

The family *Orthomyxoviridae* comprises the genus *Influenzavirus A and B*, which contains two species, influenza A virus and influenza B virus, and the genus *Influenzavirus C*, which contains one species, influenza C virus. Influenza A virus is of considerable interest to veterinarians, as different strains cause influenza in swine, equines, and avian species, as well as in humans. The mammalian influenza viruses cause local infections, usually restricted to the respiratory tract, whereas infections by avian influenza viruses occur as intestinal infections, with virulent strains (also called fowl plague) producing generalized infections. Avian strains of low virulence are endemic in many species of aquatic birds; all other forms of influenza usually occur as epidemics. Although influenza viruses are among the best studied of all animal viruses, efficient control of the diseases they cause has not yet been achieved. Influenza B and influenza C viruses cause disease in humans but not in species of veterinary importance; they will not be further discussed.

Swine influenza virus was isolated in 1931 and human influenza A virus in 1933. Although fowl plague had been known in Europe since the nineteenth century, the causative virus was not identified as an influenza A virus until 1955. Equine influenza virus was first isolated in 1956.

PROPERTIES OF INFLUENZA A VIRUS

Typical virions of influenza A virus are spherical and about 100 nm in diameter (Fig. 29-1), but larger, more pleomorphic forms are commonly seen (Table 29-1). There are eight virion proteins, five of which are structural and three associated with the RNA polymerase. The most abundant is the matrix protein (M1), which is composed of many identical small monomers associated with the inner surface of the lipid bilayer of the envelope. A second small protein M2 occurs in a small number of copies and projects as a pore through the membrane; it is the site of action of the drug amantidine. There are two kinds of peplomers, rod-shaped hemagglutinin (H) molecules, which are trimers, and mushroom-shaped neuraminidase (N) molecules, which are tetramers. Both H and N are glycoproteins and carry subtype-specific antigenic determinants. Antibodies to the hemagglutinin confer immunity to reinfection with any viral strain containing the same hemagglutinin. The RNA polymerase proteins PB1, PB2, and PA are associated with the ribonucleoprotein NP. The NP and M1 proteins determine species specificity, that is, they

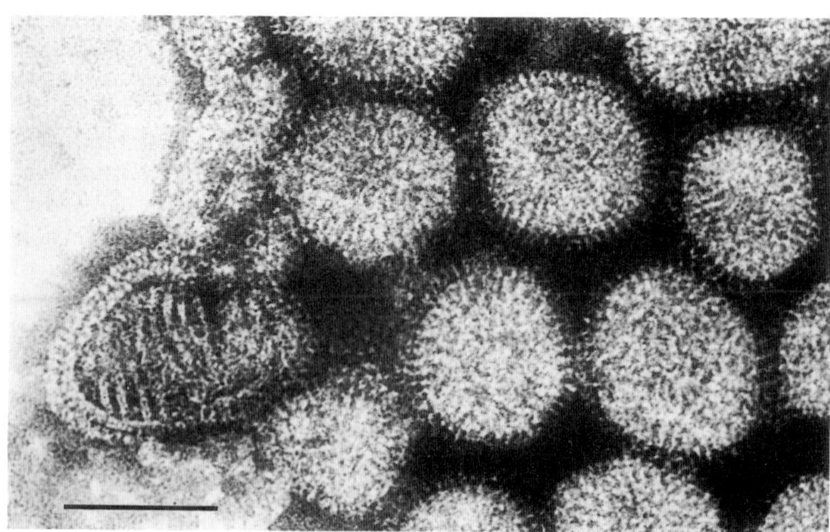

FIG. 29-1. Orthomyxoviridae. *Negatively stained preparation of virions of influenza A virus. Bar: 100 nm.*

TABLE 29-1
Properties of Influenza A Virus

Pleomorphic spherical or filamentous virion, diameter 80–120 nm
Envelope containing hemagglutinin (H) and neuraminidase (N) peplomers, a matrix protein (M1) on the inner surface, and a small number of pores composed of protein M2
Nucleoprotein of helical symmetry
Linear minus sense ssRNA genome, 13.6 kb, with 8 segments coding for 10 proteins: 5 structural, 3 associated with polymerase, and 2 nonstructural
Transcription and RNA replication in the nucleus; maturation by budding from plasma membrane; capped 5′ termini of cellular RNAs cannibalized as primers for mRNA transcription
Defective interfering particles and genetic reassortment frequently occur

distinguish between influenza A and B viruses, but antibodies to them are not protective, although both evoke cell-mediated immunity.

The minus sense ssRNA genome occurs as eight separate molecules, six of which code for a single protein and two (genes 7 and 8) for two proteins each (M1, M2, and NS1, NS2, respectively). Because of the segmented genome, genetic reassortment can occur in cells infected with two different strains of influenza A virus (see Chapter 4). Reassortment of the genes for hemagglutinin or neuraminidase produces antigenic shift. Mutations in these genes cause antigenic drift. Both of these processes occur in nature and generate the diversity which is responsible for the occurrence of epidemics.

The three influenzavirus species, A, B, and C have no shared antigens. Influenza A virus is divided into subtypes, all of which share related nucleoprotein and matrix proteins but differ in their hemagglutinin (H) and/or neuraminidase (N). So far, 14 subtypes of H (H1–H14) and 9 of N (N1–N9) have been described in birds, some of which have been found in various combinations of H and N in various species of mammals. Because any novel gene constellation can arise by genetic reassortment, any combination of H and N subtypes is theoretically possible; however, only a limited range of subtypes has so far been found in each mammalian species, although the full range occurs in birds. Viral isolates are codified as type (A or B), animal species, place, number of the isolate, year of isolation, followed in parentheses by the H and N subtypes. Thus the virus first isolated from horses in Prague in 1956 is designated as A/equi/Prague/1/56(H7N7).

Influenza viruses are sensitive to heat (56°C, 30 minutes), acid (pH 3), and lipid solvents. They are thus very labile under ordinary environmental conditions.

VIRAL REPLICATION

The influenza virus hemagglutinin (HA) adsorbs to glycoprotein receptors whose oligosaccharide side chains terminate in sialic acid, and the virion is taken up by endocytosis. In permissive cells, the HA is activated by cleavage into two parts, HA1 and HA2, which remain linked by disulfide bonds. A conformational change in the HA at the pH within the endosomes (pH 5) facilitates membrane fusion, thus triggering penetration. The nucleocapsid migrates to the nucleus where viral mRNA is transcribed by a unique mechanism, by which a viral endonuclease associated with the PB2 protein cleaves the 5′-methylguanosine cap plus 8–15 nucleotides from heterogeneous nuclear RNA, and this serves as a primer for transcription by the viral transcriptase. Of the eight primary RNA transcripts so produced, six are monocistronic mRNAs and are translated directly into the proteins representing H, N, NP, and the three components of the viral polymerase, PB1, PB2 and PA. The other two primary RNA transcripts undergo splicing, each yielding two mRNAs which are translated in different reading frames to produce M1, M2 and NS1, NS2.

The H and N polypeptides become glycosylated and acylated, and the virus matures by budding from the apical surface of the cell. It is not known by what mechanism one copy of each of the eight RNA segments is selected for incorporation into a virion and linked into a single nucleocapsid. Defective interfering particles, originally known as "incomplete virus," are often produced following infection at high multiplicity (see Chapter 4).

PATHOGENESIS AND IMMUNITY

The pathogenesis of swine and equine influenza virus infections resembles that in man (see Chapter 9). Infection occurs via the respiratory tract, by way of droplets generated by coughing and sneezing. Virions attach to the cilia of epithelial cells of the nose, trachea, and bronchi, or may be introduced directly into the alveoli, and within 2 hours viral antigen can be demonstrated in these cells. The virus spreads throughout the respiratory tract within 1 to 3 days. Transient viremia has been detected in equine influenza but appears to be rare. Necrosis of the epithelial cells coincides with the most severe clinical signs, fever and pneumonia. Influenza virus infection lowers resistance to secondary bacterial infection, which may cause bronchopneumonia.

The pathogenesis of avian influenza is quite different from that of influenza in mammals in that the virus replicates in the intestinal tract as well as the respiratory tract; virus is most readily isolated from the cloaca. In infections with virulent strains of influenza virus (fowl plague strains) viremia occurs, leading to a generalized infection. Hemorrhagic lesions may occur in the visceral organs as well as in the combs and wattles of chickens and turkeys. Avian influenza is often complicated by opportunistic secondary bacterial or viral infections.

In all species, serum antibodies detectable by hemagglutination–inhibition and neutralization tests appear 3 to 7 days after infection, reaching peak values during the second week. They may persist for up to 18 months. The antibody response in young animals is slower and less pronounced than in adults. Antibodies transferred from the dam to newborn piglets or foals via colostrum protect them for 30–35 days after birth. Secretory antibodies (IgA) are produced in the respiratory tract, appearing 8 days after infection and reaching maximal titers 1 week later. IgA titers decrease more rapidly than do the titers of antibodies in the serum. During the second week after infection, local and systemic cell-mediated responses can also be detected.

Antibody assays in birds are complicated by the fact that adult birds may have experienced infections with a variety of subtypes. Antibody titers are often low, especially in ducks.

LABORATORY DIAGNOSIS

All influenza viruses replicate well in 10-day-old embryonated hen's eggs, using either the amniotic or the allantoic route of inoculation and incubating at 35° to 37°C for 3–4 days. Viral replication is detected by the demonstration of hemagglutinating activity in the harvested amniotic or allantoic fluid. Cell culture systems used for research include chick embryo fibroblasts and the Madin-Darby canine kidney cell line (MDCK).

The best material for viral isolation from swine and horses is nasal mucus taken early in the course of the infection, or lung material obtained at necropsy. Avian influenza virus is often best isolated from cloacal swabs. Isolates from mammals can be identified by hemagglutination–inhibition tests, using a panel of subtype-specific sera. However, because birds may be infected with a variety of subtypes with different neuraminidase as well as different hemagglutinin antigens, isolates from birds should also be characterized by neuraminidase–inhibition tests.

Retrospective serologic diagnosis can be made in swine, horses, and humans, using the hemagglutination–inhibition test with paired serum samples, which must be suitably treated to eliminate nonspecifc inhibitors. Serologic methods are not of much value in birds, because of frequent infections with multiple serotypes.

SWINE INFLUENZA

Swine influenza was first observed in the north central United States at the time of the catastrophic 1918–1919 epidemic of human influenza, and for a long time it was reported only from this area, where annual outbreaks occurred each winter. It is one of the most prevalent respiratory diseases in swine in North America. In Europe, swine influenza was observed in the 1950s in Czechoslovakia, the United Kingdom, and West Germany; then the virus apparently disappeared. An outbreak was recorded again in 1976 in northern Italy and spread to Belgium and southern France in 1979. Since then swine influenza has spread rapidly to other European countries. Outbreaks have also been reported in Canada, South America, Asia, and Africa, beginning in 1968.

Swine influenza virus isolates made in Europe during and after 1979 are related to but are clearly distinct from the classic strains found in the United States. Antigenically and genetically recent European isolates, except those from Italy (which are similar to the strain from the United States), are closely related to H1N1 virus isolates from ducks. Thus two distinct antigenic variants of swine influenza virus, both of subtype H1N1, are currently cocirculating in swine in different parts of the world. Swine may also be infected with H3N2 strains of influenza virus, either from humans or birds, but such infections are inapparent. Reassortants have been detected in parts of Japan where both the H1N1 and H3N2 strains occur among swine, but so far these have not spread among humans or caused serious disease in swine.

Clinical Features

After an incubation period of 1–3 days, clinical signs, mainly restricted to the respiratory tract, appear suddenly in the majority of swine within a herd. Affected swine do not move freely and tend to huddle together. Rhinitis, nasal discharge, sneezing, and conjunctivitis develop, and weight loss is apparent in all sick swine. Infected swine have a paroxysmal cough, often associated with an arched back; breathing is rapid, labored, and often of abdominal type. Marked apathy, anorexia, and prostration are common, and the temperature rises to 41° to 41.5°C. After 3 to 6 days the swine usually recover quickly, eating normally by 7 days after appearance of the first clinical signs. If sick swine are kept warm and free of stress, the course of disease is benign with very few complications and a case–fatality rate of less than 1%, but some cases develop severe bronchopneumonia, which may result in death. Even when the swine recover, the economic consequences of swine influenza are considerable, in that sick swine either lose weight or their weight gains are reduced.

Epidemiology and Control

Swine influenza generally appears with the introduction of new swine from an infected into a susceptible herd. Frequently the disease appears simultaneously on several farms within an area, outbreaks being explosive, with all swine in a herd becoming sick at the same time. Outbreaks commence during late fall and are worst during the winter. Virus is shed in the nasal secretions, and pig-to-pig transmission probably occurs through droplets and small-particle aerosols.

The problem of the interepidemic survival of swine influenza virus has been a matter of intensive investigation for many years but it is still unsolved. Recent investigations suggest that the virus circulates in swine throughout the year and that some swine become carriers, manifesting disease only when the weather becomes colder.

Swine influenza virus (H1N1) also infects turkeys and humans. The infection in turkeys may induce clinical signs with respiratory disease or a decline in egg production and an increase in the number of abnormal eggs. Infections of humans with swine influenza virus is relatively common among slaughterhouse workers and may cause respiratory disease, but person-to-person spread is limited. However, the isolation of swine influenza virus from military recruits at Fort Dix in the United States in 1976 led to a massive immunization campaign among humans throughout the United States.

Symptomatic treatment may help prevent complications due to secondary infections. Recovery is more rapid if stress is avoided. Vaccines have been developed, but they have not been widely applied.

EQUINE INFLUENZA

Epidemics of influenza-like disease affecting horses and probably also donkeys and mules have been reported for centuries. The differentiation of equine influenza from other respiratory diseases was established in 1956 when influenza A virus (H7N7) was isolated from an epidemic among horses. A second equine virus, (H3N8), was first recovered from horses in the United States. The hemagglutinin of the first of these viruses (subtype 1) is related to that of some strains of fowl plague virus, whereas the hemagglutinin of the second (subtype 2) is antigenically related to human and some avian H3 strains. Neither subtype has undergone significant antigenic change since it was first isolated, except that antigenic drift has been detected in subtype 2, first in 1972 in South America and then in 1980 in the United States and Europe. A dramatic virgin-soil epidemic of subtype 2 influenza occurred in South Africa in 1988 following importation of horses from the United States.

In 1989 a severe outbreak of influenza A occurred in horses in northeast China, with a morbidity of 80% and a mortality of 20%; a second outbreak 1 year later was associated with a morbidity of about 50% but no mortality, probably because of the immune status of horses in the region. Of particular interest is the discovery that although the causative virus was the same antigenic composition as subtype 2 (H3N8), now circulating among horses in other parts of the world, sequence analysis of the eight genes showed that five were certainly and the other three possibly of recent avian origin. Thus, like outbreaks in swine influenza in Europe in 1979, this virus represents the transfer of an avian influenza virus to a mammal without reassortment.

Clinical Features

Signs of illness appear after an incubation period of 1–3 days, with reddening of the nasal mucosa, conjunctivitis, and increased nasal and conjunctival exudate. Usually there is transient swelling of the pharyngeal lymph nodes before a sudden elevation of temperature to between 39.5° and 41°C. The fever persists for up to 36 hours, and there is a dry, harsh, paroxysmal cough. Recovery begins after 1–2 weeks, provided sick horses are kept at rest and free of stress. Secondary bacterial or mixed viral infections may occur, with intervals of normal temperature alternating with periods of fever. Such chronic cases are characterized by purulent nasal exudate and catarrhal bronchopneumonia. In some outbreaks of equine influenza subtype 2, uncomplicated cases may also show a more severe, prolonged course.

Clinical diagnosis of acute cases is straightforward. Diagnosis in partially immune horses is more difficult, however, since equine influenza in such horses must be differentiated from other respiratory infections including equine herpesvirus 4, adenovirus, and rhinovirus infections.

Epidemiology

Equine influenza viruses are highly contagious and are spread rapidly in stables or studs by infectious exudate that is aerosolized by frequent coughing. Virus is excreted during the incubation period, and horses remain infectious for at least 5 days after clinical disease begins. Close contact between horses seems to be necessary for rapid transmission. Equine populations that are frequently moved, such as racehorses, breeding stock, show jumpers, and horses sent to sales, are at special risk. The rapid international spread of equine influenza is caused by year-round transport of horses for racing and breeding purposes, both in western Europe and between Europe and North America. Although clinical manifestations of equine influenza normally begin in the cold season, epidemics occur mostly during the main racing season, that is, between April and October in the northern hemisphere. Outbreaks are usually caused by one subtype. Apart from the recent outbreak in China, which appears to have been derived form an avian source, horses are the only known reservoir of equine influenza viruses.

Control

Stables and courses where equine influenza outbreaks occur should be put under quarantine for at least 4 weeks. Movement of persons associated with diseased horses should also be limited. After all horses have recovered, cleaning and disinfection of boxes and stables, equipment, and transport vehicles is necessary.

Prevention of equine influenza can be achieved by vaccination with a bivalent, inactivated vaccine, which is administered three times, the first two vaccinations 8–12 weeks apart, the third 6 months later. Revaccination is carried out at 9-month intervals. However, immunity to subtype 2 is weak and lasts only a short time. The experience following revaccination of racehorses every 3–6 months is excellent, and outbreaks of influenza no longer occur in such populations.

AVIAN INFLUENZA

Avian influenza viruses occur worldwide, and it seems likely that such viruses are the ultimate source of influenza viruses of mammals, either by direct transfer or via reassortment. Various species of wild birds, mainly waterfowl, constitute an important reservoir. Outbreaks of disease after infection with avian influenza viruses have been reported in various domestic and wild birds, chickens and turkeys being the most susceptible species. The clinical signs, course, and pathology in domestic birds are extremely variable. Infections can remain subclinical, develop into a mild, self-limiting disease, or induce severe acute generalized disease with high morbidity and mortality. The classic clinical signs of infection with highly virulent viruses, which belong to the subtypes H5 and H7, are the sudden onset and the occurrence of a generalized disease that is often lethal. Most avian influenza viruses are by themselves nonpathogenic, but if birds are coinfected with other microorganisms or if the environmental conditions are adverse severe disease may occur.

Avian influenza may cause tremendous economic losses. An outbreak in Pennsylvania and Virginia in 1983–1984, caused by an H5N2 virus (see Chapter 4), cost in indemnity alone approximately US$40 million. Since the 1980s influenza infection of turkeys has become economically the most important disease in this species in many parts of the United States. Losses arise from the high mortality rate, the drastic drop in egg and meat production, and the cost of control measures that include depopulation.

Properties of the Virus

A large number of different strains of influenza A have been isolated from birds, comprising all 14 known hemagglutinin subtypes and all 9 neuraminidase subtypes, in all possible combinations, from poultry as well as from wild birds. Highly pathogenic strains that produce fowl plague contain a hemagglutinin which is activated by proteolytic cleavage in a wide host cell spectrum both *in vitro* and *in vivo*. In countries where turkeys and ducks are reared for meat production, numerous isolations have been made from them, comprising almost all hemagglutinin subtypes including H1, H5, and H7. At times avian strains infect mammals; recent examples include swine in Europe in 1979 (H1N1), horses in China in 1989–1990 (H3N8), seals in waters of the northeastern United States in 1979–1980 and later years (H7N7), and mink in Sweden in 1984 (H10N4).

Clinical Features

The incubation period varies from a few hours to a few days, depending on the virus dose, the virulence of the strain, and the host species. Infection of chickens and turkeys with highly virulent viruses is characterized by the sudden onset of high mortality and also by cessation of egg laying, respiratory signs, excessive lacrimation, sinusitis, edema of the head and face, cyanosis, especially visible on the combs and wattles, and diarrhea. Less virulent viruses, although less lethal, may also cause considerable losses, particularly in turkeys, because of decreased egg production, respiratory disease, anorexia, depression, and sinusitis. Sometimes only some of these signs are seen. However, the clinical signs may be greatly exacerbated by concurrent infections (e.g., with Newcastle disease virus and various bacteria and mycoplasmas), the use of live-virus vaccines, or environmental stress (e.g., poor ventilation and overcrowding). In domestic ducks the most frequent signs are sinusitis, diarrhea, and increased mortality.

Laboratory Diagnosis

Clinical diagnosis is usually not possible except in an epidemic, because of the variability of signs and the resemblance to other avian diseases. Virus isolation is essential to establish the cause of an outbreak, since serologic diagnosis is unreliable. The widespread occurrence of avian influenza viruses of varying virulence makes it essential to determine the virulence of isolates from domestic birds in order to assess their significance. Of the various tests suggested, the intracerebral pathogenicity index and intravenous pathogenicity index tests, in 1-day-old chicks and 6-week-old chickens, respectively, are commonly used, although not without problems. Since the virulence of avian influenza viruses is in large part associated with the ability of a wide range of host cells to cleave the viral hemagglutinin, the production of plaques in a cell type permissive for virulent viruses but not permissive for avirulent viruses can also be used to assess virulence.

Epidemiology

The epidemiology of avian influenza is poorly understood because of the role of wild birds, the great variety of different strains, and the variable effects in different host species. Wild ducks and geese are regarded as refractory to disease, but wild ducks probably represent the most important reservoir of avian influenza viruses. Among domestic birds, chickens and turkeys are the species most likely to develop disease, but pheasants, quail, guinea fowl, and partridges also develop clinical illness.

The virus is shed with secretions from the respiratory tract and conjunctiva, and in feces. Transmission requires very close contact between birds, and airborne spread does not seem to play an important role. Since virus is excreted in large amounts with feces in which it can survive for long periods, mechanical spread may occur via birds, man, fomites, water, and food. Avian influenza viruses appear to be introduced into susceptible flocks periodically by interspecies transmission between chickens and turkeys, and from wild birds, especially wild ducks. Influenza in turkeys is seen principally in countries where the birds are kept in an environment to which wild birds have access.

Control

Initial control is aimed at preventing the introduction of avian influenza viruses. Legislative measures, including quarantine and trade limitations for birds and products, are provided by many countries to prevent their introduction. However, such measures do not affect wild birds, particularly migratory species, and in high-risk areas measures are therefore taken to prevent access of wild birds to poultry farms. These are not always successful, as evidenced by the Pennsylvania outbreak of 1983–1984, described in Chapter 4.

In the United States, Australia, and most European countries, virulent avian influenza virus is handled as an exotic virus; once diagnosed, quarantine and removal programs are implemented. To minimize secondary spread, strict hygienic measures must be introduced which include cleaning and disinfection, an interval between slaughter and repopulation, and controlled movement of people and animals. Vaccination has also been employed, but as with influenza in other animals there are problems in selecting the appropriate vaccine strain. Because of the risk of reassortment with "wild" viruses, only inactivated vaccines should be used, and because of the diversity of serotypes these must be polyvalent. However, experimental polyvalent vaccines are expensive and not very efficient. Local quarantine and depopulation of affected farms remain the only effective way to eradicate virulent influenza viruses from chicken and turkey farms.

FURTHER READING

Alexander, D. J., Beard, C. W., and Easterday, B. C., eds. (1987). "Proceedings of the Second International Symposium on Avian Influenza." Extension Duplicating Services, University of Madison, Wisconsin.

Kilbourne, E. D., ed. (1987). "Influenza." Plenum, New York.

Kingsbury, D. W. (1990). *Orthomyxoviridae* and their replication. *In* "Fields Virology" (B. N. Fields, D. M. Knipe, R. M. Chanock, M. S. Hirsch, J. L. Melnick, T. M. Monath, and B. Roizman, eds.), 2nd ed. p. 1075. Raven, New York.

Klenk, H.-D., and Rott, R. (1988). The molecular biology of influenza virus pathogenicity. *Adv. Virus Res.* **34,** 247.

Krug, R. M., ed. (1989). "The Influenza Viruses." Plenum, New York.

Murphy, B. R., and Webster, R. G. (1990). Orthomyxoviruses. *In* "Fields Virology" (B. N. Fields, D. M. Knipe, R. M. Chanock, M. S. Hirsch, J. L. Melnick, T. M. Monath, and B. Roizman, eds.), 2nd Ed., p. 1091. Raven, New York.

Stuart-Harris, C. H., and Potter, C. W., eds. (1984). "The Molecular Virology and Epidemiology of Influenza." Academic Press, London.

CHAPTER 30

Bunyaviridae

The largest family of mammalian viruses, *Bunyaviridae,* was one of the last to be recognized; the family now contains more than 200 viruses. Nearly all member viruses are arthropod-borne, replicating in and being transmitted by either mosquitoes, ticks, sandflies, or midges (*Culicoides*) in life cycles involving mammalian or avian vertebrate hosts. Member viruses of one genus, *Hantavirus,* are transmitted by urine and saliva (via bites) between reservoir rodent hosts, and also to humans. Two important zoonotic bunyaviruses, Rift Valley fever virus and Crimean–Congo hemorrhagic fever virus, command particular attention from national and international disease control agencies (Table 30-1).

Many bunyaviruses persist in their arthropod vectors via transovarial transmission: virus infects arthropod eggs so that larvae, nymphs, and adults of succeeding generations are infected and capable of transmission to vertebrate hosts.

PROPERTIES OF BUNYAVIRUSES

The virions of member viruses of the family *Bunyaviridae* (African place name: Bunyamwera) are spherical, approximately 90–100 nm in diameter (Fig. 30-1), and are composed of a lipid bilayer envelope with glycopro-

TABLE 30-1

Bunyaviruses Affecting Domestic Animals and Humans

Virus/genus	Geographic distribution	Arthropod vector	Animals affected	Diseases in domestic animals
Rift Valley fever/*Phlebovirus*	Africa	Mosquito	Sheep, cattle, buffalo, humans	Hepatitis, abortion, zoonosis
Akabane/*Bunyavirus*	Australia, Japan, Israel, Africa	Mosquito	Cattle, sheep	Congenital arthrogryposis–hydranencephaly
Cache Valley/*Bunyavirus*	United States	Mosquito	Cattle, sheep	Congenital infection
Nairobi sheep disease/*Nairovirus*	Eastern Africa	Mosquito	Sheep, goats	Hemorrhagic enteritis
Crimean hemorrhagic fever/*Nairovirus*	Africa, Asia	Tick	Sheep, cattle, goats, humans	Nil, zoonosis
Hantaan/*Hantavirus*	Asia	Nil	Rodents, humans	Nil, zoonosis
Belgrade/*Hantavirus*	Balkans	Nil	Rodents, humans	Nil, zoonosis
Puumala/*Hantavirus*	Northern Europe	Nil	Rodents, humans	Nil, zoonosis
Seoul/*Hantavirus*	Asia, North America	Nil	Rodents, humans	Nil, zoonosis

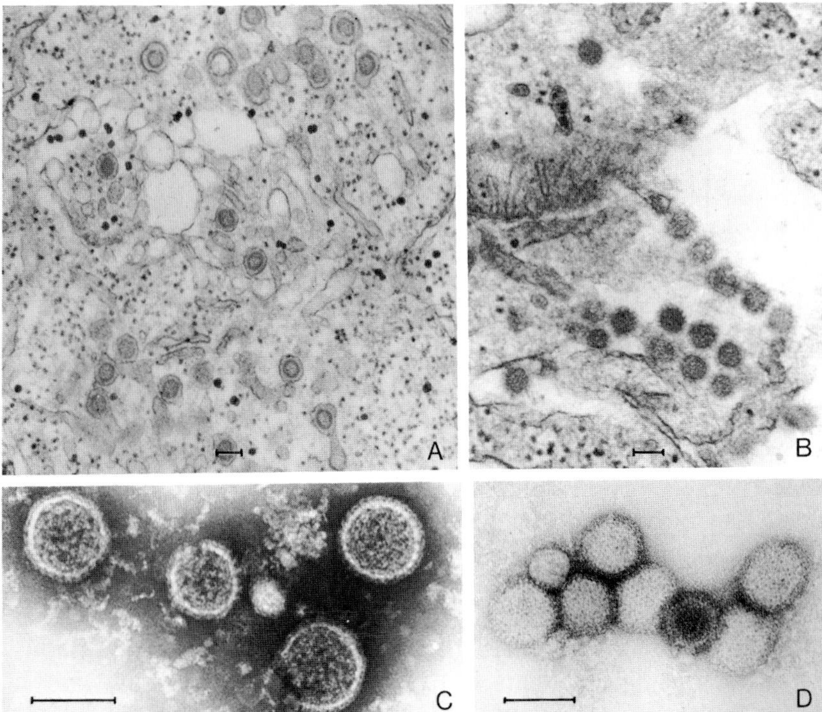

FIG. 30-1. Bunyaviridae. *(A and B) Sections of cultured cells. (A) Virions in Golgi vesicles. (B) Extracellular virions. (C and D) Negatively stained preparations. (C) Hantaan virus. (D) Rift Valley fever virus. Bars: 100 nm. (C, courtesy Drs. J. McCormick and E. L. Palmer; D, courtesy Dr. E. L. Palmer.)*

tein peplomers surrounding an interior containing three circular, helical nucleocapsids (Table 30-2). The genome consists of three linear segments of ssRNA, large (L), medium (M), and small (S), which differ in size in each genus but for *Bunyavirus* are 7, 4, and 0.9 kb, respectively, each formed into a circle by hydrogen bonding of the ends. The genome of the member viruses is primarily of minus sense, but remarkable differences in coding strategies of genes in the S segment have been found in viruses of some genera, leading to the coining of the term ambisense (see below). Virions contain four major proteins: a transcriptase (designated L, 150K–200K), a nucleoprotein (N, 25K–50K), and two glycoproteins (G1 and G2, 40K–120K) which form the surface peplomers. Epitopes for the complex antigenic interrelationships among the bunyaviruses are expressed on the glycoproteins as well as on the nucleoprotein.

TABLE 30-2
Properties of Bunyaviruses

Four genera of veterinary importance: *Bunyavirus, Nairovirus,* and *Phlebovirus,* which are arboviruses, and *Hantavirus,* which is non-arthropod-borne
Spherical, enveloped virion, 90–100 nm in diameter
Glycoprotein peplomers but no matrix protein in envelope
Three circular nucleocapsids with helical symmetry
Segmented minus sense ssRNA genome, total size 13.5–21 kb, three segments with complementary 3′ and 5′ termini; S segment of *Phlebovirus* genome is ambisense
Cytoplasmic replication; maturation by budding into Golgi vesicles
Genetic reassortment occurs between closely related viruses

Classification

The member viruses of the family *Bunyaviridae* are placed into genera on the basis of genetic relatedness (nucleotide sequence), mode of replication, size of genome segments, size of structural proteins, and antigenic relatedness (judged via indirect immunofluorescence, ELISA, and plaque-reduction neutralization tests). Five genera of vertebrate viruses (and one genus of plant viruses) have been defined. With few exceptions, viruses within a given genus are antigenically related to each other but not to viruses in other genera. As in other virus families, individual viruses are defined on the basis of unique specifity in cross-neutralization tests. There are four genera of vertebrate bunyaviruses that contain members of veterinary importance.

Bunyavirus. The genus *Bunyavirus* contains 18 serogroups and more than 160 viruses, most of which are mosquito-borne, but some of which are transmitted by sandflies or *Culicoides.* The genus includes more than 30 pathogens of domestic animals and humans, including Akabane, Cache Valley, La Crosse, Bunyamwera, and Oropouche viruses.

Phlebovirus. The genus *Phlebovirus* contains more than 60 viruses, all of which are transmitted by sandflies or mosquitoes. The genus contains important pathogens, including Rift Valley fever virus and the sandfly fever viruses.

Nairovirus. More than 33 viruses belong to the genus *Nairovirus,* mostly tick-borne, including the pathogens Crimean–Congo hemorrhagic fever, Nairobi sheep disease, and Dugbe viruses.

Hantavirus. The genus *Hantavirus* contains six viruses, none of which are arthropod-borne. All are transmitted via urine and saliva from their persistently infected reservoir rodent hosts in nature or from rats in laboratory colonies. Three of the hantaviruses cause human hemorrhagic fever with renal syndrome and similar diseases.

VIRAL REPLICATION

Bunyaviruses replicate well in many kinds of cell cultures, for instance, Vero (African green monkey) cells, BHK-21 (baby hamster kidney) cells, and mosquito (*Aedes albopictus*) cells (hantaviruses do not replicate in mosquito cells). Many also replicate to high titer in suckling mouse brain.

Viral entry into the host cell is via fusion of the viral envelope with the cell membrane; all steps in replication take place in the cytoplasm. After penetration of the host cell, the virion transcriptase is activated and transcribes subgenomic mRNAs from each of the three circular virion RNA species. After translation of these mRNAs, replication of the virion RNA and a second round of transcription occurs. The L RNA segment codes for the virion transcriptase, and the M segment codes for the G1 and G2 glycoproteins. In the genus *Bunyavirus,* the S RNA segment codes for two proteins from overlapping reading frames, the nucleoprotein and a nonstructural protein.

In the genus *Phlebovirus,* the S RNA segment also codes for two proteins, but a remarkable ambisense transcription strategy is employed (Fig. 30-2). The nucleocapsid protein (N) is encoded in the 3′ half of the viral RNA, and another protein (NSs) is encoded in the 5′ half, transcribed in the opposite direction via a complementary strand. Thus, in the transcription of the S segment, the minus sense 3′ half of the virion RNA species is transcribed into mRNA which is then translated into the nucleocapsid protein. The 5′ half of the S segment is not translated directly; instead, following replication of the whole RNA molecule, its complementary strand is transcribed into mRNA, which codes for the NSs protein. Translation of the *Phlebovirus* S segment RNA also involves overlapping reading frames. The hantaviruses have a single open reading frame in each segment (L, M, S) and no ambisense or overlapping strategies.

Genetic reassortment is a common feature but only among very closely related bunyaviruses. The viruses mature by budding into Golgi vesicles (see Fig. 30-1A) and are released by fusion of the vesicle membrane with the plasma membrane and exocytosis, or by cytolysis.

DISEASES CAUSED BY BUNYAVIRUSES

Viruses belonging to four genera, *Phlebovirus, Bunyavirus, Nairovirus,* and *Hantavirus,* cause diseases of veterinary importance.

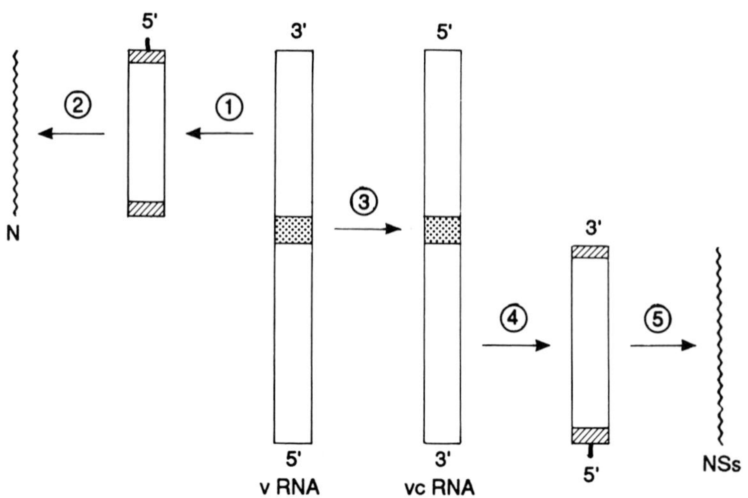

FIG. 30-2. *Ambisense gene expression of the S segment of the phlebovirus genome. The genomic RNA (vRNA) contains two open reading frames of about the same size that are read in opposite directions. (1) The vRNA is transcribed from the 3′ end to produce an mRNA of complementary sense that is translated into the N protein (2). After genomic replication (3), the full-length vcRNA is transcribed to produce a second mRNA of viral sense (4), which is translated into NSs (5). The hatched box in the center of the full-length RNAs represents the intergenic region between the two open reading frames (open boxes).*

Rift Valley Fever

Epidemics in sheep, goats, and cattle have been recognized in southern and eastern African countries from the time when intensive livestock husbandry was introduced at the beginning of the twentieth century. Between 1950 and 1976 there were at least 16 major epidemics in livestock at various places in sub-Saharan Africa. An exceptionally devastating epidemic of this mosquito-transmitted *Phlebovirus* infection occurred in Egypt in 1977 and 1978, resembling the biblical description of one of the plagues of ancient Egypt. There were many hundreds of thousands of cases in sheep and cattle and more than 200,000 human cases with 600 deaths. The extent and severity of this epidemic may have been due to the high population densities of fully susceptible animals and humans. In 1988–1989, further virus activity was detected in eastern Africa and in western Africa, with hundreds of human deaths in Senegal and Mauritania.

Clinical Features. Infected sheep develop fever, inappetence, vomiting, mucopurulent nasal discharge, and bloody diarrhea. Under field conditions, 90–100% of pregnant ewes abort, and there is a mortality rate of 90% in lambs and 20–60% in adult sheep. The clinical disease and outcome are similar in goats. In cattle the disease is somewhat less severe, with mortality rates in calves and cows of 10–30%, but pregnant cows always abort.

Pathogenesis and Immunity. After viral entry by mosquito bite or through the oropharynx, there is an incubation period of 30–72 hours, during which virus invades the parenchyma of the liver and reticuloendothelial organs, leading to widespread severe cytopathology. At necropsy of terminally affected sheep, it is not uncommon to find nearly total hepatocellular destruction. The spleen is enlarged, and there are gastrointestinal and subserosal hemorrhages. Encephalitis, evidenced by neuronal necrosis and perivascular inflammatory infiltration, is a late event, seen in a small proportion of animals surviving the hepatic infection. Recovery from encephalitis is quick, there are no sequelae, and immunity is long-lasting.

Rift Valley fever virus is a typical arbovirus, with an extrinsic incubation period of about 1 week. Virus produced in sex organs invades eggs as they are formed, thereby initiating a transovarial transmission cycle.

Laboratory Diagnosis. Because of its broad geographic distribution and its explosive potential for invading new areas of Africa where livestock farming is extensive, the laboratory confirmation of the presence of Rift Valley fever virus is treated as a diagnostic emergency. The virus, isolated in mice or in cell culture, is usually identified serologically. Retrospective serologic diagnosis is possible by demonstrating a rise in antibody titer in surviving animals.

Epidemiology. In eastern, western, and southern Africa, Rift Valley fever virus survives in a silent or minimally evident endemic cycle for many years and then, when there is exceptionally heavy rainfall, explodes in epidemics of great magnitude. Although such outbreaks had been studied for many years, it was not until recently that there has been any satisfactory explanation of this phenomenon. In an epidemic, Rift Valley fever virus is transmitted by many species of *Culex* and *Aedes* mosquitoes; important vector species have been proven by epidemiologic and laboratory studies. These mosquitoes are very numerous after heavy rains or when improper irrigation techniques are used; they are infected when feeding on viremic sheep and cattle (and humans). A very high level of viremia is maintained for 3–5 days in infected sheep and cattle, allowing many mosquitoes to become infected. This amplification of the transmission cycle, together with mechanical transmission by biting flies, results in infection and disease in a very high proportion of animals (and humans) at risk.

The epidemic cycles are started by infected mosquitoes occupying an unusual ecologic niche. Throughout the grassy plateau regions of eastern, western, and southern Africa, there are dry depressions in which floodwater *Aedes* species live, surviving long periods of drying as eggs and emerging only when the depressions are filled by exceptional rainfall. These mosquitoes are transovarially infected with Rift Valley fever virus and are capable of transmitting the virus to a few sheep, cattle, and wild ruminants, and thus starting epidemics which are maintained and amplified by other mosquito species.

In its epidemic cycles Rift Valley fever virus may also be spread directly by fomites, by direct contact, and mechanically by arthropods such as tabanid flies. Infected sheep have a very high level of viremia, and transmission at the time of abortion via contaminated placenta and fetal and maternal blood is a particular problem. Abattoir workers and veterinarians (especially those performing necropsies) are often infected directly.

The capacity of Rift Valley fever virus to be transmitted without the involvement of an arthropod vector raises clear concerns over the possibility for its importation into nonendemic areas via infected, viremic animals or humans or even via animal products. Although the virus has never appeared outside Africa, it is not clear why this is so. The source of the virus which initiated the 1977 epidemic in Egypt was never found. As was the case in Egypt, mosquito species capable of efficient transmission are present in most of the livestock-producing areas of the world.

Prevention and Control. Vaccination is used for the protection of sheep and cattle; vector control may be used to attempt to control severe epidemics in farm animals or in humans.

Vaccination. Attenuated live-virus Rift Valley fever vaccines for use in sheep, produced in mouse brain and in embryonated eggs, are effective and inexpensive, but they cannot be used in pregnant animals because they cause abortions. Inactivated virus vaccines produced in cell cultures avoid the problem of abortion. Both types of vaccines have been produced in Africa in large quantities, but, to be effective, vaccines must be delivered in a systematic way to entire animal populations, preferably on a regular schedule before the start of the mosquito season, or at least at the first indications of viral activity. These requirements make control very expensive and demanding of a skilled disease control infrastructure, an almost impossible proposition in the areas of the world where the disease exists. Even if vaccines are used only in the face of an epidemic, outbreaks occur with such explosive speed that it is difficult to deliver enough vaccine fast enough. Moreover, even when vaccine is delivered quickly, there is often not enough time for protective immunity to develop.

Vector Control. Insecticide use must be comprehensive because of the involvement in epidemics of a wide range of vectors, and it must be distributed over large areas and throughout vector breeding seasons. This is virtually impossible in Africa, but would be done if Rift Valley fever were to occur outside that continent.

Disease in Humans. Rift Valley fever virus is zoonotic and causes an important human disease that occurs coincidentally with outbreaks in ruminants. The human disease is marked by fever, chills, severe headache, "back-breaking" myalgia, diarrhea, vomiting, and hemorrhages, usually with a course of 4–6 days followed by complete recovery. In a small proportion of cases there is meningoencephalitis, hemorrhagic lesions, and/or retinitis. The overall case–fatality rate in humans is about 0.1%, but in the rare hemorrhagic fever syndrome it may reach 10%.

Akabane Disease (Congenital Arthrogryposis–Hydranencephaly Syndrome)

Seasonally, in some years, in Australia, Japan, and Israel, there are epidemics in cattle of fetal or newborn arthrogryposis and hydranencephaly, abortions, and fetal death, caused by Akabane virus, a mosquito-borne member of the genus *Bunyavirus* (for history, see Chapter 14). The virus can cause the same disease in sheep and goats. There is evidence that the virus is present in other countries of the southwest Pacific region, and in Turkey, Kenya, and South Africa. In Japan more than 42,000 bovine cases were recorded between 1972 and 1975.

Following the bite of an infected mosquito, the virus infects the pregnant cow without producing clinical signs and reaches the fetus from the maternal circulation. The primary fetal infection is an encephalomyelitis and polymyositis. Severely affected fetuses die and are aborted, but survivors develop hydranencephaly and neurogenic arthrogryposis (Fig. 30-3). Calves infected between the third and fourth months of gestation show hydranencephaly at birth; those infected between the fourth and sixth months develop arthrogryposis.

Diagnosis is suggested by clinical, pathologic, and epidemiologic observations, and may be confirmed by detection of specific antibody in serum taken from aborted fetuses or presuckle serum from deformed calves, or by detection of a titer rise between paired maternal sera. Virus is difficult to isolate after calves are born, but it can be recovered from placenta or fetal brain or muscle of calves taken by cesarian section or after slaughter of the cow by inoculation of cell cultures or by intracerebral inoculation of suckling mice.

In Japan, Akabane virus is transmitted by *Aedes* and *Culex* mosquitoes, and in Australia by the midge, *Culicoides brevitarsis.* It is not known

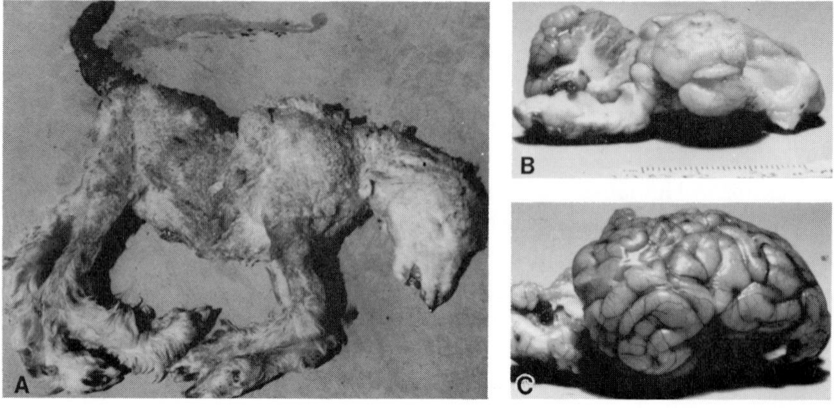

FIG. 30-3. *Akabane virus infection. (A) Arthrogryposis in a lamb born during an outbreak of Akabane infection in Australia. (B) Microencephaly, which involves mainly the cerebral hemispheres. (C) Normal brain (part of the cerebellum has been removed). (A, courtesy of Dr. I. M. Parsonson.)*

whether the virus is transmitted transovarially in any of these vectors. An inactivated virus vaccine produced in cell culture has proved safe and efficacious in Japan and Australia. In the United States, outbreaks of arthrogryposis–hydranencephaly have been seen in sheep associated with infections with another member of the genus *Bunyavirus,* Cache Valley virus.

Nairobi Sheep Disease

Nairobi sheep disease virus (genus *Nairovirus*) is the cause of disease in sheep and goats in eastern Africa. Related viruses occur in Nigeria (Dugbe virus of cattle) and India (Ganjam virus in sheep and goats). The virus is transmitted by all stages of the tick *Rhipicephalus appendiculatus,* in which transovarial infection occurs. The vertebrate reservoir host of the virus remains unknown; the virus has not been found in wild ruminants or other animals in the area.

In Kenya, sheep and goats acquire the infection when they are transported from northern districts to the Nairobi area. After a short incubation period there is high fever, hemorrhagic enteritis, and prostration. Affected animals may die within a few days, and pregnant ewes abort. Subclinical infections also occur, and recovered animals are immune. Control depends primarily on dipping to control the tick vector *Rhipicephalus,* which is also the vector of the economically important protozoal disease, East Coast fever. Vaccines are effective in preventing the disease in sheep.

Crimean–Congo Hemorrhagic Fever

Crimean hemorrhagic fever has been recognized for many years in central Asia and eastern Europe as a severe zoonotic disease affecting farmers and other people coming in contact with livestock, as well as woodcutters and other people coming in contact with ticks. The hemorrhagic fever in humans is marked by fever, prostration, and subcutaneous, gastroenteric, and genitourinary hemorrhage. There is a necrotizing hepatitis and damage to the heart and central nervous system; the case–fatality rate is about 10%. The causative virus is identical to a virus, originally named Congo virus, which causes a nonfatal febrile disease in humans in central Africa. The distribution of Crimean–Congo hemorrhagic fever virus is now known to extend from China through central Asia to India, Pakistan, Afghanistan, Iran, Iraq, other Persian Gulf countries, the Middle East, eastern Europe, to most of Saharan and sub-Saharan Africa.

The virus is maintained by a cycle involving transovarial transmission in *Hyalomma* ticks and tick transmission to domestic and wild ruminants and humans. There is no evidence that there is a clinical disease in animals other than man. The virus is also transmitted to man by direct contact with subclinically infected viremic animals, for example, during sheep shearing or veterinary procedures, and it is also transmitted from man to man, especially nosocomially. This is an emerging problem, with more and more cases being reported each year from many parts of the world and more and more antibody being found in animal populations. For example, about 8% of cattle in parts of Africa have evidence of having been infected. Prevention, which involves vector control, is difficult because of the large areas of wooded and brushy tick habitat involved.

Hemorrhagic Fever with Renal Syndrome

During the Korean war of 1950–1952, thousands of United Nations troops developed a disease marked by fever, headache, hemorrhagic manifestations, and acute renal failure with shock; the mortality rate following infection was 5–10%. The etiologic agent of this disease remained a mystery until 1978 when a virus, named Hantaan virus, was isolated in Korea from the field rodent *Apodemus agrarius* and identified as a unique bunyavirus. Recently, six related viruses have been found in other parts of the world in association with other rodents; these viruses comprise the genus *Hantavirus*. Four of these viruses have been associated with human diseases with varying clinical manifestations and a variety of local names.

The hallmark of the natural history of the hantaviruses is their lifelong inapparent infection of the reservoir rodent hosts, and their persistent shedding from these hosts in urine and saliva. Human disease involves close contact with the rodents, usually in winter when human–rodent contact is facilitated.

Epidemiologically, there are three disease patterns: rural, urban, and laboratory-acquired; from a clinical standpoint there are two disease patterns: severe (with significant mortality) and mild (without mortality). Each pattern is determined by the rodent/virus combination involved. The rural severe disease caused by Hantaan virus is widespread in the Far East (Korean hemorrhagic fever; China: epidemic hemorrhagic fever); a similar disease is caused in Greece and the Balkans by Belgrade virus. The rural mild disease caused by Puumala virus in common in northern Europe, especially in Scandinavia (Scandinavia: nephropathia epidemica; Russia: epidemic hemorrhagic fever). The urban disease, of variable severity, is associated with house rats (*Rattus rattus* and *Rattus norvegicus*) and is caused by Seoul virus; it occurs in Japan, Korea, China, South America, and the United States. Control of the rural and urban patterns of disease depends mainly on avoidance of contact between man and rodents.

From the veterinary point of view, the most important pattern of disease is that involving laboratory rats (and wild reservoir host rodents brought into laboratories) and transmission to animal caretakers and research personnel. There have been episodes of human disease in Belgium, Korea, the United Kingdom, and Japan, totalling more than 100 cases acquired in laboratories and 1 death. Prevention of introduction of the virus into laboratory rat colonies requires quarantined entry of new stock (or entry only of known virus-free stock), prevention of access by wild rodents, and serologic testing. Prevention of further distribution of these viruses involves the testing of all rat-origin cell lines before release from cell culture collections.

FURTHER READING

Bishop, D. H. L. (1990). *Bunyaviridae* and their replication. Part I: *Bunyaviridae*. *In* "Fields Virology" (B. N. Fields, D. M. Knipe, R. M. Chanock, M. S. Hirsch, J. L. Melnick, T. P. Monath, and B. Roizman, eds.), 2nd Ed., p. 1155. Raven, New York.

Calisher, C. H. (1993). Family *Bunyaviridae*, genus *Bunyavirus* (the bunyaviruses). *In* "Handbook of Infectious Diseases" (E. H. Kass, T. H. Weller, S. M. Wolfe, and D. A. J. Tyrrell, eds.), (in press).

Gonzalez-Scarano, F., and Nathanson, N. (1990). Bunyaviruses. *In* "Fields Virology"

(B. N. Fields, D. M. Knipe, R. M. Chanock, M. S. Hirsch, J. L. Melnick, T. P. Monath, and B. Roizman, eds.), 2nd Ed., p. 1195. Raven, New York.

Kolakofsky, D., ed. (1991). *Bunyaviridae. Curr. Top. Microbiol. Immunol.* **169.**

Le Duc, J. (1987). Epidemiology of Hantaan and related viruses. *Lab. Anim. Sci.* **37,** 413.

Meegan, J. M. (1979). The Rift Valley fever epizootic in Egypt 1977–1978. I. Description of the epizootic and virological studies. *Trans. R. Soc. Trop. Med. Hyg.* **73,** 618.

Parsonson, I. M., and Patterson, J. L. (1985). Bunyavirus pathogenesis. *Adv. Virus Res.* **30,** 279.

Schmaljohn, C. S., and Patterson, J. L. (1990). *Bunyaviridae* and their replication. Part II. *In* "Fields Virology" (B. N. Fields, D. M. Knipe, R. M. Chanock, M. S. Hirsch, J. L. Melnick, T. P. Monath, and B. Roizman, eds.), 2nd Ed., p. 1175. Raven, New York.

CHAPTER 31

Reoviridae

The family *Reoviridae* (named from respiratory enteric orphan viruses) includes three genera of veterinary importance: *Orthoreovirus, Orbivirus,* and *Rotavirus.* Colorado tick fever virus, which causes disease in humans but not in domestic animals, is the prototype of a fourth genus, *Coltivirus.* Three other genera in this family that infect plants and insects will not be discussed further. Although ubiquitous, most orthoreoviruses are nonpathogenic, but the genera *Orbivirus* and *Rotavirus* contain several important pathogens of domestic animals (Table 31-1).

PROPERTIES OF REOVIRUSES

Members of the family *Reoviridae* have nonenveloped spherical virions 60–80 nm in diameter, which consist of one or two outer protein coats and an inner protein coat; particles with the outer coat(s) removed are termed cores (Table 31-2). The genera differ in the number and size of segments of dsRNA in the genome and in the structure of the outer capsid (Fig. 31-1).

TABLE 31-1
Diseases of Veterinary Importance Caused by Reoviruses

Genus	Viruses, including serotype numbers	Principal species affected	Disease
Orthoreovirus	Mammalian orthoreovirus 1–3	Isolated from many species of mammals and birds	Hepatoencephalomyelitis in mice
	Avian orthoreovirus 1–11	Chickens, turkeys, and geese	Arthritis, nephrosis, enteritis, chronic respiratory disease, myocarditis
Orbivirus[a]	Bluetongue virus 1–24	Sheep, cattle, and deer	Bluetongue
	Ibaraki virus	Cattle	Acute febrile disease similar to bluetongue
	Epizootic hemorrhagic disease of deer virus 1–7	Deer	Epizootic hemorrhagic disease
	Palyam virus 1–6	Cattle	Abortion, congenital abnormalities
	African horse sickness virus 1–9	Horses, donkeys, mules, and zebras	African horse sickness
	Equine encephalosis virus 1–5	Horses	Abortion and encephalitis
Rotavirus	Rotavirus: many types, often host-specific	Most animals (including fish)	Enteritis

[a] Besides those listed, there are several other serogroups within the *Orbivirus* genus, none of which is known to cause diseases of domestic animals.

TABLE 31-2
Properties of Reoviruses

Nonenveloped spherical virion, diameter 60–80 nm

Two concentric capsids; outer capsid differs in appearance in different genera, inner capsid (core) is icosahedral in all genera

dsRNA genome, 10–12 segments, total size 18–27 kb; four genera infect vertebrates: *Orthoreovirus*, 10 segments, 23 kb; *Orbivirus*: 10 segments, 23 kb; *Rotavirus*, 11 segments, 18 kb; *Coltivirus*, 12 segments, 27 kb

Five enzymes including transcriptase in core

Cytoplasmic replication; after entry and degradation to a core, transcriptase and capping enzymes transcribe and cap early mRNAs; later genes are derepressed by an early protein, and more dsRNA molecules are synthesized, from which late uncapped mRNAs for structural proteins are transcribed

Genetic reassortment occurs between species within each genus

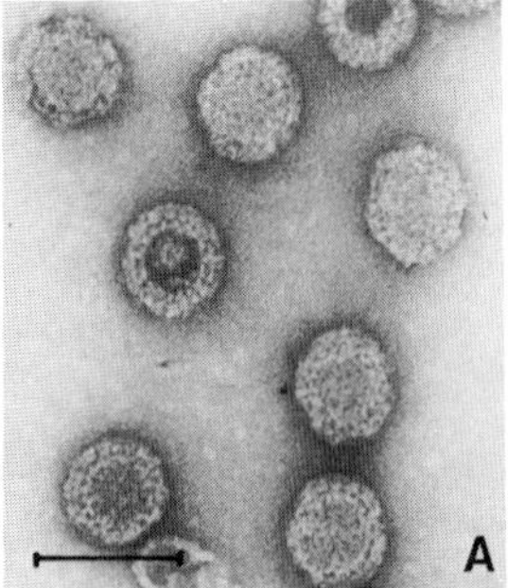

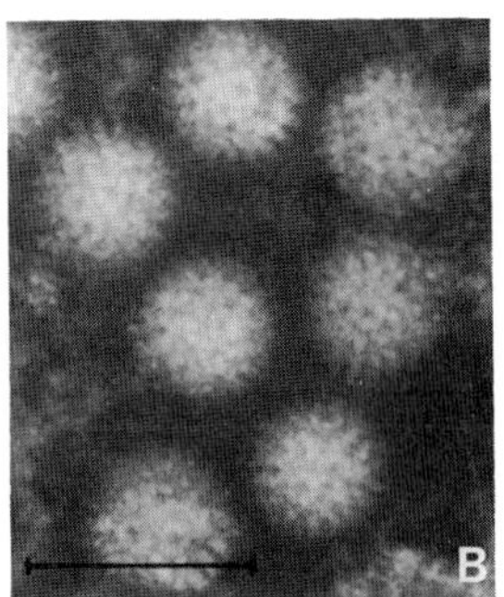

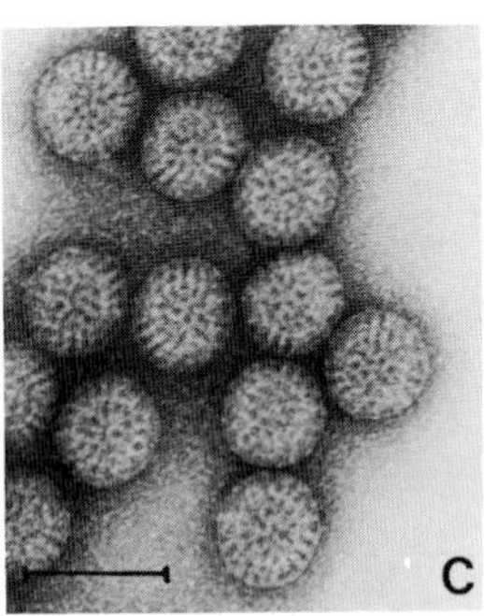

FIG. 31-1. Reoviridae. *(A)* Orthoreovirus. *(B)* Orbivirus *(bluetongue virus). (C)* Rotavirus. *Bars: 100 nm. (Courtesy Dr. E. L. Palmer).*

Orthoreovirus. The outer capsid forms a nearly spherical icosahedron composed of hexagonal and pentagonal subunits, consisting predominantly of complexes of the proteins $\sigma3$ and $\mu1C$ (see Fig. 7-1). The viral hemagglutinin, $\sigma1$, is a minor component of the outer capsid that is located close to the 12 core spikes. The inner capsid (core) consists of three major proteins, $\lambda1$, $\lambda2$, and $\sigma2$, and several minor proteins. The RNA of orthoreoviruses consists of three size classes, which can be further differentiated by polyacrylamide gel electrophoresis into ten discrete segments. These code for ten species of protein, one of which is cleaved during translation.

Orbivirus. The outer capsid of orbiviruses consists of a diffuse layer formed by two proteins but lacking any clear morphologic units, which is readily dissociated from the core. The genome is in ten segments, with a different size distribution from those of orthoreoviruses, each encoding a distinct polypeptide. Seven structural proteins and three nonstructural proteins have been identified.

Rotavirus. The outer capsid of rotaviruses contains 132 capsomers, each containing small holes; it consists of VP4 and, as a major component, a glycoprotein VP7. The inner capsid, composed of VP6, is readily dissociated from the core, which is composed of three proteins VP1, VP2, and VP3. The genome of rotaviruses has 11 segments, which, after posttranslational modification, code for 13 proteins, of which 8 are structural proteins.

Orthoreoviruses and rotaviruses are resistant to lipid solvents and are stable over a wide pH range, but orbiviruses have a narrow zone of pH stability (pH 6–8), and lose some infectivity on exposure to ether. Proteolytic enzymes, in general, increase the infectivity of orthoreoviruses and rotaviruses; for example, chymotrypsin, which is found in the small intestine, leads to loss of the outer capsid of orthoreoviruses, enhancing infectivity.

In the presence of protein orbiviruses are remarkably stable; bluetongue virus has been reisolated from blood held for 25 years at room temperature. Not all disinfectants are active against rotaviruses; although iodophors and phenolic compounds inactivate the virus, hypochlorite is ineffective.

VIRAL REPLICATION

The replication cycle has been studied in most detail with orthoreovirus 3. The intact virion may enter the cell by receptor-mediated endocytosis; alternatively, intermediate subviral particles (ISVPs) (Fig. 31-2), resulting

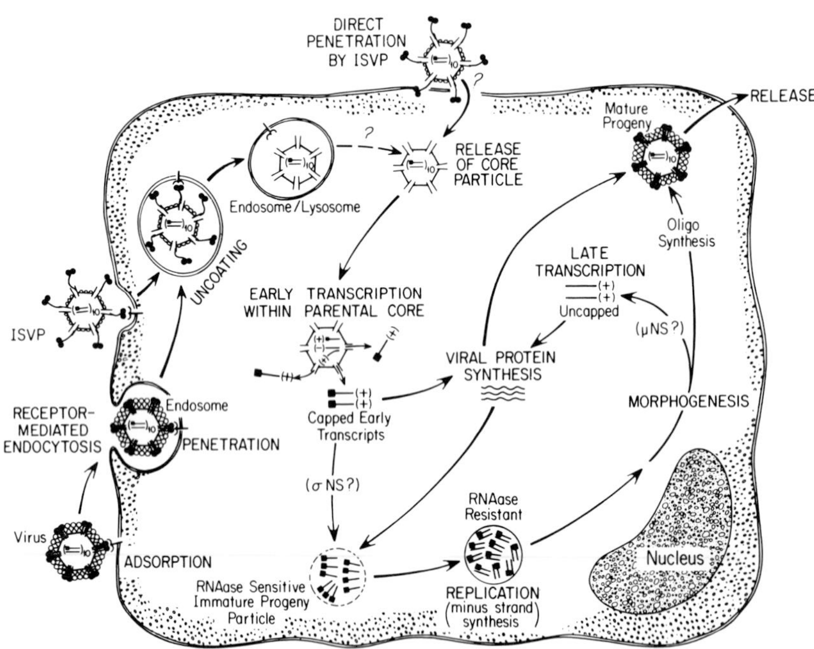

FIG. 31-2. *Diagram of the orthoreovirus replication cycle. After entry by receptor-mediated endocytosis or as an intermediate subviral particle (ISVP) produced outside the cell by intestinal proteases, a viral core is released, mRNAs are transcribed and capped, and early protein is synthesized. After synthesis of new dsRNAs, late, uncapped mRNAs for structural proteins are produced. Maturation occurs by self-assembly, and virions are released by cell lysis. [From L. A. Schiff and B. N. Fields,* In *"Fields Virology" (B. N. Fields, D. M. Knipe, R. M. Chanock, M. S. Hirsch, J. L. Melnick, T. P. Monath, and B. Roizman, eds.), 2nd Ed., p. 1275. Raven, New York, 1990].*

from digestion with chymotrypsin in the intestine, may enter directly into the cytoplasm, without entering coated vesicles or lysosomes. Both types of particles are then degraded to become "core particles," and the virion-associated transcriptase and capping enzymes transcribe 5′-capped mRNA molecules, which are not polyadenylated at their 3′ termini. Only certain genes are transcribed initially; the others are derepressed following the synthesis of an early viral protein. Protein associates with each mRNA molecule, and minus sense RNA strands are synthesized within subviral particles, producing dsRNA molecules. These in turn serve as templates for the transcription of more mRNA, which this time is uncapped. These uncapped reovirus mRNA molecules are then translated preferentially to yield a large pool of viral structural proteins, which self-assemble to form the viral core and outer capsid, the new virions being released by cell lysis.

Rotavirus Replication. Distinctive features of rotavirus replication are (1) rotaviruses enter the cytoplasm directly through the plasma membrane, penetration depending on specific cleavage of VP4 by trypsin, and (2) subviral particles bud through the membrane of the rough endoplasmic reticulum, where they briefly acquire an envelope. After separate secretion of the outer capsid glycoprotein VP7 into the endoplasmic reticulum, the temporary envelope breaks down, and VP7 assembles to complete the thin layer of protein that ultimately comprises the outer capsid of the mature virion.

DISEASES CAUSED BY ORTHOREOVIRUSES

Orthoreoviruses are generally considered to be nonpathogenic, the important exceptions being infections of rodents and poultry. There are three serotypes of mammalian orthoreovirus, all of which infect a wide range of species and are found worldwide. In mouse colonies, orthoreovirus 3 can cause natural disease, sometimes called hepatoencephalomyelitis, which is characterized by jaundice, ataxia, oily hair, and growth retardation.

Avian orthoreoviruses, of which 11 serotypes have been identified, cause disease in some flocks but are associated with only subclinical infection in others. They cause chronic respiratory disease in chickens, turkeys, and geese. They have also been associated with tenosynovitis and arthritis, usually in meat-producing birds over 5 weeks old. Bilateral swelling of the digital flexor and the tarsometatarsal extensor tendons produces lameness and can lead to rupture of the gastrocnemius tendon. Articular erosions may be recognized in chronic cases. Morbidity is often 100%, usually with a mortality of less than 2%.

Avian orthoreoviruses are most easily isolated in avian cell cultures and produce vacuoles in cells prior to syncytium formation. Identification of an isolate as being an orthoreovirus can be made by fluorescent antibody techniques; a serum neutralization test is used for typing.

DISEASES CAUSED BY ORBIVIRUSES

Bluetongue and African horse sickness have been diseases of economic importance in South Africa since the early days of European settlement. The importance of these two diseases in Africa and their ability to cause periodic but extensive epidemics in the Middle East and parts of Europe stimulated scientific inquiry into similar viruses in other parts of the world. It has now emerged that many orbiviruses exist that are nonpathogenic for domestic animals. Isolates have been made from many different families of arthropods (mosquitoes, midges, sandflies, and ticks), and from birds and terrestrial mammals. All orbiviruses so far discovered appear to be arthropod-borne.

The orbiviruses are differentiated into 13 distinct serogroups and one unclassified group, of which six include viruses that produce disease in domestic animals (see Table 31-1). No genus-specific antigen has been detected, but viruses within a serogroup have a common antigen demonstrable by immunofluorescence, immunodiffusion, and complement fixation tests. Low-level cross-reactions among individual viruses, normally considered members of distinct serogroups, have been reported, causing some uncertainty in serologic classification. Reassortment of genome segments between serologically related viruses has been described for the bluetongue and other serogroups, and a classification system based on genetically interacting groups has also been advanced.

Bluetongue

Bluetongue is an arthropod-borne virus disease of ruminants characterized by congestion, edema, and hemorrhage. The disease is of most importance in sheep, in which its severity varies from subclinical to severe depending on the strain of virus, the breed of sheep, and the local ecology. Economic losses result from death and loss of condition in sheep that survive. Convalescence may be protracted and wool growth may be impaired, leading to the production of poor fleeces. Infection of cattle and goats is often inapparent, but disease can be severe in some wildlife species, particularly white-tailed deer (*Odocoileus virginianus*) in North America. The virus can cause congenital infection in cattle and sheep, resulting in abortions and fetal abnormalities.

Until the 1940s bluetongue was recognized only in Africa, then its presence was confirmed in the countries of the eastern Mediterranean. In 1956–1957 a major epidemic occurred in Portugal and Spain in which hundreds of thousands of sheep were affected. This epidemic generated a worldwide escalation in the recognition of bluetongue as an "emerging disease" likely to cause severe economic losses. The virus was first isolated in the western hemisphere from sheep in California in 1952 and from cattle in Oregon in 1959. By the late 1970s it was realized that bluetongue virus was more widely distributed than had previously been thought, and it is probable that some livestock in most, if not all, countries in the tropics and subtropics are infected with bluetongue or closely related viruses.

The inclusion of a virus within the bluetongue group is based on the detection of a group antigen; 24 bluetongue virus types are currently recognized. As mentioned earlier, orbiviruses do not always fit neatly into serogroups, and the terms "bluetongue-like virus" and "bluetongue-related virus" have emerged to confuse the nomenclature. Classification of viruses may appear to be a topic of esoteric interest, but in fact a diagnosis of "bluetongue" has a profound effect on international livestock trade. Veterinarians responsible for international disease control usually err on the side of caution when they become aware of "bluetongue-related" or "bluetongue-like" viruses in the exporting country.

Clinical Features. In sheep, the disease is characterized by fever which may last several days before hyperemia, excess salivation, and frothing at the mouth are noticed; a nasal discharge, initially serous but becoming mucopurulent and speckled with blood, is common. The tongue may become cyanosed, hence "bluetongue." There is a marked loss of condition, and the sheep may die, often through aspiration pneumonia. The coronary bands of the feet exhibit hyperemia and are painful. Edema of the head and neck is not uncommon; animals with coronitis are often reluctant to walk and tend to be recumbent (Fig. 31-3). Hyperemia of the skin may occur, leading to "wool break" some weeks later. Muscle degeneration occurs, and in many animals convalescence is protracted. Morbidity may be as high as 80% and mortality 50%.

The disease in deer is similar. In contrast, the disease in cattle is usually inapparent and rarely acute. Some strains of bluetongue (possibly of modified-live virus vaccine origin, but transmitted by arthropod vectors) may cause abortion and congenital abnormalities (Fig. 31-3D). In calves and lambs infected *in utero,* viremia may be present at birth and persist for several weeks.

Pathogenesis. Bluetongue virus replicates in hemopoietic cells and endothelial cells of the blood vessels. Adult sheep sometimes remain viremic for 14 to 28 days, and in cattle the virus can persist for as long

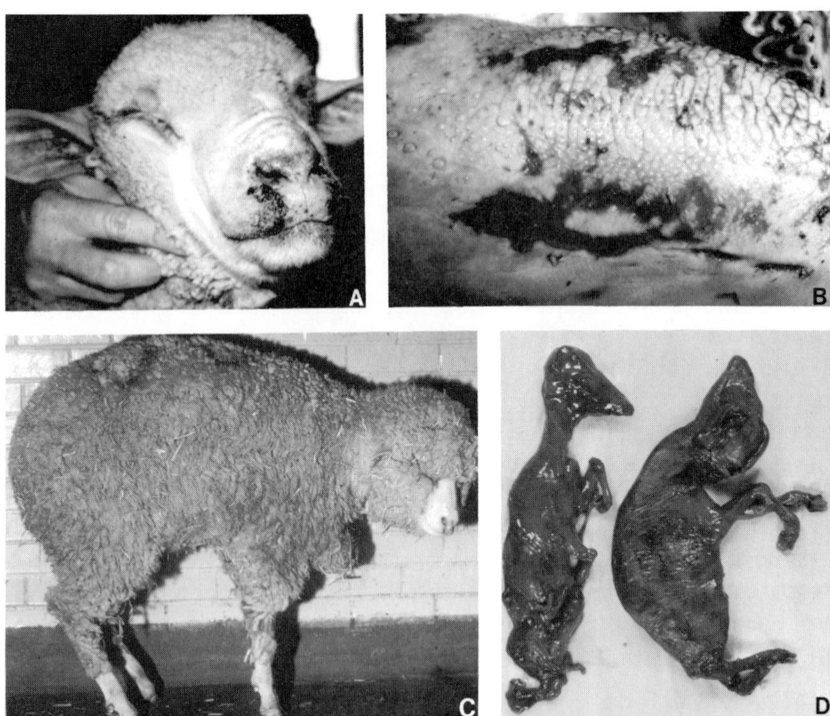

FIG. 31-3. *Bluetongue in sheep. (A) The muzzle is swollen and has erosions. (B) Erosion of the lateral margins of the tongue, which is greatly swollen and cyanosed. (C) Lameness due to hyperemia of the coronary band of the hoofs. (D) Mummified fetal lambs aborted at 135 days of gestation. (A, B, and D, courtesy Dr. B. Erasmus; C, courtesy of the United States Department of Agriculture.)*

as 10 weeks. Rarely, and only when the bull is viremic, bluetongue virus may be recovered from semen. To the extent that this might lead to the transmission of virus to cows and their offspring, this route offers an alternative to arthropod transmission for the perpetuation of the virus, but it probably occurs infrequently.

Diagnosis. Clinical diagnosis of the disease in sheep should not present a problem, but the diagnosis in cattle is more difficult. Bluetongue can be confused with the vesicular diseases, bovine virus diarrhea/mucosal disease, mild cases of rinderpest, infectious bovine rhinotracheitis, and malignant catarrh. In both cattle and sheep, photosensitization should be excluded from the diagnosis. Postmortem, apart from hemorrhage at the base of the pulmonary artery, there is no pathognomonic gross pathology.

Bluetongue virus is often difficult to isolate in the laboratory. The chances of virus isolation are enhanced if blood is collected from animals showing early clinical signs or a pronounced pyrexia, and viral isolation is most likely to be successful if the buffy coat is inoculated intravenously into 10- or 11-day-old chick embryos. Virus can be adapted to cell culture, but this system is generally considered insensitive for primary isolation. A range of serologic techniques are used for diagnosis. Techniques for using the PCR to both identify and type bluetongue virus have been described, but their value for routine diagnosis has yet to be evaluated.

Epidemiology. Bluetongue virus is transmitted by arthropods. Transplacental transmission may occur, but the virus is not transmitted by contact or through infected animal products. The epidemiology of bluetongue depends on interactions of host, vector, climate, and virus. It occurs most commonly in late summer, when the vectors, *Culicoides* species ("no-see-ums" or biting midges), are most numerous. *Culicoides* breed in many habitats, particularly in damp muddy areas and in cow dung. Moisture is important for their life cycles, but some species may be found in apparently arid areas and others can breed in highly saline water.

Female *Culicoides* take a blood meal every 3–4 days until the end of their life, which can be as long as 70 days. If the blood contains virus, it infects the cells in the hemocoel and salivary glands of the vector. After an extrinsic incubation period of 7–10 days, the virus is excreted in the saliva and can be transmitted. There is no evidence of transovarial transmission in arthropods. Not all species of *Culicoides* are vectors, and different species constitute the principal vectors in different parts of the world. Long-range, wind-borne dispersal of infected *Culicoides* may sometimes occur and constitutes a mechanism by which bluetongue virus can be introduced to a distant area.

Prevention and Control. Bluetongue viruses are now recognized to infect ruminants in every continent where livestock species are reared. Geography and climate predispose certain areas to epidemics of bluetongue, depending on the temporary introduction of efficient insect vectors into an area where livestock are susceptible. When the climate changes, the vector is no longer able to survive and virus "dies out."

The attenuated live-virus vaccines available for the control of bluetongue in South Africa have several disadvantages, in that live-virus vaccines have been associated with fetal death and cerebral abnormalities in sheep in the United States, and the use of multivalent live vaccines may lead to the emergence of genetic reassortants. In addition, *Culicoides* transmission of attenuated vaccine virus can occur, with possible reversion to virulence. Research on recombinant vaccines using the baculovirus expression system has progressed to a stage which suggests that a safe vaccine that will protect sheep and cattle from infection can be developed.

Control by vaccination is necessary where virulent bluetongue viruses are endemic. However, it is important to minimize the possibility of viral introduction into the new areas. In view of the widespread distribution of bluetongue virus in the tropics and subtropics, the control of its movement between countries by examination and testing and certification of livestock and germ plasm may not appear, at first glance, to have been effective. However, this impression is probably erroneous. In retrospect, most of the geographic expansion of bluetongue probably occurred before animals were examined for that infection by other than clinical examination. The limited number of types of bluetongue virus the United States, a country that until recently has had a very restrictive attitude to the importation of livestock from countries infected with bluetongue virus, testifies to the probable success of the policy.

Ibaraki and Epizootic Hemorrhagic Disease

Two viruses closely related to bluetongue virus, Ibaraki virus and epizootic hemorrhagic disease of deer virus, belonging to the epizootic hemorrhagic disease virus group of the orbiviruses, have been isolated from cattle and deer, respectively, affected with a disease clinically indistinguishable from bluetongue. Epizootic hemorrhagic disease virus has also been isolated from cattle, which appear to be its reservoir host. Ibaraki disease was first recorded as an acute, febrile disease of cattle in Japan in 1959, and the virus is present in many parts of Southeast Asia. Epizootic hemorrhagic disease of deer was first associated with a virus in 1955 in the United States. In 1964, the disease was seen in Alberta, Canada, and the virus has been isolated from cattle and arthropods in the United States and from arthropods in Africa. Similar viruses exist in Australia. Outbreaks of bluetongue and epizootic hemorrhagic disease are uncommon, but they are regarded as the most important diseases of Cervidae in North America.

Palyam Virus Infections

Abortions in cattle in southern Africa and an epidemic of congenital abnormalities of calves in Japan, characterized by hydranencephaly and cerebellar hypoplasia, have been shown to be caused by orbiviruses of the Palyam group. Similar diseases associated with Palyam viruses have been recorded in Australia.

African Horse Sickness

African horse sickness virus causes disease in horses, mules, and donkeys with up to 95% mortality. Apart from Venezuelan equine encephalitis, it is the most important viral disease capable of causing widespread mortality in horses. Epidemics of African horse sickness have been recognized in South Africa since 1780. More recently, major epidemics have occurred in the Middle East and Indian subcontinent in 1959–1961 and in North Africa and southern Spain in 1965–1966. Traditionally, the virus is considered endemic only in sub-Saharan Africa, but since 1987, when the disease reappeared in the Iberian Peninsula, the virus appears to have become endemic in this region. In this recent epidemic the number of horses dying has been relatively low, owing, in part, to the use of vaccines. However, in the earlier epidemic in the Middle East and Indian subcontinent, over 300,000 horses, donkeys, and mules were reported to have died. African horse sickness has never been recognized in the western hemisphere or Australia.

Nine serotypes of African horse sickness virus are recognized in South Africa, and additional serotypes are suspected to occur elsewhere in Africa. There is no significant serologic or genetic relationship between African horse sickness and other orbiviruses of veterinary importance.

Clinical Features

The severity of clinical disease in horses, donkeys, and mules varies with the strain of virus. Horses are generally the most susceptible, with high morbidity and mortality rates; there is also high morbidity in mules but mortality is low, while donkeys are the least sensitive, usually developing only a mild febrile response. In acute cases, the disease is characterized by severe and progressive respiratory disease leading to death. After an incubation period of 3–5 days, the animal develops fever for 1–2 days (40°–41°C); the breathing rate then increases, often to 70 per minute, and the affected animal stands with its forelegs apart, head extended, and nostrils dilated. Spasmodic coughing may occur terminally, accompanied by profuse sweating and discharge of frothy fluid from the nostrils. This pulmonary form is most commonly seen in completely susceptible animals infected with a highly virulent strain of the virus.

In contrast, some cases are mild and easily overlooked. Apart from fever, which may last for 5–8 days, other clinical signs are unusual, although the conjunctiva may be slightly congested. This type of disease is most commonly seen in donkeys and vaccinated horses infected with a heterologous virus type. Disease of intermediate severity is seen in some animals. The incubation period is 7–14 days, followed by fever, which persists for 3–6 days. As the temperature falls, characteristic edema appears involving the supraorbital fossae and eyelids (Fig. 31-4). Subsequently the edema extends to affect the lips, tongue, intermandibular space, and the laryngeal region. Subcutaneous edema may also track down the neck toward the chest. Mortality rates for such cases may be as high as 50%; death occurs within 6–8 days of the onset of fever. Terminally, the affected animal has signs of colic. This syndrome is sometimes referred to as the cardiac form; it is usually associated with virus strains of low virulence or is seen in vaccinated horses exposed to a heterologous type. Excess pericardial and pleural fluid may be found at necropsy.

Pathogenesis. The clinical signs of African horse sickness and bluetongue in sheep may have similarities, and it may be assumed that the pathogenesis is similar. After the bite of an infective arthropod, the virus replicates in the local lymph node before producing a transient primary viremia, which leads to infection of other tissues and organs in the reticuloendothelial system and then to a secondary viremia. As with bluetongue, the precise mechanisms by which the virus causes disease are unknown, but they involve vasculitis of small and medium-sized blood vessels.

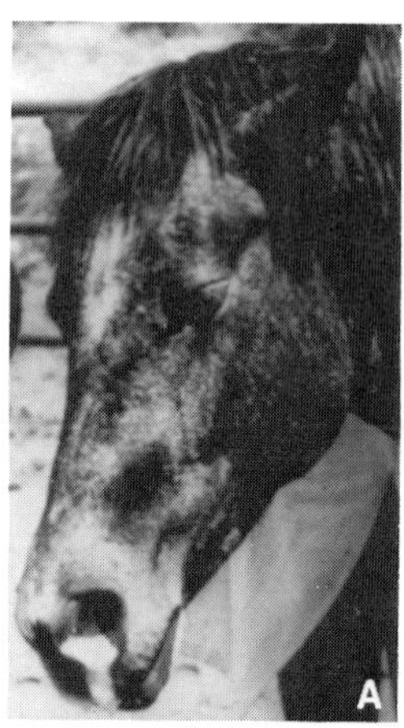

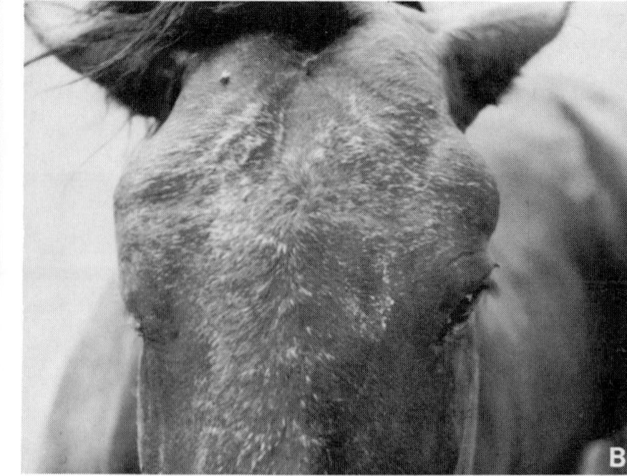

FIG. 31-4. *African horse sickness. (A) Respiratory form, with profuse frothy nasal discharge. (B) Characteristic edema of the supraorbital fossae and eyelids. (Courtesy Dr. B. Erasmus.)*

Diagnosis. African horse sickness is considered an exotic disease outside Africa. Clinical diagnosis of the pulmonary and cardiac forms is not difficult; the edema of the supraorbital fossa is characteristic of the disease. Excess pleural and pericardial fluid at postmortem provides a further reason to suspect the diagnosis, especially in endemic areas and in the appropriate season.

The virus is most easily isolated by intracerebral inoculation of 2- to 6-day-old mice with blood or a spleen suspension, using washed cell fractions. The serotype of virus isolates is determined by serum neutralization assays in mice or cell cultures.

Epidemiology. African horse sickness is usually seasonal, occurring in the late summer on swampy low-lying farms and affecting especially horses that are not stabled at night. This indicates that crepusculid and night-flying insects are the vectors. The virus infects mosquitoes, but *Culicoides* spp. are thought to be the principal vectors.

The original reservoir host of African horse sickness virus may be the zebra. Clinical disease in zebras is unusual, but the virus persists for longer than in horses.

Prevention and Control. Attentuated live-virus vaccines have been used in South Africa for many years. The polyvalent vaccine containing all nine serotypes is generally unsatisfactory since it fails to protect all horses and can cause neurologic disease. An inactivated vaccine to type 4 is available.

Vigilance in monitoring the worldwide incidence of African horse sickness is important. The explosive epidemics of the disease outside continental Africa in the 1960s and its recent reintroduction to Spain and Portugal demonstrate its invasive potential. Recognition that the related virus of bluetongue has established endemic infection in the Americas, Asia, and Australia serves as a reminder that, contrary to previous experience in the Middle East and Mediterranean areas, African horse sickness virus could become endemic if introduced to a new area such as the Americas.

Equine Encephalosis

Prior to 1967, African horse sickness virus was the only orbivirus known to cause clinical disease in horses. In that year, sporadic cases of peracute deaths, preceded by alternating periods of hyperexcitement and depression, hence the name encephalosis, occurred in horses in various parts of South Africa. At necropsy, general venous congestion, fatty liver degeneration, brain edema, and catarrhal enteritis were observed, and isolations of an orbivirus were made from various organs and blood collected from affected horses.

Serum neutralization tests have shown that there are at least five serotypes; serologic surveys have revealed a high incidence of infection with each of them. The encephalosis viruses have been recognized only in South Africa; further work is needed to define their origin, geographic distribution, and veterinary importance.

DISEASES CAUSED BY ROTAVIRUSES

Rotaviruses are a major cause of diarrhea in intensively reared farm animals throughout the world. The clinical signs, diagnosis, and epidemiology of disease are similar in all species; its severity ranges from subclinical, through enteritis of varying degrees, to death. Disease is usually seen only in young animals, 1–8 weeks old, but rarely during the first week after birth. The serologic classification of the rotaviruses is complex; there are at least six major groups and several serotypes within the groups.

Clinical Features

Rotaviruses are a main cause of a widespread and common type of diarrhea in young animals (especially calves, piglets, foals, and lambs) referred to as "white scours" or "milk scours." The incubation period is 16–24 hours. Ingestion of a large volume of milk may be a contributory factor if there is a concurrent reduction in the production of lactase caused by rotavirus infection. Other factors, primarily reduced colostrum intake, but also pathogenic *Escherichia coli,* poor hygiene, chilling, and overcrowding, may contribute to the severity of the disease. Young animals may die as a result of dehydration or secondary bacterial infection, but most recover within 3–4 days.

Pathogenesis

Rotaviruses infect the epithelial cells at the aspices of the villi of the small intestine, causing atrophy (see Fig. 9-3). The villi become shortened and covered with cuboidal epithelial cells from the crypts, which have reduced levels of disaccharidases, such as lactase, and impaired glucose-coupled sodium transport. Undigested lactose in the milk promotes bacterial growth and exerts an osmotic effect; both features exacerbate the damage to villi caused by the virus and lead to diarrhea.

Laboratory Diagnosis

Demonstration of the virus particles in feces by negative staining and electron microscopy is the most widely used diagnostic technique. Negative-contrast electron microscopy has several advantages for diagnosing rotavirus and other enteric infections. It detects a number of different viruses that are difficult to isolate and also demonstrates combined viral infections, but the major advantage is simplicity and speed, as a diagnosis can be reached within 10 minutes of receipt of the sample in the laboratory. The main disadvantage is that a high concentration of viral particles is required (at least 10^5 per gram of feces), but this can be offset by using immunoelectron microscopy (see Chapter 12).

Not all diagnostic laboratories have immediate access to an electron microscope. A range of serologic procedures for examination of feces employing antigen capture techniques, such as ELISA, are available. Rotavirus infection can also be diagnosed rapidly and simply by polyacrylamide gel electrophoresis, which separates the dsRNA genome segments. The method utilizes silver staining of subanogram amounts of nucleic acid in feces and is as sensitive as electron microscopy and ELISA. Most bovine, porcine, and avian rotaviruses are not cytopathic initially, but they can be serially passaged if grown in the presence of low concentrations of trypsin, which cleaves one of the proteins of the outer capsid, promoting uncoating in the cell.

Epidemiology

Rotaviruses are excreted in the feces of infected animals in high titer (10^{11} viral particles per gram); maximum shedding occurs on the third and fourth days. Rotaviruses survive in feces for several months, so gross contamination of the rearing pens can occur, which explains why intensively reared animals are more commonly affected. Some rotaviruses are high resistant to chlorination and can survive for long periods in water supplies, so that waterborne transmission is also possible. Rotavirus groups can be distinguished by serologic tests and polyacrylamide gel electrophoresis analysis of genome segments, but meaningful correlations of such groupings with pathogenicity have yet to be developed.

Prevention and Control

Although the management of intensive rearing units can be improved to reduce the incidence of disease, there is little likelihood that improved hygiene alone will completely control rotavirus infections. Local immunity of the small intestine is more important than circulating antibody in providing resistance to infection. In domestic mammals, rotavirus antibodies present in the colostrum are particularly important in protecting neonatal animals. Although much of the colostral antibody enters the circulation, serum antibody levels are not critical for protection; far more important is the presence of antibody in the gut lumen. Ingestion of large volumes of colostrum for a short period gives protection for only 48 hours after suckling ceases, whereas continuous feeding of smaller amounts of colostrum can provide protection for as long as it is available. Inoculation of the dam with inactivated rotavirus vaccine promotes higher levels of antibody in the colostrum and milk and a longer period of antibody secretion, with a corresponding decrease on the incidence of disease in neonates.

Recovery in affected calves can be helped by feeding them water instead of milk for 30 hours at the onset of diarrhea. Antibiotics to control the secondary bacterial diarrhea and oral electrolyte solutions containing glucose to offset dehydration may also be useful.

FURTHER READING

Bellamy, A. R., and Both, G. M. (1990). Molecular biology of rotaviruses. *Adv. Virus Res.* **38,** 1.

Gibbs, E. P. J., and Greiner, E. C. (1988). Bluetongue and epizootic hemorrhagic disease. *In* "The Arboviruses: Epidemiology and Ecology" (T. P. Monath, ed.), Vol 2, p. 39. CRC Press, Boca Raton, Florida.

Hess, W. R. (1988). African horse sickness. *In* "The Arboviruses: Epidemiology and Ecology" (T. P. Monath, ed.), Vol 2, p. 1. CRC Press, Boca Raton, Florida.

Holmes, I. H. (1988). *Reoviridae:* The rotaviruses. *In* "Laboratory Diagnosis of Infectious Diseases. Principles and Practice" (E. H. Lennette, P. Halonen, and F. A. Murphy, eds.), Vol 2, p. 384. Springer-Verlag, New York.

Kapikian, A. Z., and Chanock, R. M. (1990). Rotaviruses. *In* "Fields Virology" (B. N. Fields, D. M. Knipe, R. M. Chanock, M. S. Hirsch, J. L. Melnick, T. P. Monath, and B. Roizman, eds.), 2nd Ed., p. 1353. Raven, New York.

Matsui, S. M., Mackow, E. R., and Greenberg, H. B. (1989). Molecular determinants of rotavirus neutralization and protection. *Adv. Virus Res.* **36,** 181.

Ramig, R. F., and Ward, R. L. (1990). Genomic segment reassortant in rotaviruses and other *Reoviridae. Adv. Virus Res.* **39,** 163.

Roy, P., and Gorman, B. M., eds. (1990). Bluetongue viruses. *Curr. Top. Microbiol. Immunol.* **162,** 1.

Saif, L. J., and Thiel, K. W. (1989). "Viral Diarrheas of Man and Animals." CRC Press, Boca Raton, Florida.

Schiff, L. A., and Fields, B. N. (1990). Reoviruses and their replication. *In* "Fields Virology" (B. N. Fields, D. M. Knipe, R. M. Chanock, M. S. Hirsch, J. L. Melnick, T. P. Monath, and B. Roizman, eds.), 2nd Ed., p. 1275. Raven, New York.

Walton, T. E., and Osborn, B. I., eds. (1992). "Bluetongue, African Horse Sickness and Related Orbiviruses." CRC Press, Boca Raton, Florida.

CHAPTER 32

Birnaviridae

Infectious bursal disease was recognized as a disease of chickens in 1957, and a virus was identified as the causal agent in 1962. The viral etiology of infectious pancreatic necrosis of fish was recognized in 1960. In 1973 it was noted that these two viruses had a similar and distinctive morphology. Their assignment to a new family was clinched by the recognition in the 1970s that the genome of each consisted of two pieces of dsRNA, but it was not until 1984 that the family was officially designated *Birnaviridae*. Other members of the family affect insects and molluscs.

Several viruses with a similar genomic structure have been identified as a possible cause of diarrhea in humans, pigs, and rodents. These viruses are smaller than birnaviruses (35 nm diameter compared with 60 nm) and have provisionally been called "picobirnaviruses."

Infectious bursal disease occurs worldwide, and few commercial flocks are free of the virus. It is of considerable economic importance and is of scientific interest because of the nature of the virus and its special affinity for pre-B lymphocytes of the bursa of Fabricius, leading to acquired B-lymphocyte deficiency in affected birds.

PROPERTIES OF BIRNAVIRUSES

The nonenveloped, icosahedral virions are 60 nm in diameter, with a single shell (Fig. 32-1). They are relatively heat stable, and their infectivity is resistant to exposure at pH 3 and to ether and chloroform. There are four structural polypeptides, none of which is glycosylated, and the genome consists of two segments of dsRNA; segment A of 3.1 kbp and segment B of 2.9 kbp (Table 32-1). The coding arrangements are similar, although different names have been applied to the proteins of infectious bursal disease virus and infectious pancreatic necrosis virus. For infectious bursal disease virus segment A contains a single large open reading frame, represented as N-VP2-VP5-VP4-VP3-C, that is cleaved to yield four proteins. VP2 is a 62K precursor of the 54K major structural protein, VP5 is a 17K protein of unknown function whose sequence overlaps that of VP2, VP4 is a 29K nonstructural protein, and VP3 is a 31K minor structural protein. The smaller segment B encodes a single gene product VP1 of 90K which is presumed to be the viral RNA polymerase. VP2 determines serotype specificity and is responsible for eliciting protective antibody, the epitopes being highly conformation-dependent.

There are two serotypes of infectious bursal disease virus (IBDV), which show minimal cross-protection, and three serotypes of infectious pancreatic necrosis virus. Variant strains of IBDV serotype I have been recognized in the United States.

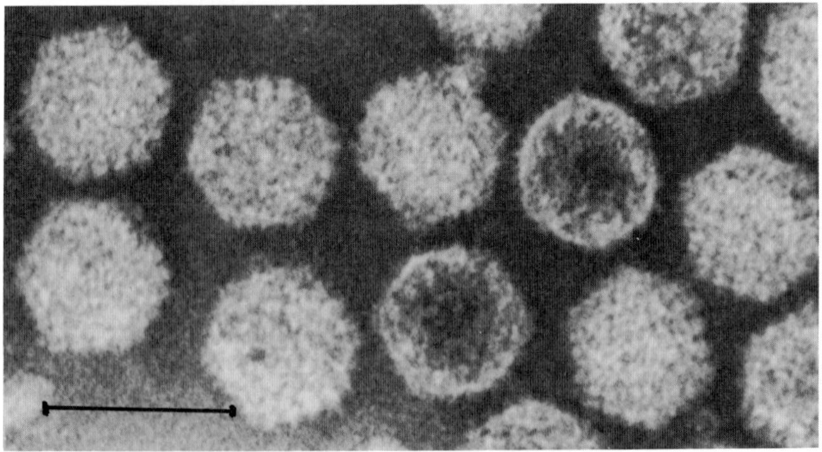

FIG. 32-1. *Negatively stained virions of infectious bursal disease virus. Bar: 100 nm. (Courtesy Dr. E. L. Palmer.)*

TABLE 32-1
Properties of Birnaviruses

Nonenveloped icosahedral virion, 32 capsomers, 60 nm diameter
dsRNA genome, with two segments: A, 3.1 kbp; B, 2.9 kbp
Four structural proteins, one nonstructural protein, virion transcriptase
Cytoplasmic replication
Survives 60°C for 60 minutes; stable at pH 3–9
Member viruses occur in chickens (infectious bursal disease virus), fish (infectious pancreatic necrosis virus), molluscs, and insects

VIRAL REPLICATION

Infectious bursal disease virus replicates in both chicken and mammalian cells; however, highly pathogenic strains are often difficult to cultivate. Infectious pancreatic necrosis virus replicates in fish cell lines incubated below 24°C. Both viruses produce cytopathic effects 1–2 days after inoculation.

Birnaviruses replicate in the cytoplasm without greatly depressing cellular RNA or protein synthesis. The viral mRNA is transcribed by a virion-associated transcriptase. Replication of the birnavirus RNA is thought to be initiated independently at the ends of the segments and to proceed by strand displacement, the inverted terminal repeats in each segment playing a role in replication and/or packaging.

INFECTIOUS BURSAL DISEASE OF CHICKENS

Clinical Features

When infectious bursal disease virus is newly introduced into a flock, morbidity approaches 100% and mortality may be up to 90%. Disease is most severe in chicks 3–6 weeks old, when the target organ, the bursa of Fabricius, reaches its maximal stage of development. Accordingly, chicks 1–14 days old are less sensitive; in addition they are usually protected by maternal antibodies. Birds older than 6 weeks rarely develop signs of disease, although they produce antibodies to the virus. After an incubation period of 2–3 days, chicks show depression, ruffled feathers, anorexia, diarrhea, trembling, and dehydration; usually 20-30% die. The clinical disease lasts for 3–4 days, then surviving birds recover rapidly.

Naturally occurring strains of infectious bursal disease virus vary in virulence, and attenuated live-virus vaccines have been developed. Infectious bursal disease virus serotype II causes inapparent infections in chickens and turkey poults.

Pathogenesis and Immunity

The most striking feature of the pathogenesis and pathology is the selective replication of infectious bursal disease virus in the bursa of Fabricius, which is enlarged (up to five times its normal size), edematous, hyperemic, and cream-colored, with prominent longitudinal striations. Hemorrhages occur beneath the serosa, and there are necrotic foci throughout the bursal parenchyma. At the time of death the bursa may be atrophied and gray, and the kidneys are usually enlarged, with accumulation of urates due to the dehydration and possibly with immune complexes in the glomeruli. Histologically there is severe depletion of lymphocytes from the bursal follicles. Lysis of B lymphocytes also occurs in other lymphoid tissues such as the spleen, but to a lesser extent.

Following oral infection, virus replicates in gut-associated macrophages and lymphoid cells from which it enters the portal circulation, leading to primary viremia. Within 11 hours of infection, viral antigen is detectable in the bursal lymphoid cells, but not in lymphoid cells of other tissues. Large amounts of virus released from the bursa produce a secondary viremia resulting in localization in other tissues. Chicks that are surgically bursectomized before infection with a normally lethal dose of virus exhibit no clinical signs, but produce high levels of neutralizing antibody, whereas nonbursectomized chicks die within 3 or 4 days. Recovered birds develop high levels of antibody to infectious bursal disease virus because their mature peripheral B lymphocytes are still functional. *In vitro* studies confirm the results of fluorescent antibody staining of tissues of affected chicks (Fig. 32-2). *In vitro,* virus replicates to a high titer in suspensions of pre-B lymphocytes from the bursa but poorly in lymphocyte suspensions from spleen, lymph nodes, or thymus.

The predilection of the virus for bursal lymphocytes leads to an important immunopathological result in birds that recover from the infection. The occurrence of what has been called "viral bursectomy" results in a diminished antibody response and increased susceptibility to a wide range of infectious agents, including several such as *Salmonella* spp. and *E. coli* which are not highly pathogenic in normal chicks. The immunosuppression leads to a variety of intercurrent infections which are most obvious in the weeks immediately following recovery from infection with the virus. There is a correlation between the variety and severity of intercurrent infections and the age of the bird; the younger birds are at the time of infection (within the period of high susceptibility between 3

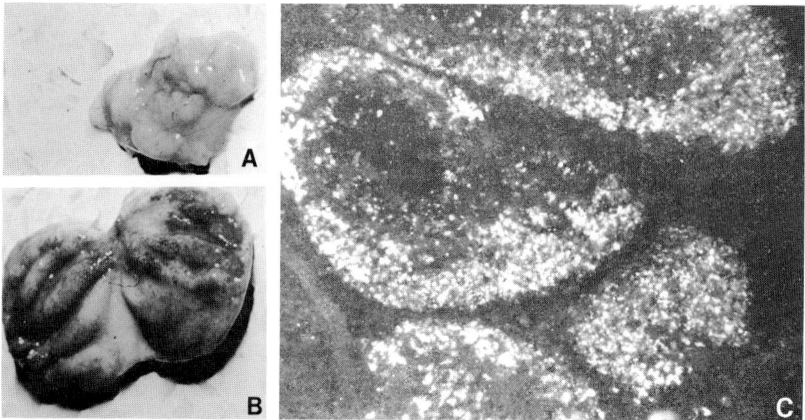

FIG. 32-2. *Infectious bursal disease. (A) Normal bursa of Fabricius. (B) Enlarged, hemorrhagic bursa of a diseased chick. (C) Specific immunofluoresence in the follicles of the bursa of Fabricius in a chick infected with infectious bursal disease virus 24 hours earlier. (C, courtesy Dr. H. Becht.)*

and 6 weeks of age), the wider the range of intercurrent infections. In addition, the immunosuppression leads to diminished antibody production after vaccination.

Laboratory Diagnosis

Immunofluorescence of impression smears of bursal tissue, gel diffusion tests with infected bursal tissue as the antigen, electron microscopy of bursal specimens, and viral isolation in embryonated eggs are all useful in confirming the clinical diagnosis. The presence of virus or viral antigen can be detected in bursal tissue by immunofluorescence for 3–4 days after infection, for 5–6 days by immunodiffusion, and for up to 14 days by viral isolation. Neutralization tests and ELISA are reliable methods for serodiagnosis.

Epidemiology

Infectious bursal disease virus is excreted in the feces for 2–14 days. It is highly contagious, and transmission occurs directly through contact and oral uptake. The virus is extremely stable and persists for over 4 months in pens and for some 7 weeks in feed. The usual cleaning and disinfection measures often do not lead to elimination of the agent in contaminated premises; hence, indirect transmission via contaminated feed, water, dust, litter, and clothing or mechanical spread through insects further spread the virus. Vetrical transmission probably occurs via the egg.

The disease is most severe when the virus is introduced into a "clean" flock. If the disease then becomes endemic, the course is much milder and spread occurs more slowly.

Control

No fully satisfactory regimen of vaccination is yet available. Breeding stock is vaccinated by adding vaccine virus to drinking water, in the hope that passively transferred maternal antibody will prevent infection of the newly hatched chicks at the time of their maximum susceptibility. An increasingly common practice is to follow oral live-virus vaccination of breeding stock, after they have reached the age of about 18 weeks, with an injection of inactivated vaccine in oil adjuvant just before they begin laying. Vaccination is repeated 1 year later. This results in a well-maintained high level of neutralizing antibody throughout the laying life of the birds. Maternal antibody provides effective protection for chicks for between 4 and 7 weeks after hatching. In situations where chicks have low or inconsistent levels of maternal antibodies, vaccination should be carried out with attenuated virus, starting at 1–2 weeks of age. The gene for VP2 has been expressed in yeast, and experimentally the product induces high titers of neutralizing antibody.

INFECTIOUS PANCREATIC NECROSIS OF FISH

Infectious pancreatic necrosis is a highly contagious and lethal disease of salmonid fish reared in hatcheries. The virus produces a subclinical infection in pike, carp, and barbels. First recognized in North America in 1941, it now occurs in many countries, probably because of worldwide shipment of eggs and live fish.

Disease is usually observed in trout fingerlings shortly after they commence to feed. With increasing age, the infection becomes subclinical. Affected fish are dark in color, with a swollen abdomen, exophthalmus, and cutaneous hemorrhages, and they are described as frantically whirling on their long axis and then lying quietly on the bottom. The mortality varies between 10% and 90%. Histologically, pancreatic necrosis involving both ascinar and islet cells is a constant finding.

Surviving fish become lifelong carriers of the virus, which they shed in feces, eggs, and sperm. Since no effective vaccine has been developed, efforts at control are based on hygiene, water disinfection, and, if an outbreak occurs, complete destocking.

Because international commerce in live fish and eggs is an important mode of spread of infection, the Code Zoosanitaire International has established guidelines for export. The guidelines specify freedom from clinical disease or pathologic changes in the farm of origin for at least 12 months, and negative results from attempts to isolate infectious pancreatic necrosis virus from pond water, eggs, sperm, and fish.

FURTHER READING

Dobos, P., Hill, B. J., Hallet, R., Kells, D. T. C, Becht, H., and Teninges, D. (1979). Biophysical and biochemical characterization of five animal viruses with bisegmented, double stranded RNA genomes. *J. Virol.* **32,** 593.

Kibenge, F. S. B., Dhillon, A. S., and Russel, R. G. (1988). Biochemistry and immunology of infectious bursal disease virus. *J. Gen. Virol.* **69,** 1757.

Lukert, P. D., and Saif, Y. M. (1991). Infectious bursal disease. *In* "Diseases of Poultry" (B. W. Calnek, ed.), 9th Ed. p. 648. Iowa State Univ. Press, Ames.

Wolf, K. (1988). "Fish Viruses and Fish Viral Diseases," p. 115. Cornell Univ. Press, Ithaca, New York.

CHAPTER 33

Retroviridae

The veterinarians Ellerman and Bang in Denmark in 1908 and the medical pathologist Rous in the United States in 1911 demonstrated that avian leukosis and avian sarcoma could be transmitted from one chicken to another by inoculation of cell-free filtrates derived from the respective tumor tissues obtained from diseased birds. The two related viruses, avian leukosis and avian sarcoma viruses, are prototypic of the etiologic agents of similar infectious malignant tumors now recognized in many other animal species, including cattle, cats, mice, and primates. These viruses are now classified as members of the family *Retroviridae,* a large family that includes many viruses of veterinary importance (Table 33-1). The name *retro* (meaning reverse) derives from the reverse transcriptase (RNA-dependent DNA polymerase) that is found within the virions of all members of the family.

The family *Retroviridae* is subdivided into seven genera, only two of which, namely, *Lentivirus* [human immunodeficiency virus (HIV)-like viruses; maedi/visna-like viruses] and *Spumavirus* (foamy viruses), have

TABLE 33-1

Diseases of Domestic Animals Caused by Retroviruses

Genus	Host	Virus	v-*onc*	Diseases
Avian type C retrovirus group	Chicken	Avian leukosis viruses	–	Lymphomas, leukemias, anemia, osteopetrosis
		Avian sarcoma viruses	+	Sarcomas
Mammalian type C retrovirus group (MLV-related viruses[b])	Chicken	Reticuloendotheliosis viruses	–[a]	Lymphomas, anemia, sarcoma
	Swine	Porcine sarcoma virus	–	Sarcoma
	Cat	Feline leukemia viruses	–	Leukemia
		Feline sarcoma viruses	+	Sarcoma
HTLV/BLV group[c]	Cattle	Bovine leukemia virus	–	Leukemia
Lentivirus	Sheep	Maedi/visna virus	—[d]	Maedi/visna, progressive pneumonia
	Goat	Caprine arthritis–encephalomyelitis virus	—	Arthritis, encephalomyelitis
	Cattle	Bovine immunodeficiency virus	—	Lymphocytosis
	Horse	Equine infectious anemia virus	—	Anemia
	Cat	Feline immunodeficiency virus	—	Acquired immunodeficiency
Spumavirus	Cattle	Bovine foamy virus	—	None known
	Cat	Feline foamy virus	—	None known

[a] Reticuloendotheliosis virus-T is a recombinant that contains a v-*onc*.

[b] MLV, Murine leukemia virus.

[c] HTLV/BLV, Human T-cell lymphotropic virus/bovine leukemia virus.

[d] Not applicable.

been given official names. The unnamed genera include the mammalian type B retroviruses, mammalian type C retroviruses, avian type C retroviruses, mammalian type D retroviruses, and the human T-cell leukemia virus/bovine leukemia virus (HTLV/BLV)-like viruses. The lentiviruses cause important chronic diseases in sheep, goats, and horses, and this genus also includes the human, bovine, feline, and simian immunodeficiency viruses. The spumaviruses are not known to be pathogenic and have been recognized only when they are found in cultured cells.

PROPERTIES OF RETROVIRUSES

Retrovirus virions are spherical, 80–130 nm in diameter, and have a unique three-layered structure (Table 33-2). Innermost is the genome–nucleoprotein complex, which includes about 30 molecules of reverse transcriptase and has helical symmetry. This structure is enclosed within an icosahedral capsid, which in turn is surrounded by a host cell membrane-derived envelope from which project glycoprotein peplomers (Fig. 33-1).

The retroviral genome is unique among viral genomes in several respects. (1) It is the only diploid genome. (2) It is the only viral RNA that is synthesized and processed by the mRNA-processing machinery of the host cell. (3) It is the only genome associated with a specific tRNA whose function is to prime replication. (4) It is the only plus sense ssRNA genome that does not serve as mRNA soon after infection. The reverse transcriptase molecule is multifunctional in that it acts as an RNA-dependent DNA polymerase, as a DNA-dependent DNA polymerase, as an RNase H, and as an integrase, the distinctive functions being

TABLE 33-2
Properties of Retroviruses

Enveloped spherical virion, 80–130 nm diameter, with peplomers 8 nm long
Helical ribonucleoprotein in central nucleoid (concentric in type C viruses; truncated cone in lentiviruses) within icosahedral capsid; surrounded by envelope
Linear plus sense ssRNA genome, diploid (inverted dimer), total size 7–10 kb; some defective, some may carry oncogene
Reverse transcriptase transcribes DNA from virion RNA; circular dsDNA is formed and integrated into cellular chromosomes as provirus
In productive infections, virions bud from plasma membrane
Some retroviruses produce malignancies, particularly leukemias and sarcomas; viruses of genus *Lentivirus* produce slow demyelinating neurologic disease, arthritis, a generalized chronic debilitating disease, or acquired immunodeficiency syndrome

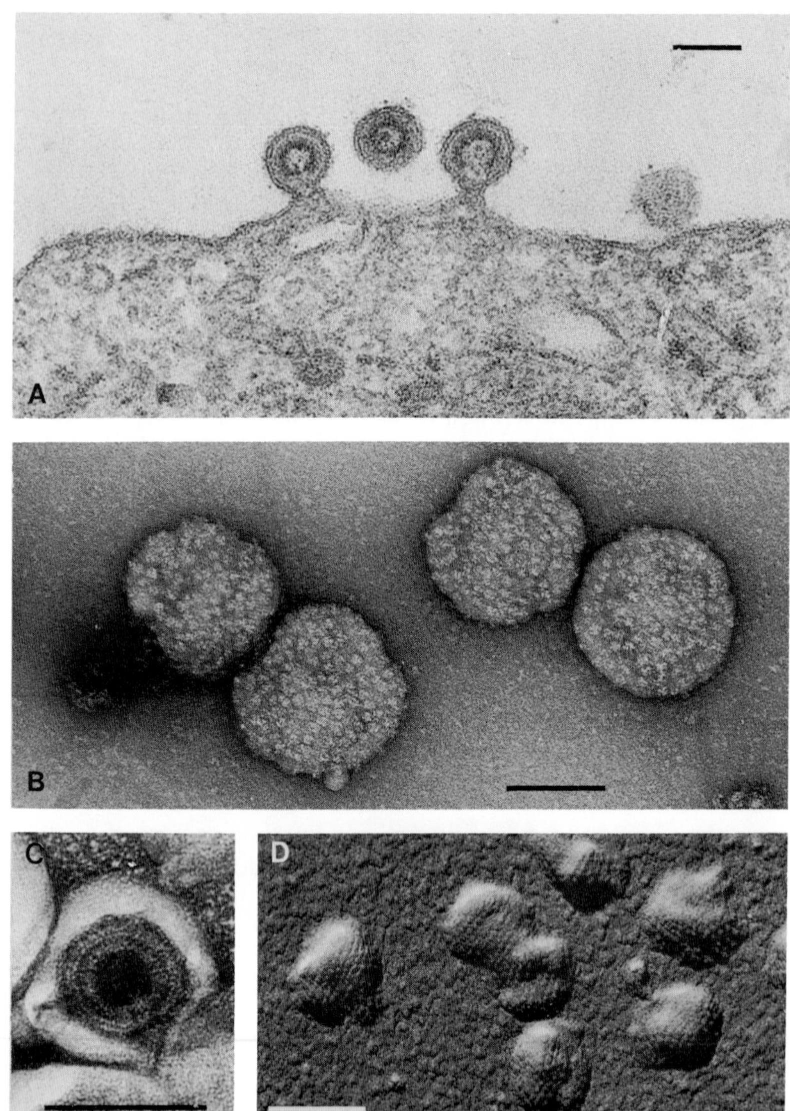

FIG. 33-1. Retroviridae, *murine leukemia virus, a typical type C retrovirus. (A) Budding of virions from a cultured mouse embryo cell. (B) Virions negatively stained with uranyl acetate, showing peplomers on the surface. (C) Virion somewhat damaged and penetrated by uranyl acetate, so that the concentric arrangement of core, shell, and nucleoid becomes visible. (D) Cores isolated by ether treatment of virions, freeze-dried, and shadow-cast. The hexagonal arrangement of the subunits of the shell around the core is recognizable. Bars: 100 nm. (Courtesy Drs. H. Frank and W. Schafer.)*

carried out by different parts of the protein molecule. Only the integrase is virus-specific; the other three functions can be carried out with any RNA, hence the importance of reverse transcriptase as a tool in recombinant DNA technology.

Each haploid segment of the genome is a linear, single-stranded, plus sense molecule of 7–10 kb, with a 3′-polyadenylated tail and a 5′ cap. The genome of nondefective retroviruses contains three major genes, each coding for two or more polypeptides. The *gag* gene (standing for group-specific antigen) encodes the virion core (capsid) proteins, the *pol* gene encodes the reverse transcriptase (polymerase), and the *env* gene encodes the virion peplomer proteins (envelope). The genome termini have several distinctive components, each of which is functionally important (Fig. 33-2).

The genome of the rapidly transforming retroviruses contains a fourth major gene, the viral oncogene (v-*onc*) (see Chapter 11). The presence of the v-*onc* gene is usually associated with deletions elsewhere in the genome, usually in the *env* gene, so that most v-*onc*-containing viruses are unable to synthesize a complete envelope and are therefore replication-defective. They are always found associated with other nondefective leukosis viruses that are replication-competent; the latter act as helpers for sarcoma virus replication (see below). Rous sarcoma virus is an exception; it contains complete *gag, pol,* and *env* genes and is therefore replication-competent, although its genome also contains the viral oncogene v-*src*.

The virion RNAs of different oncogenic retroviruses from the same species of animal show extensive homologies; those of different species (e.g., chicken, cow, cat, and mouse) show virtually no identity. The first classification of the oncogenic retroviruses was based on their host species and on the virion morphology and morphogenesis. Four types

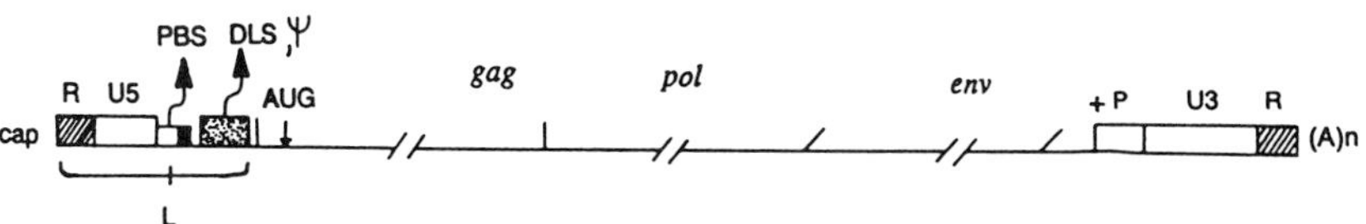

FIG. 33-2. *Features of the retrovirus genome. R, Terminal redundancy, at both termini; U5, unique 5′ sequence; PBS, primer binding site; DLS, dimer linkage site; ψ, packaging signal; AUG, initiation for* gag *protein synthesis; +P, plus strand primer region; U3, unique 3′ sequence; L, leader region;* gag, pol, env, *the three major genes. [Modified from "Microbiology" (B. D. Davis* et al., *eds.), 4th Ed., p. 1125. Lippincott, Philadelphia, Pennsylvania, 1990].*

of particles, categorized as A, B, C, and D, were recognized and the viruses classified accordingly. All oncogenic retroviruses of veterinary importance belong to the type C subgroup. Type C retrovirus morphogenesis involves the formation on the cell membrane of distinctive electron-dense, crescent-shaped (hence "type C"), nascent nucleocapsids surrounded by nascent envelope (Fig. 33-1).

Lentiviruses differ from the other retroviruses in the detailed structure of their genomes, which contain several regulatory regions not found in other retroviruses, and in their virion morphogenesis and morphology. The plasma membrane is greatly thickened at the site of budding (Fig. 33-3), and the nucleocapsid within the mature virions has the appearance of a dense cylinder, often with a concentration of electron-dense material at one end.

The antigenic relations between different retroviruses are complicated. Envelope glycoprotein epitopes are type-specific and strain-specific, and antibodies to the envelope glycoproteins neutralize viral infectivity. Core protein epitopes specified by the *gag* gene are common to the retroviruses of particular animal species, that is, they are group-specific. Some epitopes, for example, those of reverse transcriptases, are shared by viruses associated with several animal species (interspecies antigens) but distinguish avian from mammalian type C retroviruses. The internal proteins of different lentiviruses (the *gag* and *pol* gene-products) show extensive cross-reactivity but do not cross-react with the equivalent proteins of other retroviruses.

Retroviruses are inactivated by lipid solvents and detergents and by heating at 56°C for 30 minutes. However, they are more resistant than other viruses to UV light and X-irradiation, probably because their genome is diploid.

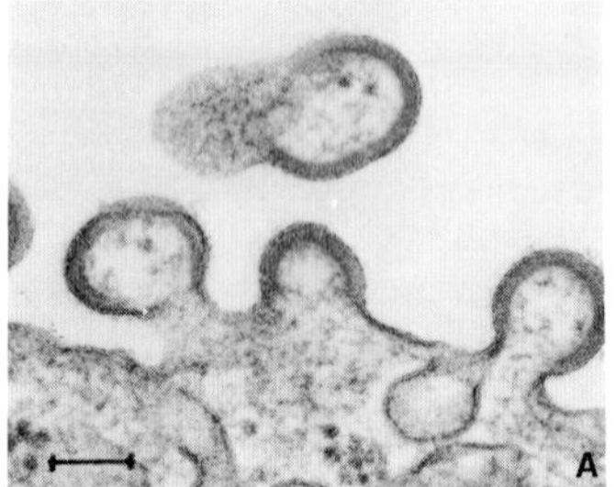

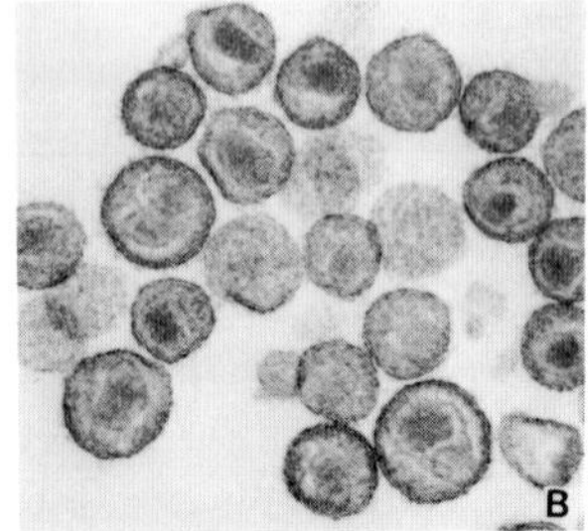

FIG. 33-3. Retroviridae, *genus* Lentivirus, *maedi/visna virus, a typical lentivirus. (A) Budding of virions. (B) Mature extracellular virions. (Courtesy R. J. Munn.)*

VIRAL REPLICATION

The essential features in the replication cycle of a nondefective retrovirus are shown in Fig. 33-4. The molecular biological aspects of retrovirus replication that relate to the role of the integrated provirus in oncogenesis have been discussed in Chapter 11. Many retroviruses (but not lentiviruses) replicate only in dividing cells. Most retroviruses are not cytopathic and do not dramatically alter the metabolism of the cells that they infect. In cell cultures, infected cells continue to divide while releasing virus.

Reverse Transcription, Integration, and Replication

Virions adsorb to specific cell receptors via envelope glycoprotein. After fusion, penetration, and uncoating, a dsDNA copy of the virion RNA is produced by the virion-associated reverse transcriptase. In the process it is increased in size by 500–600 bp at each terminus, producing long terminal repeats (LTRs), each of which consists, in a 5′ to 3′ direction, of a U3, R, and U5 region (see Fig. 11-2B). The dsDNA moves to the nucleus and circularizes with the two LTRs connected end to end, and several such molecules become integrated as provirus at different sites in the cell DNA. Transcription by cellular RNA polymerase, initiated in the 5′ LTR and ending in the 3′ LTR, generates new virion RNA.

Viral Protein Synthesis

Synthesis of viral proteins occurs at the same time as virion RNA synthesis. Two major mRNAs are transcribed: (1) a 35 S RNA, which is probably the same as full-length virion RNA, makes the *gag* protein (the same 35 S RNA is translated in a different frame for *pol*), and (2) a 25 S mRNA, spliced from the 35 S RNA, is translated to give the *env* precursor; this is read in a different frame. The three polyproteins are cleaved by a viral protease.

Maturation

The *env* protein enters the cisternae of the endoplastic reticulum during synthesis and moves to the Golgi complex where it is glcosylated. It then moves to the plasma membrane. Most of the *gag* polyprotein remains in the cytosol, but a fraction follows the same pathway as the *env* polyprotein and is glycosylated and reaches the outer side of the plasma membrane. Together with viral RNA, *gag* and *gag–pol* precursors begin to assemble nucleocapsids on the inner side of the plasma membrane and budding proceeds, the polyproteins being cleaved during the process. The nucleocapsids bind to the *env* polyprotein which is then cleaved to

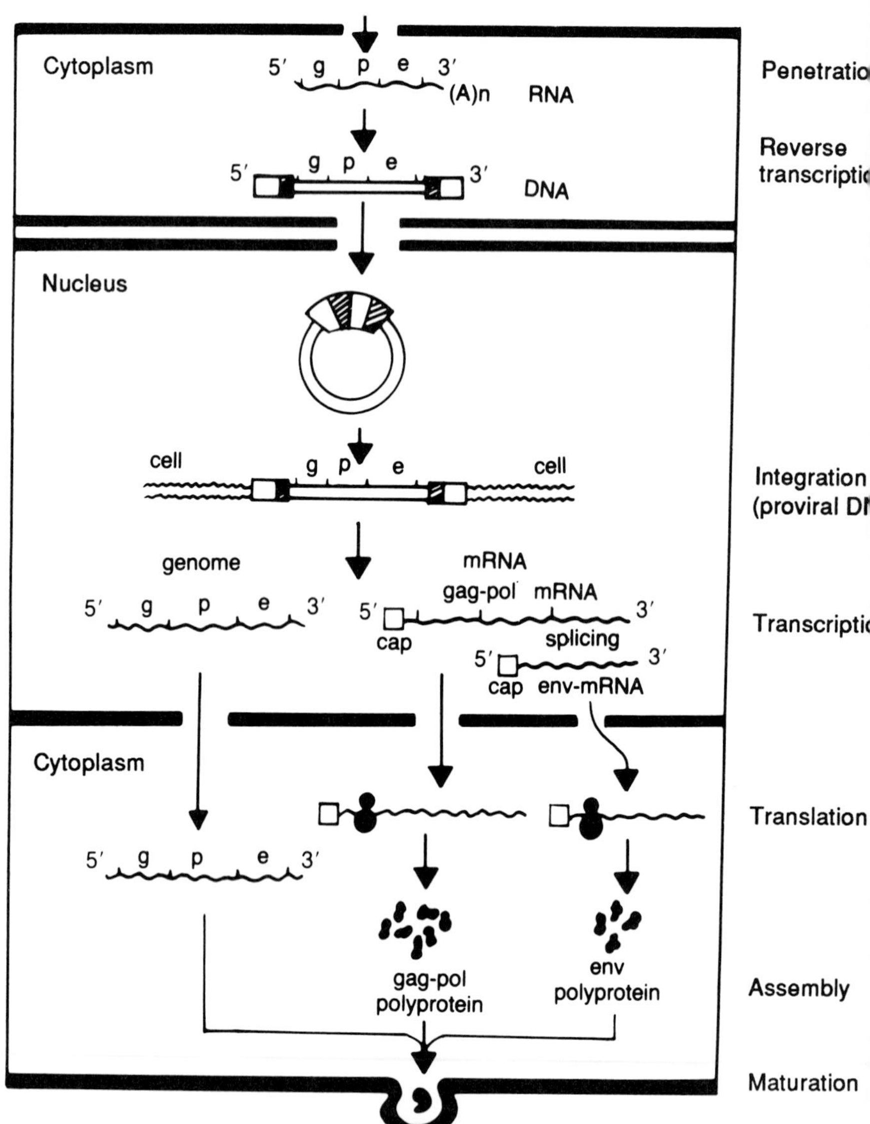

FIG. 33-4. *Replication cycle of avian leukosis virus, an exogenous replication-competent retrovirus. Virions are taken up by receptor-mediated endocytosis (top) and mature by budding through the plasma membrane (bottom). [Modified from I. Verma,* In *"Replication of Viral and Cellular Genomes" (Y. Becker, ed.), p. 275. Martinus Nijhoff, Boston, 1983.]*

the transmembrane matrix protein p15E and the external gp70 which remains bound to p15E by disulfide bonds. The packaging sequence Ψ of the viral RNA is essential; if it is spliced out of the 25 S RNA this RNA is not packaged.

Replication of retroviruses is accompanied by a high mutation frequency (10^{-4} to 10^{-5} per generation), suggesting frequent errors by reverse transcriptase. The observed sites of mutation are unevenly distributed: *gag*, *pol*, and *onc* genes are conserved as are certain parts of *env* genes; other parts of *env*, particularly those to which antibody binds, are highly variable. There is a high frequency of recombination with other retrovirus genomes in doubly infected cells. Together, the mutation and recombination frequencies far exceed those of any other animal virus. This variability accounts for the variation in the types of tumors produced by the acutely transforming oncogenic retroviruses. It makes classification of viral species difficult, a feature which is compounded by the occurrence of phenotypic mixing of the envelope proteins, to produce pseudotypes, which have the genome of one species or subtype and the envelope antigens of another. Pseudotypes have the ability to invade cells according to the receptor specificity of their envelope, but their progeny behave according to their genome specificity (see Chapter 4).

TRANSMISSION OF RETROVIRUSES

Retroviruses may be transmitted from one animal to another horizontally or vertically, and vertical transmission may occur through infectious virus (complete virions) or as provirus integrated into the DNA of the host germ plasm (Fig. 33-5). For the chicken all routes of transmission occur, although genetic transmission is restricted to nonpathogenic endogenous retroviruses. If chickens are infected horizontally when more than 5 or 6 days of age they are unlikely to develop leukemia; instead they develop a transient viremia and become immune by developing virus-neutralizing antibody. If the virus is transmitted congenitally via the egg (or in the case of mammalian viruses via the placenta) or within the first few days of life via the milk or by horizontal modes, the animal becomes viremic. The viremia persists for life, because of the induction of immunological tolerance. Such animals may appear to grow normally but frequently develop leukemia and associated diseases and are a major source of exogenous virus that is continuously shed and horizontally transmitted. Genetic (germ line) transmission occurs when germ cells, ova and sperm, contain endogenous virus. Presumably it may also occur if provirus is acquired by germ cells following horizontal transmission.

Lentiviruses are transmitted horizontally, never in the germ plasm.

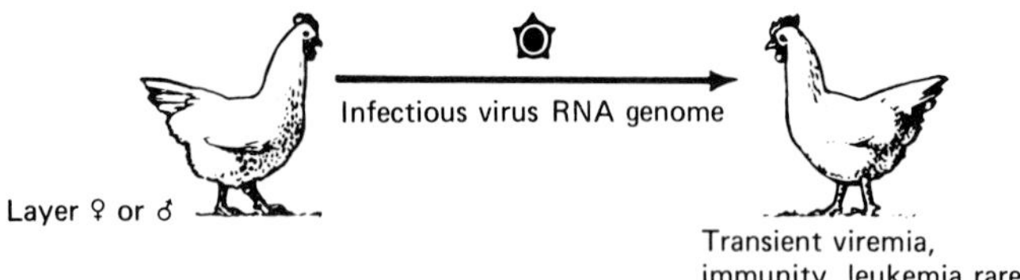

HORIZONTAL TRANSMISSION

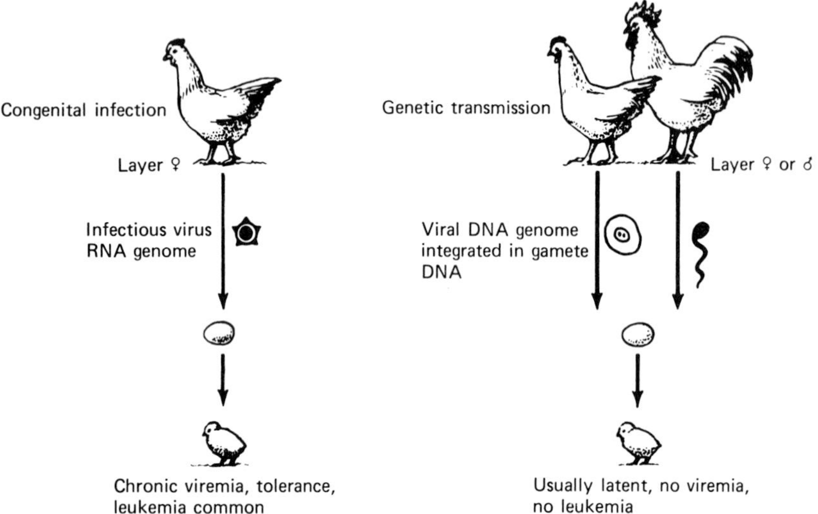

VERTICAL TRANSMISSION

FIG. 33-5. *Horizontal and vertical transmission of avian leukosis viruses. [From R. A. Weiss,* In *"Virus Persistence" (B. W. J. Mahy, A. C. Minson, and G. K. Darby, eds.), 33rd Symposium Soc. Gen. Microbiol., p. 267. Cambridge Univ. Press, Cambridge, 1982.]*

Caprine arthritis–encephalomyelitis virus is often transmitted in colostrum or milk. Little is known of the mode of transmission of spumaviruses.

DISEASES CAUSED BY AVIAN RETROVIRUSES

Since much of our understanding of the biology of the retroviruses derives from research on those affecting birds, we shall depart from the usual order of animal species and discuss them first. Retrovirus infections of chickens fall into two distinct groups: the avian leukosis viruses, which belong to the avian type C retrovirus group, and the avian reticuloendotheliosis viruses, which are currently classified within the murine leukemia virus (MLV)-related virus genus (see Table 33-1). Each of these groups of viruses, especially the first, is large and complex, and the diseases they cause are of considerable economic importance.

Avian Leukosis/Sarcoma Viruses

In considering avian retroviruses we need first recall some facets of their biology that were described earlier in this chapter and in Chapter 11, namely, that there are three classes of virus involved: endogenous, exogenous replication-competent, and exogenous replication-defective. Endogenous avian leukosis viruses occur in the genome of every chicken as DNA provirus. They are rarely expressed, but if induced by various manipulations they are nonpathogenic. Exogenous avian leukosis viruses are replication-competent and have a standard complement of *gag*, *pol*, and *env* genes. For the most part they are nonpathogenic, but in the course of lifetime infection a small percentage of infected birds develop leukemia or lymphoma. Finally, some exogenous viruses acquire a c-*onc* gene and then rapidly induce malignant tumors. The great majority of such rapidly transforming viruses lose part of their genome when they acquire the oncogene, so that they become replication-defective and depend on the helper activity of another oncovirus for productive replication. A small minority, however, like Rous sarcoma virus, have a full complement of viral genes plus a v-*onc* gene and are then rapidly oncogenic and also capable of replication without a helper virus.

Assay Methods. Rous sarcoma virus and other replication-competent acutely transforming avian retroviruses are assayed directly by focus-formation assays in chick fibroblasts. Because the assays produce infectious virions these are readily recovered and can then be studied in detail. Replication-defective rapidly transforming viruses, which carry v-*onc* genes, can also be assayed by focus formation, but virions can only be obtained in cells carrying a replication-competent leukosis virus; the yield always consists of a mixture. The replication-competent leukosis viruses, on the other hand, do not transform cells *in vitro*. Instead, they interfere with transformation by viruses with the same envelope antigen that carry a v-*onc* gene, and assay is carried out by an interference test. Assays of leukosis viruses and of the corresponding antigens can also be carried out by serologic methods, using complement fixation, ELISA, or radioimmunoassay tests.

Clinical and Pathologic Features. Avian leukosis viruses are endemic in virtually all flocks of chickens, and most chickens in a flock will have been infected within a few months of hatching. If rapidly transforming viruses are not present, disease occurs sporadically in birds over 14 weeks of age, with an overall incidence of about 3%, but sometimes as great as 20%. The variety of syndromes produced by avian leukosis/sarcoma viruses is shown in Table 33-3.

Diseases due to Exogenous Nondefective Avian Retroviruses. Exogenous nondefective avian retroviruses cause tumors only in birds that are congenitally infected and have a persistent viremia. Over the course of their life proviral DNA is integrated into many different kinds of cells, sometimes, by chance, in a location where the activity of a c-*onc* gene is disturbed in such a way as to initiate tumor production (see Chapter 11). Since lymphoid cells represent 10% of all the cells in the animal and have a very high rate of cell division, particularly in the early weeks of life, the probability that lymphoid cells are infected and transformed by leukosis viruses is higher than for most other cell types.

Lymphoid Leukosis. Lymphoid leukosis (also known as visceral lymphomatosis) is the commonest form of avian leukosis and occurs in chickens 14 to 30 weeks of age. Clinical signs are nonspecific. The comb may be pale, shriveled, and occasionally cyanotic. Inappetence, emaciation, and weakness occur, and the abdomen may be enlarged. Tumors may be present for some time before clinical illness is recognized, though with the onset of the first signs the course may be rapid. Hematologic changes are inconsistent; leukemia is uncommon, and lymphoblastoid cells are rarely seen in the circulating blood.

Tumors are usually present in the liver, spleen, and bursa and may occur in other internal organs. Microscopically the lesions are focal, multicentric aggregates of lymphoblasts with B-lymphocyte markers. They may secrete large amounts of IgM, but their capacity to differentiate into IgG-, IgA-, or IgE-producing cells is arrested. The primary target cells are post-stem cells in the bursa, within which the transformed cells invade blood vessels and metastasize hematogenously. Bursectomy, even up to 5 months of age, abrogates the development of lymphoid leukosis.

Osteopetrosis. In the osteopetrosis or "thick leg" form of the disease the bones are affected by a uniform or irregular thickening of the diaphyseal or metaphyseal regions. In advanced cases osteoma, osteogenic sarcoma, and chondrosarcoma may occur. Lesions are usually most obvious in the long bones of the leg but may also be present in the pelvis, shoulder girdle, and ribs. Birds with osteopetrosis frequently also have anemia, and they often have lesions of lymphoid leukosis.

Renal Tumors. Renal tumors are usually found coincidentally at slaughter, but they may be associated with emaciation and weakness before death. Two forms occur: nephroblastomas, which originate from

TABLE 33-3

Syndromes Produced in Chickens by Avian Type C Retroviruses

Type of virus[a]	Syndrome	Rate of development	Viral oncogene	Cell first affected	Types of lesion
Replication-competent (avian leukosis viruses)	Lymphoid leukosis	Slow	–	Lymphoblast	Lymphoid cell infiltrations of various organs
	Osteopetrosis	Slow	–	Osteoclast or osteoblast	Thickened long bones
	Renal tumors	Slow	–	Renal cells	Nephroblastoma, carcinoma
Replication-defective (avian erythroblastosis, avian myeloblastosis, avian myelocytomatosis viruses)	Erythroblastosis	Rapid	v-*erbB*	Erythroblast	Anemia
	Myeloblastosis	Rapid	v-*myb*	Myeloblast	Anemia, leukemia
	Myelocytomatosis	Rapid	v-*myc*	Myelocyte	Carcinoma, sarcoma
	Hemangioma	Rapid	?	Capillary endothelium	Hemangioma
	Sarcomas	Rapid	v-*fps*, v-*yes*	Various mesenchymal cells	Sarcoma, carcinoma
Replication-competent rapidly transforming (Rous sarcoma virus)	Sarcoma	Very rapid	v-*src*	Various mesenchymal cells	Sarcomas

[a] In addition to these exogenous viruses, all chickens carry endogenous retroviral DNA as part of their genome.

embryonic rests or nephrogenic buds in the kidneys, and carcinomas. Numerous retrovirus particles can be seen budding from transformed renal cells.

Diseases Due to Defective Avian Leukemia Viruses. A variety of neoplasms are generated by replication-defective leukemia viruses propagated by coinfection with a nondefective helper, which is usually an exogenous avian leukemia virus. These defective viruses can be divided into three groups: avian erythroblastosis, avian myeloblastosis, and avian myelocytomatosis. Their different pathogenic potential is due to the different v-*onc* genes they carry (see Table 33-3).

Erythroblastosis. The incubation period for avian erythroblastosis may be as short as 21 days. Two patterns are recognized: a proliferative form characterized by the presence of many erythroblasts in the blood and an anemic form in which the predominant feature is anemia with few circulating erythroblasts. The primary target cells are erythroblasts; infected cells resemble normal erythroblasts in appearance except that retrovirus particles can be demonstrated either within cytoplasmic vacuoles or budding from the plasma membrane. Lesions are mainly attributable to hemostatis because of the accumulation of erythroblasts in the blood vessels, particularly the capillaries and sinusoids.

Myeloblastosis. The clinical signs of avian myeloblastosis are similar to those of erythroblastosis and develop after an incubation period that may be as short as 10 days. The target cell is the myeloblast in the bone marrow. The pathologic features of myeloblastosis and erythroblastosis overlap. In myeloblastosis, leukemia is a major feature; up to 10^9 myeloblasts per milliliter are present in the blood, and in a hematocrit there may be more buffy coat than red cells. Bone marrow displacement may result in secondary anemia.

Myelocytomatosis. Signs similar to those seen in erythroblastosis develop in avian myelocytomatosis after an incubation period of 3–11 weeks. The target cells, which are nongranulated myelocytes (morphologically distinct from myeloblasts), proliferate to occupy much of the bone marrow, and tumor growth may extend through the bone and periosteum. The tumors are distinctive and characteristically occur on the surface of bone, in association with the periosteum, and near the cartilage, although any organ or tissue may be affected. Visceral organs may be infiltrated with myelocytes. Histologically, the tumors consist of compact masses of strikingly uniform myelocytes with very little stroma, similar to normal bone marrow myelocytes.

Hemangioma. After an incubation period of less than 3 weeks, a hemangioma develops, usually as a single tumor in the skin or on the surface of the viscera, as a "blood blister," which may rupture with birds then possibly bleeding to death. The visibility of a hemangioma in the skin encourages cannibalism. The target cell is located in the blood vessel wall.

Connective Tissue Tumors. A variety of malignant tumors including fibrosarcoma, fibroma, myxosarcoma, myxoma, histiocytic sarcoma, osteoma, osteogenic sarcoma, and chondrosarcoma are caused by avian oncoviruses containing v-*onc* genes. Most are replication-defective, but some, for example, Rous sarcoma virus, are replication-competent.

Diagnosis. History, clinical signs, the location of tumors, and gross and histopathologic postmortem findings are usually enough to make a diagnosis of avian leukosis. The most important disease, as far as differential diagnosis is concerned, is Marek's disease, a distinction which is important because Marek's disease can be controlled by vaccination. Viral isolation is rarely required in veterinary practice but is used for research purposes.

Epidemiology. Transmission may occur horizontally or vertically (see Fig. 33-5). Horizontal transmission is relatively inefficient requiring prolonged, close contact, and was not of major significance in the natural transmission of the disease until intensive chicken production began in the 1940s. This led to the appearance of lymphoid leukosis as an economically important disease, since horizontal transmission via saliva led to conditions which promoted egg-borne transmission. Individual infected hens may transmit virus via ova either continuously or intermittently, although some known infected hens do not transmit virus at all, and transmission is less efficient in hens more than 18 months old. Congenitally infected chickens may be immunologically tolerant, and their blood may contain up to 10^9 ID_{50} units per milliliter. They excrete virus in saliva and feces but are otherwise healthy, although some eventually develop leukosis. These birds transmit virus horizontally throughout their lives; more importantly, however, such hens transmit virus via ova, the virus infecting cells of the blastocyst from the 8-cell stage. During embryogenesis the pancreas is particularly favored as a site of replication, and large amounts of virus accumulate in the albumen. At hatching large amounts of virus are shed in the meconium, resulting in heavy environmental contamination.

Most 1-day-old chicks have maternal antibody titers between 1% and 10% of those of their dams. Thus the efficiency of passive antibody transfer is low, and the titer declines so that chicks are negative by 4–7 weeks of age. Then, if they have not been congenitally infected, they become infected by horizontal transmission and develop a transient viremia followed by high levels of antibody; virus is usually eliminated, and the antibody persists for life. However, some birds remain persistently infected and act as a source of virus for both horizontal and vertical transmission.

Roosters may be involved in the germ-line transmission of endogenous (nonpathogenic) oncoviruses, but they play no part in congenital infection.

Control. Eradication of horizontally transmitted virus has been accomplished in experimental flocks and in those used as a source of eggs for human, domestic mammal, and particularly avian virus vaccine production. Establishment and maintenance of leukosis-free flocks, which still carry endogenous avian retrovirus genes, are expensive and are not practiced commercially.

Hygiene is important in minimizing the level of virus contamination, particularly in the immediate posthatching period when the age, population density, and levels of virus are highly conducive to horizontal transmission. The "all-in all-out" principle and thorough cleaning and disinfection of incubators, hatcheries, brooding houses, and equipment is standard practice. The risk of introducing additional strains of virus is minimized if stock are obtained from a single source.

The introduction of intensive methods for broiler and egg production in the 1940s was followed by an increased incidence of leukosis, in part related to the unwitting selection of genetically susceptible chicken lines. Most modern commercial flocks have been built up with genetically resistant strains, and accordingly there has been a sharp reduction in the incidence of leukosis. Resistance correlates with viral subgroup and with the absence of receptors for viral envelope glycoproteins, the genes for virus receptors being located on an autosomal chromosome. It is possible to select for genetically resistant birds by challenging chorioallantoic membranes or chick embryo fibroblast cell cultures, derived from leukosis-free birds, with appropriate pseudotypes of Rous sarcoma virus. Failure to produce foci of cell transformation correlates with resistance, and lines of chickens can be bred that are homozygous for the resistance allele. Viral mutants able to bypass resistance frequently emerge, so that in practice genetic resistance as a basis for control requires an on-going program.

Immunization, using either inactivated or attenuated live-virus vaccines, has met with limited success.

In addition to eliminating the occurrence of tumors, eradication of leukosis viruses has a number of other benefits which include reduced mortality from other causes, improved growth rate, and improved production, quality, fertility, and hatchability of eggs.

Diseases Caused by Avian Reticuloendotheliosis Viruses

Reticuloendotheliosis viruses are pathogenic avian retroviruses that are antigenically and genetically unrelated to the avian leukosis/sarcoma retroviruses. They are now classified as a subgroup of the MLV-related group. Four member viruses have been recognized. The prototype of the group, reticuloendotheliosis virus-T, was isolated from an adult turkey that died of visceral reticuloendotheliosis and infiltrative nerve lesions. Reticuloendotheliosis virus-T is replication-defective and carries a v-*onc* gene, v-*rel*. The other avian reticuloendotheliosis viruses, namely, reticuloendotheliosis-associated virus, Trager duck spleen necrosis virus, and chick syncytial virus, are replication-competent.

When inoculated into 1-day-old chicks, reticuloendotheliosis virus-T produces severe hepatosplenomegaly with either marked necrosis or lymphoproliferative lesions. Reticuloendotheliosis virus-T pseudotypes with avian leukosis virus envelopes are produced in chickens which carry the latter viruses. Some major outbreaks of reticuloendotheliosis virus-T disease, involving the deaths of several million chickens, have occurred at a consequence of contamination of turkey herpesvirus Marek's disease vaccine with reticuloendotheliosis virus-T. There is some evidence that the virus may be mechanically transmitted by mosquitoes.

BOVINE LEUKEMIA

Now classified with the human T-cell lymphotropic viruses (HTLV), the bovine leukemia viruses cause both leukemia and lymphosarcoma, diseases which attracted attention early in the twentieth century in several European countries, notably Denmark, where clusters of herds with a high incidence of these diseases suggested a viral etiology. Bovine leukemia virus was not isolated, however, until 1969. Herds and areas characterized by a high prevalence of bovine leukemia virus are recognized in most countries. Overall prevalence figures for individual countries vary between 4 and 165 per 100,000 cattle per year, reflecting the number of low and high prevalence herds.

Pathogenesis

The course of bovine leukemia virus infection suggests a multistage process. The major target cells are B lymphocytes. Infection may be clinically inapparent or may progress to a persistent lymphocytosis and finally to tumor production, which is marked by enlarged lymph nodes and leukemic infiltrations into a variety of organs and tissues. Some tumors, particularly those from terminal cases, do not contain bovine leukemia virus or viral antigens. However, cocultivation of lymphocytes with susceptible cell cultures, with or without mitogens, results in production of infectious bovine leukemia virus. The range of susceptible cells in culture includes human, canine, and bat cells, in which the virus produces syncytia.

In contrast to the situation with chickens and cats, neither endogenous nor defective (v-*onc*-bearing) bovine oncoviruses have been recognized. Leukemogenesis probably depends on an influence on bovine c-*onc* genes by integrated bovine leukemia virus provirus.

Epidemiology and Control

Virus is shed in the urine and milk; it may also be transmitted by blood-sucking insects or iatrogenically by common equipment. Virus is transmitted horizontally within herds but does not extend readily to neighboring herds, suggesting that close and prolonged direct exposure is required. Congenital infection via the placenta also occurs. The incidence of infection is much higher than that of recognized disease, the occurrence of which is influenced by both genetic and environmental factors.

Agar gel diffusion, ELISA, and syncytium-inhibition tests are used for diagnosis. Test and removal programs have been adopted by several European countries, including Denmark and Germany, and these countries require that imported cattle be test-negative. In other countries, including the United States and Canada, individual owners have undertaken test and removal programs on a voluntary basis, but national programs have not been promulgated. An inactivated vaccine that prevents disease following bovine leukemia virus challenge has been used on an experimental basis.

OVINE RETROVIRUS DISEASES

The most important retrovirus diseases of sheep are those due to lentiviruses (see below), but viruses of the HTLV/BLV group also occur. Ovine leukemia is associated with a retrovirus closely resembling bovine leukemia virus antigenically, and outbreaks of leukemia–lymphosarcoma, in which there is evidence for both congenital and horizontal transmission, are recognized in sheep. However, little more is known about the ovine virus, and there is no evidence that the virus is naturally transmitted between sheep and cattle.

A more common retroviral disease in sheep, ovine pulmonary adenomatosis, produces signs similar to those of the lentiviral disease ovine progressive pneumonia (see below). However, the causative agent does not appear to be a lentivirus, but little is known of its molecular biology. Originally described in South Africa, where it was called jaagsiekte, ovine pulmonary adenomatosis occurs widely in the Americas and in some countries in Europe. In Peru it is responsible for about one-quarter of the annual mortality in sheep. In affected sheep, pea-sized, nodular lesions are found scattered through the lungs. Histologically these lesions are adenomas and adenocarcinomas, which metastasize to regional lymph nodes.

PORCINE LYMPHOSARCOMA

A retrovirus has been isolated from porcine lymphosarcomas, which are detected in 0.3 to 5 swine per 100,000 at slaughter and account for 25% of all porcine tumors. The tumors are found in swine from 3 to 4 months of age. Most porcine cell lines contain spontaneously produced virions of the porcine type C virus, which is highly host-specific. Viral sequences are present in multiple copies in wild Old World but not in New World species of the family Suidae, suggesting that the virus occurs as an endogenous virus in Old World wild pigs.

FELINE LEUKEMIA AND FELINE SARCOMA

Feline retroviruses of the MLV-related group may be endogenous, exogenous replication-competent (feline leukemia virus), or exogenous defective (feline sarcoma virus), producing no pathologic effects, leukemia, and sarcoma, respectively. Neoplastic and nonneoplastic disease due to feline leukemia virus occur worldwide and are the most common nonaccidental cause of death in cats. In a California survey the incidence of feline leukemia virus neoplasms was estimated to be 41.6 per 100,000 cats per year, and it has been estimated that deaths from all feline leukema virus-related diseases are 250 per 100,000 cats annually. The prevalence of antibody to feline leukemia virus varies from 6% in sparse, isolated populations to 50% in urban and colony cats.

Feline leukemia virus was first recovered in 1964, and a few other isolates have been made; however, it has proved impossible to isolate the virus from the majority of tumors that would be expected to contain it. Nevertheless, the presence of the viral genome is demonstrable by hybridization and transfection. It has therefore been suggested that viral replication and release are not required to produce disease. The discovery in 1987 of feline immunodeficiency virus has called into question many of the disease associations formerly attributed to feline leukemia virus where the associations have been made on clinical case material. Feline immunodeficiency virus (see below) has a prevalence rate in some populations of 30%, and many of the immunopathologic diseases formerly associated with feline leukemia virus must now be reassessed.

Feline sarcoma virus is known to be defective, carrying the v-*onc* gene v-*fms* and lacking an *env* gene. All strains that have been recovered from fibrosarcomas are pseudotypes with envelopes provided by feline leukemia virus, and all feline sarcoma virus stocks contain feline leukemia virus. Besides being important as pathogens of cats, feline leukemia virus/feline sarcoma virus have attracted the attention of research workers concerned with human medicine. There is no evidence that these viruses can infect humans, but it is prudent to advise that women of child-bearing age and children should avoid close contact with cats showing signs of disease associated with feline leukemia virus.

Clinical Signs and Pathologic Features

The feline oncogenic retroviruses are responsible for a variety of disease syndromes, some neoplastic and others relating to effects on hemopoietic cells and the immune system. Three types of neoplasias are recognized, namely, lymphosarcoma, myeloproliferative disease, and fibrosarcoma, and two types of nonneoplastic "antiproliferative" diseases, namely, anemia and immunopathologic disease and its consequences.

Feline Leukemia Virus Lymphosarcoma. Feline leukemia virus lymphosarcoma is the most common naturally occurring mammalian lymphosarcoma and accounts for some 30% of all feline tumors. About one-third of cats with lymphosarcoma have no demonstrable feline leukemia virus antigens (see Diagnosis), and the virus can rarely be isolated. Nevertheless, epidemiologic studies support the view that feline leukemia virus causes the vast majority of cases of feline lymphosarcoma.

Four major forms of lymphosarcoma are recognized based on the location of the primary tumor: (1) multicentric, in which tumors occur in various lymphoid and nonlymphoid tissues; (2) a thymic form, occurring particularly in kittens; (3) an alimentary form, usually occurring in older cats in which lymphoid tissues of the gastrointestinal tract and/or mesenteric lymph nodes are affected; and (4) an unclassified form, which is uncommon and in which tumors are found in nonlymphoid tissues such as skin, eyes, and central nervous sytem. The lymphosarcomas are predominantly T-lymphocyte tumors, except the alimentary tract form which is a B-lymphocyte tumor.

Feline Leukemia Virus Myeloproliferative Diseases. In the feline leukemia virus myeloproliferative diseases transformation of one or a combination of bone marrow cell types is induced by the virus. Four types are recognized: (1) erythromyelosis, in which the target is an erythroid cell; (2) granulocytic leukemia in which a granulocytic myeloid cell, usually a neutrophil, is targeted; (3) erythroleukemia, in which both erythroid and granulocytic myeloid precursors become neoplastic; and (4) myelofibrosis, a proliferation of fibroblasts and cancellous bone resulting in medullary osteosclerosis and myelofibrosis. These diseases, which are similar to those produced by the acutely transforming avian oncoviruses, are characterized by the presence of large numbers of neoplastic cells in the bone marrow, a nonregenerative anemia, and immunosuppression.

Feline Sarcoma Virus Fibrosarcoma. Feline sarcoma virus fibrosarcoma accounts for 6–12% of all feline tumors, usually as solitary tumors in older cats. In young feline leukemia virus-infected kittens, feline sarcoma virus may on rare occasions induce a multifocal subcutaneous fibrosarcoma, which is anaplastic, rapidly growing, and frequently metastatic. One strain of feline sarcoma virus induces melanoma as well as fibrosarcoma. There is no evidence that feline sarcoma virus is transmitted horizontally; the tumors and the virus appear to arise *de novo* following feline leukemia virus infection.

Anemia and Immunopathologic Disease. Transformation of erythropoietic cells may produce erythroblastosis, erythroblastopenia, or pancytopenia, all of which are associated with anemia. This group includes both immune complex diseases and immunodeficiency diseases. Sometimes persistent, high levels of feline leukemia virus antigens are produced, which when bound in immune complexes produce glomerulonephritis. In other cases lymphoid cells are greatly depleted, in party by antibody-dependent cytotoxicity, with feline oncovirus membrane-associated antigens being the target. This leads to a variety of secondary infections, in which the cat fails to thrive, growth is stunted, the hair coat is harsh, and there is intercurrent and repeated infection, chronic stomatitis and gingivitis, nonhealing skin lesions, subcutaneous abscesses, chronic respiratory disease, and a high incidence of feline infectious peritonitis (see Chapter 26). Toxoplasmosis and infection with *Hemobartonella felis* are much more common in feline leukemia virus-infected cats than in normal animals. Poor reproductive performance, including infertility, fetal deaths, and abortions, is also attributed to feline leukemia virus infection.

Pathogenesis and Immunity

There are three antigenic types of feline leukemia virus, A, B, and C, which are based on differences in the envelope antigens. Cells transformed by either feline leukemia virus or feline sarcoma virus, unlike infected, nontransformed cells, express a novel viral antigen in their plasma membrane [feline oncovirus membrane-associated antigen (FOCMA)], antibodies to which, like antibodies to the envelope antigens, protect cats against disease. The cytoplasm of feline leukemia virus-infected cells contains the envelope protein and several internal proteins. Antibodies to the internal proteins and the reverse transcriptase are not protective but may be involved in immune complex disease.

Within 6 weeks of infection with feline leukemia virus, one of two host–virus relationships develops: persistent active infection or a self-limiting infection. Persistent active infection is recognized by the presence of persistent viremia. The serum of persistently infected cats lacks both neutralizing and FOCMA-related antibodies. Viremia persists for months and is usually terminated by feline leukemia virus-related disease. Persistently infected cats shed virus in secretions and represent the most important source for the dissemination of feline leukemia virus. Immunosuppression is the most common sequel to persistent feline leukemia virus viremia and accounts for most feline leukemia virus-related deaths. Viremic cats have suppressed blastogenic responses to T-cell mitogens, suppressed antibody responses, prolonged allograft rejection times, hypocomplementemia, thymic atrophy, depletion of the paracortical zones of lymph nodes, and an almost total failure of interferon production. Age appears to have some influence on the disease pattern, perhaps because of an association between the virus and dividing cells.

The vast majority of cats exposed to infection with feline leukemia virus develop a self-limiting infection. They remain nonviremic, develop neutralizing and FOCMA-related antibodies, do not shed virus, and do not develop feline leukemia virus-related disease. Sometimes there is a transient viremia, which disappears with the development of neutralizing and FOCMA-related antibodies.

Finally, in some cats persistent viremia is initially accompanied by high FOCMA-related antibody. This is an unstable condition; either such cats develop neutralizing antibody, or the FOCMA-related antibody declines and the cats develop feline leukemia virus-related disease.

Diagnosis

Viral isolation is rarely possible, but a number of diagnostic tests have been developed based on detecting viral proteins in cells in the blood, either by indirect immunofluorescence or ELISA. The indirect immunofluorescence test is performed on blood smears on glass slides, which may be mailed to an appropriate laboratory. ELISA is performed on plasma or buffy coat cells; it is available commercially in kit form. Both tests detect a group-specific antigen within the core.

Epidemiology

Only the nonpathogenic endogenous type of feline leukemia virus is transmitted vertically, via the germ plasm. Although many cats are exposed to horizontally transmitted, pathogenic feline leukemia virus, relatively few become infected, in spite of the fact that the saliva of persistently infected and viremic cats may contain 10^6 infectious virions per milliliter. Prolonged, direct exposure is usually required for transmission, which may occur by mutual grooming or possibly via fleas. Circumstantial evidence suggests that biting, such as occurs during fighting, is probably the most important method of transmission, which may also occur iatrogenically via blood transfusion, multiple-use syringes, and surgical instruments.

The prevalence of feline leukemia virus infection and disease parallels the opportunities for exposure. The prevalence in single, confined, household cats is about 1%; infection rates progressively rise if cats also go outside (particularly to shows), live in a multiple cat household, or live in breeding colonies. Infection rates may be as high as 33% in colonies in which the virus is endemic

Control and Treatment

Using immunofluorescence or ELISA procedures for detecting viral antigens, it is possible with a test and removal program to establish feline leukemia virus-free cat colonies. Such programs may be undertaken by large catteries, particularly where the incidence of infection is high and there is clinical evidence of disease due to feline leukemia virus. The laboratory tests aid in identifying preclinical or subclinical infections and confirming clinical diagnosis.

In 1985 an inactivated vaccine was licenced in the United States. Clinical trials suggest that this vaccine reduces the incidence of disease by 70%. A subunit vaccine has been described that protects cats. The antigen is a nonglycosylated protein derived from the envelope protein gp70, expressed in *E. coli*, and administered with two adjuvants. Various antiviral drugs used in cancer therapy in humans have been tried in particularly valuable cats, with limited success.

DISEASES CAUSED BY LENTIVIRUSES

In 1933, 20 karakul sheep were imported into Iceland from Germany, and within 2 years two diseases, called maedi (=dyspnea) and visna (=wasting), emerged, which in the following years were responsible for the deaths of 105,000 sheep. A further 600,000 sheep were slaughtered in 1965, when the diseases were declared eradicated. These diseases have an incubation period of over 2 years, an insidious onset, and a protracted clinical course, lasting 6 months to several years, unless terminated by intercurrent disease. Sigurdsson, who demonstrated that both Icelandic diseases were transmissible with cell-free filtrates, described the diseases as "slow virus infections," thus introducing into virology a term that has since been widely used for other infections as well (see Chapter 10). Maedi and visna appear to have been caused by the same or very closely related lentiviruses (*lentus* = slow). Other lentiviruses have been found to cause diseases in goats, cattle, horses, and cats.

Since the discovery in 1983 that the human acquired immunodeficiency syndrome (AIDS) was caused by the human immunodeficiency virus (HIV), and the virus found to be a lentivirus, the lentiviruses have become the most intensively studied viruses of all time, and there has been remarkable progress in defining their basic properties. HIV now serves as a model system, and while there are substantial similarities between it and the lentiviruses of veterinary importance, some differences are evident. Some of the animal diseases, especially those caused by the simian and the feline immunodeficiency viruses, are used as models for the study of the pathogenesis of human AIDS and in the testing of drugs and vaccines.

Properties of Lentiviruses

In many of their properties, including virion structure and replication cycle, the lentiviruses resemble the other retroviruses, but there are some important differences. The nucleocapsid of the virion is cylinder-shaped rather than icosahedral (see Fig. 33-3). The genome is larger than that of other retroviruses, about 10 kb, and in addition to the *gag*, *pol*, and *env* genes, there are six small, nonstructural genes not found in other retroviruses that regulate various events in the replication cycle (Fig. 33-6). The *pol* and *env* genes are separate in lentiviruses, whereas they overlap in other retroviruses. The genomes of lentiviruses have homology with each other but not with other retroviruses.

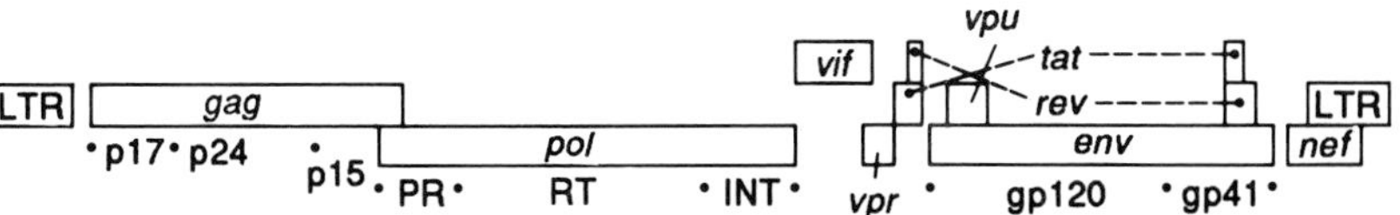

FIG. 33-6. *The genome of human immunodeficiency virus type 1. The* tat *and* rev *genes have two separate exons. The* gag *polyprotein is cleaved to yield the proteins p17, p24, and p15. The* pol *protein is cleaved to produce protease (PR), reverse transcriptase (RT), and integrase (INT). The* env *polyprotein (gp160) is cleaved to produce gp120 and gp41. [From "Microbiology" (B. D. Davis* et al., *eds.), 4th Ed., p. 1146. Lippincott, Philadelphia, Pennsylvania, 1990.]*

Replication

Since HIV has been studied in much greater detail than other lentiviruses, the account of the replication cycle is based on work with that virus. The envelope glycoprotein gp120 binds to the 54K CD4 protein on the plasma membranes of macrophages and their bone marrow precursors as well as dendritic cells of lymph nodes, astroglia, B lymphocytes, and colonic epithelial cells. T helper lymphocytes are important target cells infected secondarily by contact with these cells. Any cell expressing CD4, even if acquired by transfection, can be infected. In addition to gp120, the N terminus of gp41, which is a fusion protein, is required for infection, possibly by binding to a second receptor molecule. CD4 synthesis is down-regulated in infected cells, with profound impairment of function; down-regulation is probably due to *env*–CD4 complex formation in the cytosol. Both gp160–CD4 and gp120–CD4 complexes can be immunoprecipitated from infected cell extracts.

All infected cells may remain latently infected for prolonged periods. Triggers for productive infection such as antigen or other mitogens which stimulate the cells to cycle and divide are of critical importance in initiating productive infection and the progression of clinical disease. Cell death appears to be due to the insertion of many copies of gp41 across the cell membrane and to the accumulation of nonintegrated DNA.

Mutation

As with other retroviruses, mutation rates are very high, and point, deletion, and insertional mutations occur. The *env* protein gp120 has five hypervariable regions, while *gag* and *pol* genes are less variable. It is likely that the mutation rate per nucleotide is uniform across the whole genome, but the mutations that are found are those essential for survival of the virus such as *env* mutations that give rise to immune response escape mutants. Antibody-resistant mutants emerge frequently, often as a consequence of point mutations. Mutations during progression of the disease may also change and broaden the tropism of the virus.

Pathogenesis

Entry of the virus followed by infection of antigen-presenting cells, especially macrophages and dendritic cells, is followed by infection of Th ($CD4^+$) lymphocytes. There follows a latent period, which is usually long, during which the lentivirus genome can be detected in a small fraction of peripheral blood leukocytes, typically about 1 in 10,000, by *in situ* DNA hybridization using viral probes. Activation of Th lumphocytes so that they begin to cycle, an essential prequisite for viral replication, may be caused by a variety of mechanisms. Alloantigens introduced with the infecting inoculum, or transfusions or continued unprotected sex, are probably important for activating HIV, and infections with various herpesviruses and adenovirus up-regulate transcription of HIV.

The close confinement of Icelandic sheep that provided opportunities for the spread of visna/maedi also facilitated the spread of respiratory pathogens; for the feline immunodeficiency virus there is evidence that coinfection with feline leukemia virus may be significant in precipitating clinical immunodeficiency disease. Some lentiviruses, such as bovine immunodeficiency virus and equine infectious anemia virus, may remain latent throughout the life of the animal without serious clinical disease being observed, creating a major dilemma for disease control, especially when individual animals may have high sentimental or monetary value.

Immune Response

Antibody-dependent and cell-mediated immune responses develop both to external virion proteins, such as gp120 and gp41 and to internal virion proteins such as the reverse transcriptase and p24. Antibody positivity to lentiviruses develops more slowly than for other viral infections, which is of considerable epidemiologic significance in that seronegative individuals may be infectious. Antibodies to gp41 and p24 epitopes appear first, but with the onset of clinical disease the level of these antibodies decreases rapidly. Cell-mediated immune responses are strong to p24 but weak to gp120. Tc lymphocytes restricted by either class I or II MHC are recognized. Macrophages present viral antigen in association with class II MHC. $CD4^+$ cells bind gp120, endocytose the complex, and present it in association with MHC class II. Natural killer cells and antibody-dependent cell-mediated cytoxicity mechanisms operate.

None of these mechanisms succeeds in controlling the infection, however, and the immune responses decline sharply with the onset of clinical disease. The causes for the decline include the following: (1) Th cell death; (2) death of antigen-presenting cells (macrophages, dendritic cells, and B lymphocytes); (3) Tc killing of Th cells and antigen-presenting cells that adsorb, process, or express viral antigens; (4) virus-induced down-regulation of CD4; (5) reduced lymphokine production (e.g., of interleukin 2 and interferon γ); (6) production of suppressor factors; and (7) genetic variation affecting critical viral epitopes.

Transmission

Lentiviruses are transmitted by a variety of body fluids, including blood, semen, bronchial secretions, tears, saliva, and milk, which contain either free virus or infected cells. There are important differences between different lentivirus species in relation to the importance of different body fluids. For example, blood and semen are significant in human HIV transmission, blood (including blood transferred by biting flies) in equine infectious anemia, milk in caprine arthritis–encephalomyelitis, and saliva in feline immunodeficiency virus infection.

Diagnosis

The most widely used diagnostic tests for the detection of antibody are ELISAs in which either or both core and surface antigens are present, but Western blots are more sensitive and may be used to confirm diagnosis. Antigen may be detected in peripheral blood leukocytes by ELISA, and viral DNA may be detected in these cells by *in situ* hybridization, directly or following the polymerase chain reaction. Virus can be isolated by cocultivation of gradient-purified peripheral blood leukocytes with mitogen-stimulated donor purified peripheral blood leukocytes in the presence of interleukin 2. Reverse transcriptase assays performed at various times on the supernatants from these cultures provide a basis for diagnosis and virus isolation. The reverse transcriptase of lentiviruses is Mg^{2+}-dependent whereas that of other retroviruses is Mn^{2+}-dependent.

Ovine Lentivirus Diseases (Maedi/Visna)

Visna, in which the lesions occur in the central nervous system, has been rarely recorded in sheep outside Iceland, although a few cases have been described in Holland. However, a disease very like maedi occurs in several countries in Europe and in the United States, where it is called ovine progressive pneumonia, but it does not occur in Australia or New Zealand, which have large sheep populations.

Visna. Following experimental infection, the incubation period of visna varies from a few months to 9 years. The onset of clinical signs is insidious and usually begins with slight weakness of the hind legs. Affected sheep may straggle the flock and stumble and fall for no apparent reason. There is progressive weight loss, and trembling of facial muscles and lips may occur. The paresis eventually leads to paraplegia. There is no fever, the appetite is maintained, and sheep remain alert. The clinical course may last several years, with periods of remission. The cerebrospinal fluid contains up to 200 mononuclear cells per milliliter (normal 50/ml).

Maedi/Progressive Pneumonia. The onset of clinical signs in the pulmonary lentivirus diseases of sheep is insidious and is seldom detected in sheep less than 3 years old. Incubation periods of up to 8 years have been recorded. There is progressive weight loss, and dyspnea, initially detectable only after exercise, becomes progressively more apparent. Affected sheep straggle when the flock is driven. The head may jerk rhythmically with each inspiration, nostrils are flared, and there may be a slight nasal discharge and a cough. Severely dyspneic sheep spend much time lying down. The clinical course may last 3 to 8 months; it may be prolonged by careful nursing or shortened by pregnancy, stress such as occasioned by inclement weather or poor nutrition, or intercurrent disease, particularly pneumonia due to *Pasteurella* spp. Pregnant ewes may abort or deliver weak lambs.

Arthritis and lymphoid tumors of the mammary gland in addition to pneumonia have been observed in sheep following experimental infection with strains of virus recovered in the United States.

Pathogenesis and Pathology. Prior to 1933, Icelandic sheep were genetically isolated for 1000 years, and it has been suggested, but not proven either for them or for other breeds of sheep, that there may be a genetic predisposition to lentivirus disease, especially visna. The ovine lentiviruses are probably most commonly acquired by droplet infection via the respiratory tract. Experimentally, visna can be produced by intracerebral inoculation of sheep. A lymphocyte-associated viremia occurs, in which about 1 in every 10^6 peripheral blood leukocytes is infected.

Lentiviruses are exceptionally resistant to interferon, and despite a diverse range of immune responses, including the production of neutralizing antibodies and a cell-mediated immune response, neither virus nor infected cells are eliminated. Immune suppression abrogates or delays the progress of degenerative changes, indicating that immune mechanisms are significant in the inflammatory changes in both the lung and central nervous system. In an infected sheep, antigenic variation in the envelope antigens (see Chapter 10) may be an important mechanism for circumventing viral elimination.

Apart from neurogenic muscle atrophy, no gross lesions are found in visna, and histologically lesions are usually confined to the central nervous system; occasionally slight lung pathology may be present. The characteristic lesion of the central nervous system is a demyelinating leukoencephalomyelitis. The meninges and subependymal spaces are infiltrated with mononuclear cells, mainly lymphocytes with some plasma cells and macrophages. There is perivascular cuffing, neuronal necrosis, malacia, and demyelination scattered patchily throughout the central nervous system.

Gross findings in maedi and ovine progressive pneumonia are restricted to the lungs and associated lymph nodes. The lungs show extensive consolidation and do not collapse when the thoracic cavity is opened. Bronchial and mediastinal lymph nodes are greatly enlarged. Histologically there is hyperplasia of the fibrous tissue and muscle of the alveolar septa, along with mononuclear cell inflammatory infiltration.

Epidemiology and Control. Droplet transmission is facilitated by housing and close confinement and was important in Iceland, where sheep were housed for 6 months during the winter. Transmission is usually direct, although infection via drinking water or from fecal or urine contamination may occur. Asymptomatic sheep are rarely a source of virus for infection of other sheep, with the possible exception of ewe to lamb transmission via milk. Evidence for transplacental infection and infection via semen is conflicting. Biting arthropods and surgical equipment could readily transmit virus mechanically from viremic sheep.

Visna/maedi was eradicated from Iceland by a drastic slaughter policy before the availability of any diagnostic test. Test and removal programs are used in Norway and Holland. Gel diffusion, complement fixation, ELISA, and a syncytial plaque reduction assay are used for antibody detection.

Caprine Arthritis–Encephalomyelitis

First recognized in the United States in 1974, caprine arthritis–encephalomyelitis is now known to occur worldwide. Two syndromes are recognized: encephalomyelitis in kids 2–4 months old and more commonly arthritis in goats from about 12 months of age onward. In the United States, caprine arthritis–encephalomyelitis is now the most important disease of goats; infection rates as high as 80% have been reported in some herds, and the economic loss from the disease is substantial. The virus is not known to be naturally transmitted to other animal species. Experimentally, the virus infects sheep and causes arthritis. However, despite the high incidence of infection of goats in Australia and New Zealand, infection of sheep has not been reported in these countries.

Clinical Features and Pathology. The central nervous system disease is a progressive leukoencephalomyelitis associated with ascending paralysis. Affected goats also show progressive wasting and trembling, and the hair coat is dull; however, they remain afebrile, alert, and usually maintain good appetite and sight (Fig. 33-7). Terminally there is paralysis, deviation of the head and neck, and paddling. At necropsy, lesions may be visible as focal malacia in the white matter but are more reliably identified microscopically as foci of mononuclear cell inflammation and demyelination.

The onset of arthritis is usually insidious and progresses slowly over months to years, but in some cases disease may appear suddenly and remain static. The joints are swollen and painful, particularly the carpal joints (Fig. 33-7) but also hock, stifle, shoulder, fetlock, and vertebral joints. Cold weather exacerbates the signs. Bursae, particularly the atlanto-occipital, and tendon sheaths are thickened and distended with fluid. Thickening of the joint capsules results in restricted movement and flexion contracture. The basic lesion is a proliferative synovitis of

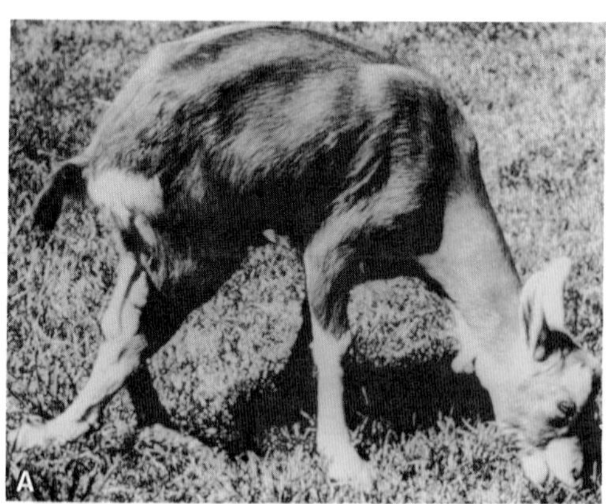

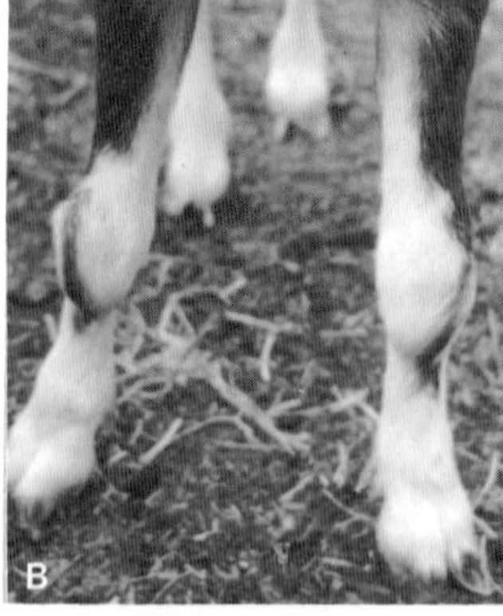

FIG. 33-7. *Caprine arthritis–encephalomyelitis. (A) Kid goat with paralyzed hindquarters, but alert and attempting to graze. (B) Enlarged carpal joints in a 5-year-old goat. (Courtesy J. R. Gorham and Dr. T. H. Crawford.)*

joints, tendon sheaths, and bursae characterized by villous hypertrophy, synovial cell hyperplasia, and infiltration with lymphocytes, plasma cells, and macrophages. Progression is accompanied by degenerative changes including fibrosis, necrosis, mineralization of synovial membranes, and osteoporosis. Mild interstitial pneumonia and hyperplasia of pulmonary lymphoid tissue may be seen at postmortem.

Epidemiology and Control. Virus is acquired during the neonatal period, via colostrum or milk. The cycle of infection can be broken if kids are delivered by cesarian section and fed cow's milk or milk from caprine arthritis–encephalomyelitis virus-free does.

Antibodies can be detected by gel diffusion, indirect immunofluorescence, or ELISA tests. Such assays underlie voluntary control programs based on test and removal.

Bovine Immunodeficiency Virus

Bovine immunodeficiency virus was isolated from peripheral blood leukocytes in 1972; its genome has been sequenced and is similar to that of other lentiviruses. It can be grown in monolayer cell cultures from a variety of bovine embryonic tissues, producing a cytopathic effect characterized by syncytium formation. When virus is transmitted to calves by intravenous inoculation, there is an immediate leukopenia followed within 15–20 days by lymphocytosis which persists. Virus persists in naturally infected cows for at least 12 months, but neither the prevalence of the infection nor its economic significance has been determined.

Equine Infectious Anemia

Equine infectious anemia is an important chronic disease of horses that occurs worldwide.

Clinical Signs and Pathogenesis. Following primary infection, most horses develop fever after an incubation period of 7–21 days. The disease is recognized as four interchanging, overlapping syndromes. In acute equine infectious anemia there is a marked fever, weakness, severe anemia, jaundice, blood-stained feces, tachypnea, and petechial hemorrhages of the mucosae. Perhaps as many as 80% of acute cases die; others pass into the subacute form, in which continuing moderate fever is followed by recovery. Recovery from either the acute or subacute disease is followed by lifelong persistent infection. Recovered viremic horses may appear and perform well, but some experience recurrent episodes of disease associated with the emergence of antibody-escape mutants, while others develop chronic disease that varies from mild signs of illness and failure to thrive to episodic or persistent fever, cachexia, and ventral edema.

The disease is due to infection of lymphocytes, in which degenerative or proliferative responses may occur. Lifelong, cell-associated viremia develops in all infected horses. It is uncertain whether anemia develops as a consequence of bone marrow suppression, increased clearance of red cells from the circulation, or autoimmune destruction of erythrocytes. Vasculitis, including glomerulonephritis, is mediated by immune complexes.

Epidemiology and Control. Tabanid flies and stable flies (*Stomoxys* spp.), mosquitoes, and possibly biting midges (*Culicoides*) can serve as mechanical vectors for equine infectious anemia virus. Transmission occurs particularly in the summer months in low-lying, humid, swampy areas such as occur in the Mississippi delta region of the United States and in parts of South and Central America, South Africa, and northern Australia. National prevalence figures are geographically uneven and reflect the importance of insect transmission. On farms on which infection has been endemic for many years the prevalence may be as high as 70%. Iatrogenic transmission by the use of nonsterile equipment has been responsible for some major outbreaks. Transplacental infection has been recognized; colostrum and milk, saliva, urine, and semen are other unproven but possible modes of transmission.

In endemic areas the rate of transmission may be reduced by insect-proof stabling of horses during those times of the year (summer) and that time of the day (dusk) when insects are most active. Iatrogenic transmission is avoided by careful hygiene.

The development in 1970 of a gel diffusion test for detecting antibodies to equine infectious anemia virus was followed in the United States by regulations, promulgated by federal and state agencies and some breed societies, to limit the movement of seropositive horses. In some instances, a negative test has been required as a condition of entry to racetracks, saleyards, and shows. Buyers of horses have also increasingly sought negative test certification. The U.S. Department of Agriculture introduced regulations relating to the licensing and operation of laboratories authorized to conduct the gel diffusion (Coggins) test, and horses imported into the United States and some other countries are required to have a negative test certificate. For horses remaining within a state, testing is not compulsory, nor is it compulsory for an owner to destroy a horse giving a positive test.

Feline Immunodeficiency Virus

Since its first isolation in California in 1987 and the availability of ELISA diagnostic tests, feline immunodeficiency virus (FIV) has been identified in many countries and probably has a worldwide distribution; it has occurred at least since 1968 and probably much earlier. Although all isolates of FIV have come from domestic cats, antibodies have been found in the African lion, jaguar, tiger, bobcat, and puma. The seroprevalence varies from 1% in random surveys to 30% in sick cats. It is now clear that many of the signs of disease in cats formerly associated with aging or more recently with feline leukemia virus infection may have been due to FIV infection, and it is likely that the account of the clinical features of feline leukemia virus infection given earlier in this chapter will need to be revised. Various disease associations derived from retrospective studies need to be confirmed by statistically valid prospective studies.

Clinical Features. The precise clinical importance of FIV has yet to be determined, but it is known that the incubation period lasts for several years, followed by an insidious onset of clinical disease, which is assumed to resemble the syndromes found at various stages of human AIDS. To the veterinarian, the usual presenting signs are recurrent fevers of undetermined origin, leukopenia, lymphadenopathy, anemia, lethargy, weight loss, and nonspecific behavioral changes. At this stage opportunistic infections are not evident, but in more advanced cases there are secondary bacterial and fungal infections, especially in the mouth, peridontal tissue, cheeks, fauces, and tongue, and about 25% have chronic respiratory disease and a lesser number chronic enteritis, urinary tract infection, dermatitis, and neurologic signs. The final picture resembles that of advanced human AIDS, with a variety of opportunistic infections including some due to viruses, bacteria, fungi, protozoa, and helminths. At this stage about 5% of the cats have serious neurologic disease, although histologic studies reveal that a higher proportion have lesions of the central nervous system.

Diagnosis. In experimental infections, antibodies can be detected within 2–4 weeks of infection, using ELISA, immunofluorescence, or Western blotting. In cats brought to the veterinarian's office, false-positive ELISAs range from 2% to 20%, probably because of the use in cats of vaccines that have been produced in feline cell cultures; vigorous attempts are under way to improve the specificity of ELISA. In peripheral blood leukocytes FIV antigen can be detected by ELISA or proviral DNA by the polymerase chain reaction.

Transmission. Horizontal transmission by contact can occur but is inefficient. Bite wounds appear to be the major mode of transmission, accounting for the higher incidence of infection in male cats. Neither venereal, *in utero,* colostrom/milk, or maternal grooming are significant modes of transmission.

Control. Nonspecific treatment of signs and specific drugs directed against reverse transcriptase, such as azidothymidine, may be used. Appropriate test and removal programs and certification at the point of sale can be applied to control the infection. No human public health risks have been identified.

FURTHER READING

Anonymous. (1991). Colloquium on feline leukemia virus/feline immunodeficiency virus: Tests and vaccination. *J. Am. Med. Vet. Assoc.* **199,** 1271.

Cheevers, W. P., and McGuire, T. C. (1985). Equine infectious anemia virus: Immunopathogenesis and persistence. *Rev. Infect. Dis.* **7,** 83.

Dulbecco, R. (1990). Oncogenic viruses II. RNA-containing viruses (retroviruses). *In* "Microbiology" (B. D. Davis, R. Dulbecco, H. N. Eisen, and H. S. Ginsberg, eds.), 4th Ed., p. 1123. Lippincott, Philadelphia, Pennsylvania.

Kakoma, I., Ristic, M., and Essex, M., eds. (1988). Animal retroviruses. *Vet. Microbiol.* **17** (special issue), 195.

Narayan, O., and Clements, J. E. (1989). Biology and pathogenesis of lentiviruses. *J. Gen. Virol.* **70,** 1617.

Neil, J. C., Fulton, R., Rigby, M., and Stewart, M. (1991). Feline leukemia virus: Generation of pathogenic and oncogenic variants. *Curr. Top. Microbiol. Immunol.* **171,** 67.

Payne, L. N., and Purchase, H. G. (1991). Leukosis/sarcoma group. *In* "Diseases of Poultry" (B. W. Calnek, ed.), 9th Ed., p. 386. Iowa State Univ. Press, Ames.

van der Masten, M. J., and Miller, J. M. (1990). Bovine leukosis virus. *In* "Virus Infections of Ruminants" (Z. Dinter and B. Morein, eds.), p. 419. Elsevier, Amsterdam.

Witter, R. L. (1991). Reticuloendotheliosis. *In* "Diseases of Poultry" (B. W. Calnek, ed.), 9th Ed., p. 439. Iowa State Univ. Press, Ames.

Wong-Staal, F. (1990). Human immunodeficiency viruses and their replication. *In* "Fields Virology" (B. N. Fields, D. M. Knipe, R. M. Chanock, M. S. Hirsch, J. L. Melnick, T. P. Monath, and B. Roizman, eds.), 2nd Ed., p. 1529. Raven, New York.

CHAPTER 34

Other Viruses

In the preceding chapters diseases of veterinary importance caused by viruses belonging to 18 families have been described. There are several other virus families or genera with members that cause diseases of domestic animals, and there are a few other viruses and viruslike infectious agents of domestic or laboratory animals whose taxonomic status is as yet uncertain. These viruses are described in this chapter.

ARENAVIRIDAE

The prototype arenavirus, lymphocytic choriomeningitis virus, which produces a clinically inapparent lifelong infection in mice, has been known for over 50 years and has provided an important model for studies of persistent infections (see Chapter 10) and immunological tolerance. More recently, four other arenaviruses have been discovered in Africa and ten in the Americas; four of these cause hemorrhagic fever in humans (Table 34-1).

The family *Arenaviridae* derives its name from the presence within virions of ribosome-like particles, which in electron micrographs resemble grains of sand (*arenosus* = sandy) and are incorporated into virions coincidentally during budding. Arenaviruses are pleomorphic, 110–130 nm (rarely up to 300 nm) in diameter (Fig. 34-1), and are composed of a lipoprotein envelope covered with glycoprotein peplomers surrounding two nucleocapsid segments which appear as finely helical circles. The genome comprises two linear segments of ssRNA, 7.2 and 3.4 kb in size, each formed into a circle by hydrogen bonding of the ends. Most of the genome is of minus sense, but the 5′ half of the small genome segment and a short sequence at the 5′ end of the large segment are of plus sense: the term ambisense has been coined to describe this and the similar genome of some members of the family *Bunyaviridae* (see Chapter 30). Arenaviruses replicate to high titer in cell cultures, for example, in the E-6 cloned line of Vero (African green monkey) cells. The viruses replicate in the cytoplasm and mature via budding from the plasma membrane.

Each arenavirus is maintained in nature by a rodent species in which persistent infection and chronic virus shedding in urine and oral secretions result in transmission to each new generation. Vertical (transplacental) transmission of lymphocytic choriomeningitis virus also occurs and leads to immunological tolerance in offspring. The relevant reservoir hosts of the zoonotic arenaviruses are listed in Table 34-1. The natural history of the human diseases is determined by the pathogenicity of the virus, the geographic distribution, habitat and habits of the rodent reservoir host, and the nature of the human–rodent interaction. Human infection with lymphocytic choriomeningitis virus presents as one of three syndromes: (1) most commonly as an influenza-like illness with

TABLE 34-1
Distribution and Rodent Hosts of Arenaviruses That Are Human Pathogens

Virus/disease	Geographic distribution	Natural host
Lymphocytic choriomeningitis virus/ influenza-like disease, meningitis	Europe, Americas	*Mus musculus*
Junin virus/Argentinian hemorrhagic fever	Argentina	*Calomys musculinus*
Machupo virus/Bolivian hemorrhagic fever	Bolivia	*Calomys callosus*
Guanarito virus/Venezuelan hemorrhagic fever	Venezuela	*Sigmodon* sp.
Lassa virus/hemorrhagic fever	West Africa	*Mastomys natalensis*

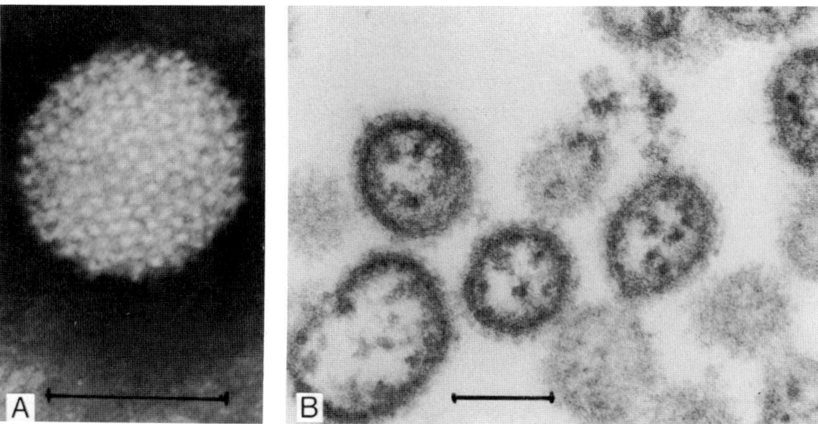

FIG. 34.1 Arenaviridae. *(A) Tacaribe virus, negatively stained. (B) Lassa virus, thin section of infected cell. Bars: 100 nm.*

fever, headache, myalgia, and malaise; (2) less often as an aseptic meningitis with severe headache, papilledema, and elevated cerebrospinal fluid pressure; (3) rarely as an encephalomyelitis with depression, coma, and disturbed nerve function. The other four arenaviruses listed in Table 34-1 produce a severe hemorrhagic fever in humans.

Lymphocytic choriomeningitis virus is distributed throughout Europe and the Americas in the common house mouse (*Mus musculus*), where it is highly focal in mouse populations. For this reason the distribution of human cases is also focal; the distribution of human cases is seasonal as well, probably because mice move into closer contact with man in houses and barns in cold weather. The same circumstances that introduce lymphocytic choriomeningitis virus into houses and barns serve to introduce the virus into laboratory and commercial mouse, rat, hamster, guinea pig, and rhesus monkey colonies. In the United States, the virus has been a particular problem in hamster colonies and immunocompromised [nude, severe combined immunodeficient (SCID), etc.] mouse colonies, resulting in contaminated diagnostic reagents, failed research protocols, and clinical disease in laboratory and animal care personnel. The increasing popularity of hamsters as pets has also resulted in many human disease episodes, some involving hundreds of cases. Nevertheless, in many circumstances wild mouse entry into laboratory animal colonies is still not effectively prevented.

Recently, it has been realized that an important lethal disease of marmosets or tamarins, called marmoset (callitrichid) hepatitis, is caused by a virus that is very closely related to lymphocytic choriomeningitis virus.

Some marmosets, such as the golden lion tamarin, are endangered species; programs to breed the animals and release them back into their natural habitats are confounded by diseases such as this.

Past human infection with arenaviruses is usually diagnosed serologically, by indirect immunofluorescence, using inactivated cell culture "spotslides" as antigen substrate. Such tests may be set up to measure IgM antibody so as to indicate recent infection. Lymphocytic choriomeningitis in rodent colonies is diagnosed serologically, with confirmation by virus isolation in cell culture. Lassa, Machupo, Guaranarito, and Junin viruses are classified as Biosafety Level 4 pathogens, that is, they must be handled only in maximum security laboratories. Lymphocytic choriomeningitis virus isolates from nature, including those from laboratory rodent colonies, also require adequate containment facilities, usually at Biosafety Level 3. Specimen transport must be arranged in keeping with national and international regulations.

ARTERIVIRUSES

Morphologically, the arteriviruses resemble the togaviruses, with which the genus *Arterivirus* was formerly classified. The name of the group derives from the major pathologic finding observed in horses infected with equine arteritis virus. All species grow quickly, and the macrophage is their primary target of infection. All have the capacity to establish asymptomatic persistent infections in their natural hosts and to cause severe disease in certain circumstances (Table 34-2). Equine arteritis virus replicates in primary equine kidney cells; however, not all strains cause cytopathology in these cells, so viral growth must be detected indirectly, for example, by immunofluorescence.

Properties and Replication

The properties of the arteriviruses are summarized in Table 34-3. The genome of equine arteritis virus consists of a single strand of plus sense RNA 12 kb in size. Full-length genomic RNA is synthesized via a minus sense complementary strand. Transcription involves the synthesis of a nested set of seven 3′-coterminal mRNAs, each reflecting a single open reading frame. The subgenomic RNAs are composed of leader and body sequences which are not encoded contiguously on the viral genome (the leader sequence is derived from the extreme 5′ end of the genome). The arteriviruses also employ ribosomal frameshifting in their translation. Nucleotide sequencing indicates that the RNA polymerase gene takes up about 75% of the 5′ end of the genome; the genes which encode the

TABLE 34-2
Diseases Caused by Arteriviruses

Virus	Transmission	Host animal	Disease	Distribution
Equine arteritis virus	Contact	Horse	Respiratory disease, congenital disease, generalized infection, abortion	Worldwide
Simian hemorrhagic fever virus	Contact/fomites	Macaques	Hemorrhagic fever	Worldwide
Lactate dehydrogenase-elevating virus	Contact	Mouse	Model of persistent viral infection	Worldwide
Lelystad virus	Contact, congenital	Swine	Respiratory disease, infertility, congenital disease	North America, Europe

viral structural proteins are located in the 3′ end of the genome, the part that is transcribed as a coterminal nested set. This replication strategy (gene order, transcription as a nested set of mRNAs, ribosomal frame-shifting, etc.) resembles that of coronaviruses and toroviruses. Four virion proteins have been described in equine arteritis virus: a nucleocapsid protein (14K), two envelope proteins (18K and 28K–42K), and a 21K protein of unknown function.

TABLE 34-3
Properties of Arteriviruses

Spherical virion, enveloped, with peplomers, diameter 60–70 nm
Icosahedral capsid, diameter 28–35 nm
Linear, plus sense ssRNA genome, 12 kb, 5′ end capped, 3′ end polyadenylated, infectious; genes for nonstructural protein located at 5′ end of genome
Seven 3′-coterminal mRNA transcripts; transcribed as a nested set, each reflecting a single open reading frame encoding one protein
Two envelope proteins, one nonglycosylated (18K) and one glycosylated (28K–42K), one nucleocapsid protein (14K), and a 21K protein of unknown nature
Cytoplasmic replication, budding from membranes of cytoplasmic organelles
Genus *Arterivirus* includes equine arteritis virus, simian hemorrhagic fever virus, and lactate dehydrogenase-elevating virus

Equine Arteritis

Equine arteritis is a systemic febrile disease, usually observed only on breeding farms. However, serologic studies indicate that infection is usually subclinical and is widespread in equine populations worldwide. The clinical features of overt infections are acute depression with fever, leukopenia, anorexia, palpebral edema, conjunctivitis, catarrh, and edema of legs, genitalia, and abdomen. The disease is rarely fatal, but 40% to 80% of infected pregnant mares abort. Infection may lead to a carrier state, with stallions transmitting the virus chronically via semen. The basic lesion caused by the virus is a segmental necrosis of small arteries throughout the body. Transmission is via aerosol and contact with infected horses or aborted fetuses and placentas. Immunization of horses with an attenuated live-virus vaccine prepared in cell cultures produces long-lasting immunity and no untoward effects. In view of the very rare occurrence of clinical outbreaks of disease the need to immunize equine populations is disputable, but because of the effect of infections on reproductive outcome, immunization of valuable breeding mares is commonly undertaken.

Simian Hemorrhagic Fever

Simian hemorrhagic fever virus was first isolated in 1964 during devastating epidemics in macaques imported from India into the Soviet Union and the United States. Nearly all infected animals die. Similar epidemics have occurred frequently since then; for example, in the United States in 1989 there were epidemics at three primate colonies resulting in the death of more than 600 cynomolgous macaques (*Macaca fascicularis*). The onset of disease in macaques is rapid, with early fever, facial edema, anorexia, adipsia, dehydration, skin petechia, diarrhea, and hemorrhages. Death occurs between 5 and 25 days, and mortality approaches 100%. Within a colony, infection spreads rapidly, probably via contact and aerosol. Pathologic lesions include hemorrhages in the dermis, nasal mucosa, lung, and intestine and other visceral organs. Shock is suspected as the underlying cause of death.

All species of macaques (genus *Macaca*) are highly susceptible to simian hemorrhagic fever virus, and macaques are the only animals the develop severe, usually fatal disease. Epidemics in macaque colonies originate from accidental introduction of the virus from other primate species that are persistently infected without showing clinical signs. In captivity, Patas monkeys (*Erythrocebus patas*) have often been implicated as the source of virus, but in the wild African green monkeys (*Cercopithecus aethiops*) and baboons (*Papio anuibus* and *P. cyanocephalus*) also carry the virus in their blood persistently. Transmission in primate colonies is facilitated by poor practices, such as reuse of syringes and needles and tattooing equipment and inadequate cage sterilization. It is not known how virus is transmitted among non-macaques, nor whether the virus exists in nature in macaques (obviously, however, natural transmission of the virus from persistently infected African monkeys, such as Patas monkeys, to macaques which come from Asia is not possible because of the geographic separation). Control is based on species separation in colonies and on proper containment facilities and practices.

Porcine Epidemic Abortion and Respiratory Syndrome

In 1987 a new disease characterized by abortion, infertility, and respiratory signs appeared in swine herds in the United States and Canada, and in 1990–1991 the same syndrome was recognized in several countries in Europe. Dutch research workers, who propose the name "porcine epidemic abortion and respiratory syndrome" for the disease, have reported that the causal virus is an arterivirus, and similar isolates have been made in North America.

The clinical signs, which are somewhat similar to those of pseudorabies, occur in sows and their piglets. After an incubation period of 4–7 days, infected sows become listless and exhibit a transient blue discoloration of the ears, abdomen, and vulva. Some sows abort; others give birth to weak, stillborn, or mummified piglets. Young piglets, infected *in utero* or shortly after birth, often develop neurologic and respiratory disease and die; fattening pigs are less severely affected. The origins, ecology, and epidemiology of the virus have yet to be determined.

The causal agent, called the Lelystad virus, can be isolated by inoculating cultures of swine alveolar macrophages with material from the lungs or tonsillar tissues of sick piglets or with the serum of diseased sows.

FILOVIRIDAE

In 1967 a previously unknown hemorrhagic fever occurred in Germany and Yugoslavia among laboratory workers and veterinarians engaged in processing kidneys from African green monkeys (*Cercopithecus aethiops*) that had been imported from Uganda to prepare cell cultures for poliovirus vaccine production; there were 7 deaths among 31 cases. Many of the monkeys from the same shipments died of a similar hemorrhagic disease. A virus isolated from patients, named Marburg virus, was found to be morphologically unique, antigenically unrelated to any known human or animal virus, and uniformly lethal when inoculated into several species of monkeys.

In 1976, epidemics of hemorrhagic fever occurred in hospitals in Zaire and the Sudan; there were more than 500 cases and 430 deaths. In these epidemics there were many iatrogenic nosocomial infections, caused by the reuse of contaminated needles and syringes in hospitals, and there was community spread associated with intimate patient contact. A virus, named Ebola virus, was isolated in these epidemics and found to be morphologically identical but antigenically distinct from Marburg virus. Since these initial outbreaks, sporadic human cases of Marburg and Ebola hemorrhagic fever have been recognized in eastern and southern Africa.

In 1989 and 1990, several shipments of monkeys imported from Asia into the United States were found to have been infected with a filovirus related to Ebola virus. Monkey infection was associated with illness, and there were substantial numbers of death. Virus was isolated from cynomolgus monkeys (*Macaca fascicularis*), and antibody was detected in cynomolgus, African green, and rhesus (*Macaca mulatta*) monkeys. Virus isolates were morphologically identical to but biologically, antigenically, and genetically distinct from prototype filoviruses; the virus has been named Reston virus. Infections, determined by seroconversions and in one case by virus isolation, occurred in some persons occupationally exposed to actively infected cynomolgus monkeys. Although severe hemorrhagic fever had marked past human filovirus infections, there were no illnesses noted in association with any of these infections. Sera from a large number of persons with varying levels of exposure to monkeys were tested for filovirus antibody; approximately 14% of persons having close occupational contact with monkeys were positive to filovirus test antigens.

To avoid risks associated with the importation of monkeys, most countries have import quarantine procedures in place. In this context it is relevant that wild-caught monkeys are no longer being widely used for vaccine production, partly because of export prohibitions established by source countries for conservation purposes. In 1990, additional local, national, and international primate transport and import restrictions were imposed. Protocols to prevent filovirus infection in workers in primate facilities were improved; these actions have resulted in substantial improvement in facilities and work practices.

The origins and the natural histories of Marburg, Ebola, and Reston viruses have remained a mystery. It has always been presumed that the viruses are zoonotic, that is, transmitted to humans from ongoing life cycles in animals, probably primates. However, all attempts to backtrack from the monkeys involved in the original European Marburg disease episode or from Ebola index cases in Africa failed to uncover a reservoir. Backtracking from the monkeys invovled in the Reston virus emergence in the Philippines has not yet been done. Whatever the source, person-to-person transmission and nosocomial transmission have been the means by which outbreaks have progressed.

Marburg and Ebola viruses cause fulminant hemorrhagic fever in humans and severe disease in most of the monkey species that have been infected experimentally; disease is marked first by fever and depression, then by diarrhea, petechial rash, prostration, shock, and death. If these viruses are suspected as the cause of disease in humans or in monkeys, consultation and laboratory diagnosis are available from the maximum containment laboratories that operate in several countries. Specimen transport must be arranged in conformance with national and international regulations.

The virions of members of the family *Filoviridae* (*filum* = thread) are very long, filamentous rods or more compact convoluted forms, each composed of a lipid bilayer envelope covered with peplomers surrounding a helically wound nucleocapsid (Fig. 34-2). The virions are 80 nm in diameter and have a unit nucleocapsid length of 800–1000 nm, but particles as long as 14,000 nm have been seen. The genome is a single molecule of minus sense ssRNA, 12.7 kb in size. The virions contain seven proteins, designated L (putative transcriptase), G (glycoprotein peplomers), N (nucleoprotein), VP40, VP35, VP30 (associated with virion RNA), and VP24 (membrane protein). Marburg and Ebola viruses are distinguishable by small differences in genome size and protein profiles,

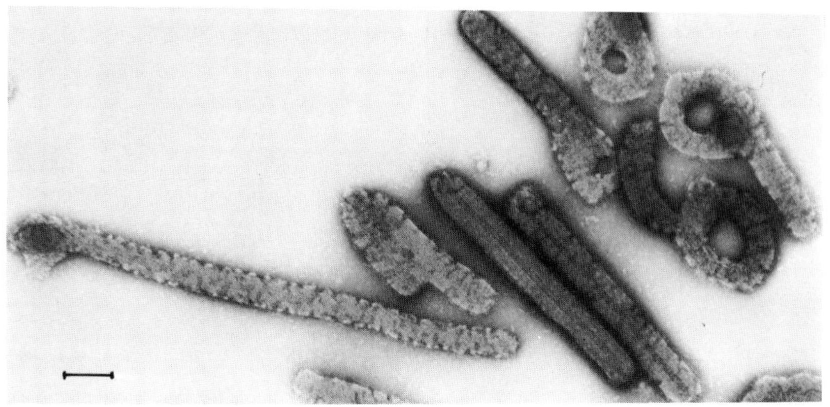

FIG. 34-2. Filoviridae. *Ebola virus, negatively stained. Bar: 100 nm.*

as well as by the absence of antigenic cross-reactivity. The viruses replicate well in cell cultures, for example, in Vero (African green monkey) cells, as well as in guinea pigs, hamsters, and monkeys. Viral replication in the cytoplasm of host cells is marked by the formation of large inclusion bodies, and maturation occurs via budding from the plasma membrane.

"TOROVIRIDAE"

The family name *Toroviridae* has been proposed for a group of previously unclassified RNA viruses (*torus* = lowest convex molding at the base of a column). The prototype member is Berne virus, which was recovered in 1972 from a horse in Switzerland and shown by a serologic survey to occur among horses and cattle in that country. Another member, Breda virus, has been recovered from the feces of diarrheic calves in the United States. Serum neutralization tests have revealed antibodies in ungulates, lagomorphs, and wild rodents, and typical virions have been seen in stools of cats and humans with diarrhea. The Berne virus grows in secondary horse kidney cells.

The virions of Berne and Breda viruses have a similar and characteristic morphology, containing an elongated nucleocapsid of helical symmetry coiled into a hollow tube and tightly surrounded by an envelope. The capsid may be bent into an open torus, conferring a disk- or kidney-shaped morphology to the virion (largest diameter 120–140 nm), or may be straight, resulting in a rod-shaped particle (35 × 170 nm), with club-shaped peplomers 20 nm long (Fig. 34-3). The genome consists of a single

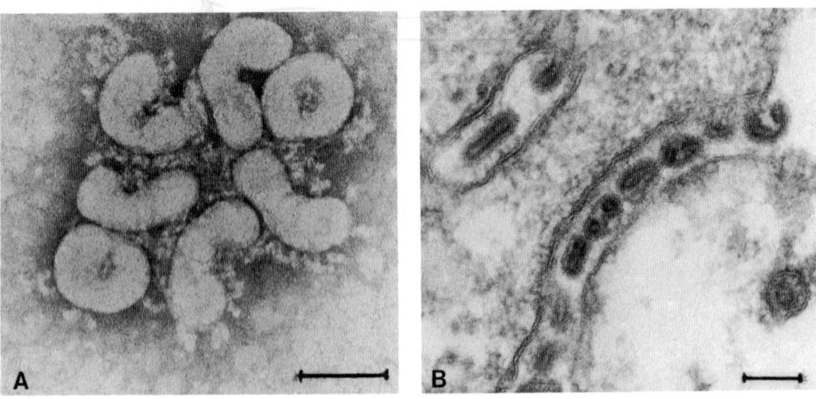

FIG. 34-3. "Toroviridae." *(A) Berne virus, negatively stained, showing characteristic virion morphology. (B) Berne virus, thin section of infected cell, showing accumulation of virions in the Golgi complex. Bars: 100 nm. (Courtesy Dr. M. Weiss.)*

molecule of plus sense ssRNA, more than 20 kb in size. The genome possesses multiple open frames which occur in the same order as in the coronaviruses (5′-polymerase, peplomer glycoprotein, nonglycosylated envelope protein, nucleocapsid protein-3′), and, as in the coronaviruses, these genes are expressed through the synthesis of a 3′-coterminal nested set of mRNAs 5 to 8 kb in size. Major structural proteins of 80K–100K (peplomer glycoprotein), 22K (nonglycosylated envelope protein), and 20K (nucleocapsid protein) have been identified. The glycoprotein peplomers are recognized by both neutralizing and hemagglutination-inhibiting monoclonal antibodies. Replication is dependent on some nuclear function of the host cell, and maturation occurs by budding into the lumen of Golgi cisternae.

ASTROVIRUSES

Astroviruses were first described in 1975, when they were found by electron microscopy in the feces of children with diarrhea. They have also been identified in the feces of calves, lambs, piglets, dogs, cats, deer, mice, turkeys, and ducks. The virions are spherical, 27–30 nm in diameter, and have a distinctive star-shaped surface structure when seen by negative-contrast electron microscopy (Fig. 34-4). There are four structural proteins; the genomes consist of a single molecule of plus sense ssRNA, 7.2–7.9 kb in size, and they produce subgenomic mRNA.

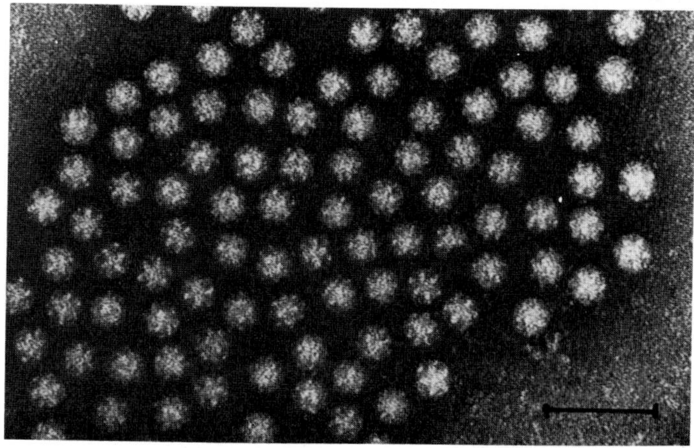

FIG. 34-4. "Astroviridae." *Astrovirus, negatively stained. Bar: 100 nm. [From D. R. Snodgrass and E. W. Gray,* Arch. Virol. **55,** *287 (1977); courtesy Dr. D. R. Snodgrass.]*

Overall, these characteristics suggest that they constitute a new family, but this proposal has not yet been formally advanced.

The astroviruses of humans, calves, and pigs can be cultivated in primary embryonic kidney cells and a colon carcinoma cell line if trypsin is added to the growth medium, but they are usually noncytopathic. There are no antigenic cross-reactions between isolates from different animal species.

The astroviruses mainly effect the villi of the small intestine, where they replicate in mature epithelial cells and also in subepithelial macrophages, producing partial villus atrophy. Lactase levels in the small intestine are reduced during infection. Apart from producing abnormally colored and soft feces, most animals remain normal; few clinical signs are seen in experimentally infected gnotobiotic animals, and hence astroviruses, although often associated with diarrhea especially in very young animals, are considered relatively unimportant pathogens. The duck astrovirus was found in association with a fatal hepatitis, but further study of this syndrome is needed.

HEPADNAVIRIDAE

Although the prototype virus of the family, *Hepadnaviridae*, hepatitis B virus, is of major importance in human medicine, these viruses are of limited veterinary importance. Viruses closely related to hepatitis B virus have been discovered in Pekin and other ducks, woodchucks (*Marmota monax*), and tree and ground squirrels (*Spermophilus beecheyi*), and there is less well documented evidence of similar viruses in marsupials, rodents, and cats. There is also a suspicion that there is a similar virus and associated hepatocellular carcinoma of dogs. Hepatitis B virus in humans causes acute hepatitis, chronic hepatitis, liver cirrhosis, and primary hepatocellular carcinoma. Hepatic carcinoma is found in hepadnavirus-infected Pekin ducks; infected woodchucks develop acute hepatitis and, commonly, hepatic carcinoma, but not cirrhosis. Infected ground squirrels rarely develop hepatitis.

Although hepadnaviruses are extremely difficult to propagate in tissue culture, much is known of their structure and mode of replication. Hepadnavirus virions are 40–48 nm in diameter and composed of an inner icosahedral nucleocapsid (core) surrounded by an envelope (Fig. 34-5). The genome of hepadnaviruses consists of a single molecule of circular (via base pairing of cohesive ends), partially double-stranded DNA. The complete strand is negative-sense and 3.0–3.2 kb in size; the other strand varies between 1.7 and 2.8 kb, leaving 15–50% of the molecule single-stranded. The complete strand contains a nick at a unique site, and it has

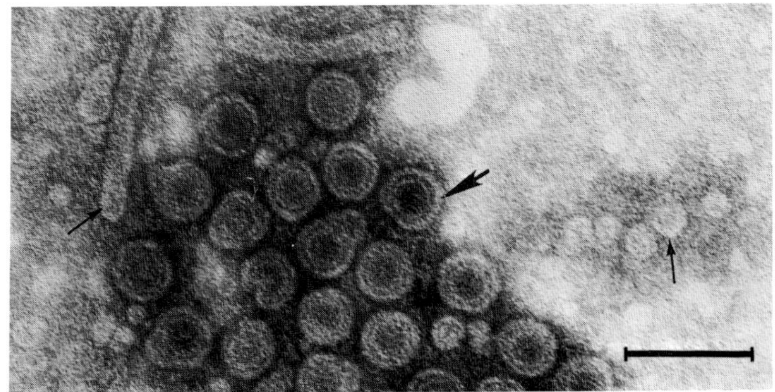

FIG. 34-5. Hepadnaviridae. *Hepatitis B virus (large arrow) and HBsAg particles (small arrows), negatively stained. Bar: 100 nm. (Courtesy Dr. I. D. Gust and J. Marshall.)*

a protein molecule covalently attached to its 5′ end. The hepadnavirus genome has three (avian viruses) or four (mammalian viruses) open reading frames.

The hepadnaviruses have a unique mode of replication involving a reverse transcriptase. (1) Following infection, the virus genome is converted to a complete dsDNA closed circle by a DNA polymerase carried in the core. (2) The minus strand of this DNA is used as the template for the synthesis of a full-length plus strand RNA transcript, which is packaged in viral core particles in the cytoplasm of the infected cell. (3) The viral reverse transcriptase, utilizing a protein primer, then transcribes a minus strand DNA from the RNA template, the latter being simultaneously degraded. (4) The viral DNA polymerase utilizes the minus DNA strand as template for the synthesis of the plus strand of the DNA. Newly synthesized dsDNA is packaged into virions before this last step is complete, so viral DNA is only partially double-stranded. Integration of viral DNA into cellular DNA occurs and leads to persistent infection and to the eventual development of primary hepatocellular carcinoma in humans, ducks, and woodchucks.

The envelope of the hepatitis B virion is composed of three viral proteins, each of which occurs in glycosylated and nonglycosylated forms, and some host cell lipid. Envelope material is also formed into noninfectious spherical (22 nm in diameter) or filamentous (22 nm in width, varying in length) particles called hepatitis B surface antigen (HBsAg) particles; these particles express at least five antigenic specificities. The icosahedral nucleocapsid core of the virion is made up of one antigenically distinct protein (HBcAg) which is phosphorylated by a protein kinase present in the core. HBcAg in serum can be modified, thereby expressing a second antigenic specificity known as HBeAg. Each of these antigenic specificities is used in diagnostic tests and in tests to judge the status of human patients with regard to persistent virus carriage, the presage of chronic liver disease and hepatocellular carcinoma.

Virions present in the serum of chronic carriers of the hepadnaviruses are accompanied by a large excess of noninfectious HBsAg particles, up to 10^{13} per milliliter. These particles serve as the antigen for the most common diagnostic tests, and they have been used to produce a vaccine for human hepatitis B, although this has now been largely replaced by recombinant DNA vaccines expressed in yeast cells.

DELTA VIRUS

Hepatitis B virus serves as helper for delta virus (also called heptatitis D virus), which is a satellite virus in that it requires the presence of hepatitis B virus for its replication and assembly. The delta virus virion is 35–37 nm in diameter and consists of a shell made of HBsAg surrounding a core structure containing delta antigen and a circular ssRNA genome with a size of 1.75 kb. Delta virus has not yet been classified, but it shares features with certain satellite viruses of plants. When delta virus is present along with hepatitis B virus infection, disease is more severe and there is increased mortality. The mechanisms involved in this interaction are unknown.

"CIRCOVIRIDAE"

A new family that we have provisionally called the *"Circoviridae"* has been proposed to include porcine circovirus and psittacine beak and feather disease virus. Although somewhat larger, chicken anemia virus has a similar genome and virion structure and will also be described in this section. The icosahedral virions, with a diameter of 15–17 nm (24 nm for chicken anemia virus), enclose covalently closed circular minus sense ssDNA genomes of 1.76 kb (2.12 kb for chicken anemia virus). There appears to be a single structural protein of 30K in porcine circovirus, whereas the chicken anemia virus virion contains three structural proteins, of which only a 50K protein reacts with hyperimmune serum. There are no common antigenic determinants and no sequence homology between the three viruses. Viral infectivity resists heating at 60°C for 30 minutes.

Viral replication occurs in the nucleus and depends on cellular proteins produced during the S phase of the cell cycle. The dsDNA replicative intermediate of chicken anemia virus has been cloned and is infectious. There are three partially overlapping reading frames coding for putative peptides of 52K, 24K, and 14K.

Porcine Circovirus

Porcine circovirus was first isolated in Germany in 1974, from a pig kidney cell line (PK15) persistently infected with the virus. The virus appears to be nonpathogenic for pigs and for the several laboratory animals tested. Of various animals tested, only pigs have antibodies; specific antibodies have been found widely among domestic pigs, mini-pigs, and wild boars in Germany.

Psittacine Beak and Feather Disease

It has long been known that, when in captivity, many species of Australian parrots undergo permanent loss of feathers and develop beak and claw deformities. In 1984 thin section electron microscopy of affected tissues from such birds revealed cells containing large numbers of virions which were later found to resemble those of the porcine circovirus in size and genome structure. Psittacine beak and feather disease is usually seen in young birds during first feather formation, and the feathers become necrotic and dystrophic and are symmetrically lost. Beak and claw deformation are not always seen; when present beak deformation is characterized by palatine necrosis, abnormal elongation, and fractures. Some birds die after the first appearance of malformed feathers, whereas others may live for years in a featherless state.

Chicken Anemia Virus

First recognized in Japan in 1979, chicken anemia virus is now known to occur worldwide; only a single serotype has been recognized. The icosahedral virions (Fig. 34-6) contain a circular minus sense ssDNA 2.12 kb in size.

Clinical Features. Disease occurs in chicks hatched to breeder hens that are infected with chicken anemia virus after they come into lay, the virus being vertically transmitted. Although there is no disease in the hens, at 2–3 weeks of age the chicks show anemia, bone marrow aplasia, and atrophy of the thymus, bursa of Fabricius and spleen. Disease is often most severe in chicks that are mixedly infected with the chicken anemia virus and other viruses such as reovirus (anemia–dermatitis syndrome of broiler chickens) and adenovirus (inclusion body hepatitis/

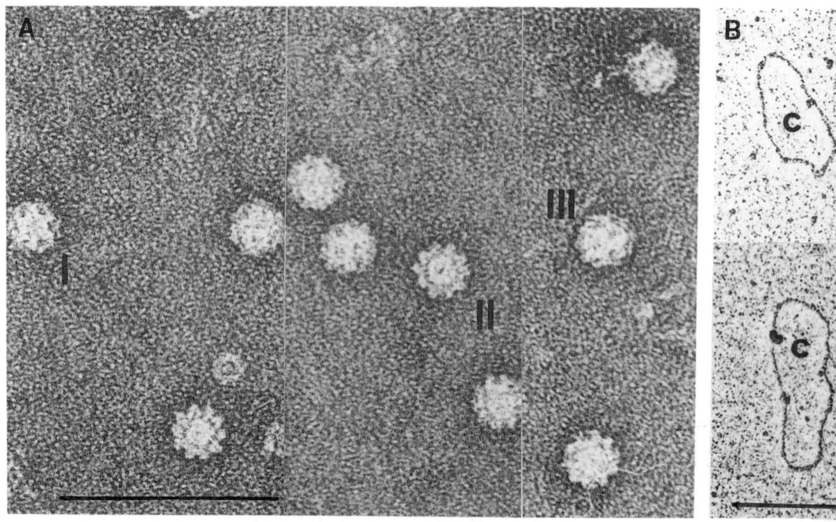

FIG. 34-6. *(A) Virions of chicken anemia virus as seen by negative staining. Bar: 100 nm. (B) Kleinschmidt preparation showing the circular DNA molecules of the genome of chicken anemia virus. Bar: 1 kb; magnification: ×50,000. (Courtesy Dr. R. Lurz and Dr. H. Gelderblom.)*

aplastic anemia syndrome). Dual infections with immunosuppressive viruses such as reticuloendotheliosis virus, virulent Marek's disease virus, and infectious bursal disease virus also enhance the severity of chicken anemia virus infection, resulting in higher mortalities and more persistent anemia.

Diagnosis. There is no satisfactory rapid method of laboratory diagnosis. Virus can be isolated in lymphoblastoid cell lines, but up to 10 passages may be required to detect cytopathology. Neutralization or immunofluorescence tests can be used for the serologic diagnosis, but they are time-consuming and insensitive.

Control. It is difficult to maintain breeder flocks free of chicken anemia virus for the duration of their lives. Although most infections are subclinical, isolated flocks may not be infected until they commence to lay, with disastrous consequences for their progeny. No satisfactory vaccine has been developed.

SUBACUTE SPONGIFORM ENCEPHALOPATHIES

Scrapie is the prototype of a group of degenerative neurologic diseases called the subacute spongiform encephalopathies, which includes the human diseases kuru, Creutzfeldt-Jakob disease, and Gerstmann-Sträussler disease, mink encephalopathy, "wasting disease" of mule deer and elk, and bovine spongiform encephalopathy. Spongiform encephalopathies can be transmitted with varying success to many experimental animals, including mice, ferrets, hamsters, rats, mink, sheep, goats, pigs, cattle, monkeys, and chimpanzees; disease usually occurs after very long incubation periods.

Causative Agent

What makes the subacute spongiform encephalopathies different from all other infectious diseases is the nature of the infectious agent. Filtration suggests a diameter of 30–50 nm for the infective agent, yet electron microscopy of fractions of high infectivity obtained from infected brains (10^7–10^8 LD_{50} units/ml) reveal no structures resembling virions. Further, the infectivity associated with such preparations shows extremely high resistance to inactivation by heating, UV irradiation, and many chemicals. Analogies were made with the "viroids" found to cause certain infectious diseases of plants, which are small circular RNA molecules which neither code for nor require a protein coat. However, the subacute spongiform encephalopathy agents differ in many respects from plant viroids, not least in the fact that all attempts to demonstrate a nonhost nucleic acid, by all available techniques, have been negative. From this kind of uncertainty and much experimental work have come three principal theories about the nature of spongiform encephalopathy agents.

Virus Theory. Since there are viruses that have not yet been visualized nor had their nucleic acid isolated and characterized, one key unresolved question is whether the subacute spongiform encephalopathy agents contain a nucleic acid moiety. One view is that the demonstrated hydrophobicity of the agents, their strong tendency to aggregate and to associate with fragments of plasma membrane (as judged by infectivity), and the inaccuracy of available assays, which depend on the production of disease after long incubation periods, tend to obscure the fact that the infectious agent is indeed a small but otherwise conventional virus; the small target size measured by radiation inactivation and other methods of inactivation could reflect a highly aggregated infectious entity. Few scientists working in the field now accept this view.

Virino Theory. The virino theory suggests that the nucleic acid of the subacute spongiform encephalopathy agents is too small to code for any protein but that it does serve a regulatory function. In this theory the protein component of the agent is host-derived. Again, there is no convincing evidence to support this hypothesis.

Prion Theory. A third view is that a pure protein particle, the prion, containing no nucleic acid, could "infect" a host, "replicate," and cause irreparable neurologic damage. Careful examination of scrapie brain material containing high-titer infectivity has revealed the presence of *prion protein* (PrP^c), which is a cell-surface constituent of neurons that is encoded by a single chromosomal gene. A fraction of prion protein from scrapie-infected brain (called Prp^{sc}) differs from PrP^c in that it is less soluble and largely resistant to proteases; it is suggested that PrP^{sc} (Fig. 34-7) is the infectious agent. Recently it was found that a proline-to-leucine mutation at position 102 in the human PrP gene is linked to the rare familial Gerstmann-Sträussler syndrome, a spongiform encephalop-

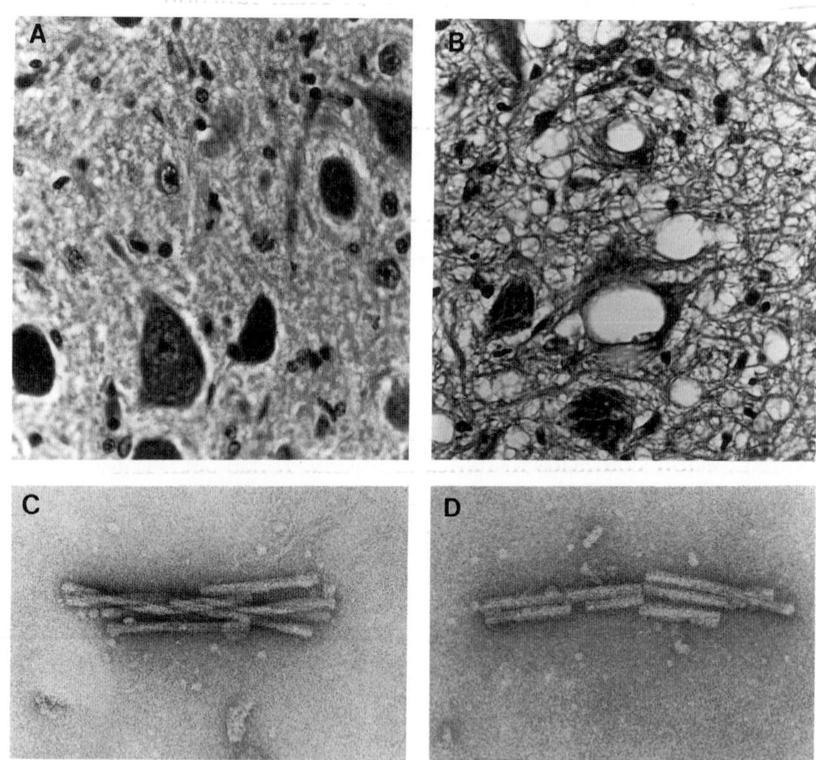

FIG. 34-7. *Scrapie. (A) Section of brain of a normal sheep. (B) Section of brain of a sheep that died of scrapie. Note the extensive spongiform changes but the lack of evidence of an inflammatory or immune response. Hematoxylin and eosin stain; magnification: ×420. (C and D) Electron micrographs of extensively purified prion protein rods from a case of Creutzfeld-Jakob disease, negatively stained with uranyl formate. Bar: 100 nm. (A, B, courtesy Dr. J. D. Foster; C, D, courtesy Dr. S. B. Prusiner.)*

athy which is thus both hereditary in humans and transmissible to subhuman primates.

There are two hypotheses as to the role of the prion protein. One suggests that the infectious agent is a small nucleic acid that is replicated conventionally and provided with a PrP-derived coat by the host cell; this hypothesis suffers from the fact that all attempts to demonstrate nucleic acid have been negative. In the other, "protein only" hypothesis, it is proposed that a mutation(s) in the gene encoding the normal prion protein, PrP, or the introduction of abnormal prion protein molecules from another animal, such as PrP^{Sc}, causes an aberrant conformation of the normal cellular protein. This aberrant conformation causes normal PrP molecules to aggregate in neuronal tissue, forming protease-resistant amyloid deposits that ultimately disrupt brain function. For scrapie, these fibrillar structures are called scrapie-associated fibrils. Recent experimental evidence supporting this theory includes the experimental insertion of a mutated PrP gene into mouse eggs and the finding that the resultant transgenic mice developed spongiform encephalopathy. The question is whether the protein isolated from the transgenic mice can "infect" other mice, that is, produce spongiform encephalopathy. Such studies are underway. Needless to say, this theory of transmissible infectivity in the absence of nucleic acid, although the most attractive at this time, is the most heretical.

Scrapie

Scrapie is a chronic fatal ataxic disease of sheep and occasionally of goats, which is widely distributed in Europe and North America and occurs in a few countries in Africa and Asia. It has been known since the 1940s that scrapie was transmissible from sheep to sheep, with an incubation period of several years, but research on the nature of the etiological agent lagged until it was shown in 1965 that it could be transmitted to mice. With adaptation to mice and hamsters the incubation period was reduced to about 3 months. Even so, such long incubation periods and the difficulty in defining the nature of the scrapie agent greatly hamper research.

Clinical Features. The earliest clinical sign is pruritus, manifested by rubbing the affected parts against fence posts and biting the flanks. Muscular tremors, elicited by rubbing the skin over the flanks, led to the French name for the disease, "tremblant du mouton." Later motor disturbances develop, with a weaving gait, staring eyes, and eventually hindquarter paralysis. There is never any fever, but affected sheep rapidly lose weight and die, usually within 4–6 weeks from the onset. There is a strong genetic predisposition in the susceptibility of sheep, but not among goats.

Pathology. The infectious agent has been transmitted to goats, mice, hamsters, ferrets, and monkeys; most experimental study is based on the use of mice, in which there is host genetic control of the length of the incubation period and the distribution of lesions, which is also dependent on the strain of scrapie agent used. The only pathologic lesions occur in the central nervous system, in which there is hypertrophy of astrocytes, vacuolation of the neurons, and neuronal degeneration; there is a complete absence of any signs of an inflammatory reaction or an immune response (Fig. 34-7B).

Diagnosis. The diagnosis is usually based on clinical signs and histopathologic findings at postmortem, particularly vacuolation of neurons, supplemented by detection of scapie-associated fibrils in brain material by electron microscopy, or the detection of PrP^{sc} by Western blot analysis. Attempts to devise a live animal test by detection of PrP^{sc} in lymph node biopsy material have met with limited success.

Epidemiology. The mechanism of spread among sheep remains uncertain. The agent may spread horizontally from naturally infected sheep to uninfected sheep or goats, but this has not been observed among experimentally infected sheep. Susceptible sheep have developed the disease in pastures previously occupied by scrapie-affected sheep. The scrapie agent is transmitted from ewes to lambs even without suckling, but it is not yet certain whether this is due to transplacental or perinatal infection. The first appearance of the agent in naturally infected lambs occurs in the intestine, tonsils, spleen, and lymph nodes. This early tropism suggests infection by the oral route. Experimentally, susceptible species have been infected by oral and intracerebral routes.

Control. Scrapie was recognized in the United States in 1947 and in 1952, all introductions being traced to importations from Canada and before that to the United Kingdom. Attempts have been made to eradicate the disease from the United States, infected flocks being slaughtered and the owners indemnified from public funds. However, the long incubation period of the disease and the extensive interstate movement of sheep have made eradication unfeasible. At present, a "certified flock" program is being developed for the United States, so that the movement of sheep among such flocks can be done without risk, and the movement of sheep among other flocks is not constrained. In some European countries few control measures have been taken, although the disease is controlled in other countries. Under the European Community Charter, scrapie will become a notifiable disease and subject to control regulations throughout the Community. Successful efforts have been made to exclude scrapie from some countries with large sheep populations (Australia, New Zealand) by strict control of importations and slaughter of any imported animals that may develop disease during the long period of quarantine.

Bovine Spongiform Encephalopathy

Bovine spongiform encephalopathy (BSE) was first diagnosed in the Great Britain in 1986. It has since reached epidemic proportions there and has been identified subsequently in Northern Ireland, the Republic of Ireland, Oman, Switzerland, France, and probably several other European countries. In Great Britain, by 1991, there had been more than 26,000 cases (up to 300 suspect cases reported per week) on more than 9000 farms. More than 98% of cases were in dairy cows; by 1991, 22% of dairy herds but only 2.2% of beef herds had experienced at least one case. There have also been cases of spongiform encephalopathy in a small number of zoo animals and in cats in the United Kingdom, and one of ten pigs developed the disease following experimental inoculation of BSE material. Comprehensive research and public information programs have been set in place to deal with this situation.

Diagnosis. As with scrapie, diagnosis is impossible until the disease develops; in Britain it was found useful to distinguish between "suspicion" and "conviction" to allow development of obvious signs before making a decision to slaughter. Confirmation of the clinical diagnosis is currently based on histologic examination of a paraffin-embedded section of brain material obtained via the foramen magnum, thus obviating the need to open the cranial cavity.

Epidemiology. Epidemiologic investigation has determined that the disease was caused by feeding cattle ruminant protein supplements in the form of meat and bone meal produced by rendering animal waste, including waste derived from sheep carrying the scrapie agent. A major change in the rendering process in most parts of the United Kingdom in the early 1980s resulted in a large increase in the amount of scrapie agent remaining in the rendered product, and hence a greatly increased exposure of cattle to the agent. As the number of infected cattle increased, the infection rate may have been further amplified by inclusion in rendered products of waste from BSE-infected cattle. There is no significant horizontal spread; each case represents part of an extended common source epidemic.

Control. In 1988 a plan was adopted to control and eliminate BSE from the United Kingdom by banning the feeding of ruminant protein to ruminants. In the absence of transmission other than by this means, this regimen would be expected to lead to a decline in the incidence of disease by 1993 and to its disappearance by the turn of the century. However, it is not certain that there are no other means of transmission. It is known that scrapie can pass from ewe to lamb congenitally or via milk. Calves born after the ban on ruminant protein feeding are therefore being watched carefully for evidence of BSE. To date, one case has been found in a calf born after the feeding ban went into effect. One case of spongiform encephalopathy has also been found in a Greater Kudu born in the London Zoo after the feeding ban; this animal's dam had died earlier of suspected BSE.

The BSE epidemic has raised much public concern about possible human health hazards associated with eating beef, drinking milk, using fetal calf serum in vaccine manufacture, etc. There is no evidence that BSE has been responsible for causing disease in humans, but, as noted by an official investigative committee in the United Kingdom, the evidence does not exclude the possibility. Measures were introduced in the United Kingdom to prevent any part of a suspect BSE-infected animal from entering the food chains of other animals or humans. The agriculture departments of several European countries and the United States have commissioned research on the epidemiology and natural history of BSE to try to determine whether it constitutes a human health hazard.

Transmissible Mink Encephalopathy

Transmissible mink encephalopathy was first recognized on mink farms in Wisconsin in 1947, carcasses of scrapie-infected sheep having been fed to the mink. The pathology and pathogenesis of the disease are similar to those of scrapie. There seems no doubt that it is due to infection of mink with the scrapie agent. It spreads between mink by fighting and cannibalism; transplacental or perinatal infection from the mother does not occur.

Wasting Disease of Mule Deer and Elk

Workers in the United States have described a chronic wasting disease in mule deer and elk in Colorado and Wyoming, with behavioral changes and progressive weight loss over a period of weeks or months. The histopathologic changes are similar to those seen in scrapie, and transmission to animals following experimental infection has been achieved.

BORNA DISEASE

Borna disease is a rare progressive encephalopathy of horses and occasionally of sheep that occurs sporadically in Germany and in Switzerland but has not been diagnosed with certainty elsewhere. After an incubation period varying from a few weeks to many months, there are disturbances in coordination and sensory functions followed by lethargy, paralysis, and death. Ninety percent of affected animals die within 3 weeks of the onset of signs. Clinically inapparent infections have also been described.

Histopathologic lesions include perivascular cuffing and degeneration of ganglion cells, as seen in other forms of viral encephalitis. Pathognomonic of Borna disease are round or oval intranuclear inclusion bodies in neurons of the hippocampus and olfactory lobes, readily visualized after staining with Giemsa stain. The disease is mediated by a T-cell-dependent immunopathologic reaction, in which $CD4^+$ cells play a major role.

Antibodies in serum and cerebrospinal fluid can be demonstrated by binding assays, but they do not neutralize infectivity. Diagnosis is based on assays of virus-specific antibodies by ELISA or by immunofluorescence with persistently infected cells. Postmortem diagnosis is verified by immunohistologic demonstration of viral antigen in brain sections.

The causative virus has never been visualized in spite of the fact that it is present in the brains of affected animals in relatively high concentrations, but virus-specific antigens can be demonstrated, mainly in the nuclei of infected cells. The viral genome appears to consist of ssRNA; because infectivity is lipid-sensitive, the virion is thought to be enveloped.

The virus is noncytocidal and cell-associated. It replicates in embryonic brain cells, and cocultivation of these with various cell lines results in persistent, slowly progressive infections.

Animals of many species can be infected by intracerebral or intranasal inoculation of brain homogenates or cerebrospinal fluids obtained from animals harboring the virus. The clinical manifestations depend on the host species and virus strain, varying from inapparent, in mice and hamsters, to alterations in behavior, or obesity, disturbances in fertility, blindness, or paralysis followed by death in other species. Antibodies against Borna disease virus have been found in sera and cerebrospinal fluids from human patients with psychiatric disorders.

FURTHER READING

Bishop, D. H. L. (1990). *Arenaviridae* and their replication. *In* "Fields Virology" (B. N. Fields, D. M. Knipe, R. M. Chanock, M. S. Hirsch, J. L. Melnick, T. P. Monath, and B. Roizman, eds.), 2nd Ed., p. 1231. Raven, New York.

Bradley, R., and Matthews, D. (1992). Transmissible spongiform encephalopathies of animals. *Off. Int. Epiz. Sci. Tech. Rev.* **11,** 333.

Chesebro, B. W., ed. (1991). Transmissible spongiform encephalopathies. *Curr. Top. Microbiol. Immunol.* **172,** 1.

Dealler, S. F., and Lacey, R. W. (1990). Transmissible spongiform encephalopathies: The threat of BSE to man. *Food Microbiol.* **7,** 253.

Gibbs, C. J., Jr., Bolis, C. L., Asher, D. M., Bradley, R., Fite, R. W., Johnston, R. T., Mahy, B. W. J., and McKhann, G. M. (1992). Recommendations of the International Round Table Workshop on BSE. *J. Am. Med. Vet. Assoc.* **200,** 164.

Horzinek, M. C., Flewett, T. H., Saif, L. J., Spaan, W. J. M., Weis, M., and Woode, G. N. (1987). A new family of vertebrate viruses: *Toroviridae. Intervirology* **27,** 17.

Jordan, F. T. (1990). "Poultry Diseases," 3rd Ed. Bailliere Tindall, London.

Kimberlin, R. H. (1990). Unconventional "slow" viruses. *In* "Topley and Wilson's Principles of Bacteriology, Virology and Immunity" (L. H. Collier and M. C. Timbury, eds.), 8th Ed., Vol. 4, p. 671.

Kurtz, J. B., and Lee, T. W. (1987). Astroviruses: Human and animal. *In* "Novel Diarrhea Viruses" (G. Bock and J. Whelan, eds.), CIBA Foundation Symposium No. 128, p. 92. Wiley, New York.

Ludwig, H., Bode, L., and Gosztonyi, G. (1988). Borna disease: A persistent virus infection of the central nervous system. *Prog. Med. Virol.* **35,** 107.

McCormick, J. B. (1990). Arenaviruses. *In* "Fields Virology" (B. N. Fields, D. M. Knipe, R. M. Chanock, M. S. Hirsch, J. L. Melnick, T. P. Monath, and B. Roizman, eds.), 2nd Ed., p. 1245. Raven, New York.

Murphy, F. A., Kiley, M. J., and Fisher-Hoch, S. (1990). *Filoviridae:* Marburg and Ebola viruses. *In* "Fields Virology" (B. N. Fields, D. M. Knipe, M. S. Hirsch, J. L. Melnick, T. P. Monath, and B. Roizman, eds.), 2nd Ed., p. 933. Raven, New York.

Noteborn, M. H. M., de Boer, G. E., van Roozelaar, D. J., Karreman, C., Kranenburg, O., Vos, J. G., Jeurissen, S. H. M., Hoeben, R. C., Zanlema, A., Koch, G., van Ormondt, H., and van der Eb, A. J. (1991). Characterization of chicken anemia agent virus DNA that contains all elements for the infectious replication cycle. *J. Virol.* **65,** 3131.

Prusiner, S. B. (1991). Molecular biology of prion diseases. *Science* **252,** 1515.

Ritchie, B. W., Niagro, F. D., Lukert, P. D., Steffens, W. L., and Latimer, K. S. (1989). Characterization of a new virus from cockatoos with psittacine beak and feather disease. *Virology* **171,** 83.

Robinson, W. S. (1990). Hepadnaviridae and their replication. *In* "Fields Virology" (B. N. Fields, D. M. Knipe, M. S. Hirsch, J. L. Melnick, T. P. Monath, and B. Roizman, eds.), 2nd Ed., p. 2137. Raven, New York.

Tischer, I., Gelderblom, H., Vettermann, W., and Koch, M. A. (1982). A very small porcine virus with circular single-stranded DNA. *Nature (London)* **295,** 64.

Todd, D., Creelan, J. L., Mackie, D. P., Rixon, F., and McNulty, M. S. (1990). Purification and biochemical characterization of chicken anemia agent. *J. Gen. Virol.* **71,** 819.

Wells, G. A. H., and McGill, I. S. (1992). Recently described scrapie-like encephalopathies of animals: Case definitions. *Res. Vet. Sci.* **53,** 1.

Wensvoort, G., Terpstra, C., Pol, J. M. A., ter Laak, E. A., Bloemraad, M., de Kluyver, E. P., Kragten, C., van Buiten, L., den Besten, A., Wagenaar, F., Broekhuijsen, J. M., Moonen, P. L. J. M., Zetstra, T., de Boer, E. A., Tibben, J. H., de Jong, M. F., van't Veld, P., Groenland, G. J. R., van Gennup, J. A., Voets, M. T., Verheijden, J. H. M., and Braamskamp, J. (1991). Mystery swine disease in The Netherlands: The isolation of Lelystad virus. *Vet. Q.* **13,** 121.

CHAPTER 35

Viral Diseases by Domestic Animal Species

In the preceding chapters the contribution of individual viruses to animal disease has been examined in the context of the families of viruses. In this final chapter important diseases and syndromes caused by viruses in each domestic animal species are listed together with their etiologic associations. The aim is to provide a bird's-eye view of the commonest viral diseases and syndromes in each animal species. A practicable way of doing this in a concise form is to provide one or two tables for each major domestic animal species, and one for small laboratory animals.

EXPLANATION OF THE TABLES

Such a tabulation inevitably involves oversimplification, but page numbers have been provided to direct the reader to appropriate pages for detailed coverage of each of these viral infections. Nevertheless, in these tables we have attempted to ascribe to each disease a measure of its importance (+ to ++++), as viewed from the perspective of veterinary medicine in countries with modern agricultural practices. When considering diseases that have been eliminated from these countries, we have incorporated into our assessment the relative risk of these exotic diseases should they be reintroduced. For example, foot-and-mouth disease, which is given a ++++ rating in cattle, is an important disease even in countries in which it does not currently occur, because of its potential impact on beef exports and the rapidity with which this virus can spread from herd to herd. In contrast, rinderpest, although one of the most important disease of ruminants in countries where it has not been eliminated, is only given a ++ rating, because there is little chance of the virus being reintroduced in countries with modern veterinary services and, even if it were to be introduced in these countries, its elimination would present few difficulties. Had these tables been written from the perspective of the developing countries, then some diseases considered important in areas where intensive husbandry systems predominate would have been rated as inconsequential. For example, infectious bovine rhinotracheitis deserves a high rating in the intensive cattle production environment (dairy or beef) but is not important in developing countries.

There is an arbitrary element in relation to the group of diseases (generalized, respiratory, etc.) to which certain infections are allocated. For example, most generalized skin diseases result from blood-borne infection, but they have been listed as skin diseases. Where viruses cause generalized signs and also signs of particular importance in some system, or in the newborn, they have been entered in both categories. The other headings in the tables have been selected to draw attention to the classification of the causal virus and whether it is persistent, the geographic distribution of the disease, and the availability of vaccines.

The Further Reading list incorporates the more recent textbooks and monographs on viral diseases of veterinary importance.

FURTHER READING

Appel, M. J., ed. (1987). "Virus Infections of Carnivores." Elsevier Science, Amsterdam.

Bhatt, P. N., Jacoby, R. O., Morse, H. C., and New, A. E. (1986). "Viral and Rickettsial Infections of Laboratory Rodents." Academic Press, Orlando.

Blood, D. C., and Radostits, O. M. (1989). "Veterinary Medicine, a Textbook of the Diseases of Cattle, Sheep, Pigs, Goats and Horses," 7th Ed. Bailliere Tindall, London.

Blowey, R. W., and Weaver, A. D. (1991). "A Colour Atlas of Diseases and Disorders of Cattle." Wolfe Publ., London.

Calnek, B. N., Barnes, H. J., Beard, C. N., Reid, W. N., and Yoder, H. W., eds. (1991). "Diseases of Poultry," 9th Ed. Iowa State Univ. Press, Ames.

Castro, A. E., and Heuschle, W. P., eds. (1992). "Veterinary Diagnostic Virology—A Practitioner's Guide." Mosby Yearbook, New York.

Darai, G., ed. (1987). "Virus Diseases in Laboratory and Captive Animals." Kluwer, Academic Publ., Boston, Massachusetts.
Dinter, Z., and Morein, B., eds. (1990). "Virus Infections of Ruminants." Elsevier Science, Amsterdam.
Fowler, M. E., ed. (1986). "Zoo and Wild Animal Medicine," 2nd Ed. Saunders, Philadelphia, Pennsylvania.
Fraser, C. M., ed. (1991). "The Merck Veterinary Manual," 7th Ed. Merck, Rahway, New Jersey.
Greene, C. E. (1990). "Infectious Diseases of the Dog and Cat." Saunders, Philadelphia, Pennsylvania.
Harrison, G. J., and Harrison, L. R. (1986). "Clinical Avian Medicine and Surgery." Saunders, Philadelphia, Pennsylvania.
Howard, J. L., ed. (1992). "Current Veterinary Therapy 3, Food Animal Practice." Saunders, Philadelphia, Pennsylvania.
Martin, W. B., and Aitken, I. D., eds. (1991). "Diseases of Sheep," 2nd Ed. Blackwell, Oxford.
NRC (National Research Council). (1991). "Infectious Diseases of Mice and Rats." National Academy Press, Washington, D.C.
Pensaert, M. B., ed. (1990). "Virus Infections of Porcines." Elsevier Science, Amsterdam.
Petrak, M. L., ed. (1982). "Diseases of Cage and Aviary Birds," 2nd Ed., Lea & Febiger, Philadelphia, Pennsylvania.
Randall, C. J. (1991). "A Colour Atlas of Diseases and Disorders of the Domestic Fowl and Turkey," 2nd Ed. Wolfe Publ., London.
Smith, W. J., Taylor, D. J., and Penny, R. H. C. (1990). "A Colour Atlas of Diseases and Disorders of the Pig." Wolfe Publ., London.
Timoney, J. F., Gillespie, J. H., Scott, F. N., and Barlough, J. E. (1988). "Hagan and Bruner's Infectious Diseases of Domestic Animals," 8th Ed. Cornell Univ. Press, Ithaca, New York.
Wolf, K. (1988). "Fish Viruses and Fish Viral Diseases." Comstock Publ. Associates (Cornell Univ. Press), Ithaca, New York.

Tables 35–1 through 35–12 follow.

TABLE 35-1

Generalized and Respiratory Diseases of Cattle

Disease	Importance	Virus family (genus or subfamily)	Number of serotypes	Geographical distribution	Vaccines	Persistence	Page
Generalized Diseases, Including Central Nervous System Involvement							
Bluetongue	++	*Reoviridae* (*Orbivirus*)	24	Tropics and subtropics; temperate areas of North America	Attenuated but used only in sheep	±	542
Bovine ephemeral fever	++	*Rhabdoviridae* (*Lyssavirus*)	1	Africa, Asia, Australia	Inactivated and attenuated	−	504
Bovine immunodeficiency	?	*Retroviridae* (*Lentivirus*)	?	Worldwide	None	+	591
Bovine leukemia	++	*Retroviridae* (HTLV/BLV group)	1	Worldwide; control and eradication programs in Europe	None	+	577
Bovine spongiform encephalopathy	+	Unclassified (scrapie agent)	None	United Kingdom	None	+	615
Bovine virus diarrhea	++	*Flaviviridae* (*Pestivirus*)	1	Worldwide	Inactivated and attenuated	+	448
Foot-and-mouth disease	++++	*Picornaviridae* (*Aphthovirus*)	7	Eradicated in North and Central America, Australia, Japan; controlled in European countries; common elsewhere	Inactivated	+	409

Malignant catarrhal fever	+	*Herpesviridae* (*Gammaherpesvirinae*)	1	Worldwide	None	+	366
Rabies	+	*Rhabdoviridae* (*Lyssavirus*)	1	Central and South America	Inactivated and attenuated	+	493
Rift Valley fever	++	*Bunyaviridae* (*Phlebovirus*)	1	Africa	Attenuated and inactivated	−	528
Rinderpest	++	*Paramyxoviridae* (*Morbillivirus*)	1	Eradicated except in Africa and parts of Asia	Attenuated	−	481
Respiratory Diseases[a]							
Bovine respiratory syncytial virus infections	+++	*Paramyxoviridae* (*Pneumovirus*)	1	Worldwide	Attenuated	−	486
Infectious bovine rhinotracheitis[b]	+++	*Herpesviridae* (*Alphaherpesvirinae*)	1	Worldwide	Attenuated	+	345
Malignant catarrhal fever	+	*Herpesviridae* (*Gammaherpesvirinae*)	1	Worldwide	None	+	366
Parainfluenzavirus 3 infection	+	*Paramyxoviridae* (*Paramyxovirus*)	1	Worldwide	Inactivated and attenuated	−	477

[a] Rhinoviruses (p. 422) and adenoviruses (p. 330) have been associated with respiratory disease in cattle but are of little clinical importance.
[b] Caused by same virus (bovine herpesvirus 1) as infectious pustular vulvovaginitis.

TABLE 35-2

Diseases of Cattle Affecting Intestinal Tract, Reproductive System, and Skin

Disease	Importance	Virus family (genus or subfamily)	Number of serotypes	Geographical distribution	Vaccines	Persistence	Page
Enteric Diseases[a]							
Bovine coronavirus diarrhea	+	*Coronaviridae (Coronavirus)*	1	Worldwide	Inactivated, given to dam	−	461
Bovine rotavirus diarrhea	++	*Reoviridae (Rotavirus)*	Several	Worldwide	Attenuated, given to dam	−	550
Bovine virus diarrhea	++	*Flaviviridae (Pestivirus)*	1	Worldwide	Inactivated and attenuated	+	448
Reproductive and Neonatal Diseases							
Akabane disease	+	*Bunyaviridae (Bunyavirus)*	1	Africa, Asia, Australia	Inactivated	−	531
Bluetongue	++	*Reoviridae (Orbivirus)*	24	Tropics, subtropics, and temperate areas of North America	Attenuated but used only in sheep	+	542
Bovine virus diarrhea	++	*Flaviviridae (Pestivirus)*	1	Worldwide	Inactivated and attenuated	+	448
Infectious pustular vulvovaginitis[b]	++	*Herpesviridae (Alphaherpesvirinae)*	1	Worldwide	Attenuated	+	366
Palyam virus infection	+	*Reoviridae (Orbivirus)*	6	Worldwide	None	−	546

Skin Diseases, Including Stomatitis							
Bovine herpes mammillitis and pseudo-lumpyskin disease	+	*Herpesviridae (Alphaherpesvirinae)*	1	Worldwide	None	+	349
Bovine papillomatosis	+	*Papovaviridae (Papillomavirus)*	6	Worldwide	Autogenous	+	325
Bovine papular stomatitis	+	*Poxviridae (Parapoxvirus)*	1	Worldwide	None	–	380
Cowpox	+	*Poxviridae (Orthopoxvirus)*	1	Europe	None in use	–	375
Lumpyskin disease	+	*Poxviridae (Capripoxvirus)*	1	Africa	Attenuated	–	383
Mucosal disease[c]	++	*Togaviridae (Pestivirus)*	1	Worldwide	Inactivated and attenuated	+	448
Pseudocowpox	+	*Poxviridae (Parapoxvirus)*	1	Worldwide	None	–	378
Vesicular stomatitis	+	*Rhabdoviridae (Vesiculovirus)*	7	Americas	Inactivated and attenuated	–	500

[a] Caliciviruses (p. 425), astroviruses (p. 605), and toroviruses (p. 604) are associated with enteric infection and diarrhea in cattle but are of little clinical importance.

[b] Caused by the same virus as infectious bovine rhinotracheitis.

[c] Caused by the same virus as bovine virus diarrhea.

TABLE 35-3

Generalized and Respiratory Diseases of Sheep and Goats

Disease	Importance	Virus family (genus or subfamily)	Number of serotypes	Geographical distribution	Vaccines	Persistence	Page
Generalized Diseases, Including Central Nervous System Involvement							
Bluetongue	++	*Reoviridae (Orbivirus)*	24	Tropics, subtropics, and temperate areas of North America	Attenuated	±	542
Caprine arthritis–encephalomyelitis	++	*Retroviridae (Lentivirus)*	1	Most countries	None	+	589
Foot-and-mouth disease	+	*Picornaviridae (Aphthovirus)*	7	See Table 35-1 for details		–	411
Goatpox	+	*Poxviridae (Capripoxvirus)*	1	Africa and Asia	Inactivated and attenuated	–	381
Louping ill	+	*Flaviviridae (Flavivirus)*	1	United Kingdom	Inactivated	–	446
Nairobi sheep disease	+	*Bunyaviridae (Nairovirus)*	1	Africa	None in use	–	532

Peste des petits ruminants	++	*Paramyxoviridae* (*Morbillivirus*)	1	Africa and Middle East	Attenuated	–	483
Rift Valley fever	++	*Bunyaviridae* (*Phlebovirus*)	1	Africa	Attenuated and inactivated	–	528
Scrapie	+	Unclassified (spongiform encephalopathy)	Unknown	Most countries	None	+	613
Sheeppox	++	*Poxviridae* (*Capripoxvirus*)	1	Africa and Asia	Inactivated and attenuated	–	382
Respiratory Diseases[a]							
Ovine pulmonary adenomatosis	++	*Retroviridae* (mammalian type B retrovirus group)	1	Most countries	None	+	579
Parainfluenza-virus 3 infection	+	*Paramyxoviridae* (*Paramyxovirus*)	1	Worldwide	Inactivated and attenuated	–	477
Ovine progressive pneumonia (maedi)	+	*Retroviridae* (*Lentivirus*)	1	Most countries	None	+	588

[a] Adenoviruses (p. 333) and respiratory syncytial viruses (p. 486) have been associated with respiratory disease in sheep and goats but are of little clinical importance.

TABLE 35-4

Diseases of Sheep and Goats Affecting Intestinal Tract, Reproductive System, and Skin

Disease	Importance	Virus family (genus or subfamily)	Number of serotypes	Geographical distribution	Vaccines	Persistence	Page
Enteric Diseases[a]							
Nairobi sheep disease[b]	+	*Bunyaviridae (Nairovirus)*	1	Africa	None in use	–	532
Peste des petits ruminants[b]	++	*Paramyxoviridae (Morbillivirus)*	1	Africa and Middle East	Attenuated	–	483
Reproductive and Neonatal Diseases							
Akabane disease	+	*Bunyaviridae (Bunyavirus)*	1	Africa, Asia, Australia	Inactivated	–	628
Bluetongue	++	*Reoviridae (Orbivirus)*	24	Tropics, subtropics, and temperate areas of North America	Attenuated	±	542

Border disease[c]	+	*Flaviviridae (Pestivirus)*	1	Worldwide	None in use	+	451
Rift Valley fever	++	*Bunyaviridae (Phlebovirus)*	1	Africa	Attenuated and inactivated	–	528
Wesselsbron disease	+	*Flaviviridae (Flavivirus)*	1	Africa	Attenuated	–	447
Skin Diseases							
Goatpox	+	*Poxviridae (Capripoxvirus)*	1	Africa and Asia	Inactivated and attenuated	–	382
Orf (contagious pustular dermatitis)	++	*Poxviridae (Parapoxvirus)*	1	Worldwide	Wild-type virus, atypical site	–	381
Sheeppox	++	*Poxviridae (Capripoxvirus)*	1	Africa and Asia	Inactivated and attenuated	–	382

[a] Rotaviruses (p. 550), astroviruses (p. 605), and adenoviruses (p. 330) have been associated with enteric disease in sheep and goats but are of little clinical importance.

[b] Generalized diseases which often present as enteric diseases.

[c] Probably caused by the same virus as bovine virus diarrhea.

TABLE 35-5

Generalized and Respiratory Diseases of Swine

Disease	Importance	Virus family (genus or subfamily)	Number of serotypes	Geographical distribution	Vaccines	Persistence	Page
Generalized Diseases, Including Central Nervous System Involvement							
African swine fever	++++	Unclassified	Unknown	Sub-Saharan Africa, Spain, Portugal, and Sardinia	None	+	395
Foot-and-mouth disease	++++	*Picornaviridae (Aphthovirus)*	7	See Table 35–1 for details		–	410
Encephalomyocarditis	+	*Picornaviridae (Cardiovirus)*	1	Worldwide	None	–	422
Hog cholera	++++	*Flaviviridae (Pestivirus)*	1	Eradicated in North and Central America, Australia, Japan; controlled in European countries, common elsewhere	Attenuated	+	452
Porcine epidemic abortion and respiratory syndrome	+++	*Arterivirus*	1	North America, Europe	None	?	601

Porcine hemagglutinating virus encephalomyelitis	+	*Coronaviridae* (*Coronavirus*)	1	Worldwide	None	–	463
Porcine lymphosarcoma	+	*Retroviridae* (MLV-related virus)	1	Worldwide	None	+	579
Porcine polioencephalomyelitis	+	*Picornaviridae* (*Enterovirus*)	1	Worldwide	Inactivated, used in eastern Europe	–	418
Pseudorabies	+++	*Herpesviridae* (*Alphaherpesvirinae*)	1	Worldwide, except Australia and Japan	Inactivated and attenuated	+	351
Swine vesicular disease	+	*Picornaviridae* (*Enterovirus*)	1	Sporadic in Asia and Europe	None used	–	417
Vesicular exanthema of swine	+	*Caliciviridae* (*Calicivirus*)	Many	Eradicated in swine worldwide	None used	–	427
Vesicular stomatitis	+	*Rhabdoviridae* (*Vesiculovirus*)	7	Sporadic in the Americas	Inactivated	–	500
Respiratory Diseases							
Cytomegalic inclusion body disease of swine	+	*Herpesviridae* (*Betaherpesvirinae*)	1	Worldwide	None	+	364
Porcine epidemic abortion and respiratory syndrome	+++	*Arterivirus*	1	North America, Europe	None	?	601
Swine influenza	+	*Orthomyxoviridae* (*Influenzavirus A*)	2	Worldwide, sporadic	None in commercial use	–	516

TABLE 35-6

Diseases of Swine Affecting Intestinal Tract, Reproductive System, and Skin

Disease	Importance	Virus family (genus or subfamily)	Number of serotypes	Geographical distribution	Vaccines	Persistence	Page
Enteric Disease							
Porcine epidemic diarrhea	+	*Coronaviridae* (*Coronavirus*)	1	Europe	None	–	463
Rotavirus gastroenteritis	+++	*Reoviridae* (*Rotavirus*)	Many	Worldwide	Attenuated, given to dam	–	550
Transmissible gastroenteritis	++	*Coronaviridae* (*Coronavirus*)	1	Worldwide	Attenuated, given to dam	+	462
Reproductive and Neonatal Diseases							
Hog cholera	++++	*Flaviviridae* (*Pestivirus*)	1	Eradicated in North and Central America, Australia, Japan; controlled in European countries, common elsewhere	Attenuated	+	452
Japanese encephalitis virus infection	++	*Flaviviridae* (*Flavivirus*)	1	Asia	Inactivated and attenuated	–	447

Parvovirus disease	++	*Parvoviridae (Parvovirus)*	1	Worldwide	Inactivated	+	311
Porcine epidemic abortion and respiratory syndrome	+++	*Arterivirus*	1	North America, Europe	None	?	601
Pseudorabies	+++	*Herpesviridae (Alphaherpesvirinae)*	1	Worldwide, except Australia and Japan	Inactivated and attenuated	+	351
Skin Diseases, Including Stomatitis							
Swinepox	+	*Poxviridae (Suipoxvirus)*	1	Worldwide	None used	–	384
Swine vesicular disease	+	*Picornaviridae (Enterovirus)*	1	Sporadic in Asia and Europe	None used	–	417
Vesicular exanthema of swine	+	*Caliciviridae (Calicivirus)*	Many	Eradicated in swine worldwide	None used	–	427
Vesicular stomatitis	+	*Rhabdoviridae (Vesiculovirus)*	7	Sporadic in the Americas	Inactivated	–	500

TABLE 35-7
Disease of Dogs

Disease	Importance	Virus family (genus or subfamily)	Number of serotypes	Geographical distribution	Vaccines	Persistence	Page
Generalized Diseases, Including Central Nervous System Involvement							
Canine distemper	++++	*Paramyxoviridae (Morbillivirus)*	1	Worldwide	Attenuated	+	483
Canine parvovirus infection	++++	*Parvoviridae (Parvovirus)*	1	Worldwide	Attenuated and inactivated	(sometimes) +	316
Infectious canine hepatitis	++	*Adenoviridae (Mastadenovirus)*	1	Worldwide	Attenuated and inactivated	+	334
Rabies	+	*Rhabdoviridae (Lyssavirus)*	1	Worldwide except some island countries, Scandinavia, and Australia	Inactivated and attenuated	+	493

Respiratory Diseases							
Canine laryngotracheitis	++	*Adenoviridae (Mastadenovirus)*	1	Worldwide	Attenuated	−	334
Parainfluenzavirus 2 infection	+	*Paramyxoviridae (Paramyxovirus)*	1	Worldwide	None	−	476
Enteric Diseases							
Canine coronavirus infection	++	*Coronaviridae (Coronavirus)*	1	Worldwide	Inactivated	?	462
Canine parvovirus infection	++++	*Parvoviridae (Parvovirus)*	1	Worldwide	Attenuated and inactivated	+	316
Reproductive and Neonatal Diseases							
Hemorrhagic disease of pups	++	*Herpesviridae (Alphaherpesvirinae)*	1	Worldwide	None	+	356
Disease of Mucous Membranes							
Canine papillomatosis	+	*Papovaviridae (Papillomavirus)*	Several	Worldwide	None	+	327

TABLE 35-8
Diseases of Cats

Disease	Importance	Virus family (genus or subfamily)	Number of serotypes	Geographical distribution	Vaccines	Persistence	Page
Generalized Diseases, Including Central Nervous System Involvement							
Feline immunodeficiency syndrome	+++	*Retroviridae* (*Lentivirus*)	?	Worldwide	None	+	593
Feline infectious peritonitis	+++	*Coronaviridae* (*Coronavirus*)	1	Worldwide	None	+	464
Feline leukemia	++++	*Retroviridae* (MLV-related virus)	1	Worldwide	Inactivated subunit	+	579
Feline panleukopenia	+++	*Parvoviridae* (*Parvovirus*)	1	Worldwide	Attenuated and inactivated	+	412
Rabies	+	*Rhabdoviridae* (*Lyssavirus*)	1	Worldwide except some island countries, Scandinavia, and Australia	Inactivated and attenuated	+	493

Respiratory Diseases							
Feline calicivirus infection	+++	*Caliciviridae (Calicivirus)*	1	Worldwide	Attenuated and inactivated	+	428
Feline rhinotracheitis	+++	*Herpesviridae (Alphaherpesvirinae)*	1	Worldwide	Attenuated and inactivated	+	357
Enteric Diseases[a]							
Feline panleukopenia	+++	*Parvoviridae (Parvovirus)*	1	Worldwide	Attenuated and inactivated	+	412
Reproductive and Neonatal Diseases							
Feline panleukopenia	+++	*Parvoviridae (Parvovirus)*	1	Worldwide	Attenuated and inactivated	–	412
Skin Diseases							
Cowpox virus infection	+	*Poxviridae (Orthopoxvirus)*	1	Sporadic in Europe	None used	–	376

[a] A torovirus-like virus has been associated with diarrhea in the cat.

TABLE 35-9

Diseases of Poultry and Other Avian Species[a]

Disease	Species	Importance	Virus family (genus or subfamily)	Number of serotypes	Vaccines	Persistence	Page
Generalized Diseases, Including Central Nervous System Involvement							
Adenovirus infection (egg drop syndrome)	Chickens, ducks, and turkeys	+	*Adenoviridae (Aviadeno-virus)*	Unknown	Inactivated	+	336
Avian encephalo-myelitis	Chickens, ducks, and turkeys	+	*Picornaviridae (Enterovirus)*	1	Attenuated	−	419
Avian influenza	Chickens, turkeys, ducks, aquatic wild birds	++	*Orthomyxoviridae (Influenzavirus A)*	14	Inactivated	−	519
Avian leukosis	Chickens	++	*Retroviridae* (avian type C retrovirus group)	1	Inactivated and attenuated	+	571
Bluecomb	Turkeys	+	*Coronaviridae (Coronavirus)*	1	Inactivated	+	468
Chicken anemia	Chickens	+	?"*Circoviridae*"	1	None	+	619
Eastern equine encephalitis	Pheasants	+	*Togaviridae (Alphavirus)*	1	Inactivated	−	439
Gosling hepatitus	Geese	+	*Parvoviridae*	1	Attenuated	−	319

disease			*(Birnavirus)*		attenuated		
Marek's disease	Chickens	+++	*Herpesviridae (Alphaherpesvirinae)*	1	Attenuated	+	359
Newcastle disease	Chickens, pigeons, other avian species	++++	*Paramyxoviridae (Paramyxovirus)*	1	Attenuated and inactivated	–	478
Respiratory Diseases							
Avian infectious bronchitis	Chickens	+++	*Coronaviridae (Coronavirus)*	Several	Attenuated	+	466
Avian reovirus infections	Chickens and other avian species	+	*Reoviridae (Reovirus)*	11	None used	?	541
Infectious larnygotracheitis	Chickens	+++	*Herpesviridae (Alphaherpesvirinae)*	1	Attenuated	+	358
Turkey rhinopneumonitis	Turkeys	+	*Paramyxoviridae (Pneumovirus)*	1	Attenuated	–	487
Enteric Diseases							
Duck hepatitis	Ducks and turkeys	+	*Picornaviridae (Enterovirus)*	1	Attenuated	?	421
Duck plague	Ducks	+	*Herpesviridae (Alphaherpesvirinae)*	1	None used	+	363
Skin Diseases							
Avian pox	All Species	++	*Poxviridae (Avipoxvirus)*	1	Attenuated	–	387

[a] All diseases of poultry except eastern equine encephalitis (Americas) have a worldwide distribution, but fowl plague (avian influenza) and velogenic Newcastle disease are regarded as exotic viruses in most developed countries.

TABLE 35-10

Generalized and Respiratory Diseases of Horses

Disease	Importance	Virus family (genus or subfamily)	Number of serotypes	Geographic distribution	Vaccines	Persistence	Page
Generalized Diseases, Including Central Nervous System Involvement							
African horse sickness	++	*Reoviridae (Orbivirus)*	9	Africa, Spain, Portugal	Attenuated	–	547
Borna disease	+	Unclassified	1	Europe	None	+	616
Eastern equine encephalitis	++	*Togaviridae (Alphavirus)*	1	Americas	Inactivated	–	435
Equine arteritis	+	*Arterivirus*	1	Worldwide	Attenuated	+	600
Equine encephalosis	+	*Reoviridae (Orbivirus)*	Several	South Africa	None	–	549
Equine infectious anemia	+	*Retroviridae (Lentivirus)*	1	Worldwide	None used	+	591
Getah encephalitis	+	*Togaviridae (Alphavirus)*	1	Asia	None	–	432
Venezuelan equine encephalitis	+	*Togaviridae (Alphavirus)*	7	South and Central America	Inactivated and attenuated	–	435
Western equine encephalitis	+	*Togaviridae (Alphavirus)*	1	Americas	Inactivated	–	435
Respiratory Diseases[a]							
Adenovirus pneumonia	+	*Adenoviridae (Mastadenovirus)*	Unknown	Worldwide	None	–	334
Equine rhinopneumonitis	+++	*Herpesviridae (Alphaherpesvirinae)*	2	Worldwide	Inactivated and attenuated	+	354
Equine influenza	+++	*Orthomyxoviridae (Influenzavirus A)*	2	Worldwide	Inactivated	–	517

TABLE 35-11

Disease of Horses Affecting Intestinal Tract, Reproductive System, and Skin

Disease	Importance	Virus family (genus or subfamily)	Number of serotypes	Geographical distribution	Vaccines	Persistence	Page
Enteric Disease[a]							
Reproductive and Neonatal Diseases							
Equine abortion	+++	*Herpesviridae (Alphaherpesvirinae)*	1	Worldwide	Inactivated and attenuated	+	354
Equine arteritis	+	*Arterivirus*	1	Worldwide	Attenuated	+	600
Equine coital exanthema	+	*Herpesviridae (Alphaherpesvirinae)*	1	Worldwide	None	+	355
Skin Diseases, Including Stomatitis							
Equine papillomatosis and sarcoids	+	*Papovaviridae (Papillomavirus)*	Several	Worldwide	None	+	327
Vesicular stomatitis	+	*Rhabdoviridae (Vesiculovirus)*	7	Americas	None used	−	500

[a] Rotaviruses (p. 550) and toroviruses (p. 604) have been associated with enteric disease but are of uncertain clinical importance.

TABLE 35-12

Diseases of Rabbits and Laboratory Rodents[a]

Disease	Rodent species	Importance	Virus family (genus)	Persistence	Page
Generalized Diseases					
Cowpox	Rat	++	*Poxviridae (Orthopoxvirus)*	–	376
Encephalomyocarditis	Mouse	++	*Picornaviridae (Cardiovirus)*	–	422
	Rat	+			
Hemorrhagic fever with renal syndrome	Rat	+	*Bunyaviridae (Hantavirus)*	+	534
Lactate dehydrogenase-elevating virus infection	Mouse	+[b]	*Arterivirus*	+	599
Lymphocytic choriomeningitis	Mouse	+[b]	*Arenaviridae (Arenavirus)*	+	595
Mouse hepatitis	Mouse	+++	*Coronaviridae (Coronavirus)*	–	468
Mousepox (ectromelia)	Mouse	++++	*Poxviridae (Orthopoxvirus)*	–	377
Myxomatosis	Rabbit	+++	*Poxviridae (Leporipoxvirus)*	–	386
Rabbit hemorrhagic disease	Rabbit	++++	*Caliciviridae (Calicivirus)*	–	429
Rabbitpox	Rabbit	+++	*Poxviridae (Orthopoxvirus)*	–	376
Respiratory Infections					
Sendai virus infection	Mouse	++++	*Paramyxoviridae (Paramyxovirus)*	–	476
	Other species	+			
Enteric Diseases					
Reovirus 3 infection	Mouse	++	*Reoviridae (Orthoreovirus)*	–	541
	Other species	+			

[a] As a general principle, vaccination of laboratory animals should be avoided.

[b] Usually subclinical; potential contaminants of material collected from rodents and used for experimental studies.

Glossary*

abortive infection Viral infection in which some viral genes are expressed but no infectious virus is produced.

abortive transformation Situation in which cells that have undergone transformation due to integration of adenovirus DNA or polyomavirus DNA revert to normal on passage.

active immunization Specific acquired immunity resulting from immunization with viruses or viral antigens.

adjuvant Substance administered with antigen that nonspecifically enhances the immune response.

affinity Thermodynamic measure of the strength of binding of an individual Fab segment of an antibody molecule to an antigenic determinant.

affinity maturation Increase in affinity of antibodies associated with hypermutation of V_H genes in B cells and the selection of the most appropriate molecules by decreasing amounts of retained antigen.

airborne transmission Method of spread of infection by droplet nuclei or dust.

alternate complement pathway Pathway of complement activation initiated via C3 without previous activation of C1, C4, and C2, as in the classical pathway; does not require antibody.

ambisense (applied to ssRNA viral genome) Part of the nucleotide sequence is of plus sense, part is of minus sense.

amphotropic retrovirus A retrovirus that will replicate in the cells of one or more species in addition to those of the original host.

anamnestic (secondary) response Rapid rise in antibody-dependent and/or cell-mediated immunity following second or subsequent exposure to antigen.

anchorage independence Ability of a cell transformed by an oncogenic virus to grow in suspension in semisolid agar medium.

antibody (immunoglobulin) Specialized serum protein produced in response to an antigen, which has the ability to combine specifically with that antigen.

antibody–complement-mediated cytotoxicity Cell lysis mediated by antibody and complement, usually via alternate complement activation pathway.

* Many of these terms have a wide usage in biology; here they are described in terms of virology. For more detailed definitions, see K. E. K. Rowson, T. A. L. Rees, and B. W. J. Mahy, "A Dictionary of Virology," Blackwell Scientific Publications, Oxford, 1981; R. C. King and W. D. Stnafield, "A Dictionary of Genetics," 4th Ed., Oxford University Press, New York, 1990p W. J. Herbert, P. C. Wilkinson, and D. I. Stott, eds., "Dictionary of Immunology," 3rd Ed., Blackwell Scientific Publications, Oxford, 1985.

antibody-dependent cell-mediated cytotoxicity Lysis of target cells that express viral antigen on their surface, to which specific antibody binds; immunologically nonspecific killer cells bind via Fc receptors to the antibody and mediate lysis.

antigen Substance that can induce an immune response when introduced into an animal and which binds to the corresponding antibody *in vitro*.

antigen-presenting cell Dendritic cell, Langerhans cell, macrophage, or B cell which processes and presents peptide antigen to lymphocytes in association with MHC protein.

antigenic determinant (epitope) Region of an antigen that binds antibody.

antigenic drift Point mutation(s) in gene(s) specifying the surface protein(s) of a virus, resulting in antigenic change.

antigenic shift Genetic reassortment between two subtypes of a viral species that has a segmented genome, resulting in the emergence of a new subtype with a completely different surface protein.

antiseptic Chemical germicide for use on skin or mucous membranes.

arbovirus Arthropod-borne; a virus that replicates in an arthropod and is transmitted by bite to a vertebrate host in which it also replicates.

attachment Specific adsorption of virus to its receptor on the plasma membrane of the host cell.

attenuated Reduced in virulence.

avidity Measure of the firmness of the binding of antigen to antibody; influenced by affinity and valency.

B lymphocyte (B cell) Lymphocyte derived from the bursa of Fabricius in birds or its equivalent (bone marrow) in mammals, which differentiates into an antibody-producing plasma cell.

bacteriophage A virus that replicates in a bacterium.

benign tumor A circumscribed tumor (lump) produced by excessive proliferation of cells, without any tendency for invasiveness or metastasis (*see* malignant tumor).

biological transmission Transmission by an arthropod after replication in the vector.

booster Second or subsequent dose of vaccine given to enhance the immune response.

budding Mode of maturation of some viruses whereby viral peplomers (and sometimes matrix protein molecules) accumulate in localized areas of the plasma membrane; after nucleocapsids move to such areas the virion is completed and buds from the cell.

bursa of Fabricius Hindgut organ in the cloaca of birds that controls the ontogeny of B lymphocytes.

cancer Vernacular term covering all types of malignant tumors.

cap 7-Methylguanosine present in the genome of some plus sense ssRNA viruses, or added to the 5′ terminus of an RNA transcript as part of its processing into mRNA.

capsid Protein shell which surrounds the viral nucleoprotein.

capsomer Morphologic units of which the capsid is constructed, visible with the electron microscope.

carcinoma Malignant tumor of epithelial origin.

carrier An animal (often asymptomatic) carrying and often shedding infectious virus.

case–control study Attempt to identify the cause of a disease by comparing cases with matched controls.

cell-mediated immunity Immunity effected predominantly by T lymphocytes (and accessory cells) rather than by antibody.

chronic infection Infection characterized by continued presence of virus, with or without continuing signs of disease.

cis- (*trans*-) active elements Protein factors that act on regulation on the same (*cis*) or another (*trans*) DNA molecule.

classical complement activation pathway Series of sequential enzyme–substrate interactions activated by antigen–antibody complexes and involving all C components.

clathrin-coated pits Depressions in the plasma membrane coated with clathrin, a fibrous protein, which contain the receptors for viruses undergoing receptor-mediated endocytosis.

clone A population of cells or viral particles derived from a single precursor cell or viral particle and thus having essentially the same genetic constitution.

cloning (molecular) Term denoting the isolation and propagation of foreign genes in prokaryotic or eukaryotic cells by recombinant DNA technology.

cloning vector Plasmid or viral DNA into which foreign DNA may be inserted to be propagated using recombinant DNA techniques.

coding redundancy Coding of the same amino acid following substitution of one of the four nucleotides for another as the third nucleotide of the triplet (codon).

codon The triplet of nucleotides that codes for a single amino acid.

cohort study Attempt to identify the cause of a disease by comparing exposed and control populations in a prospective study.

cold-adapted mutant Mutant that replicates best at lower than body temperature.

complement system Series of serum proteins, the first of which binds to any antigen–antibody complex triggering a cascade reaction; the later components in the complement cascade exert a variety of effects including lysis of microorganisms and infected cells, phagocytosis, chemotaxis, and inflammation.

complementary DNA (cDNA) Group of DNA molecules possessing the information contained in mRNAs, but with termini related to those produced by restriction endonucleases.

complementation Occurs in doubly infected cells and involves one of the viruses providing a gene-product which the other requires but cannot make.

conditional lethal mutants Mutants which will not replicate under conditions in which the wild-type virus replicates, but will replicate under permissive conditions, such as a different temperature or in another cell line.

conformational epitope Epitope composed of nonadjacent amino acids in the same or different polypeptide chains that are brought into proximity in the native protein by folding.

consensus sequence Archetypal amino acid sequence with which all variants are compared.

critical population size Minimum size of population needed to ensure the endemic (enzootic) status of an infection.

cross-sectional study Epidemiologic method by which a population is surveyed over a limited period of time to determine the relationship between a disease and presumed etiologic factors.

cuffing Perivascular infiltration of lymphocytes around blood vessels in brain, in response to certain viral infections.

cup probang Cup on the end of a flexible rod, used for obtaining samples of pharyngeal or esophageal fluid.

cytocidal (noncytocidal) infection Virus infection resulting in (not producing) death of the infected cell.

cytokine Polypeptide that participates in intercellular signaling via secretion into the extracellular space and binding to receptors on nearby target cells.

cytopathic effect Morphologic changes in cells resulting from viral infection.

cytopathogenic Virus which causes a cytopathic effect.

cytosol Liquid medium of the cytoplasm.

cytosolic pathway (of viral antigen processing) Production of antigenic peptide by degradation of viral polypeptide produced during viral replication and its association with class I MHC protein.

cytotoxic T cell (Tc) Subset of T cells capable of antigen-specific lysis of virus-infected cells that express viral antigen on their surface in association with class I MHC protein.

defective virus A virus that cannot replicate because it is defective in some way, usually lacking some essential gene. Some defective viruses can replicate in mixed infections with a helper virus.

defective interfering particle Defective virus which interferes with the replication of homologous complete virus.

delayed hypersensitivity T-cell-mediated, antibody-independent, antigen-specific inflammatory reaction.

dendritic cell *See* antigen-presenting cell.

diploid genome Genome that contains two copies of each gene.

disinfectant Chemical germicide for use on inanimate surfaces.

double-stranded (ds) Nucleic acid that occurs as a two-strand helix. Abbreviation (ds) used throughout book.

early viral genes Genes that are transcribed before viral nucleic acid replication occurs.

eclipse period Interval between viral penetration and production of the first progeny virions.

ecotropic viruses Retroviruses that replicate only in cells from the host species from which they were originally isolated.

elimination Country-level equivalent of eradication.

endemic, enzootic (disease) Disease that is continuously present in a particular population; sometimes the word endemic is used for human populations and enzootic for populations of other animals.

endogenous retroviruses Viruses whose genome occurs as a provirus integrated into the host cell DNA and thus transmittable from parent to daughter cells during normal cell division.

endosomal pathway (of viral antigen processing) Production of antigenic peptide by degradation of exogenous viral polypeptide taken up by antigen-presenting cells and its association with class II MHC proteins.

enhancer Upstream nucleotide regulatory sequence which enhances the expression of genes under its control.

envelope Lipoprotein outer covering of virions of some viruses, derived from cellular membranes but containing virus-specific proteins, usually glycoprotein peplomers.

epidemic, epizootic (disease) Disease occurring in an unusually high number of humans or animals in a population at the same time.

epidemiology Science of the study of disease in populations.

episome Autonomous extrachromosomal genetic element; may become integrated into a chromosome.

epitope *See* antigenic determinant.

eradication "Rooting out" of an infectious disease, on a continental or global scale.

exocytosis Mode of maturation whereby enveloped virions bud into a cellular organelle (Golgi or rough endoplasmic reticulum) and are released from the cell when the membrane of the organelle fuses with the plasma membrane.

exogenous retroviruses Horizontally transmitted retroviruses.

exon Coding sequence of genome that is not deleted by splicing of the primary RNA transcript, but appears in mRNA and is translated into protein (*see also* intron).

expression vector *See* cloning vector.

exotic virus Virus not normally occurring in a particular country.

extrinsic incubation period Interval between infective feed of an arthropod and development of infectivity of that arthropod for a vertebrate.

Fab Fragment antigen-binding; portion of an immunoglobulin molecule produced by papain digestion and comprising the variable domains of light and heavy chains; carries the antigen-binding site.

Fc Fragment crystallizable; portion of an immunoglobulin molecule produced by papain digestion and comprising the constant domain of both heavy chains; does not bind to antigen, but is responsible for effector functions.

Fc receptor Receptor present on various leukocytes which binds immunoglobulin via the Fc part of the molecule.

fomites Inanimate objects that may be contaminated with viruses and transmit infection (singular: fomes).

genome Complete set of genes of a virus or organism.

haploid genome Genome that contains one copy of each gene.

helical symmetry Configuration of nucleocapsid in which the nucleic acid and protein capsomers are arranged as a helix.

helper T cells (Th) T cells which when stimulated by antigen in association with class II MHC molecules are able to enhance the function of other lymphocytes.

helper virus A virus which, in a mixed infection with a defective virus, provides some factor(s) which enables the defective virus to replicate.

hemadsorption Adsorption of erythrocytes to the surface of virus-infected cells.

hemagglutination Agglutination of red blood cells.

hemagglutinin Viral glycoprotein peplomer that binds to red blood cells.

heteropolyploid Two different viral genomes within a single virion.

hexamer (hexon) In an icosahedral capsid, those capsomers having six neighboring capsomers.

horizontal transmission Transfer of infectious virus from one animal to another by means other than vertical transmission.

host range Range of species of animals (and cells derived therefrom) susceptible to a particular virus.

humoral immunity Immunity mediated by antibodies.

hybridoma Antibody-secreting cell line formed by the fusion of a myeloma tumor cell with a particular clone of antigen-primed B lymphocytes.

iatrogenic Caused directly by human (medical, veterinary) intervention.

icosahedral symmetry Configuration of a virion in which capsomers are assembled into a symmetrical polyhedron having 20 equilateral triangular faces and 12 vertices.

idiotype The antigenic determinant represented by the unique variable region of a specific antibody molecule.

immune complexes Antigen–antibody complexes.

immune response (Ir) genes Genes which influence the immune response to a given antigen; they map within the major histocompatibility complex (MHC) genetic locus.

immunogen *See* antigen.

immunologic memory Capacity of an animal which has been exposed to a particular antigen to respond more rapidly and effectively on reexposure to that antigen.

immunologic tolerance Specific unresponsiveness to a particular antigen.

incidence (of disease) Measure of the frequency of that disease over time.

incidence rate (of a disease) Proportion of population contracting that disease during a specified unit of time.

inclusion body Area with altered cytochemical staining properties in the nucleus and/or cytoplasm of a virus-infected cell.

incubation period Interval between the time of infection and the onset of clinical signs.

infectious dose 50 (ID_{50}) Dose of virus required to infect 50% of inoculated hosts.

interference Prevention of the replication of one virus by another virus, or by products (interferons) produced by cells as a result of viral infection.

interferons Family of cellular proteins (cytokines) produced and secreted in response to foreign nucleic acid (especially viral) that protect other cells against viral infection.

interleukins Acting between leukocytes; soluble substances (cytokines) produced by leukocytes that stimulate the growth or activities of other leukocytes.

intron (intervening sequence) Sequence of DNA that has no coding function and is excised in processing of RNA transcript to produce mRNA.

killer (K) cell "Null" (non B, non T) Fc-receptor-bearing lymphocyte responsible for antibody-dependent cellular cytotoxicity.

late viral genes Genes transcribed after viral nucleic acid replication.

latent infection Persistent infection in which little or no infectious virus is detectable, despite the continued presence of the viral genome.

leader sequence Nontranslated segment of mRNA from its 5′ end to the start codon. May contain regulatory signals.

leader sequence peptide Sequence of 15–20 amino acids at the N terminus of eukaryotic proteins that determines its ultimate destination.

lethal dose 50 (LD_{50}) Dose of virus required to kill 50% of inoculated animals.

leukemia Neoplastic proliferation of leukocytes.

leukosis Condition in which there is an abnormal increase in the number of leukocytes.

ligand Receptor-binding molecule on surface of virion.

liposome Artificially constructed lipid vesicle into which viral proteins or other substances may be incorporated.

long terminal repeat (LTR) Identical sequences some hundreds of nucleotides long at the termini of proviral DNA of retroviruses, each comprising sequences from both termini of the viral RNA and including promoter and enhancer sequences.

lymphokine Soluble mediator produced by lymphocytes that influences the function of other cells. A subclass of cytokines.

lymphoma Tumor of lymphoid tissue.

lysosome Cytoplasmic organelle containing hydrolytic enzymes.

lytic infection *See* cytocidal infection.

major histocompatibility complex (MHC) Chromosomal region containing the genes for histocompatibility antigens and the genes involved in the immune response.

malignant tumor Invasive tumor resulting from uncontrolled proliferation of abnormal (transformed) cells.

marker rescue Phenomenon found if cells that are mixedly infected (transfected) with active virus and inactivated virus or viral DNA yield progeny that contain some gene(s) from the inactivated virus or viral DNA.

matrix protein Protein lining the inner surface of the envelope of many enveloped viruses.

mechanical transmission Transmission of a virus by an arthropod, without replication in the vector.

memory cells T and B lymphocytes that mediate immunologic memory.

messenger RNA (mRNA) A single plus strand of RNA produced by transcription from the genome, which, sometimes after processing, carries genetic information to the ribosomes to make protein. The genome of certain RNA viruses can act directly as mRNA.

metastasis Spread of cells of a malignant tumor to other parts of the body.

MHC protein Proteins encoded by genes of the MHC complex. Class I MHC associated with foreign (viral) peptide produced in virus-infected cells elicits a cytotoxic T-cell response; class II MHC associated with foreign (viral) peptide derived from exogenous viral proteins processed by antigen-presenting cells elicits a helper T-cell response.

MHC restriction The recognition of foreign (viral) antigen by T cells occurs only when that antigen is presented on a cell surface as a peptide in association with "self" MHC protein.

molecular cloning *See* cloning (molecular).

molecular mimicry Shared identity of sequences of genes or proteins from disparate organisms (e.g., from a virus and a vertebrate).

monoclonal antibody Antibody produced by a clone of B cells, with a specificity for a particular epitope (*see* hybridoma).

monocistronic Corresponding to a single gene (cistron).

multiplicity of infection Measure of the number of virus particles inoculated per cell.

mutation Heritable change in the nucleotide sequence of the genome of an organism.

natural killer (NK) cell Immunologically nonspecific lymphocyte with the capacity to kill virus-infected or tumor cells in absence of prior immunization.

negative stain Chemical that stains the background, outlining the object (e.g., for electron microscopy, potassium phosphotungstate).

negative, or minus sense *See* sense.

nested set Subgenomic mRNAs which have an identical 5′ leader sequence and which extend for different lengths from a common 3′ terminus; found during replication of coronaviruses, toroviruses, and arteriviruses.

nonsense mutation Mutation which produces one of the three stop codons, resulting in premature termination of the growing polypeptide chain.

nonstructural protein Virus-coded protein found in infected cells but not part of the structure of the virion, although some nonstructural proteins, such as polymerase, may be incorporated in the virion.

Northern blot Laboratory jargon derived by analogy with Southern blot; transfer of RNA fragments from polyacrylamide gels to nitrocellulose filter paper by blotting, then probing with labeled complementary DNA.

nosocomial Hospital-acquired.

nucleocapsid Viral nucleic acid surrounded by its protein capsid.

nude mouse Strain of hairless mouse that is congenitally without a thymus gland.

oncogene (cellular; c-*onc*; *syn.* protooncogene) Cellular gene that may lead to production of a malignant tumor when mutated or if expressed in an unregulated way.

oncogene (viral; v-*onc*) Viral gene that is responsible for the oncogenicity of oncogenic viruses.

oncogenesis (carcinogenesis, tumorigenesis) The process of development of a malignant tumor.

oncogenic virus Virus able to transform cells and to induce malignant tumors when inoculated into certain laboratory animals, or in nature.

Okazaki fragments Short fragments of DNA synthesized as intermediates in the discontinuous replication of DNA.

open reading frame (ORF) Nucleic acid sequence between start and stop codons (*see* reading frame).

operator Sites in genome at which repressors (regulatory proteins) bind. They are always close to the promoter sequence and sometimes overlap it.

palindrome Sequence in dsDNA with adjacent reverse repeats; the sequence of one strand read left to right is the same as that of the other strand read right to left.

pandemic (panzootic) Worldwide epidemic (epizootic).

passive immunization Transfer of antibodies to a nonimmune animal, either by maternal transfer or artificial inoculation.

pentamer (penton) The 12 capsomers located at the vertices of the virions of an icosahedral virus. Each has 5 neighboring capsomers.

peplomer (spike) Oligomer of viral glycoprotein projecting from a viral envelope.

permissive (temperature or cell) The temperature or cell type that permits the replication of a conditional lethal viral mutant.

persistent infection In animals and cells, infection that persists for a prolonged period after the primary infection.

phenotype Appearance (characteristics) of a virus or organism, resulting from the expression of its genotype.

plasma cell Antibody-secreting cell derived as the end stage of differentiation of a B lymphocyte.

plasmid Self-replicating extrachromosomal circular DNA molecule found in many bacteria.

plaque Localized region of cell lysis resulting from cell-to-cell spread of virus replicating in a cell monolayer, usually under agar.

plaque assay Assay based on the number of plaques produced when a standard volume of a viral suspension is inoculated on a cell monolayer.

point mutation Alteration in a single base in the nucleic acid of a genome.

polarity (1) Of RNA, *see* sense. (2) Of cell, referring to differences between apical and basolateral surfaces of epithelial cells.

poly(A) tail (polyadenylated RNA) Sequence of 50–200 adenylate residues present in the genome of some ssRNA viruses or enzymatically added to the 3′ terminus of an RNA transcript, in the process of formation of mRNA.

polycistronic Representing several genes.

polykaryocyte Cell with multiple nuclei (synonyms: syncytium, giant cell).

polyploid More than one copy of the genome present (e.g., in a virion).

polyprotein First product of transcription from the genome of some positive sense RNA viruses that is then cleaved into smaller proteins.

prevalence (of a disease) Number of cases of that disease at a particular point in time.

prevalence rate (of a disease) Number of cases of that disease at a particular point in time divided by the population at risk.

primary immune response Immune response following the first contact of an animal with an antigen.

prion protein Surface protein of neurons encoded by a chromosomal gene, mutations of which may produce proteins that cause subacute spongiform encephalopathy.

processing (1) Of RNA transcripts, series of posttranscriptional alterations to primary RNA transcripts, which lead to the formation of mRNA. (2) Of proteins, changes subsequent to translation of polypeptide, such as cleavage, glycosylation, or phosphorylation.

prodrug Chemotherapeutic agent which depends on a viral enzyme to convert it to its active form.

productive (or nonproductive) infection Infection of a permissive (or nonpermissive) cell by a virus resulting in the production (or failure of production) of infectious progeny virions.

promoter Region of nucleic acid molecule to which RNA polymerase binds in order to initiate transcription.

positive, or plus sense *See* sense.

prospective study Attempt to identify the cause of a disease by observing populations that are exposed to the infection over a period of time.

provirus Viral genome covalently integrated into a host cell chromosome, and thus transmissible from a cell to its daughter cells.

pseudotype Of retroviruses, genome derived from one parent virus, enclosed within a capsid specified by a second, coinfecting virus.

reactivation (cross, multiplicity) Recovery of viable virus following coinfection of a cell with two inactivated parent viruses with lesions in different genes.

reading frame A nucleotide sequence that starts with an initiation (start) codon, partitions the subsequent nucleotides into amino acid-encoding triplets, and ends with a termination (stop) codon.

reassortment Recombination between viruses with segmented genomes whereby some progeny of a doubly infected cell acquire genome segments from another virus.

receptor Structure on the surface of a cell that is recognized by a specific extracellular molecule or structure (ligand) that binds to it.

receptor-mediated endocytosis Uptake of virion (or hormone) following attachment to a specific receptor on the plasma membrane.

recombination (intramolecular) Exchange of nucleic acid sequences between molecules derived from different parents, giving rise to progeny with a different genotype.

repeat (reiterated) sequence Nucleotide sequence present in more than one copy (usually many copies).

replicative intermediate Intermediate in the replication of viral nucleic acid, consisting of one complete (template) strand on which one or several nascent strands of opposite sense are replicating simultaneously, with a polymerase molecule at each growing point.

reservoir host Animal species constituting the major source of virus in nature.

restriction endonuclease Enzyme (bacterial in origin) capable of cleaving double-stranded DNA at specific palindromes.

retrospective study Attempt to identify the cause of a disease by comparing the presence or absence of suspected etiologic factors in animals with a certain disease to their occurrence in animals without that disease.

reverse genetics Genetic studies that proceed from the recognition of a gene to the function of its product.

reverse transcriptase Enzyme carried by retroviruses and hepadnaviruses that transcribes DNA from RNA.

S phase Stage of cell cycle when DNA synthesis occurs.

sarcoma Malignant tumor of cells of mesenchymal origin.

secondary immune response *See* anamnestic response.

sense The polarity of a single-stranded nucleic acid; positive (plus) sense is that found in messenger RNA.

sentinel study Investigation of the circulation of arboviruses by testing for specific antibodies in exposed ("sentinel") animals.

sigla (acronym) Name formed from a few letters, often initial letters of descriptive words (e.g., *Reoviridae* = respiratory, enteric, orphan viruses).

signal sequence Amino-terminal sequence of 16–30 amino acids that initiates transport across membranes; subsequently cleaved off.

signal transduction Conversion of information recognized by specific cellular receptors into a new form, such as a change in activity of cellular proteins.

single-stranded (ss) Nucleic acid that occurs as a single strand. Abbreviation (ss) used throughout book.

site-directed mutagenesis Introduction of a particular point mutation or deletion at a predetermined position.

slow infection Infection with a prolonged preclinical phase (incubation period), which is followed by slowly progressive disease.

Southern blot Transfer of DNA fragments from a polyacrylamide gel to nitrocellulose filter paper by blotting, so that specific sequences can be recognized by hybridization with radioactively labeled nucleic acid probes. Named after Edward Southern.

splicing Process of excision of introns and linking of exons from RNA transcripts, to form mRNA.

start (initiation) codon Group of three adjacent ribonucleotides (AUG) in an mRNA, where translation is initiated. It is preceded by base sequences that have a high affinity for ribosomes.

stop (termination) codon Ribonucleotide triplet (UGA, UAG, UAA) in an mRNA signaling the termination of translation of a polypeptide chain.

structural proteins Virus-coded proteins that are an essential part of the structure of a virion.

suppressor mutation Compensating mutation, generally in another gene, that restores the wild-type phenotype without affecting the mutant gene.

suppressor T cell (Ts) Subclass of T lymphocytes that exerts an inhibitory control on B cells, helper T cells, and effector T cells.

surveillance (disease) The collection, collation, and analysis of data on disease incidence and its dissemination.

surveillance and containment Strategy for control of an infectious disease by which active cases are searched for and isolated, their source determined, and their contacts vaccinated.

syncytium Polykaryocyte (multinucleated giant cell) formed by fusion of adjacent cells.

T cell Thymus-derived lymphocytes responsible for cell-mediated immunity or for immune regulation.

T-cell receptor (TCR) Receptor molecule on the surface of T cells that recognizes antigenic peptide in association with MHC protein.

TATA box Consensus sequence TATAAAA that starts about 30 bases upstream from the cap site which directs RNA polymerase II to begin synthesis at the cap site.

temperature-sensitive mutation Mutation resulting in a gene-product that is nonfunctional at a certain ("nonpermissive") temperature but functional at the permissive temperature.

transcriptase RNA polymerase responsible for transcription.

transcription unit Region of genome extending from transcription initiation site to transcription termination site, including all introns and exons. May include more than one gene.

transduction Transfer by a virus of cellular genes from one organism or cell to another.

transfer RNA (+RNA) An RNA molecule that transfers an amino acid to a growing polypeptide chain during translation.

transformation (1) Transfer of genetic information into a cell via free DNA. (2) Infectious process in which a virus does not kill the host cell but induces genetic changes in it that lead to changes in growth characteristics and sometimes to tumor formation.

translocation Movement of immunoglobulin across the wall of the intestinal tract in newborn animals.

translocation cutoff Time at which translocation ceases.

transovarial transmission Transmission of virus from one generation to the next through the egg.
trans-stadial transmission Transmission of virus from one developmental stage (instar) of an arthropod to the next stage.
tumor (T) antigens Virus-specific proteins found in transformed cells; some are required to maintain transformation; others not.
tumor suppressor gene Cellular gene whose gene product is involved with regulation of growth; mutations in such genes may permit excess activity of c-*onc* genes, leading to cancer.
tumor-associated transplantation antigen Antigens found on the surface of tumor cells that are undetectable on normal cells of adult individuals and that act as transplantation antigens.
uncoating An early step in the viral replication cycle involving the removal of some or all of the viral coat, thus freeing the viral genome for expression of its functions.
vector (1) intermediate host (e.g., arthropod) that transmits the causative agent of disease from infected to noninfected hosts. (2) Plasmid or viral DNA employed in recombinant DNA technology to clone a foreign gene in prokaryotic or eukaryotic cells. (3) Virus used to incorporate gene for protective antigen from another virus for study of its function or use as vaccine.
vertical transmission Transmission of virus from parent to progeny through the genome, sperm, or ovum or extracellularly (e.g., through milk or across the placenta).
viral core Viral nucleic acid and associated proteins.
viremia Presence of virions in the bloodstream, either free (plasma viremia) or in infected leukocytes (cell-associated viremia).
virgin-soil epidemic (epizootic) Epidemic (epizootic) occurring in a totally nonimmune (naive) population.
virokine Cytokine specified by a viral gene.
virion Complete virus particle.
viroid Infectious RNA molecules which do not code for or require a coat protein, so far found only among plant viruses.
virulence Measure of the ability of an infectious agent to inflict damage on a host.
Western blot Laboratory jargon derived by analogy with Southern blot; transfer of proteins from polyacrylamide gels to nitrocellulose filter paper by blotting, then probing with labeled antibodies.
wild type The original strain of virus, from which mutants may have arisen.
xenotropic viruses Retroviruses that replicate only in cells from animals other than the species from which they were derived.
zoonosis Infectious disease transferred from animals to humans.

Index

B

D

E

J

K

L

M

N

Q

R

S

T

U

V

W

X

Y

Z

ISBN 0-12-253056-X